Cranio-Sacral Integration

· *Foundation* ·

Thomas Attlee

Illustrated by Sam Wilson

Photographs by Peter Ashworth

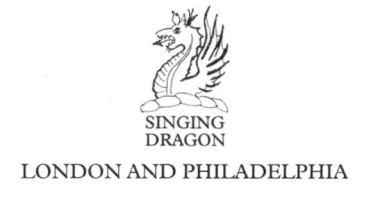

SINGING DRAGON

LONDON AND PHILADELPHIA

First published in 2012
by Singing Dragon
an imprint of Jessica Kingsley Publishers
116 Pentonville Road
London N1 9JB, UK
and
400 Market Street, Suite 400
Philadelphia, PA 19106, USA

www.singingdragon.com

Copyright © Thomas Attlee 2012
Illustrations copyright © Sam Wilson 2012
Photographs copyright © Peter Ashworth 2012

All rights reserved. No part of this publication may be reproduced in any material form (including photocopying or storing it in any medium by electronic means and whether or not transiently or incidentally to some other use of this publication) without the written permission of the copyright owner except in accordance with the provisions of the Copyright, Designs and Patents Act 1988 or under the terms of a licence issued by the Copyright Licensing Agency Ltd, Saffron House, 6–10 Kirby Street, London EC1N 8TS. Applications for the copyright owner's written permission to reproduce any part of this publication should be addressed to the publisher.

Warning: The doing of an unauthorised act in relation to a copyright work may result in both a civil claim for damages and criminal prosecution.

Library of Congress Cataloging in Publication Data
Attlee, Thomas.
  Cranio-sacral integration / Thomas Attlee.
    p. ; cm.
  Includes bibliographical references and index.
  ISBN 978-1-84819-098-6 (alk. paper)
  I. Title.
  [DNLM: 1. Manipulation, Osteopathic--methods. 2. Massage--methods. 3. Psychophysiology. 4. Sacrum--physiology. 5. Skull--physiology. WB 537]
  LC classification not assigned
  615.8'22--dc23
                            2011050175

British Library Cataloguing in Publication Data
A CIP catalogue record for this book is available from the British Library

ISBN 978 1 84819 098 6
eISBN 978 0 85710 078 0

Printed and bound in Great Britain

Thank you

to my family,
Janice, Ashley, Ruskin

to all my students at the
College of Cranio-Sacral Therapy
over the past 26 years

to all my tutors
at the college

to Sam Wilson
for the illustrations

to Peter Ashworth
for the photographs

to Alice Paton
for modelling for the photos

to Jessica Kingsley
for publishing this book

to the production team
at Jessica Kingsley Publishers

Contents

Part I Introduction: Setting the Scene

Chapter 1.	Amy	10
Chapter 2.	The Source of Life	11
Chapter 3.	A Fundamental Platform	13
Chapter 4.	Cranio-Sacral Integration	17
Chapter 5.	The Matrix: A Broad Perspective on the Cranio-Sacral System	19
Chapter 6.	Living in the Material World: Anatomy of the Cranio-Sacral System	25
Chapter 7.	Cranio-Sacral Motion	48
Chapter 8.	Treatment: Fundamental Principles – The Inherent Treatment Process	53
Chapter 9.	Stimulus	65
Chapter 10.	Responses to Treatment	69
Chapter 11.	To Treat or Not to Treat: Contra-Indications	74
Interlude 1.	A Time for Reflection: Key Concepts in Cranio-Sacral Integration	76

Part II Essential Concepts

Chapter 12.	Pigs, Elephants and Snakes: The Concept of Quality	78
Chapter 13.	Fluid Analogies	87
Chapter 14.	Fulcrums	90
Chapter 15.	Calm Quiet Presence: The State of the Practitioner	99
Chapter 16.	Stillness	107

Part III A Framework for Integrated Treatment: Basic Skills

Chapter 17.	Integrated Treatment	112
Chapter 18.	Tuning In – 1	114
Chapter 19.	Tuning In – 2	120
Chapter 20.	Opening Up the System: Settling and Grounding	126
Chapter 21.	The Suboccipital Region	136
Chapter 22.	Core Treatment: Overall Approach	145

Interlude 2.	Key Elements in the Overall Approach to Cranio-Sacral Integration	147
Chapter 23.	Core Treatment: Individual Processes	148
Chapter 24.	The Spine	150
Chapter 25.	The Occiput and Spine	155
Chapter 26.	The Sacrum and Spine	162
Chapter 27.	The Sphenoid	175
Chapter 28.	The Temporal Area	189
Chapter 29.	The Frontal Area	202
Chapter 30.	The Parietal Area	211
Chapter 31.	The Falx Cerebri and Falx Release	216
Chapter 32.	Completion	223
Chapter 33.	Still Point	225
Chapter 34.	Practice: An Integrated Treatment Framework	232

Part IV *Further Concepts*

Chapter 35.	The Return of Rhythmic Motion	238
Chapter 36.	Biodynamics, Biomechanics and the Quantum Model	244
Chapter 37.	Keep Breathing	249

Part V *Fascial Unwinding*

Chapter 38.	Fascia	256
Chapter 39.	Evaluation of the Fascia	265
Chapter 40.	Fascial Unwinding within the Trunk Region	276
Chapter 41.	Fascial Unwinding of the Arm	279
Chapter 42.	Fascial Unwinding of the Leg	290
Chapter 43.	Fascial Unwinding of the Neck	303
Chapter 44.	Key Factors in Fascial Unwinding	310

Part VI *Spheno-Basilar Patterns*

Chapter 45.	Scales and Arpeggios: Spheno-Basilar Patterns Part 1– Honing Basic Skills	316
Chapter 46.	Opus 27 Number 2: Spheno-Basilar Integration	331

Part VII The Nervous System

Chapter 47.	The Nervous System: The Basics	340
Chapter 48.	The Nervous System: Relations with the Cranio-Sacral System	346
Chapter 49.	The Autonomic Nervous System	359
Chapter 50.	Double Contacts with the Sacrum	370
Chapter 51.	Facilitated Segments and T4 Syndrome	379
Chapter 52.	Autonomic Nervous System Integration	384

Part VIII Further Contacts and Concepts

Chapter 53.	The Throat	394
Chapter 54.	Energy Drive	407
Chapter 55.	The Emotional Body	414
Chapter 56.	Personal Development	419
Chapter 57.	Further Contacts	421
Chapter 58.	Diagnosis	429

Part IX An Integrated Treatment Approach

Chapter 59.	An Integrated Treatment Approach	438

Part X Conclusion

Chapter 60.	Cranio-Sacral Integration: A Summary	446
	Glossary	*448*
	References	*456*
	Index	*457*

Part I
Introduction
SETTING THE SCENE

Chapter 1

Amy

Amy was six months old when her parents brought her to see me. She had been screaming continuously for all of those six months, day and night, night and day, all day, every day. She was screaming as she arrived, in obvious inconsolable pain.

Her parents had taken her to countless doctors, specialists and therapists. She had been given endless medications. Nothing had helped.

Her parents were at their wits' end. They were desperately concerned for their baby. They had hardly had any sleep in six months. They were exhausted. They couldn't take Amy anywhere because of her constant screaming. They couldn't invite friends round. Their life was a continuous nightmare. They were on the point of breaking up.

I placed my hands on Amy's abdomen. Within a few seconds she had stopped screaming. Within minutes she was asleep. From that moment on, she was a happy healthy little girl, no longer screaming inconsolably, but growing up contentedly just like any other child. Life became peaceful and harmonious. Her parents stayed together and had another baby. I saw Amy and her younger brother from time to time as they grew up healthy and happy – family life transformed from the nightmare of those early months.

What happened during those few minutes of treatment?

What happened was cranio-sacral integration.

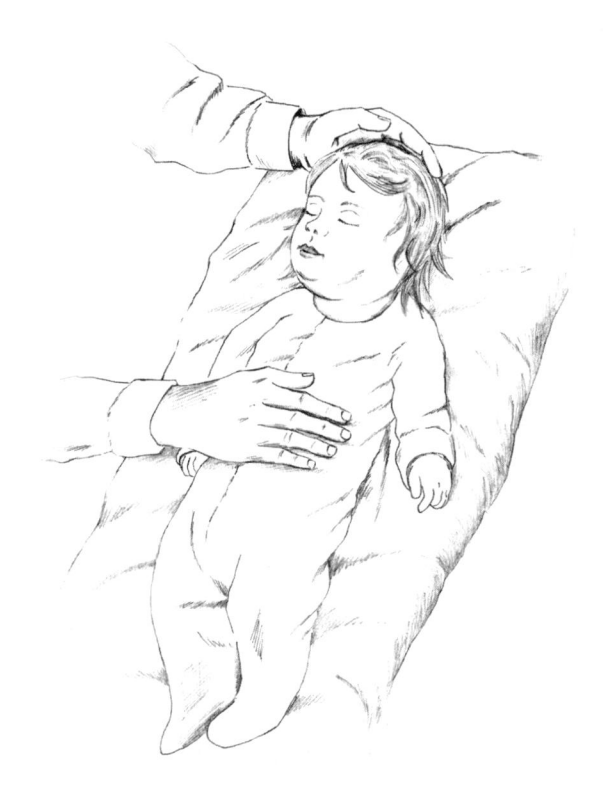

Chapter 2

The Source of Life

When we rest our hands very lightly on the body and tune in on a subtle level, we can feel rhythmic motion being expressed throughout the body, as if the whole body were gently breathing – not just the usual breathing of the lungs, but a more gentle, subtle, rhythmic motion.

Vitality

What is causing this movement? The natural world is guided by forces and rhythms which surround us and permeate us. This rhythmic motion is a reflection of a natural force, a *vital force*, which is present throughout nature and which perfuses all living things. It is what makes us alive. This inherent force is expressed within each individual as *vitality*, or aliveness. It is this natural force which determines the orderly progression of life, growth, development, health and healing and which restores and maintains balance and integration – whether in an acorn, or in a human being. This natural force and the individual vitality which it engenders are expressed in the body as *rhythmic motion*.

Resistance

Rhythmic motion is expressed as *expansion and contraction*. This expansion and contraction is present in every individual cell throughout the body. It is also expressed through the body as a whole – the whole body expanding and contracting as one complete integrated unit. This rhythmic movement can be felt throughout the whole internal *matrix* of the body and in the external matrix – in the whole person and in their surroundings. Everything that happens to us – every injury, every illness, every tension, every trauma – influences this rhythmic motion, creating disturbances to its fluent expression – twists, turns, restrictions, resistances.

Engagement

When a cranio-sacral therapist tunes in on a very subtle level, he or she can *engage* with these inherent movements and natural forces within the body. This interaction enables the patient's system to respond to the therapist's gentle contact by addressing and releasing any disturbances and resistances, thereby re-establishing a more calm, settled, balanced, integrated state where disruptive tensions and restrictions have subsided, where rhythmic motion is being expressed evenly, regularly and clearly, where the underlying vitality which maintains our health can be expressed freely, and where the body can consequently function more smoothly and fluently.

Release

How does the body resolve disturbances? As part of the body's natural day-to-day function, the rhythmic motion will, from time to time, draw to points of stillness – where the movement ceases temporarily. This is part of the body's *inherent treatment process*. These *still points* are significant moments of healing. They tend to evolve around focal points of restriction – areas of the body where rhythmic motion and the vitality which it reflects are not flowing freely. As the body draws to these points of stillness, its inner resources are focused around this fulcrum. This harnesses the healing potency of the vital forces within the system, enabling the *release* of these restrictions, allowing the system to *reorganise* and realign itself within its new-found unrestricted state, leading to a return to a more balanced and freely mobile *neutral* state, with the re-emergence of a more expansive rhythmic motion and an increasingly free flow of vitality throughout the body.

This process is a natural inherent healing process, which the body is carrying out regularly of its own accord. However, the body's healing potential can be compromised by injury and trauma. By engaging with the system, the cranio-sacral therapist can *enhance* the body's inherent healing potential, helping it to eliminate the restrictions to the free flow of vitality, restoring health.

Penetrating to the deepest levels

The cranio-sacral system and its motion are subtle. In order to engage with them, the cranio-sacral therapist needs to use an extremely light touch – barely a touch at all, simply being there with their *calm, quiet presence*. Cranio-sacral integration is therefore a very *gentle* therapy. It is through this unimposing gentleness that the body is able to relax and open up (secure in the knowledge that it is not being threatened) enabling the cranio-sacral process to penetrate to the deepest levels of our being. Cranio-sacral integration is therefore a very *profound* therapy, reaching levels which are not generally accessed by other more physical or more invasive means (which might induce the body's protective mechanisms) and is therefore able to connect with and enhance the underlying health deep within, addressing the root causes of severe and profoundly debilitating disease – as well as relieving less severe conditions.

The whole person

Cranio-sacral integration is not merely treating the body. It recognises that body, mind and feelings are absolutely and inextricably intertwined. It therefore engages with every aspect of our being – physical, mental, emotional, spiritual. So its effects are profound and widespread and can be effective over a very wide range of circumstances and conditions. Cranio-sacral integration is not treating conditions; it is treating people; it is treating *the whole person* and everything about the person at a fundamental and profound level, bringing everything into a fine-tuned, smoothly flowing, integrated state in which the body's physiology and healing powers can function optimally. In doing so, it can enable the body to address whatever symptoms, conditions or disturbances that particular individual may be experiencing – since all symptoms and conditions are a reflection of disturbances to the underlying vitality – and it can thereby restore health and fluency on all levels.

In Amy's case, her birth had been long and traumatic. The effects of this experience had been a combination of severe compression – during the prolonged process of being pushed forcefully through the birth canal – and fear, as her heartbeat fluctuated wildly, her oxygen supply came and went, and her nine months of cosy comfortable existence in her mother's womb came to a sudden and dramatic conclusion.

This had left her whole system in a state of shock – contracted, seized up – her autonomic nervous system highly overstimulated, her solar plexus intensely agitated, her digestive system constricted, her whole body locked in fear and terror at a profound and fundamental level. Nothing had been able to help her (no medication was ever going to influence that level of her being) because nothing was engaging with this deep sense of shock held in the very essence of her system. Cranio-sacral integration was able to do exactly that, and was therefore able to release that profound trauma in her system, release the blockage and restriction, the contraction, compression and overstimulation that had resulted from her traumatic experience of birth, and so enable her to settle into a peaceful natural state of ease and harmony.

Chapter 3

A Fundamental Platform

True health
What exactly is cranio-sacral integration? We have seen that it is gentle, it is profound, it is all embracing, it is powerful. It is a therapy which integrates our underlying function at a deep level, so that the healing forces within can operate smoothly and fluently and from this integrated underlying function emerges true health. True health arises from a strong freely expressed inherent vitality. Cranio-sacral integration establishes this inherent vitality and enables its free flow throughout the system, enabling the body to overcome disease and disturbance, to release tension and restriction, so that symptoms, conditions, and their underlying causes can drop away and be resolved.

Underlying strength
Cranio-sacral integration does not therefore specifically revolve around symptoms and diseases. It revolves around establishing the underlying strength of the system. As a result, cranio-sacral integration is not limited to specific types of condition. The establishment of underlying health enables the body to resolve disturbances on every level so that anyone, whatever their condition, can potentially be helped.

Wide application
Consequently, the applications of cranio-sacral integration are very wide – from simple aches and pains to the most complex chronic or persistent problems, from colic and ear infections in babies, through learning difficulties and asthma in children, to back pain, menstrual disorders, emotional stresses and the after-effects of major accidents, injuries or serious illnesses in all ages.

It can address intransigent conditions that have not responded to other forms of treatment, chronic disease that seems to have no solution, obscure and abstract conditions that seem to have no specific cause, the debilitating long-term effects of meningitis, post-viral syndrome or myalgic encephalomyelitis (ME) – all through the gentle integration of the cranio-sacral system. It can also be helpful in maintaining an overall state of balance and integration in all aspects of life.

It has a special part to play in addressing the far-reaching and potentially life-determining consequences of severe trauma and shock – whether due to severe car accidents, mugging, rape, sexual abuse, childhood abuse, birth, war, post-traumatic stress disorder, or any other cause – releasing both the physical and psycho-emotional effects of trauma, freeing the patient from restrictive patterns and habits imposed on them by their traumas and restoring tranquillity.

Ultimately, cranio-sacral integration can be beneficial in almost any circumstance, because it is concerned with establishing a fundamental platform of inner health from which the body can deal with whatever comes its way. It is concerned with enhancing health, strength and vitality at the very core of our being, thereby stimulating the body's own natural potential, helping the body to eradicate the root of any problem. It is concerned with integrating all the body's resources to function at their optimum level.

What does it involve?
Cranio-sacral treatment is most often carried out with the patient lying down, fully clothed, in a quiet and peaceful environment. Treatment involves a very gentle touch of the practitioner's hands. This light contact may be taken up on the cranium (head), the sacrum (tailbone), the feet, the trunk, or any other part of the body as appropriate.

It generally brings a feeling of deep relaxation and warmth, as the whole person – body and mind – engages with the underlying health spreading through the body, and is encouraged towards a more balanced, calm and integrated state of ease and well-being.

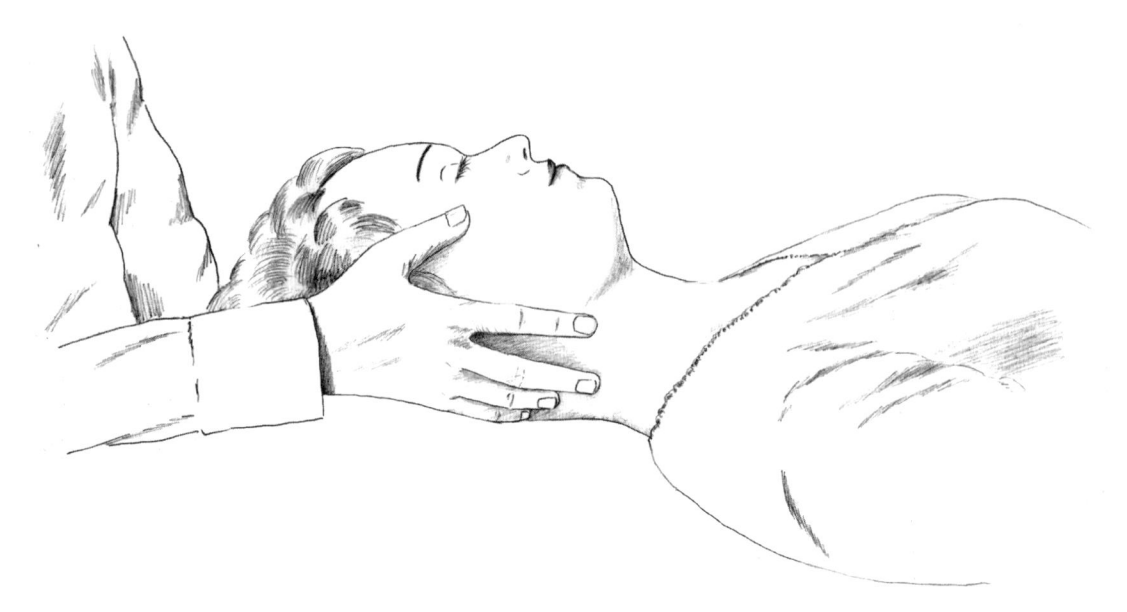

The benefits of cranio-sacral integration

Cranio-sacral integration can be of benefit at any age – for babies, children, pregnant women, elderly people and adults, in birth, in sickness or in health.

Babies

There are several reasons why cranio-sacral integration is very suitable and relevant for babies and children. It is gentle and non-invasive. Babies can be treated while asleep, or feeding, or cradled in their parents' arms, and there is no need to disturb them by removing clothing.

Cranio-sacral integration is effective at relieving many common childhood conditions which plague the majority of parents, causing endless sleepless nights and untold worry and anxiety – including colic, poor sleep, restlessness, hyperactivity and many others, most of which generally result from the stresses and strains of the birth process.

Cranio-sacral integration is uniquely effective in dealing with the effects of birth trauma (both the compressive forces exerted on the skull, and the shock effects of a traumatic birth) with its many possible consequences, physical and emotional, including nerve compressions, reduced blood supply to the brain, agitation, hyperactivity, withdrawal, shyness, dyslexia, behavioural disorders, epilepsy, autism, squint and cerebral palsy – any of which may potentially impose patterns of limited function for life.

By ironing out the various effects of injury and illness as they develop, cranio-sacral integration can create a balanced, well-integrated physical, mental and emotional state, enabling the baby not only to enjoy a happier, healthier childhood, but also to grow up with the ability to make optimum use of his or her potential.

Early treatment ensures a more complete resolution of any problems arising from the birth process, with fewer treatments needed. Regular treatment throughout babyhood and childhood helps to resolve the effects of any falls, injuries and illnesses which are an inevitable part of childhood. Together, these enable the child's early experience of life to be as positive and comfortable as possible, thereby creating positive patterns for the future.

Olivia was nine months old and she had been in hospital for the past three months. She was having epileptic fits every three minutes or so, repeatedly, 24 hours a day, and had been doing so for the past six months. Every few minutes she would start to shake, her eyes would roll, her head would pull back and her whole body would tremble for a minute or so, then it would subside, only to start up again three minutes later. She and her mother were living in the hospital so that she could be monitored and cared for constantly. Every medication for epilepsy and several others besides had been tried without any benefit. The hospital had exhausted all possibilities and had run out of ideas.

Olivia's parents heard about cranio-sacral therapy and phoned me and asked if it would be possible for me to go and see her in hospital. I arrived to find Olivia going through her regular fits every three minutes. I tuned in to her system and felt this very powerful pattern of compression as if her head and neck had been compressed forcefully down into her shoulders and twisted to the right (although there was no sign of this externally). As I engaged with her system, she continued to experience her fits every few minutes. I maintained engagement, allowing her system to release the profound effects of birth trauma that were imprinted into her. I spent two hours with Olivia that evening, allowing the treatment process to take its course.

By the end of the treatment she was fitting only every 20 minutes. The next day she came out of hospital. When the family came to see me a week later, she was just experiencing a few fits each day, and within a few more treatments, the fits had disappeared completely.

Children

It is such a joy to treat babies and children. They are a pleasure to watch and to work and play with; their systems are generally very responsive; and most of all, one can often see such substantial and significant transformation in their lives – from what might have been a life of debility and restriction to a life full of health, happiness, promise and potential.

Cranio-sacral integration can be highly effective in treating children with asthma, with its deeper understanding of the complex combination of factors which contribute to the condition. It can also, as mentioned above, be helpful in treating children with dyslexia, dyspraxia, behavioural disorders and epilepsy. It is also uniquely effective in treating the after-effects of meningitis, which are so often misdiagnosed, misunderstood or not acknowledged.

Children inevitably tend to experience a substantial number of knocks and falls as a part of everyday life, during school, games and sports, and also the inevitable infections and illnesses of childhood. Young people are generally resilient and they usually appear to recover, but all these minor knocks, falls and illnesses accumulate steadily in their systems, contributing to the gradual deterioration in health that creeps on with age, and to which children can be so blithely and fortunately oblivious. So even when the child appears to be fully recovered on the surface, clearing these effects through regular cranio-sacral integration can help to maintain a healthier, more integrated underlying state which will stand them in good stead for the future. More specifically, it is quite common for children not to fully recover from some apparently minor illness or infection, remaining lethargic, irritable, grumpy, apathetic, losing their appetite, their enthusiasm and their vitality – often dragging on for months, perhaps changing them forever. Cranio-sacral integration can be very helpful in restoring them to their former vitality.

Sophie was ten and had been a very lively, enthusiastic girl, always keen to go to school, always having friends round and going to her friends' houses, enjoying a multitude of different activities with great enthusiasm. Then she caught flu – nothing unusual about that – she was unwell for a week or two, but when the illness was over, she just wasn't the same girl any more. She was constantly tired, she didn't want to go to school, she just sat around, not wanting to do anything; she was moody and irritable, and this dragged on and on and on for months. Of course her mother took her to the doctor, but the doctor couldn't identify any cause or offer any solution.

By the time her mother brought her to me, it had been almost a year and Sophie was still lethargic and apathetic. Just one treatment cleared out the persistent effects that had lodged in her system, dragging her down into her debilitated state and Sophie was transformed. She positively bounded off the table, was raring to go to school the next day and wanted friends round after school. Her mother was overjoyed: 'I'm so delighted to have my little girl back.'

Pregnant women

Pregnancy is a very special time and a very significant time for cranio-sacral treatment – for the baby, both in immediate terms and in the future – and in preparing for the birth. Everything that can be done to enhance the pregnancy is very worthwhile.

Most significantly, regular cranio-sacral integration during pregnancy is likely to enable an easier, smoother, more natural birth, since preparing the mother for birth and ironing out any tensions, restrictions and imbalances in the mother helps the body to function as it should during labour, reducing any complications and the need for interventions such as forceps, ventouse and medication, with all the potential consequences on baby and mother.

Furthermore, regular cranio-sacral integration during pregnancy creates a more comfortable, healthy and harmonious environment for the baby during its nine month residence in the womb, thereby promoting healthy growth and development during that crucial time.

And let's not neglect mother. Cranio-sacral integration will not only help a mother to be more comfortable during the pregnancy and help her to give birth more easily, but also consequently reduce the difficulties and discomforts that so often ensue from giving birth – from chronic back pain and pelvic dysfunctions to episiotomy and pubic symphysis displacement.

Elderly people

Once again it is the gentleness of cranio-sacral integration that is so much appreciated by elderly patients. They often have a lifetime of accumulated aches and pains, restricting their mobility, disrupting their bodily functions and generally leaving them feeling debilitated. They have often been given pills for their arthritis which have given them digestive disturbances, more pills for their digestion which has given them headaches, more pills for their headaches which have made them feel sick, more pills for their nausea which leave them drowsy and vague. They come into the clinic, rattling with all those pills inside them and feeling very fed up – although often very patient and forbearing – and find that all they need to do is lie quietly on the couch and feel this very gentle touch of the therapist's hands, and their aches and pains start to dissolve away. They find that as time goes on (and with due consultation with their doctors) they no longer need the array of medications that they have been taking; and they find life looking so different – clearer, more comfortable, happier, easier. Countless times, elderly patients have told me that they feel 20 years younger.

Adults

In adults, cranio-sacral integration is effective throughout the full range of conditions that may arise, from the common conditions that affect so many people – back pain, sprains and strains, sports injuries, digestive disturbances, and stress-related disorders – to more comprehensive reintegration after car accidents and other severe injuries and traumas, or debilitating illnesses.

But it is also much appreciated for its more general effect of clearing out clutter, restoring health and vitality, establishing a more comfortable state, easing the multitude of persistent daily discomforts that affect so many people – headaches, backache, joint pains, tightness, tension, agitation, irritability, tiredness, exhaustion – and bringing the body into a more comfortable sense of ease, peace and well-being in which it can function more fluently and effectively, both physically and mentally.

Cranio-sacral integration responds to each individual according to his or her own needs, allowing and enhancing the body's inner wisdom to address whatever needs to be addressed and to resolve any disturbance accordingly.

Underlying health

Inevitably, patients tend to see their situation in terms of symptoms or a condition. They don't on the whole come to a therapist saying 'Please can you enhance my underlying vitality'. So it is appropriate to talk in terms of the various conditions that patients experience and for which they seek symptomatic relief. But ultimately, cranio-sacral integration is effective precisely because it is not merely addressing conditions. It is promoting the body's own healing ability, enhancing the inherent potential within the body to restore, maintain and enable health and healing – establishing that underlying platform of health and vitality that will enable the body to deal with the vicissitudes of life and to be healthy.

Chapter 4

Cranio-Sacral Integration

A spreading chestnut tree

The cranial concept was originally conceived by William Sutherland (1873–1954), an American osteopath, whose first insight into the cranio-sacral process came to him in 1899 and who devoted his whole life to the continuing development of the concept. From these roots it has grown and developed over the years, initially being taught within osteopathic colleges as cranial osteopathy (as practised by a small proportion of osteopaths) and subsequently expanding outside the osteopathic community as cranio-sacral therapy, branching out in different directions to form a continually evolving spreading chestnut tree of cranial work. Within this tree, there are several branches, each with its own distinctive features.

Branches

Two of the most prominent branches are:

- the approach of John Upledger, based on his 'pressurestat' conceptual model of the cranio-sacral system and expanding out to a broad application involving the use of various energetic and emotional resources
- the biodynamic model developed by James Jealous, with its predominant emphasis on the external forces of primary respiration as the principal source of health and healing.

Both these approaches, along with a wide variety of other variations, can be highly effective and profound, and each can be explored and studied elsewhere through its various texts, sources and resources.

A broad spectrum

In cranio-sacral integration, we appreciate the value and validity of all approaches, and also have our own contribution to add. Certain approaches may suit certain patients better than others. Certain approaches may suit particular circumstances or conditions better than others. Perhaps most of all, a certain approach may suit specific practitioners better than others. Cranio-sacral integration embraces the whole spectrum, maintaining a comprehensive, flexible view, appreciating how the various different concepts can be integrated to provide a broad spectrum approach that can respond to each patient according to his or her needs at an effective and profound level.

Much in common

The various approaches have their differences. They also have much in common. Essentially, all of them are utilising inherent natural forces – manifesting as rhythmic motion – as the source of the deepest and most effective healing. It is not necessary to eschew or discard different approaches. We can incorporate them all, integrate them, and use them as appropriate.

Ultimately, as we shall see, therapeutic effectiveness depends more on the individual therapist, and the inner resources which he or she has developed, rather than on the approach.

All approaches to cranio-sacral therapy involve:

- a light touch
- engaging with the inherent healing potential within the body manifesting as rhythmic motion
- the presence of a therapist
- a conceptual model.

Differences between approaches revolve primarily around:

- the exact degree of lightness of touch
- the exact degree to which the inherent forces are engaged

- the exact level of involvement by the therapist
- the different conceptual models and terminology used.

Evolution

Sutherland developed his concepts over many years, from an initial orientation to bones, membranes and a more active therapist input in the early years (an approach sometimes described as biomechanical) to an orientation to external forces and minimal therapist input in his later years (an approach sometimes referred to as biodynamic). Different branches of cranio-sacral therapy have adopted approaches from different stages of his life.

Life, science, and cranio-sacral therapy have continued to evolve since then. The evolution of new ideas can add to, rather than replace, old concepts. The development of quantum science doesn't mean that Newtonian laws no longer apply. We are still subject to gravity and would be foolish not to take it into account in our everyday life.

A broad spectrum of health care

In providing the best health care for patients, there are times when surgery, medication or hospitalisation might be appropriate (for example, following a severe car accident, or for an acute life-threatening infection), and the many different options for health care (surgery, medication, homeopathy, osteopathy, chiropractic, acupuncture, herbalism, yoga, meditation, and many others) all have their potential benefits.

In the same way, within the spectrum of cranio-sacral therapy, different resources may be suitable for different circumstances and the many options within the spectrum of cranio-sacral therapy – biodynamic, biomechanical, fascial unwinding, emotional release, etc. – all have their place and suit different people at different times.

Cranio-sacral integration:
- sees each individual as an integral part of the unified natural world around us
- addresses the whole person rather than specific symptoms, restrictions or conditions
- integrates not only the whole person – mind, body, spirit – but also the whole person within the context of their life
- integrates the deepest healing forces of nature with an informed awareness and understanding of anatomical, physiological and pathological relationships
- appreciates the value of the whole spectrum of cranio-sacral approaches:
  - integrating quantum and Newtonian concepts
  - integrating biodynamic and biomechanical concepts
  - recognising the value of working with the whole range of different levels, rhythms and tides
  - recognising that a variety of resources can be helpful in the therapeutic process
- provides a cohesive integrated treatment framework:
  - enabling each treatment to be a cohesive integration in itself
  - seeing each moment of every treatment within the context of overall integration of the whole person
  - addressing and integrating all layers and levels of the patient's being
  - integrating a range of resources to respond appropriately to each patient according to their needs.

Chapter 5

The Matrix
A Broad Perspective on the Cranio-Sacral System

The forces of nature which permeate our bodies and underlie our existence (described by William Sutherland as 'the Breath of Life'; Sutherland 1967) make us alive, creating and maintaining our individual *vitality*. This underlying vitality, pervading every cell, every tissue, every part of the body, is expressed as *rhythmic motion* – expanding and contracting, rising and falling, in wave-like, tide-like motion (described by Sutherland as primary respiration – respiration because it feels like breathing, primary because it is more fundamental to life than thoracic respiration).

Quality, symmetry and motion

As this fundamental life force is expressed through the body, the particular way in which it is expressed in each person creates an individual *quality* or qualities – combinations of characteristics – for that individual. The life force is expressed *symmetrically* through the body around the central midline. It is expressed as rhythmic *motion*.

- In a 'perfect' healthy body, the quality will be warm, soft, loose, free, vital.
- The 'perfect' body will be perfectly symmetrical.
- The motion will be expressed as an even rhythmic motion of ample amplitude expressed on various levels.

Of course no one has a 'perfect' body. Everyone has a history – genetic patterns, birth trauma, childhood falls, physical injuries, illnesses, tensions, traumas, stresses – all of which cause disturbance to their system and therefore to their function.

Disturbance to this perfect, balanced, healthy state will affect quality, symmetry and motion:

- The quality may become tight, restricted, hard, contracted, agitated, or changed in a multitude of different ways, reflecting the nature of the injury or disturbance.
- The symmetry may be disturbed, creating patterns of asymmetry – pulls, twists, focal points of restriction to the free flow of movement – reflecting the site of disturbance.
- The motion may become constricted, reduced in amplitude, slower, faster, weaker, agitated or in turmoil, reflecting the nature of the disturbance.

The cranio-sacral therapist can identify and interpret these changes in quality, symmetry and motion, and through this information can assess and address the underlying causes of any disturbances.

These disturbances of quality, symmetry and motion reflect disturbances of health on all levels:

- physical, mental, emotional or spiritual
- superficial or profound
- recent or chronic
- transient or deeply ingrained.

By tuning in to these characteristics of quality, symmetry and motion, we can:

- read the health, vitality, and nature of the person on all levels
- identify disturbances to healthy function from whatever cause
- identify the source of the disturbance.

By helping the body to release any restrictions and return to a fluent, freely mobile expression of healthy balanced quality, symmetry and motion, the cranio-sacral therapist can assist in the elimination of the underlying source of any dysfunction – thereby also eliminating symptoms – integrating the system as a whole, and restoring health and vitality.

What does this cranio-sacral system actually consist of?

The cranio-sacral system could be defined in terms of specific anatomical structures, most notably:

- the cranium (the bones of the head)
- the sacrum (the tailbone)
- the membranes, which extend from cranium to sacrum, enveloping the brain and spinal cord
- the cerebrospinal fluid, which is contained within the membranes and bathes the brain and spinal cord.

But before we examine the relevance of these anatomical structures, we first need to gain a broader perspective.

A broader perspective

The cranial concept was first inspired by looking at the bones of the cranium. William Sutherland, a student osteopath at the American School of Osteopathy in Kirksville, Missouri in the United States in 1899, looked at a skull and realised that the bones were designed for movement. Conventional anatomy books (at least in the English language) state that the bones of the adult cranium do not move, but Sutherland explored his hypothesis and felt movement in the head, a subtle rhythmic expansion and contraction.

Exploration

Sutherland's lifelong explorations took him way beyond the bones of the cranium, and we can also see beyond the bones. Conventional anatomy books *still* state that the bones of the cranium do not move, but like Sutherland we too can tune in to the head and feel subtle rhythmic movement, along with various qualities and asymmetries.

As we continue to tune in to the body, we soon realise that the movements and other characteristics that we are feeling are much softer than bone, and much more expansive than bone, so it is clearly not merely the movement of bones that we are feeling.

We can extend our awareness to consider what other softer, more pliable structures might be involved, and we can turn our attention to the membranes which line the bones and envelop the central nervous system, to see if this is where the movement is being expressed.

In doing this, we can observe that the movements and qualities that we feel have a more fluidic quality to them than any membrane. So again we can reflect on what structures within the body could be expressing such a fluidic motion and we can extend our awareness further, to the cerebrospinal fluid contained within the membranes and bathing the brain and spinal cord.

Here we might feel that at last we have a recognisable anatomical structure which matches the fluent, fluidic, fluctuating sensations that we are experiencing. But then we realise that these movements and qualities are not limited to the core of the system where the cerebrospinal fluid is located, but extend to all the soft tissues and fluids throughout the body.

So it is not just bones, or membranes, or cerebrospinal fluid that we are tuning in to, but everything in the body.

Beyond fluids

Then, with our touch so soft and light that we are barely touching the head, we can observe that, even with our hands off the body, we can still feel these movements, qualities and asymmetries; and we can come to the realisation that what we are tuning in to is the movement of something more subtle than bones, membranes, or fluids. What we are picking up through this subtle level of palpation is the movement of a universal force which pervades all the tissues of the body but which also extends beyond the tissues. We are engaging with the *matrix*.

The matrix

What we are tuning in to is not specifically bones, membranes or fluids, but the movement of subtle energy or vitality through these structures and beyond these structures, the movement of the whole energy matrix within and around the body – an energy matrix which incorporates the bones, membranes and fluids, but which does not specifically consist of them (see Figure 5.1 and Box 5.1).

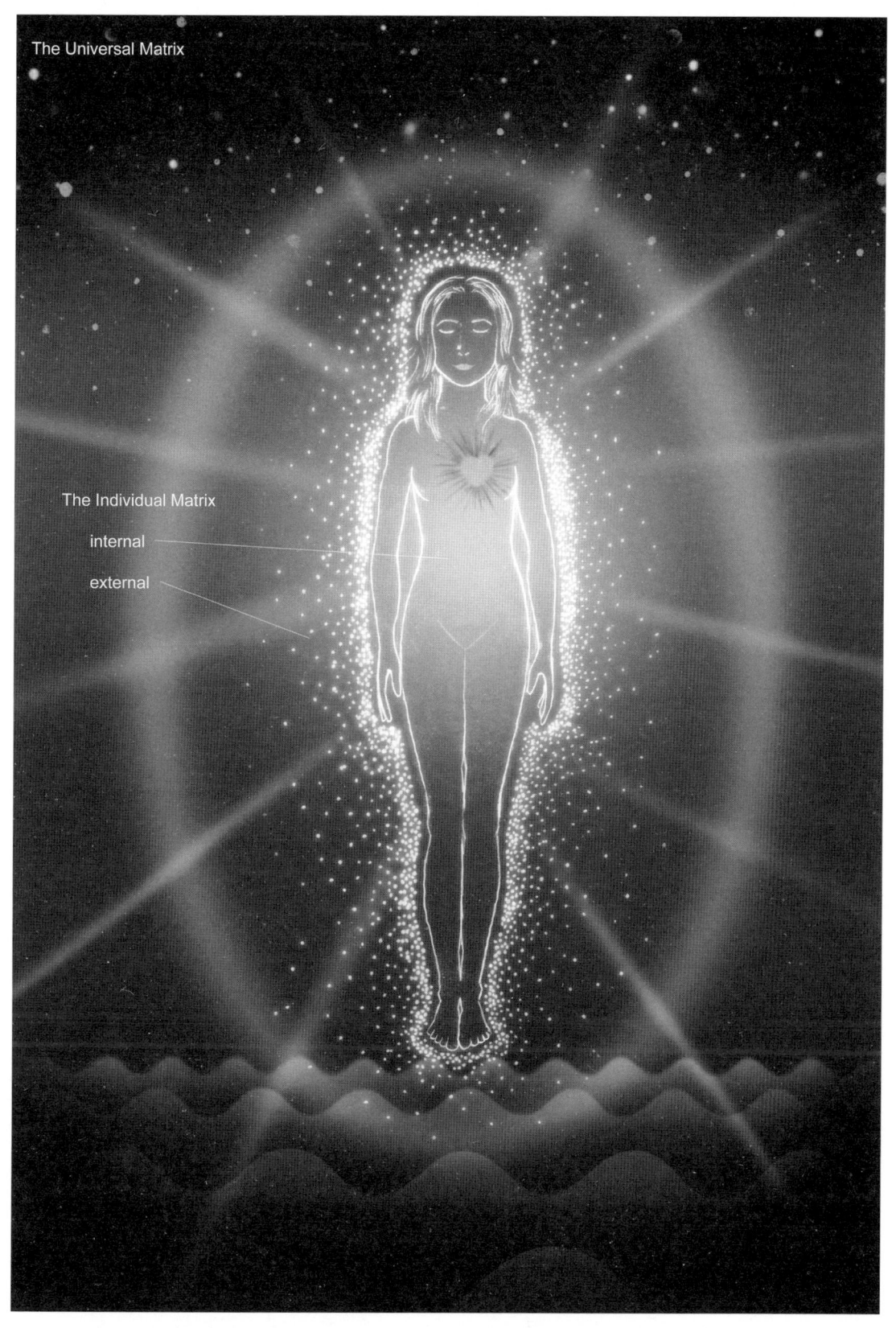

5.1 The matrix of the physical body (the internal matrix) is cocooned within the outer layers of the matrix (the external matrix) which blend into the matrix of the world around us (the universal matrix)

This matrix is present in early embryonic life, forming an energetic field or blueprint into which the physical body grows and develops. Throughout life the matrix is present as a force field within which we exist, visible to some as the aura, palpable to some as a cushion of energy or field of energy. The physical body is not simply within this matrix, it is a part of the matrix. The physical tissues are a densification of the energy of the matrix into physical form, shaped by the forces within the matrix.

Every part of the body, every tissue – every bone, muscle, fascia, membrane, fluid – is composed of subatomic particles, quantum units of energy in constant motion and vibration. The matrix of the physical body (the internal matrix) is cocooned within the outer layers of the matrix (the external matrix – the etheric body and the other layers of the aura, less dense components of the matrix). Your personal matrix (your individual matrix) blends into the matrix of the world around us (the universal matrix).

Through this continuous matrix are flowing the fundamental natural forces of the universe (the Breath of Life), the generative and regenerative forces which create and maintain life and health; and as they flow through the matrix, these natural forces generate subtle rhythmic motion.

Continuing our exploration

As we continue to explore, we can discover that this energy matrix is affected by emotions – the qualities, asymmetries and movements that we feel, change in response to emotional reaction:

The patient is lying on the couch, perhaps imagining themselves on a peaceful sunny tropical island, or dreaming of love – the quality, symmetry and motion that you experience as you engage with their system will reflect these pleasant dreams. The patient then remembers a serious accident they suffered, or remembers that they have to go to the dentist or thinks back on something that makes them sad or angry – the characteristics of their system will change accordingly.

Box 5.1 The matrix

The term *matrix* is Latin for *womb* and indicates a flexible environment within which something can develop. (Hence its use also as a flexible mathematical grid which expands and contracts as its contents develop.)

In the context of cranio-sacral integration:

- The *embryonic matrix* is the force field within which the embryo grows and develops.
- The *individual matrix* is the force field within which your physical body and its immediate surroundings (etheric body, auric field) exist. It includes all the structures within (*internal matrix*) and around (*external matrix*) your physical body and the forces operating within, between and through them.
- The *universal matrix* is the universal field of forces within which the natural world forms and develops, and within which we exist and are influenced. It comprises the whole universe and the forces of nature which bind it together, which hold the planets and galaxies in appropriate relation to each other, and which maintain the integrity and continuity of everything going on within the natural world.

Natural forces within the universal matrix flow through your body (your individual matrix) generating rhythmic motion and maintaining life, growth, development and healing. Each of us exists as a small but integral part of the wider universal matrix.

Recognising the matrix enables us to understand that everything in the body and its surroundings – bones, muscle, membrane, fascia, fluid – is composed of subatomic particles, a quantum mass of elementary particles and forces; and therefore to see the body and its surroundings, not simply as separate mechanical physical structures, but as a continuous cohesive unit, a mass of quantum particles, waves and forces in constant flux, with infinite potential for change.

Everything that you think and feel affects your body and affects your cranio-sacral system and leaves its mark to be identified by the cranio-sacral therapist.

We can also see that emotions are affected by everything around us:

You are sitting in a railway carriage, a whole compartment to yourself, contentedly engrossed in your book. Your cranio-sacral system will be quietly reflecting that peaceful contentment. Then someone else comes in – and your system immediately changes. Of course it depends who they are and how they behave. Perhaps they simply sit down in the opposite corner of the carriage and start reading their magazine and you settle back contentedly into your book. Perhaps they are loud and unruly and they sit down very close to you and stare at you intensely and persistently; you begin to feel uncomfortable and threatened. Perhaps they are drunk and disorderly. Perhaps they are the most beautiful person that you have ever seen. Whichever way, your system will change, the quality, symmetry and motion will adjust to whatever is going on within you, which in turn is adjusting to whatever is going on around you.

Through this scenario we can see how these changes to your quality, symmetry and motion are affected by every little transient event in everyday life. *How much more will they be affected by major traumas, accidents and injuries, leaving their effects deeply imprinted into our systems?*

So as we tune in to the patient, every patient, and engage with the patterns of movement and stillness within their system, we are feeling not only the effects of physical injury and disease within their bodies, but also the effects of thought and emotion – current emotions or deeply ingrained past trauma – and consequently the influence of the outside world and their whole life circumstances and surroundings upon these patterns of energy movement within their body.

So when we tune in to the cranio-sacral system, we are in fact tuning in to:

- the whole person and their response to the environment within which they are living
- the whole body-mind complex within the context of their life
- the whole matrix of the individual within the wider matrix of the world around them.

This is the cranio-sacral system.

Box 5.2 Quantum science

A *quantum* is the smallest unit of anything, such as photons of light; it was first defined by Max Planck in 1900.

Quantum theory/quantum mechanics/quantum science/quantum physics are the basis of modern scientific thinking. Initially conceived in the 1920s by Werner Heisenberg, Erwin Schrödinge and Paul Durak, they recognise that everything in the universe (galaxies, planets, mountains, rocks, plants, animals, humans, oceans, fluids, air, heat, light, thought) is composed of quanta – elementary particles, waves and forces – in a state of constant interaction, through which everything influences everything else, including the observer and the observed.

Box 5.3 The extent of the individual matrix

The external component of your individual matrix is composed of the etheric body and the other layers of the aura surrounding your physical body. It is visible to some and palpable to others as a cushion of energy and may often be felt during cranio-sacral treatment. The distance to which it extends beyond the skin is described quite specifically in various texts. For the most part they tend to give different values, ranging from a few inches to several feet. This is perhaps partly because the matrix changes from moment to moment in response to circumstances, partly because its limit is not clearly defined and tends to fade or blend into the surrounding universal matrix, partly because it is composed of various distinct layers, partly because there are various different fields around our bodies, all of which are interacting. These include a biomagnetic field extending indefinitely until it gradually fades into the surrounding atmospheric magnetic field.

Box 5.4 The matrix in science

The matrix and its associated fields are increasingly recognised within scientific circles, and incorporated into medical research, as described by the distinguished biologist and physiologist James Oschman in his comprehensive book *Energy Medicine: The Scientific Basis* (Oschman 2000).

The living matrix

The living matrix is a continuous and dynamic, supramolecular web-work, extending into every nook and cranny of the body: a nuclear matrix within a cellular matrix within a connective tissue matrix. In essence, when you touch a human body you are touching a continuously interconnected system, composed of virtually all of the molecules in the body, linked together in an intricate web-work. (*Energy Medicine: The Scientific Basis.* Oschman 2000)

Biomagnetic fields

A Superconducting Quantum Interference Device (SQUID) is a magnetometer for measuring biomagnetic fields. SQUIDs are now being used in medical research laboratories around the world to map the magnetic fields produced by physiological processes inside the human body.

Living organisms have biomagnetic fields around them. These fields change from moment to moment in relation to events taking place inside the body. These fields give a clearer representation of what is going on in the body than classical electrical diagnostic tools such as the electrocardiogram and the electroencephalogram.

All parts of the living matrix set up vibrations that move about within the organism, and are radiated into the environment. These vibrations or oscillations occur at many different frequencies, including invisible and near-visible light frequencies. These are not subtle phenomena, they are large or even gigantic in scale. Moreover, their effects are not trivial, because living matter is highly organised, and exceedingly sensitive to the information conveyed by coherent signals. (*Energy Medicine: The Scientific Basis.* Oschman 2000)

Chapter 6

Living in the Material World
Anatomy of the Cranio-Sacral System

Introduction

The fact that we are working with a matrix of subtle energy doesn't mean that anatomical structures become irrelevant. This energy pervades, perfuses and forms these structures. These structures are energy – in a more condensed form. It is a basic law of physics that all matter is energy. Everything in the body, even the most solid bone, is formed of molecules, of subatomic particles, of elementary particles in constant dynamic motion, of energy.

The physical body has grown and developed embryologically from an inner source of life. These anatomical structures – bones, muscles, organs – are the physical manifestation of the inner being, formed, developed and perfused by the inherent forces of vitality. They have developed within, and been formed by, the matrix within which they are growing. Their composition is more dense than subtle energy, but they are an integral part of the matrix, and remain a significant reflection and extension of our inner self.

Bones, membranes, fascia, soft tissues and fluids can all be adversely affected by injury and disease, leading to pain and disturbed function; and when they are adversely affected, this will be reflected in the quality of the tissues, the asymmetries within the body, and the restricted expression of rhythmic motion both locally and through the body as a whole. In order for someone to feel healthy and be healthy, vitality needs to be expressed freely in all tissues of the body.

So in order to engage with all levels of the cranio-sacral system, it is still valuable to:

- understand the various structures of the body
- see how they reflect vitality through the expression of rhythmic motion
- see how restrictions in these anatomical structures can affect the flow of energy, with consequent adverse effects on health
- assist the body's inherent potential to address the restrictions within the gross anatomy, releasing the kinetic energy locked into these body structures, enabling them to return to free and balanced mobility and free expression of rhythmic motion.

Within the wider perceptual context of force fields and the matrix, it is therefore still relevant to look at the structures which form the *anatomical cranio-sacral system*. These are:

- *the membrane system,* which surrounds and envelopes the central nervous system
- *the bones of the cranium and sacrum,* which attach to the membrane system
- *the cerebrospinal fluid,* which is contained within the membrane system
- *the fascia,* which radiates out from the membrane system to all parts of the body.

1. The membrane system

The membrane system (Figure 6.1) consists of a triple layered membrane, surrounding and enclosing the central nervous system (brain and spinal cord). These membranes are also known as the *meninges*, and are the structures affected in meningitis.

The three layers of the membrane system are:

- the pia mater
- the arachnoid mater
- the dura mater.

The term *mater* is Latin for *mother*, and reflects the motherly protective function of these membranes in enveloping the brain and spinal cord in a protective covering, impermeable to the outside environment.

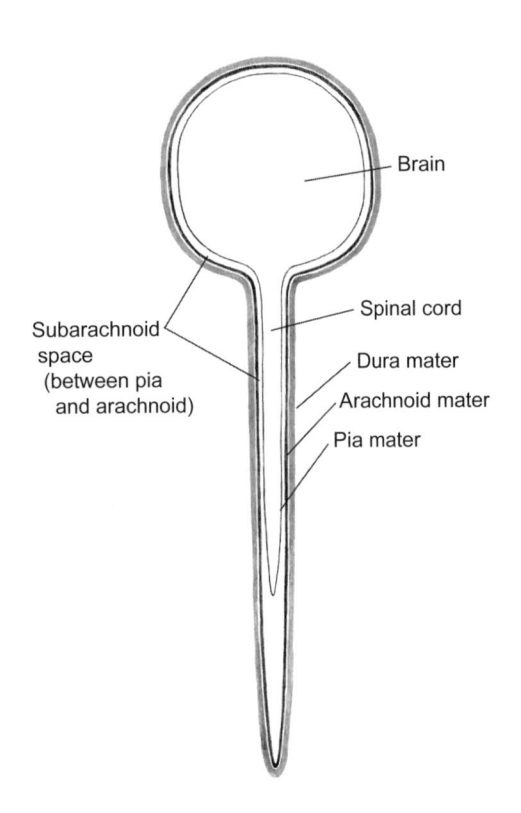

6.1   A triple layered membrane system

Pia mater

Pia mater means soft mother. This is the innermost layer and is a soft delicate inner layer of membrane closely enveloping the central nervous system, following closely every gyrus and sulcus (every bump and dip) on the surface of the brain and spinal cord.

Arachnoid mater

Arachnoid mater is the term for the middle layer of membrane. Between the arachnoid mater and the pia mater, there is a fluid filled space known as the *subarachnoid space* (inside the arachnoid mater, outside the pia mater) containing cerebrospinal fluid. The term arachnoid refers to the spider-web structure of trabeculae which form a network of fibrous connections passing between the arachnoid and the pia within the subarachnoid space. The subarachnoid space also contains a network of tiny cerebral blood vessels supplying oxygen to the cortex and penetrating into the brain tissue.

Dura mater

Dura mater means tough mother. This is the outermost layer of the three membranes, a stronger tougher layer. It forms the outer perimeter of the membrane system, protecting the central nervous system from the surrounding environment. It is impermeable to fluids and therefore prevents potentially damaging organisms and fluids from gaining access to the brain and spinal cord. As the outermost layer, it also provides attachment and connection of the membrane system to the surrounding bones, and is the layer which relates most closely to the surrounding structures and surrounding environment. Consequently it is the layer most frequently referred to, and the term dura is commonly (although imprecisely) used to refer to the whole membrane system, encompassing all three layers.

SUBDIVISIONS OF DURA

The *cranial dura* is the dura within the cranium, surrounding the brain. The *spinal dura* is the dura within the vertebral column of the spine, surrounding the spinal cord. However, these are not separate structures.

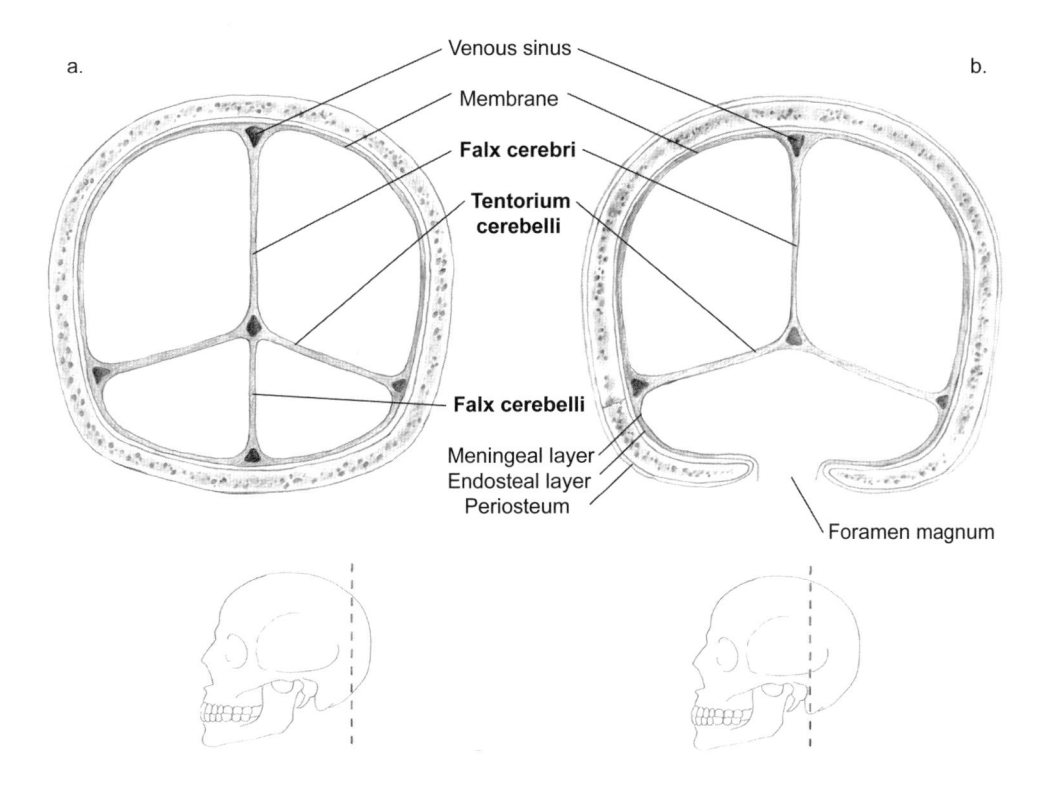

6.2 *The intracranial membranes – infoldings of membrane, partially dividing the intracranial space*
  a. Coronal section through the cranium in line with the posterior occiput
  b. Coronal section through the cranium in line with the foramen magnum
  (The falx cerebelli is not present at this point)

The dura mater and indeed all three membranous layers form a *continuous unified sheath* around the central nervous system from the top of the cranium (lining the inner surface of the skull) down to the sacrum (within the sacral canal) and the distinction between cranial dura and spinal dura is only for convenience of anatomical location.

The dura is itself further subdivided into two layers of dural membrane: an outer layer and an inner layer, with the two layers having separate blood supply, separate nerve supply and separate functions.

The outer layer of dura, known as the *endosteal* layer, forms a lining to the internal surface of the bones of the cranium. It is also continuous with the *periosteum*, the membranous layer which envelops the outer surface of the cranial bones, forming a membranous sac containing the bones of the cranium (see Figure 6.2).

The inner layer of dura, known as the *meningeal* layer, forms an inner lining, a lining within a lining, but also folds in to form several *infoldings* (together with the arachnoid mater and pia mater) partially dividing the intracranial space into sections, and creating membranous folds – also known as the *intracranial membranes* – between the different parts of the brain (see Figure 6.2).

Disturbances, asymmetries and restrictions to these infoldings can have profound effects on the balance and integration of the whole cranio-sacral system; and restoration of symmetry and free mobility of these intracranial membranes can be profoundly therapeutic. These infoldings are also significant because they form the *venous sinuses* (see Figure 6.2) and therefore determine the pathways of *venous drainage*, draining deoxygenated venous blood from the brain (thereby enabling the supply of fresh oxygenated arterial blood to the brain).

28 \ Cranio-Sacral Integration

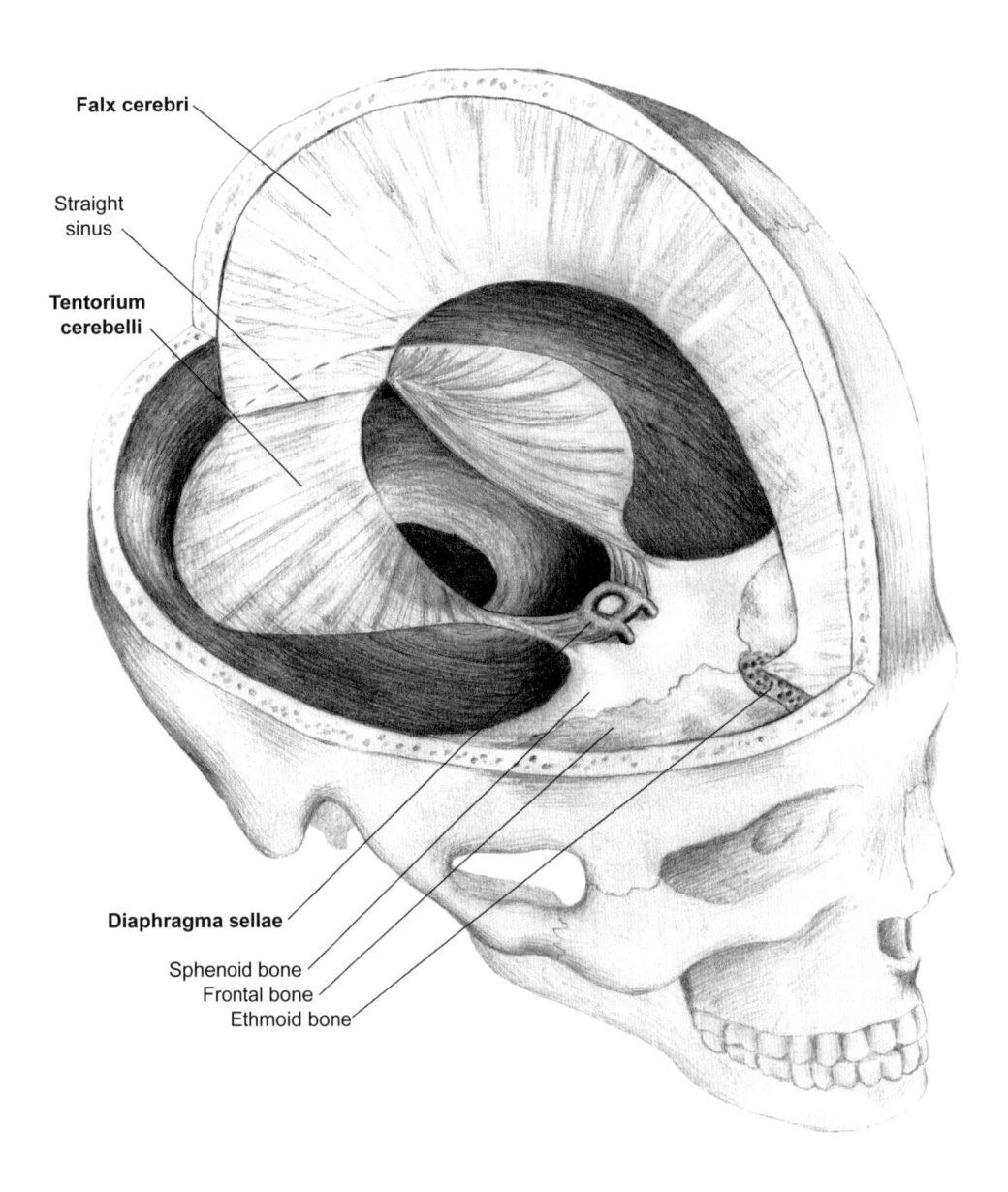

6.3   The intracranial membranes – oblique view

Membranous infoldings

There are four principal infoldings:

- *The falx cerebri:* a sickle-shaped membrane running from front to back of the cranium along the midline between the two cerebral hemispheres (see Figures 6.3 and 6.4).
- *The falx cerebelli:* a much smaller sickle-shaped membrane passing down the midline of the occipital region between the two cerebellar hemispheres (see Figure 6.4).

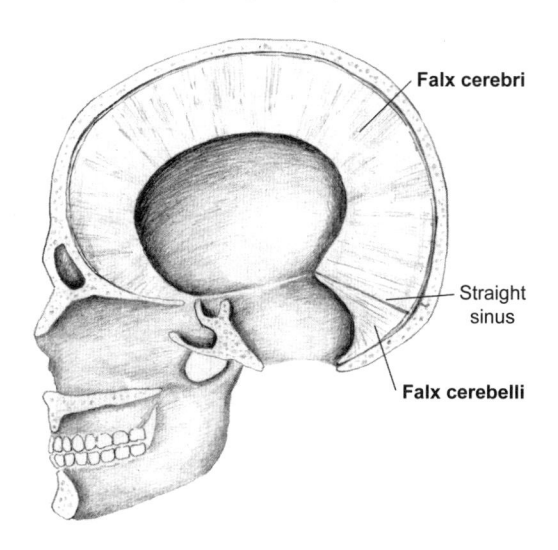

6.4   Falx cerebri and falx cerebelli – mid-sagittal section

- *The tentorium cerebelli:* a tent-shaped membranous structure passing almost horizontally across the cranium dividing the cerebrum above from the cerebellum below (see Figures 6.3 and 6.7).
- *The diaphragma sellae:* a small horizontal membrane forming a roof over the *sella turcica* of the sphenoid bone and enveloping the pituitary gland (see Figure 6.3).

These are not separate structures; they are all part of a continuous membranous sheath. Each infolding is formed as a double membrane, with the membrane from each side folding in to form this double membrane (see Figure 6.2).

At the points where the inner layer of dura separates from the outer layer of dura to form these infoldings, spaces are formed. These spaces are the *venous sinuses* mentioned above which are responsible for venous drainage from the brain.

Venous blood drains away from the brain along these venous sinuses, on its way back to the heart. Further venous sinuses are formed at the junctions between the infoldings and elsewhere. The falx cerebri, the falx cerebelli and the tentorium cerebelli all meet at the *straight sinus* (see Figures 6.2, 6.3 and 6.4).

The whole membrane system is of course expressing inherent rhythmic motion, along with all the other components of the matrix, expanding and contracting like an elongated balloon.

All parts of the membrane system, from the top of the cranium to the tip of the coccyx, are interconnected, forming a *reciprocal tension membrane system* (see Figure 6.5). This suggests that tensions or imbalances within any part of the membrane system are liable to influence all other parts of the membrane system. These reciprocal effects are clearly apparent, but since the nature of the membrane is such that these forces could not be transmitted by simple mechanical means, they must be transmitted by more subtle energetic means.

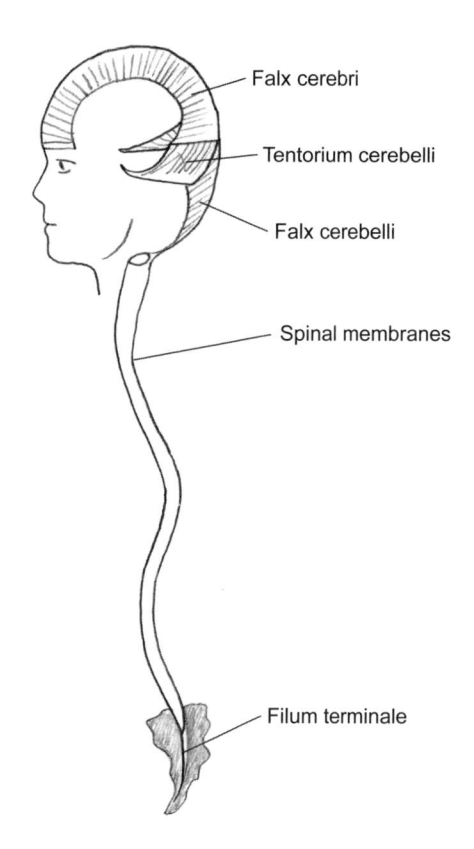

6.5   The reciprocal tension membrane system

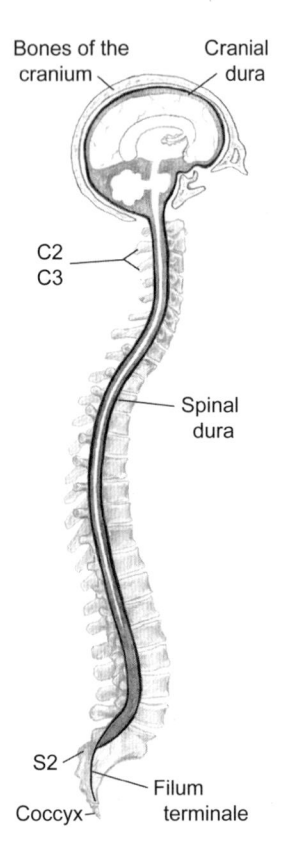

6.6 The dural membrane forms firm bony attachments to the internal surface of all the bones of the cranium, the 2nd and 3rd cervical vertebrae, the sacrum and the coccyx

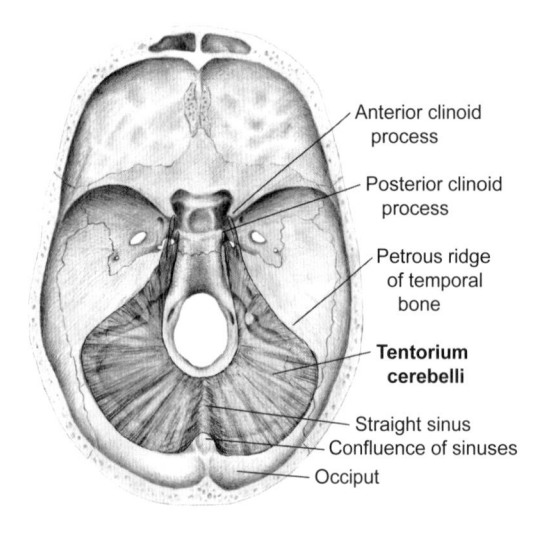

6.7 The tentorium cerebelli

Bony attachments to the membrane system

The dural membrane forms firm bony attachments to the internal surface of all the bones of the cranium: the frontal bone, the two parietal bones, the two temporal bones, the occipital bone (occiput), the sphenoid bone, the ethmoid bone, and also to the following bones: the second and third cervical vertebrae (C2 and C3), the sacrum and the coccyx (see Figure 6.6).

The infoldings form indirect attachments more specifically within the cranium to the following bones:

- *Falx cerebri:* to the ethmoid (at the crista galli), frontal, parietals and occiput.
- *Falx cerebelli:* to the occiput.
- *Tentorium cerebelli:* to the occiput, parietals, temporals, sphenoid (at the clinoid processes).
- *Diaphragma sellae:* to the sphenoid.

The *falx cerebri* (see Figures 6.3 and 6.4) runs from front to back within the cranium, partially dividing the cranium into two halves, and forming a double-layered membranous sheet between the two cerebral hemispheres. It attaches anteriorly to the crista galli of the ethmoid, passes up along the midline of the inner surface of the frontal bone, runs along the midline of the inner surface of the parietal bones on each side of the sagittal suture, and down the midline of the occiput as far as the *confluence of sinuses* and the straight sinus, where it meets and blends into the tentorium cerebelli and falx cerebelli. At its anterior attachment to the ethmoid, it blends into the surrounding membranes. Along its superior border it blends into the surrounding membranes from which it has been formed.

The *falx cerebelli* (see Figure 6.4) runs along the midline of the inner surface of the occiput, from the straight sinus and confluence of sinuses above, down to the *foramen magnum* below, where it blends into the surrounding membranes.

The *tentorium cerebelli* (see Figures 6.3 and 6.7), commonly known as the tent, forms a tent-shaped double-layered membrane passing almost horizontally across the back of the cranium, passing from the confluence of sinuses posteriorly, along the bony ridges on the inner surface of the occiput, passing forward and medially along the petrous ridges of the temporal bones, and giving out four thin projections of membrane which attach onto the clinoid processes of the sphenoid bone:

- the upper layer attaches to the anterior clinoid processes
- the lower layer attaches to the posterior clinoid processes.

The two layers of the tentorium are formed embryologically from separate sources, and have separate nerve supplies (the upper leaf from the ophthalmic branch of the trigeminal nerve and the lower leaf from the upper cervical spinal nerves) and may therefore be influenced and affected separately by different factors. The tentorium surrounds a central space anteriorly through which the brainstem passes from the cerebral hemispheres above down to the spinal cord below.

The attachment of these infoldings to the bones is described as *indirect*, because the inner layer of dura is coming into contact with the bones only indirectly through the outer layer of dura, and the outer layer is uniformly attached to the bones throughout their inner surface. However, the clearly evident ridges of bone standing out from the inner surface of the cranium along the edges of the infoldings are a clear indication of the forces transmitted through these membranes into the bone.

Box 6.1 Development of bony ridges

Bony ridges, bumps and protrusions throughout the body develop in response to the pull of muscles, ligaments, membranes and other tissues. A good example is the mastoid processes – the bony lumps behind your ears – which are not present at birth, but which develop as a baby starts to move its head, in response to the pull of the sterno-cleido-mastoid muscles that attach there. In the same way, forces exerted through the intracranial membranes stimulate the development of bony ridges on the internal surface of the cranium.

The influence of these membranous attachments plays an integral part in the rhythmic motion of the cranium, establishing fulcrums around which the individual bones express their expansive and contractive movements.

Around the foramen magnum, the dura forms a thicker, more resistant, more firmly attached ring of membrane. This is not an insignificant anatomical detail; the greater resistance of the membrane in this region can be clearly felt by the cranio-sacral therapist and influences the mobility of the system as a whole.

Spinal membranes

In the spine, the spinal dura is also subdivided into an outer and inner layer, with an endosteal layer lining the bony vertebral canal and a meningeal layer (together with arachnoid and pia) enveloping the spinal cord.

Within the vertebral column, the meninges form a membranous tube (often referred to as the dural tube, although it again includes arachnoid mater and pia mater) floating freely within the vertebral canal, except for its attachments at:

- *the foramen magnum:* throughout its circumference
- *C2 and C3:* small attachments to the anterior wall of the vertebral canal
- *the sacrum:* to the anterior wall within the sacral canal at the second sacral segment
- *the coccyx:* via the *filum terminale* – a thin filament of membrane (comprising all three layers of membrane) which passes down from the lower end of the spinal cord to attach to the posterior surface of the first coccygeal segment (see Figure 6.6).

Apart from these firm bony attachments, the dural tube is otherwise free to float within the vertebral canal – although it is loosely tethered by the nerve roots which penetrate the membrane throughout its length. The dura is also loosely attached to the pia mater internally by denticulate ligaments passing between the two membranes, particularly in the lower part of the spine.

Throughout the vertebral canal, the dural membrane is penetrated by nerves, which exit from the central nervous system to travel to the periphery and enter the central nervous system from the periphery. At these points of penetration, the dura envelops each nerve for a few millimetres of its pathway from the central nervous system before blending into the *epineurium*, the fascial sheath which envelops the nerve throughout the rest of its pathway, providing continuity between the membrane and the fascia (see Figure 6.8).

Disturbances to the membrane system

Tensions, restrictions, or disturbances of the membrane system can arise from *many different sources*. Some of the more common sources are: meningitis, meningisms, sclerosis following on from inflammation, meningeal cysts, arachnoiditis, emotional tension, sympathetic stimulation, intrinsic pulls and imbalances within the reciprocal tension membrane system as a whole – whether arising in the sacrum, the cranium, the vertebral column, or from within the membranes themselves – injury or damage from a blow to the head, a fall on the sacrum, or from birth trauma, or disturbance of the membranes from any injured or diseased part of the body through neurological input from the affected area.

Tensions within the membranes can have *widespread effects*, both locally and distantly, both within the cranium and down the spine, impingeing on nerves and nerve roots, constricting blood vessels, restricting the movement of bones – both within cranial sutures and between vertebral segments, transmitting pulls and imbalances throughout the body. These often unrecognised internal restrictions can have far reaching consequences – whether through disturbed nerve function, disrupted visceral function, or severe pain – and may be at the root of chronic debilitating ill health.

Membranous restrictions transmitted *through the spinal dura* may impinge on spinal nerve roots, as the nerves penetrate the membranes, with repercussions in any of the organs, muscles or other structures supplied throughout that nerve pathway, perhaps to the viscera, perhaps to the arms or legs, perhaps maintaining visceral disturbances or leading to sciatica.

These pulls may be transmitted to other vertebral segments, stirring up old injuries and

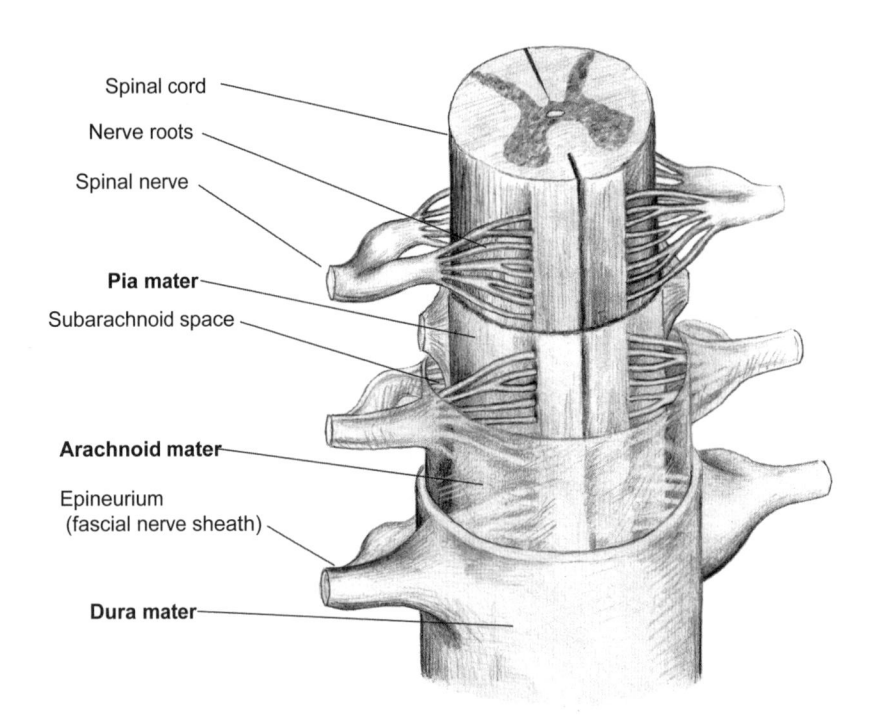

6.8 Throughout the vertebral canal, the membranes are penetrated by nerves exiting from the central nervous system and travelling to and from the periphery

weak areas (facilitated segments) in other parts of the spine. Local restrictions can therefore lead to reactions anywhere in the body. Tracing the restriction to its source, rather than treating the symptomatic area is of course essential and cranio-sacral palpation of the membranous pulls enables this where other methods are unable to do so, through engagement with the membranes.

Membranous restrictions *within the cranium* may impinge on cranial nerves as they pass out through the foramina of the cranium. Any of the cranial nerves could be affected, with consequences such as squint, Bell's Palsy (facial paralysis), trigeminal neuralgia, or in the case of the vagus nerve – widespread consequences on visceral function from colic and digestive disturbance to respiratory and cardiac dysfunction.

Membranous disturbances in the cranium may also potentially influence the drainage of venous blood within the cranium (via the venous sinuses) leading to congestion and thereby reducing the flow of fresh arterial blood and therefore oxygen to the brain. Arterial supply to the brain may also be adversely affected through damage to the network of vessels within the arachnoid mater. Meningeal restriction may also obstruct the free flow of cerebrospinal fluid interfering with its nutritive and protective functions to the brain and spinal cord. This is particularly significant in babies and children, potentially limiting brain growth and development. Membranous contraction around the brain may lead to headaches, migraine, a sense of congestion, contraction, tightness, vagueness, confusion, unclear thinking.

One common and often severely debilitating example of this is the long-term after-effects of meningitis, with its typical symptoms of persistent head pain, neck pain, pain behind the eyes, poor memory, poor concentration, vagueness. These persistent effects of meningitis, often misdiagnosed, are highly responsive to cranio-sacral treatment, often relieving conditions which have persisted for years and have not responded to other forms of treatment.

Cathy was in her mid-thirties and life was a struggle. She used to be a lively active young woman, full of the joys of life and enthusiastic about her job, but in her mid-twenties she had contracted bacterial meningitis and ever since she had felt too unwell to do anything much. She was constantly exhausted; just getting up in the morning was a huge effort; her brain felt constantly foggy; thinking was an effort; working was an effort; even the simplest task at work seemed to require so much concentration and even then she couldn't work out how to do it. But worst of all were the headaches, the intense pain behind her right eye, in the right side of her head and down the right side of her neck. Each day the pain would intensify as the day wore on, sometimes exploding with intensity.

The meningitis had of course been treated medically at the time, but when she went back to her doctor about the persistent symptoms, he assured her that they were nothing to do with the meningitis. As the years went by, she had seen countless doctors, all of whom said the same thing – nothing to do with the meningitis, no apparent cause for her symptoms. She was told again and again that it was psychosomatic and was referred for counselling and psychotherapy. She found this hard to believe and accept as it didn't fit in with her perspective at all and she felt that she was so normal in every other respect. She desperately wanted to be better, made every effort to recover and tried various other therapies. By now she had heard the psychosomatic point of view so many times and been told that there was nothing wrong with her so often that she had begun to doubt herself and to believe that she must be mad. But how could there be nothing wrong with her when she felt so bad.

Her symptoms and her story were typical of the chronic effects of meningitis. Tuning in to her system was even more convincing. The pattern of intense contraction in the membranes down that right hand side was unmistakable. There was nothing remotely psychosomatic about it. Treatment, as so often with meningitis effects, was immediately effective – even after ten years. The first session brought a dramatic improvement, and within a few more she was back to her old self – lively, enthusiastic, no longer exhausted, free of pain, able to think clearly and able to enjoy life again.

Free mobility and fully integrated function of the reciprocal tension membrane system is fundamental to health.

2. The bones

The second component of the anatomical structures of the cranio-sacral system is the bones which attach directly to the membrane system. These are:

- all the bones of the cranium
- the second and third cervical vertebrae
- the sacrum
- the coccyx.

Bones are the most evident, tangible, solid component of our bodies and therefore provide the most obvious visible framework around which to explore the cranio-sacral system. They are also the component which first attracted Sutherland's attention in developing the cranial concept, through his observation of the bones of the cranium as an osteopathic student. Consequently, much of cranial work has tended to revolve around bones. But it is helpful to keep this in proportion and recognise that the bones are not the basis of the cranio-sacral process. They are just the most dense and solidified component of the matrix and it is the matrix and the expression of vitality through the matrix which is more significant as the basis of the cranio-sacral process.

The bones, however, are a significant part of our material bodies and therefore a significant part of the cranio-sacral process, each bone expressing inherent rhythmic motion along with the rest of the matrix. The following bones are of particular significance within the cranio-sacral system because of their connection to the membrane system. They therefore exert a more significant influence on (and are in turn influenced by) the membrane system; and restrictions to the motion of these bones may play a significant part in restricting the free mobility and function of the membranes and on the integrity of the system as a whole.

The bones of the cranium (see Figures 6.9–6.13) are:

- the frontal bone
- the two parietal bones
- the two temporal bones
- the occipital bone (occiput)
- the sphenoid bone
- the ethmoid bone.

We will be exploring each bone individually in greater detail in subsequent chapters within the context of treatment.

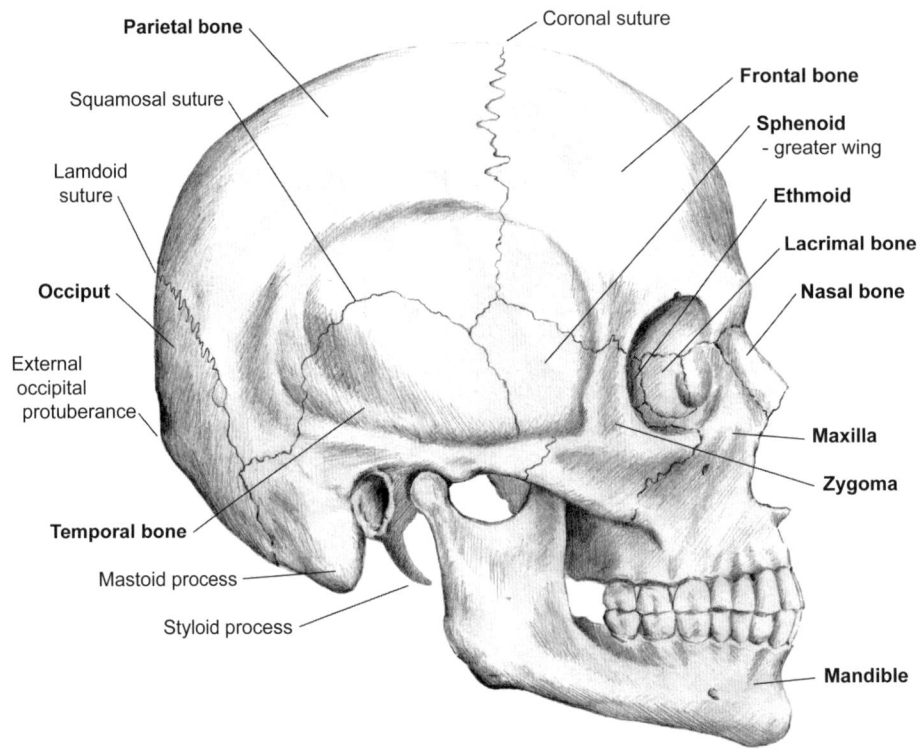

6.9   The cranium – lateral view

6.10 *The cranium – anterior view*

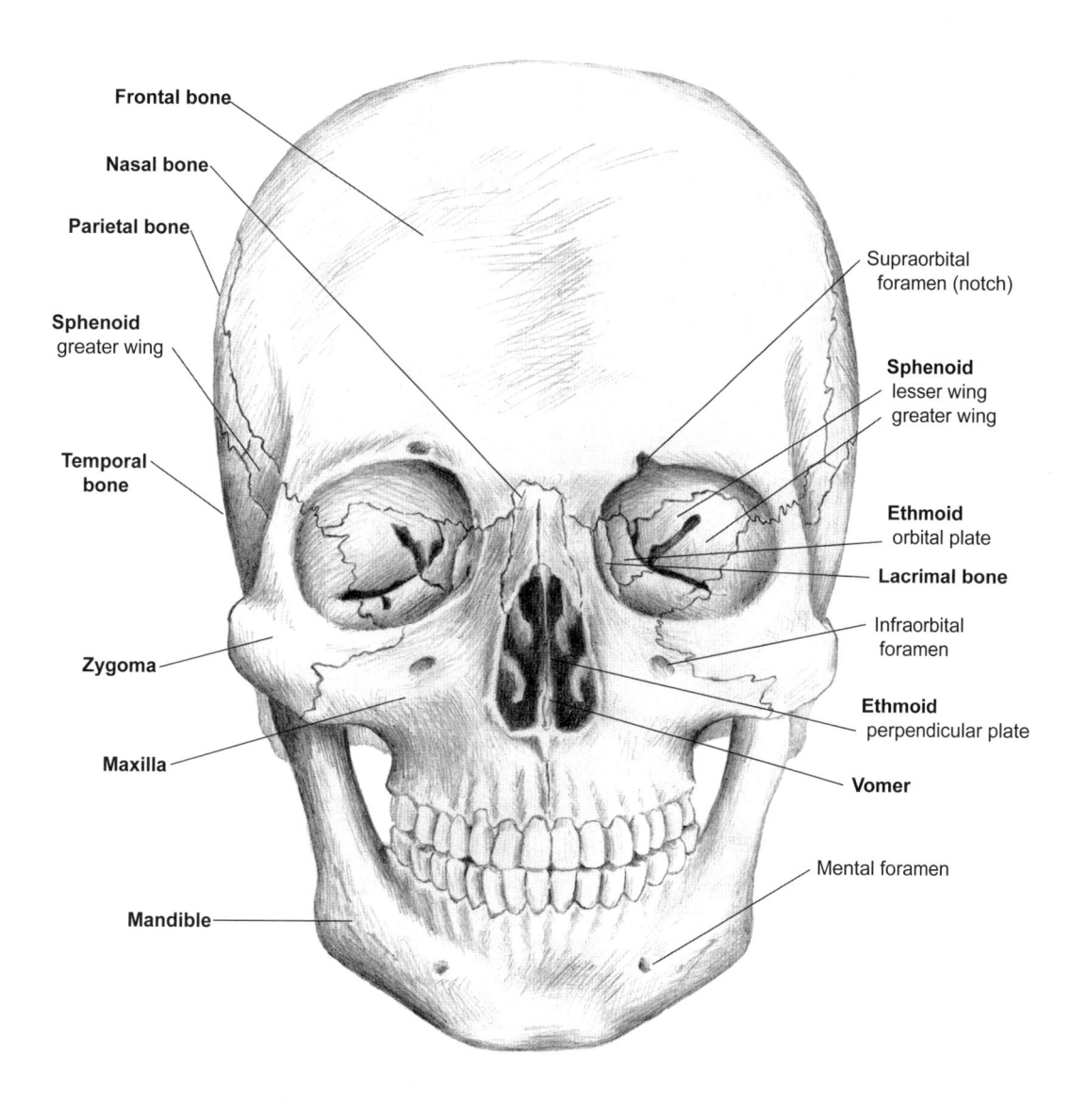

36 \ Cranio-Sacral Integration

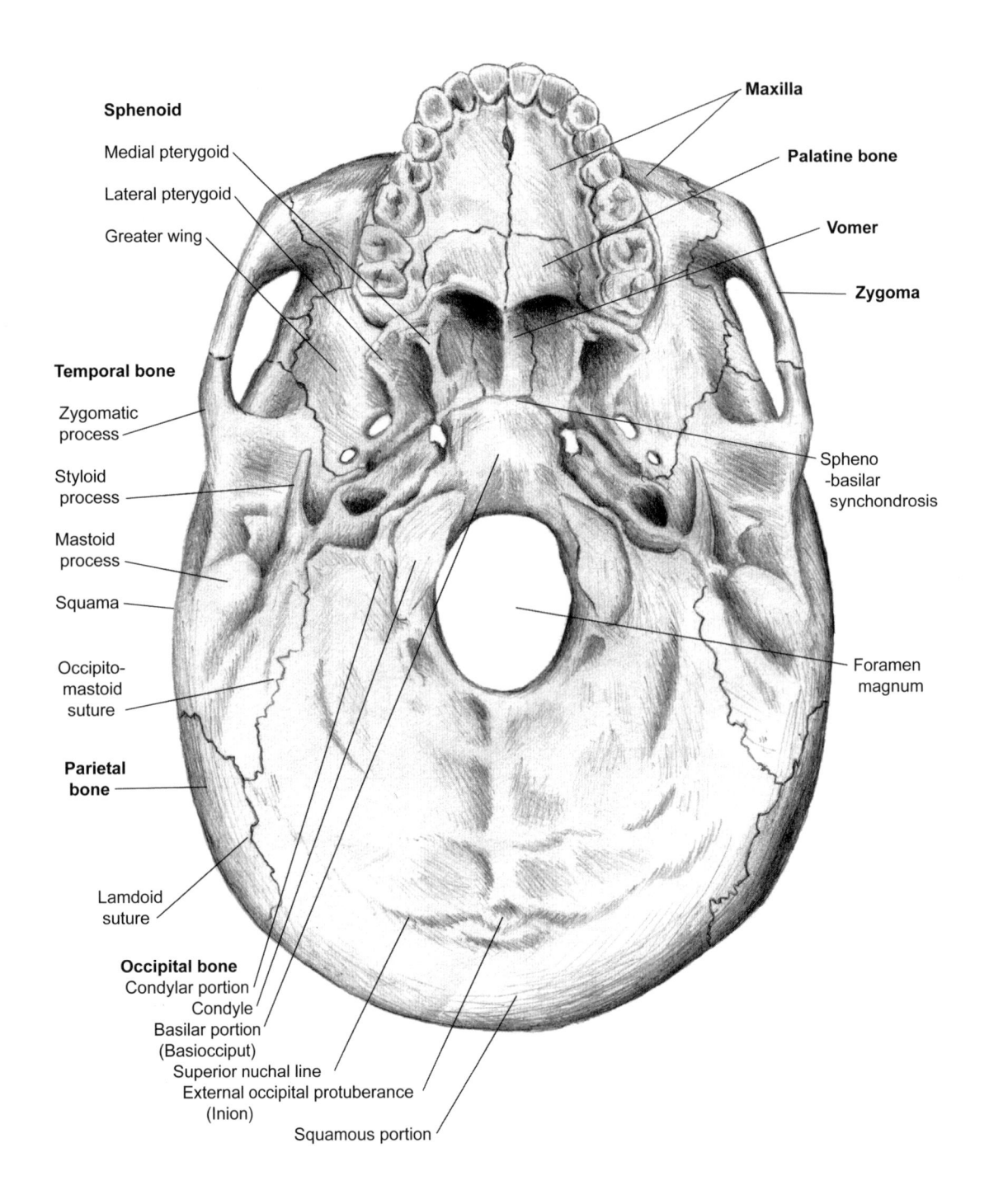

6.11 The cranial base – inferior view

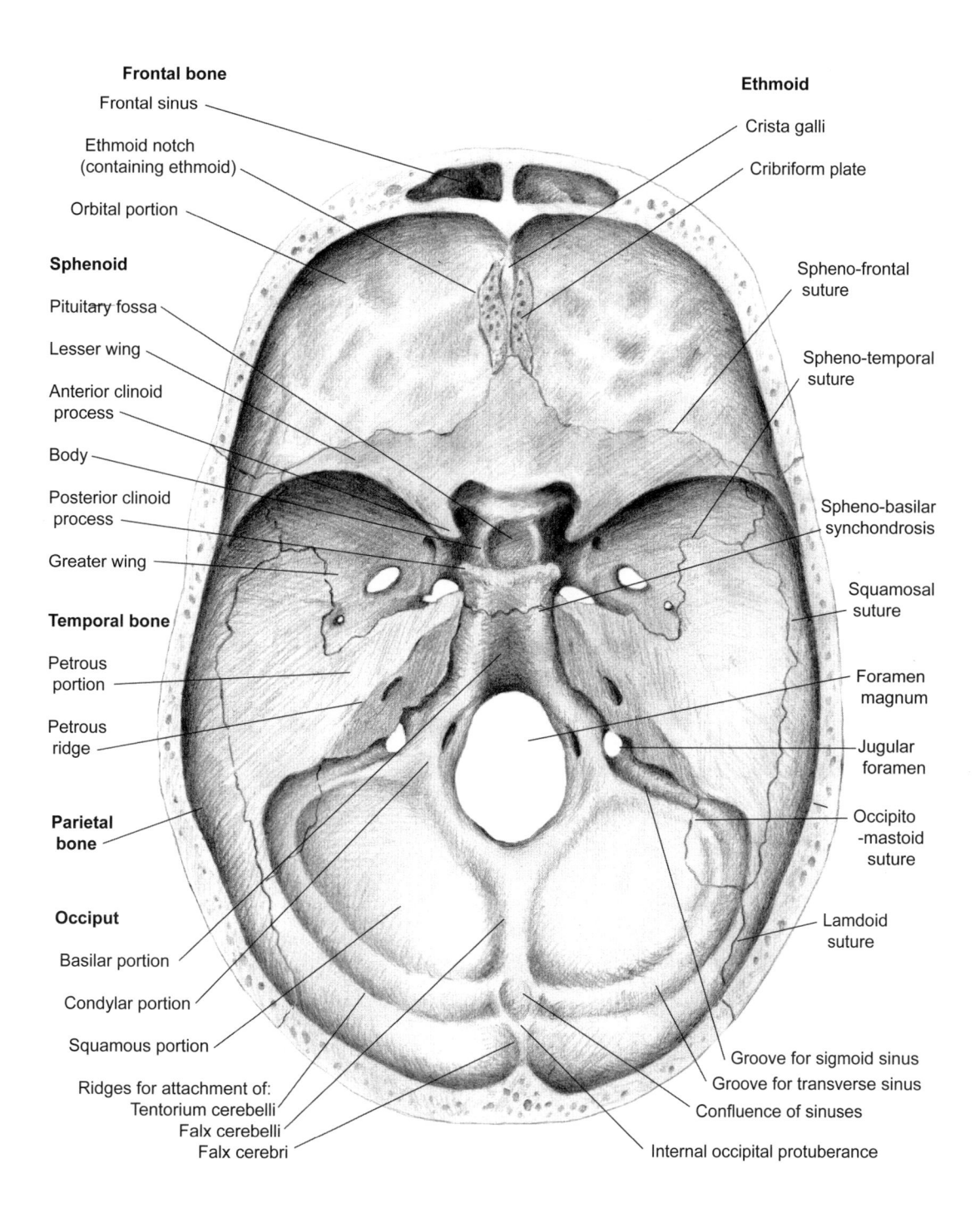

6.12 The cranial base – superior view

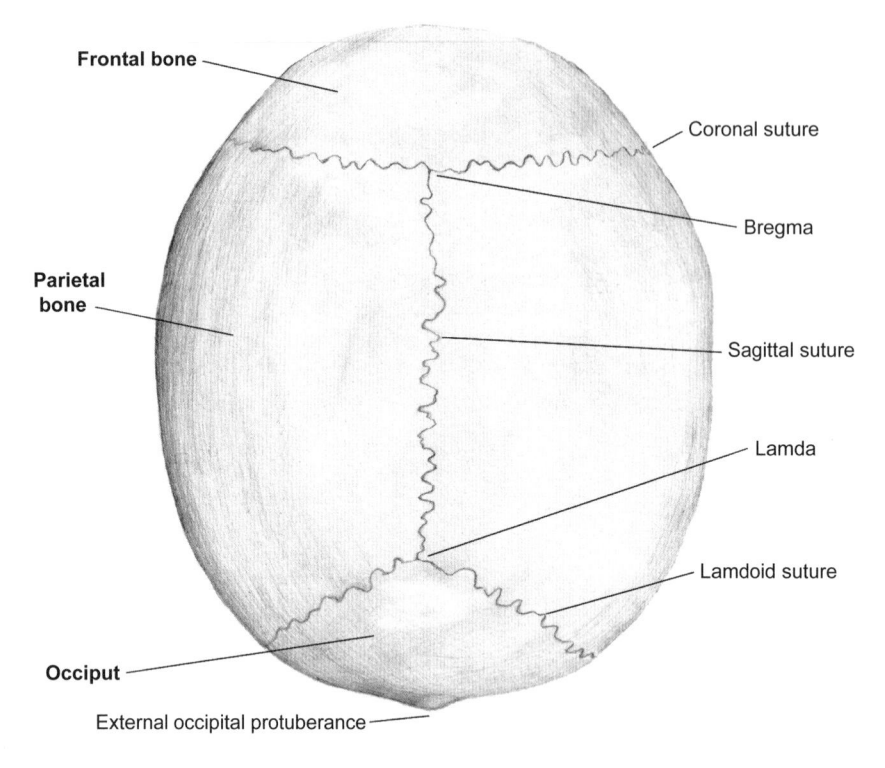

Frontal bone
Coronal suture
Bregma
Parietal bone
Sagittal suture
Lamda
Lamdoid suture
Occiput
External occipital protuberance

6.13 The cranium – superior view

Disturbances to the bones

Many of the repercussions of bony disturbances have been covered in describing the disturbances to the membrane system above – after all, they are all part of the same integrated system. Disturbances to the bones of the cranium, whether through head injuries or birth trauma, or internal forces transmitted through the membranes, may displace the cranial bones, compress the sutural junctions between cranial bones, or leave force vectors or locked kinetic energy within the bones – all of which may affect the quality, symmetry and free expression of rhythmic motion, with consequent adverse repercussions on blood supply to the brain, venous drainage from the brain, cranial nerve function, circulation of cerebrospinal fluid around the brain, or the free flow of vitality within the cranium.

Cranial bone distortions may also directly affect the membranes – perhaps causing local repercussions through damage to the many tiny blood vessels within the arachnoid mater, with potential adverse consequences on the brain including haemorrhage and stroke – but most significantly having far reaching consequences on the balance and integrity of the whole system.

Although the membrane attachments to the C2 and C3 vertebrae are small, tensions or twists in the neck may also have repercussions on the reciprocal tension membrane system as a whole.

Injury to the sacrum, for example slipping on ice and sitting down heavily, may lead to restricted mobility of the sacrum at the sacro-iliac joints or lumbo-sacral joint. This may have repercussions, not only locally, causing back pain and sciatica, but also, through the membranous attachments to the sacrum and coccyx, resulting in pulls transmitted up through the reciprocal tension membrane system, with repercussions anywhere in the body – due to effects on the spinal nerve outlets throughout the spine – and up into the cranium, perhaps highlighting any weak spots, previous injuries, or facilitated segments, or pulling the whole system into a state of imbalance and discomfort with a multiplicity of symptoms (see Figures 6.9–6.13).

> **Box 6.2 Do cranial bones move?**
> There has been much debate over the years as to whether the cranial bones are capable of movement, generally accompanied by the assumed conclusion that, if they don't, then the whole basis of cranial work is negated. The bones do move – slightly – as clearly demonstrated by various recent researches (see Chaitow 2005 for a comprehensive collation of the research) and their mobility influences health and function. But this is not the point. The point is that the movement of the bones is not the basis of the cranio-sacral process. It is not particularly significant whether the bones move or not. The movements that we are feeling in cranio-sacral integration are not the movement of the bones. They are the movement of the matrix, of the vitality, of the life force.

> **Box 6.3 Dead bones, living bones**
> In examining a real skull in isolation – dry, rigid, solid – it may be difficult to recognise that the bones of the cranium could move in relation to each other, as described in cranial texts. It is helpful to realise that living bone is different from dry dead bone. A dead branch or tree trunk is solid and immobile, but the living branches of a tree, even a solid tree trunk, can bend and sway in the wind. Similarly, living bone is more pliable and flexible than the bones of a dry skull.

3. Cerebrospinal fluid

The membrane system contains and encloses *cerebrospinal fluid*, a clear colourless fluid which surrounds and bathes the central nervous system, creating the environment within which the central nervous system grows, develops and functions.

The free flow of cerebrospinal fluid is essential to the healthy functioning of the central nervous system; and since it provides nutrition and drainage for the brain and spinal cord, it is essential that this fluid should not be static or stagnant. Cerebrospinal fluid is produced and reabsorbed continuously, providing a consistent flow of fresh fluid around the brain and spinal cord in constant motion.

Cerebrospinal fluid (CSF) is contained within:

- the ventricular system
- the subarachnoid space.

The *ventricular system* is a system of cavities and canals deep within the brain and spinal cord (see Figures 6.14 and 6.15 and Box 6.4).

The *subarachnoid space* is the fluid-filled space between the two membranous layers of the arachnoid mater and pia mater – inside the arachnoid mater and outside the pia mater (see Figure 6.15b and Box 6.4).

Formation of CSF from arterial blood

Cerebrospinal fluid enters the membrane system at the *choroid plexi* – filter-like structures located within the roofs of the four ventricles of the brain (see Figure 6.15b). Arterial blood enters these choroid plexi, and cerebrospinal fluid is the clear colourless product which is extracted from the blood and which emerges from the choroid plexi into the ventricular system, to be distributed throughout the central nervous system.

The choroid plexi are not in fact filters. They consist of a mass of convoluted tubules, from which the specific constituents required for the formation of this delicately balanced fluid are transported across the membranes of the choroid plexi by active transport into the ventricles. The resultant fluid is therefore an extract from blood, containing the perfect balance of chemical and hormonal constituents for optimum function of the central nervous system, ensuring the exclusion of bacteria, large proteins, red blood cells, and any other unwanted substances.

Distribution through the ventricular system

Cerebrospinal fluid is distributed throughout the *ventricular system*, through all four ventricles and the various canals which connect them, including the central canal of the spinal cord (see Box 6.4).

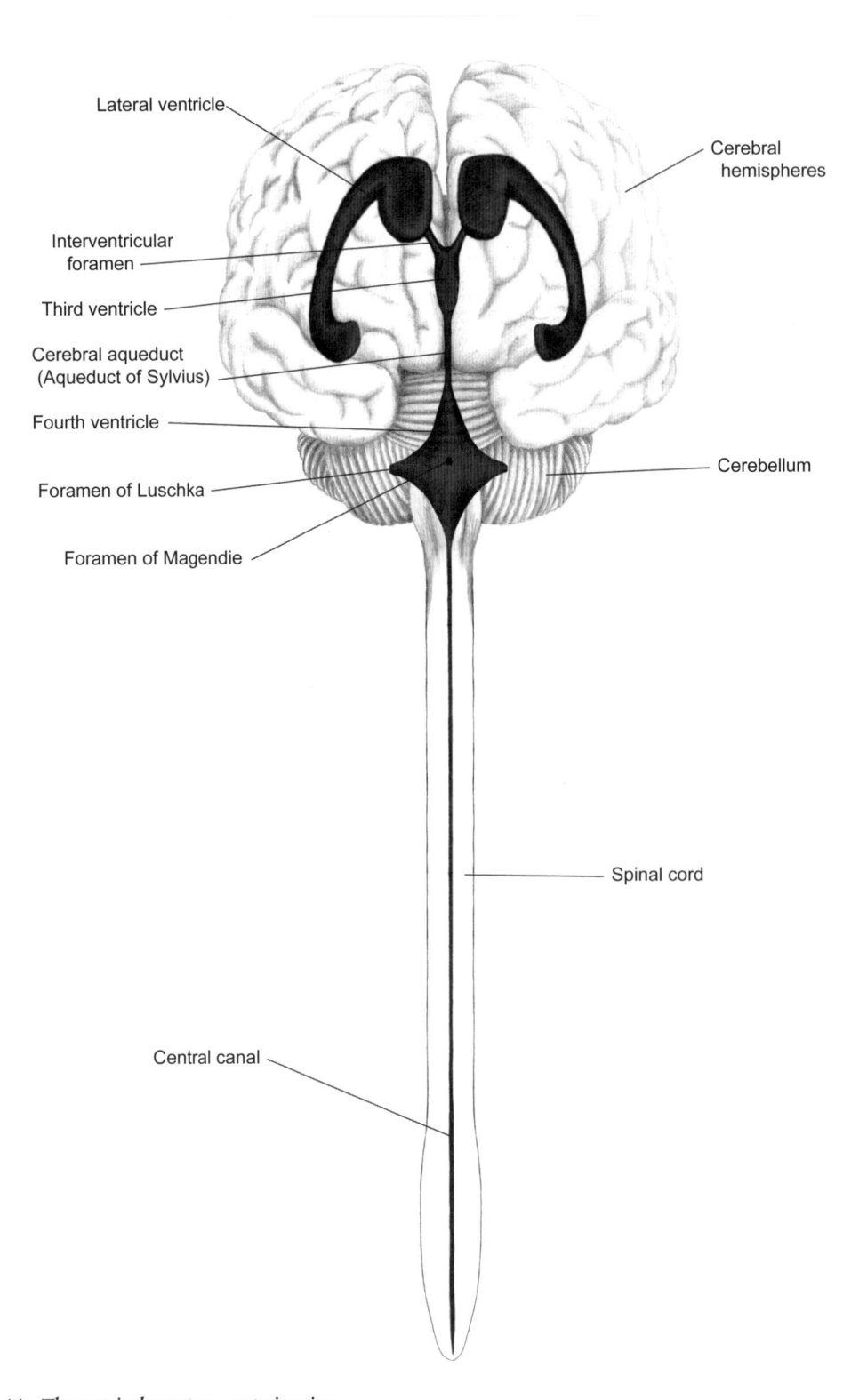

6.14 The ventricular system – anterior view

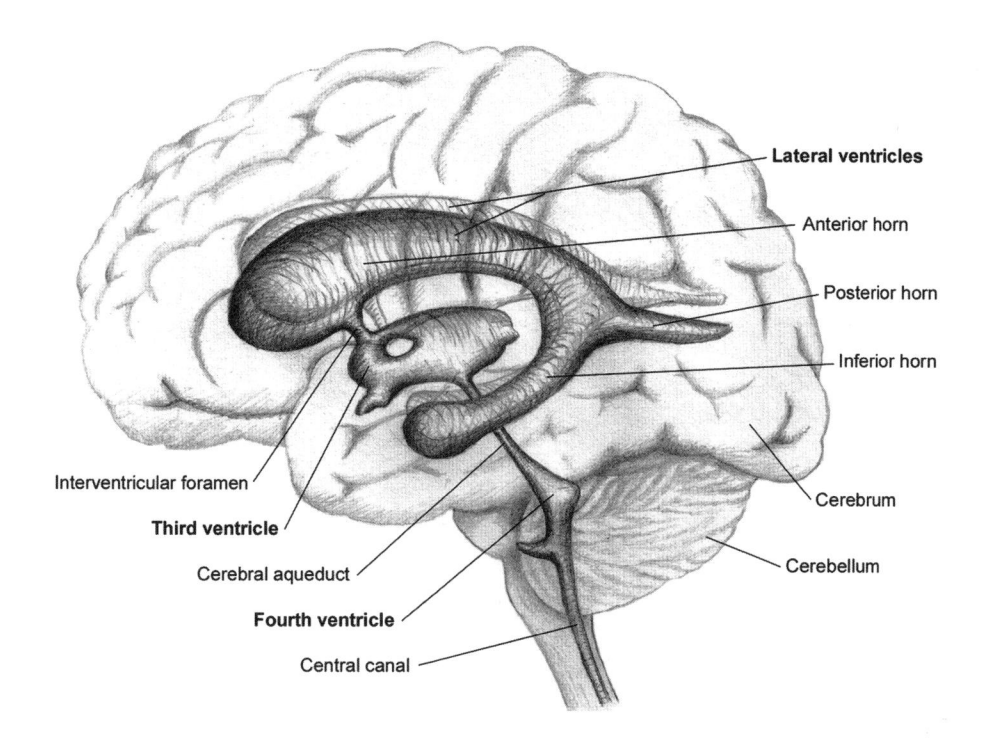

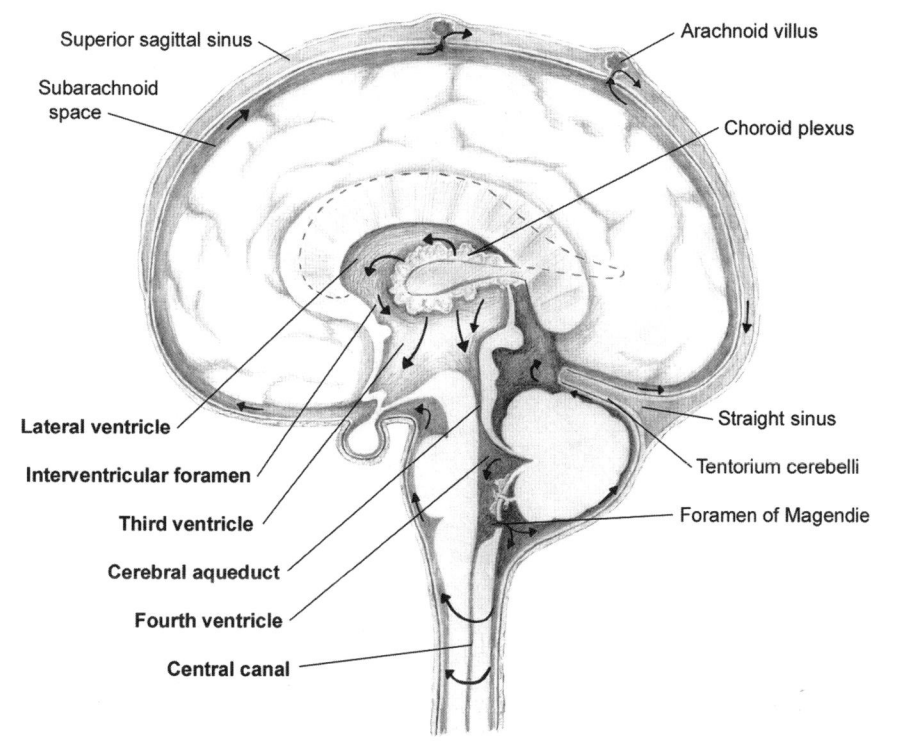

6.15 *The ventricular system*
Above – lateral view
Below – mid-sagittal section

Box 6.4 The ventricular system

The ventricular system is a system of cavities and canals deep within the central nervous system. These cavities and canals are spaces within the nerve tissue of the brain and spinal cord. They have a thin membranous lining (the *ependymal*) and the whole ventricular system is filled with cerebrospinal fluid. Cerebrospinal fluid is formed within the four ventricles of the ventricular system and also flows out to the subarachnoid space surrounding the brain and spinal cord.

The ventricular system consists of *four ventricles* connected by various *communicating channels*. Two *lateral ventricles* (the first and second ventricles) are located within the two cerebral hemispheres, each of which communicates via an *interventricular foramen* to the third *ventricle*, located centrally between the two thalami. The third ventricle communicates inferiorly via the *cerebral aqueduct* (Aqueduct of Sylvius) to the *fourth ventricle* located between the cerebellum (posteriorly) and the pons and medulla (anteriorly). The fourth ventricle is continuous inferiorly with the *central canal* passing down the centre of the spinal cord.

Choroid plexi

In the roof of each of the four ventricles are located the *choroid plexi* – filter-like structures through which the cerebrospinal fluid is extracted from arterial blood. Arterial blood enters the convoluted tubules of the choroid plexi, and cerebrospinal fluid is the clear colourless fluid which is extracted from the arterial blood within these tubules, and transported by active transport across the walls of the choroid plexi into the ventricular spaces, leaving behind the red blood cells, large proteins, bacteria and other large particles, which remain in the arterial blood.

Foramina

In the posterior and lateral walls of the fourth ventricle are three foramina:
- the foramen of Magendie (medial aperture), posteriorly
- two foramina of Luschka (lateral apertures), bilaterally.

Through these foramina, cerebrospinal fluid can pass from the ventricular system to the subarachnoid space.

Subarachnoid space

The subarachnoid space is the space between the arachnoid mater and pia mater layers of the meninges, surrounding the brain and spinal cord – inside the arachnoid mater, outside the pia mater. Cerebrospinal fluid flows throughout the ventricular system, and also passes out through the foramina of Magendie and Luschka into the subarachnoid space. Cerebrospinal fluid then circulates through the subarachnoid space around the brain and spinal cord.

Cerebrospinal fluid also seeps through the walls of the ventricles into the nerve tissue of the brain and spinal cord, and from the subarachnoid space through the pia mater into the tissues of the brain and spinal cord.

Since cerebrospinal fluid is an extract from blood, and is very similar to many other fluids in the body – extracellular fluid, intracellular fluid, lymph – it is not distinguishable as a separate entity once it dissipates out into the body fluids.

Arachnoid villi

Cerebrospinal fluid is eventually returned to the blood partially via the *arachnoid villi* (see Figure 6.16), small protrusions of arachnoid mater which project out from the subarachnoid space, through the inner layer of impermeable dura mater, into the superior sagittal sinus, thereby enabling the cerebrospinal fluid to rejoin the venous blood which then drains from the venous sinuses via the internal jugular vein to be returned to the heart.

As mentioned above, cerebrospinal fluid also drains primarily along the olfactory nerve pathways into the lymphatic system, as well as through other cranial nerve and spinal nerve roots.

Emergence from the ventricular system to the subarachnoid space

Cerebrospinal fluid is then able to pass out of the ventricular system through three tiny foramina (holes) in the roof and walls of the fourth ventricle – the foramen of Magendie and the two foramina of Luschka – thereby entering the *subarachnoid space* (see Figures 6.14 and 6.15b). The cerebrospinal fluid is then distributed throughout the subarachnoid space which surrounds the central nervous system (see Figure 6.15b). The presence of cerebrospinal fluid here provides a cushion around the brain and spinal cord, thereby protecting them from the shock of any physical blows or injuries. There are notable accumulations of cerebrospinal fluid in various *cisternae*, including the cisterna magna (behind the medulla, below the cerebellum) and the lumbar cistern (in the lower spine – the site from which cerebrospinal fluid is extracted through lumbar puncture).

Reabsorption into the venous blood

Cerebrospinal fluid is then reabsorbed back into the blood at the venous sinuses. Part of this reabsorption is enabled by the presence of *arachnoid villi* – small protrusions of arachnoid mater which penetrate the impermeable dura mater, thereby enabling the cerebrospinal fluid to pass from the subarachnoid space into the venous blood of the *superior sagittal sinus*, which runs along the superior border of the falx cerebri. This has conventionally been regarded as the principal channel of drainage for cerebrospinal fluid. However, modern research indicates that this accounts for only a small proportion of cerebrospinal fluid drainage, and that the principal channels of drainage are along the olfactory nerve pathways draining into the lymphatic system, as well as through other cranial nerve and spinal nerve roots.

The blood from the venous sinuses drains through the internal jugular vein back to the heart. There is therefore a continuous replenishment of cerebrospinal fluid – produced from arterial blood at the choroid plexi, and returning to the venous blood at the arachnoid villi (see Figures 6.15b and 6.16 and Box 6.5).

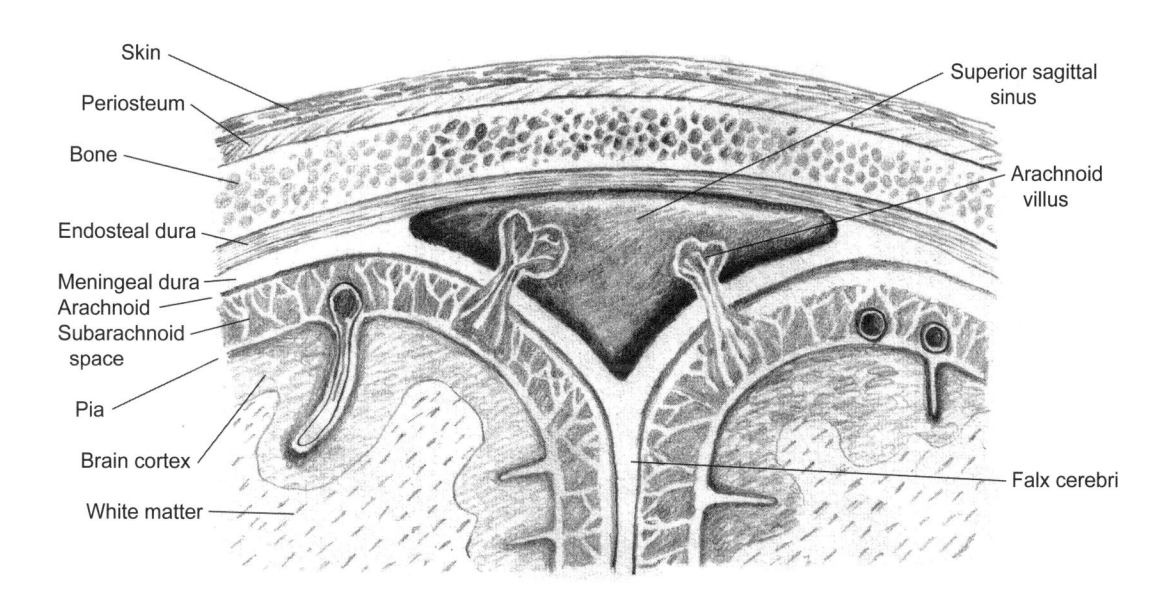

6.16 *Arachnoid villi enable the return of cerebro-spinal fluid from the subarachnoid space to the venous blood in the superior sagittal sinus*

44 \ Cranio-Sacral Integration

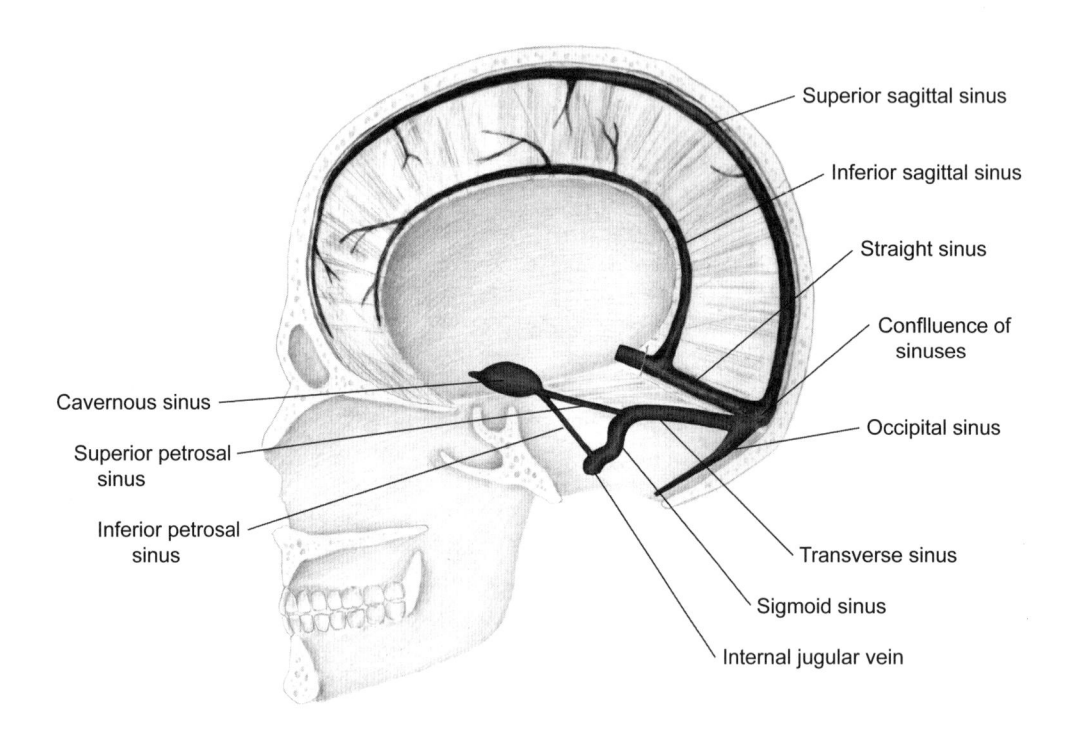

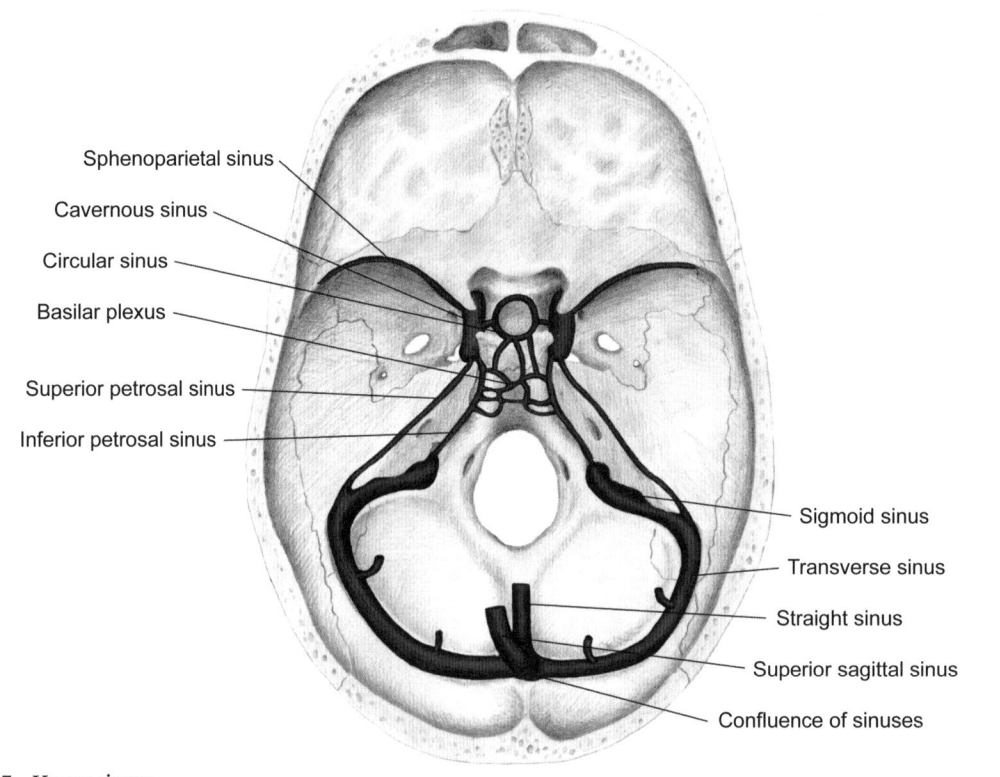

6.17 *Venous sinuses*
Above – lateral view
Below – superior view

Box 6.5 The venous sinues

The venous sinuses (see Figures 6.17 and 6.18) are the major channels for drainage of venous blood from the brain. They exist only within the cranium. The term 'sinus' means a space, and the venous sinuses are blood-filled spaces within the dura. They are formed between the two layers of dural membrane, and their proper function is therefore very much dependent upon the healthy state of the membrane system.

The venous sinuses are lined with endothelium, which is continuous with the endothelial layer of the veins. However, they differ from veins in the following ways:
- They contain no valves.
- Some of them have blind ends.
- They are formed within the dura.
- Their walls contain no muscular tissue, consisting solely of an endothelial layer (whereas veins are composed of an inner endothelial layer, a middle muscular layer and an outer connective tissue layer).

Small and large veins throughout the cranium empty into the venous sinuses, which in turn drain almost all the blood from the brain, out of the cranium via the two internal jugular veins, passing through the jugular foramina.

The venous sinuses (primarily the superior sagittal sinus) receive cerebrospinal fluid draining out from within the membrane system back to the venous system via the arachnoid villi.

The principal venous sinuses forming the major superficial channels of drainage comprise the following:
- *Superior sagittal sinus*
  - passing along the superior border of the falx cerebri
  - drains posteriorly towards the confluence of sinuses.
- *Inferior sagittal sinus*
  - passing along the free (inferior) border of the falx cerebri
  - drains posteriorly into the straight sinus.
- *Straight sinus*
  - passing along the border between the falx cerebri, falx cerebelli and tentorium cerebelli
  - drains posteriorly towards the confluence of sinuses.
- *Occipital sinus*
  - passing along the occipital border of the falx cerebelli
  - drains superiorly towards the confluence of sinuses.
- *Two transverse sinuses*
  - passing along the attached (occipital) border of the tentorium cerebelli
  - drain laterally *away* from the confluence of sinuses into the sigmoid sinuses.
- *Two sigmoid sinuses*
  - 'S' shaped sinuses twisting inferiorly along grooves in the petrous portions of the temporal bones towards the jugular foramina
  - drain inferiorly from the transverse sinuses into the internal jugular veins.

Other major venous sinuses lying deeper within the cranium include the following:
- *Two cavernous sinuses*
  - located on each side of the body of the sphenoid
  - receiving venous blood from the orbits and surrounding area
  - drain posteriorly via the superior petrosal sinuses and inferior petrosal sinuses into the sigmoid sinuses.
- *Circular sinus*
  - passing around the pituitary
  - connecting the two cavernous sinuses.
- *Two superior petrosal sinuses*
  - passing from the cavernous sinuses to the *superior* end of the sigmoid sinuses
  - drain posteriorly into the sigmoid sinuses.

- *Two inferior petrosal sinuses*
  - passing from the cavernous sinuses to the *inferior* ends of the sigmoid sinuses (the junction with the internal jugular veins)
  - drain posteriorly into the sigmoid sinuses.

Various other smaller sinuses exist deep within the cranium, for example the spheno-parietal sinuses. All veins and venous plexi within the cranium drain into the various sinuses at some point.

Volume

The total volume of cerebrospinal fluid contained within the ventricles and subarachnoid space is approximately 150 millilitres (a quarter of a pint). The choroid plexi produce around 600 millilitres of cerebrospinal fluid each day, enabling the body to replace and replenish its cerebrospinal fluid four times every day.

Seeping through the brain

As well as circulating through the ventricles and venous sinuses, cerebrospinal fluid seeps into the brain tissue, permeating the ependyma which lines the ventricles. Cerebrospinal fluid is therefore able to wash through the brain tissue, carrying out its nutritive and cleansing functions, before passing back outward through the pia mater to the subarachnoid space and consequently draining to the venous sinuses and back to the heart.

The production and absorption of cerebro-spinal fluid is a continuous process. However, cerebrospinal fluid is also, like everything else, expressing inherent rhythmic motion, which can be felt as waves of fluidic expansion and contraction, rising and falling.

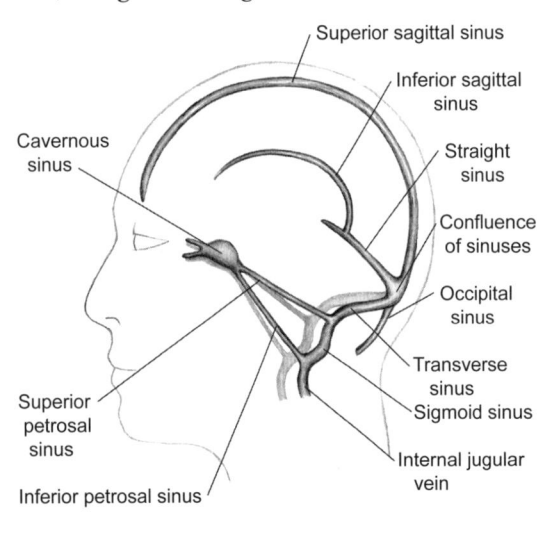

Cerebrospinal fluid provides the medium within which the central nervous system exists. It also provides nutrients and drains away unwanted waste products from the brain and spinal cord. The free unrestricted flow of cerebrospinal fluid is therefore essential to proper healthy function of the central nervous system and consequently to integrated healthy function generally.

4. The fascia

The final component of the anatomical cranio-sacral system is the fascia. *Fascia* is a connective tissue which forms a continuous sheath throughout the body from the top of the head to the soles of the feet – enveloping every organ, nerve, blood vessel, muscle, bone, and every structure throughout the body.

This continuous fascial sheath forms a close connection to the membrane system at the points where each peripheral nerve emanates from the central nervous system. Every nerve to any part of the body must penetrate the membranes as it leaves the brain or spinal cord. As it penetrates the membrane it is initially enveloped in a projection of membrane which is then continuous with the *epineurium* or fascial sheath which envelops the nerve throughout its pathway to the periphery (see Figure 6.19).

Fascia extends throughout the body, creating a unity of structure from the top of the head to the tips of the toes, enveloping everything in between. It also connects into the membrane system at the neurological outlets described above. Fascial restrictions may stem from a wide variety of causes – sprained ankles, operation scars, wounds, bruises, injuries to the arms or legs, frozen shoulders, muscular tensions, emotional tension, sympathetic stimulation. Fascial pulls, twists, restrictions and resistances resulting from such injuries may be transmitted throughout the body with repercussions elsewhere, impingeing on nerves and blood vessels, creating tensions and

6.18 Venous sinuses – schematic view

discomforts, perpetuating neurological symptoms and muscular weakness, or restricting blood supply to the head or elsewhere. The fascia has a very rich innervation of sympathetic nerve supply.

Working with the fascia is a powerful and profound aspect of cranio-sacral integration with far reaching benefits and influences on the whole body-mind complex. It is an integral and vital part of the cranio-sacral process.

Like all structures in the body, fascia exhibits inherent rhythmic motion.

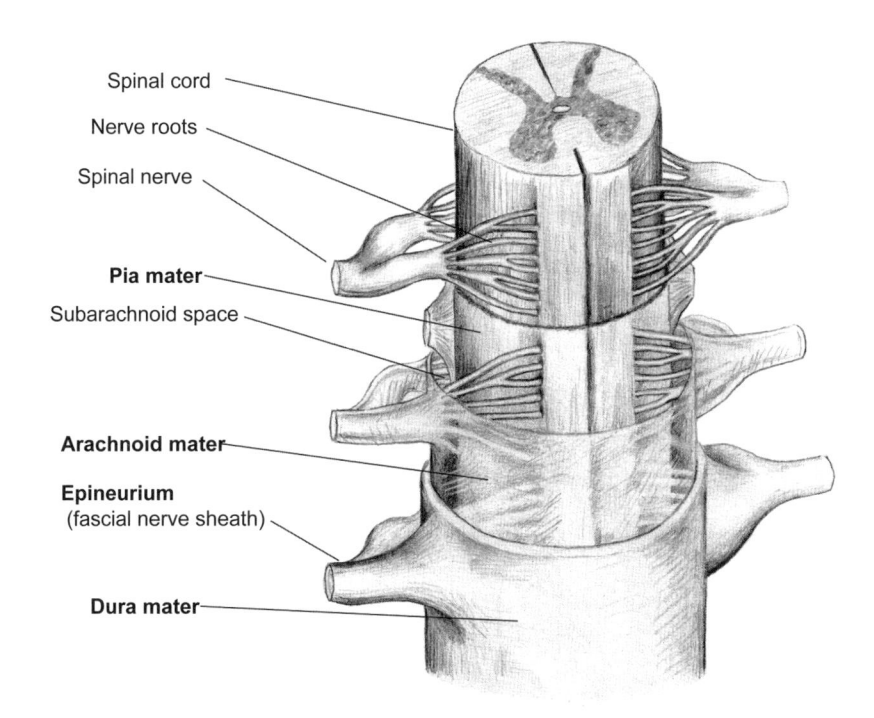

6.19 As it penetrates the membrane, each nerve is initially enveloped in a projection of membrane which is then continuous with the epineurium or fascial nerve sheath which envelops the nerve throughout its pathway to the periphery

Chapter 7

Cranio-Sacral Motion

Cranio-sacral integration is not primarily about bones, or membranes, or fluids; it is about underlying vitality – expressed as rhythmic motion – *cranio-sacral motion*.

Just as the natural forces of the universe generate the rhythmic motion of tides and waves within the oceans, so those natural forces, as they spread through the body, generate rhythmic motion on different levels, manifesting as different rhythms with different rates, reflecting different depths of our being.

There are many rhythms within the body, some readily identifiable – such as heartbeat and respiration – others more subtle – such as the rhythms of the cranio-sacral system, and others yet to be identified.

Within the cranio-sacral concept, three principal rhythms are commonly defined:
- *cranio-sacral rhythm* (also known as the cranial rhythmic impulse or CRI)
- *middle tide* (also known as the potency tide or mid-tide)
- *long tide.*

All of these rhythms are subtle and are not likely to be immediately accessible to the casual observer. But if you create an appropriately calm, quiet environment, in an atmosphere of stillness, then as the system becomes settled, you may feel the gradual emergence of the gentle rise and fall of the cranio-sacral rhythm. This is the most superficial of the three rhythms, similar to waves gently ebbing and flowing on a beach.

7.1   Layers of rhythmic motion

As you remain engaged with the system, you may feel a gradual settling and sinking into a deeper level of connection, and gradually you may feel the emergence of a deeper slower rhythmic motion, with a similar rise and fall, but a slower rate. This is the middle tide.

If you work deeply with the system, and settle into a profound stillness, where the superficial patterns of disturbance have released or subsided and both patient and practitioner have settled into a profound therapeutic space, then you may encounter the long tide. This, as its name suggests, is a much longer, deeper, tide-like.

All three rhythms are present continuously, and an experienced cranio-sacral therapist may identify any or all of them at any time, separately or simultaneously. Depending on circumstances, one or other of the rhythms is likely to be predominant at any one time.

All three rhythms are expressed throughout the body and can be identified anywhere in the body (or outside the body).

All three rhythms are relatively stable, changing little in response to circumstances, changing slightly in response to therapeutic releases and interactions. This stability and consistency are more evident at the deeper levels.

All three rhythms exhibit the same wave-like, tide-like motion of two phases:

- an expansion phase
- a contraction phase.

The *cranio-sacral rhythm* has a rate of approx *4–14 cycles per minute* (variable from person to person); in other words each complete cycle of expansion and contraction lasts approximately *5–10 seconds*.

The *middle tide* has a rate of approximately *2–2½ cycles per minute*; in other words each complete cycle of expansion and contraction lasts *20–25 seconds*.

In *long tide*, each complete cycle of expansion and contraction lasts *100 seconds*.

A state of being

The cranio-sacral rhythm is reminiscent of waves rising on to a beach and ebbing away again. It reflects a more superficial aspect of our being, more related to day-to-day life.

The middle tide has a slower deeper quality, more like waves rolling through the ocean. This level reflects deeper aspects of our being – our underlying nature – and the levels of health relating to these deeper levels.

The long tide has a profound, distant, spacious, timeless quality, like the tides rising and falling deep within the ocean. It is very constant within each individual and also from one person to another, reflecting a universal rhythmic motion that unites all living things, and reflecting our deeper spiritual nature.

Tuning in to these different expressions of rhythmic motion is not simply a matter of following movement or feeling a rhythm. It is engaging with *a state of being*.

The two phases of motion

The whole body responds to rhythmic motion as a single unified unit, expanding and contracting as one. Rhythmic motion is also expressed in every individual cell throughout the body. Every structure throughout the body – every bone, membrane, organ, cell – is expressing rhythmic motion in its own individual way, as part of the unified whole – in unison. As Sutherland (1967) expressed it, 'Every drop knows the tide.'

Expansion phase

During the expansion phase (see Figure 7.2) of cranio-sacral motion:

- the whole body expands and widens away from the midline, externally rotating out from the spine
- the head widens and slightly shortens
- the ventricles widen
- vitality rises up from the sacrum to the cranium.

Contraction phase

During the contraction phase:

- the whole body contracts and narrows towards the midline, internally rotating around the spine

- the head narrows and slightly lengthens
- the ventricles narrow
- vitality flows from the cranium down towards the sacrum.

Expression of rhythmic motion throughout the body

Because different parts of the body reflect cranio-sacral motion in different ways, terminology has evolved to describe the various expressions of rhythmic motion in various structures. During the expansion and contraction phases of motion, midline structures rock forward and back in flexion and extension, and paired structures and the body as a whole move into external rotation and internal rotation.

Flexion/extension

- *Flexion*: corresponds to the expansion phase.
- *Extension*: corresponds to the contraction phase.

The terms flexion and extension refer particularly to midline structures – sacrum, sphenoid, ethmoid, occiput – which rock forward and backward in response to the rhythmic motion of the cranio-sacral system. However, these terms may often be used more loosely to describe rhythmic motion more generally throughout the system.

(*The terms flexion and extension were first used by Sutherland because they describe the movement at the inferior angle of the spheno-basilar synchondrosis – see Chapter 45.*)

External rotation/internal rotation

- *External rotation*: corresponds to the expansion phase.
- *Internal rotation*: corresponds to the contraction phase.

These terms describe the response to cranio-sacral motion as expressed in the body generally – the arms, legs, trunk – and also specifically in certain bilateral structures such as the temporal bones and certain bones of the face. All of these structures open out into external rotation during the expansion phase and close in to internal rotation during the contraction phase.

a.

Expansion phase (Flexion)   Contraction phase (Extension)

b.

Expansion phase (Flexion)   Contraction phase (Extension)

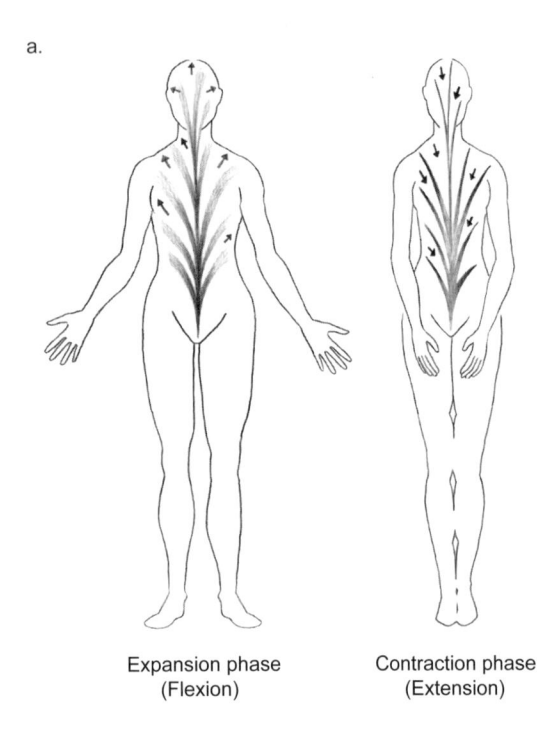

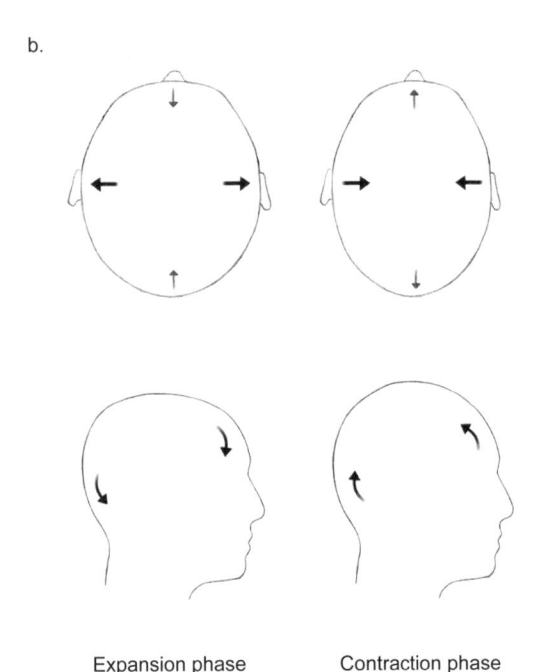

7.2 *The whole body responds to rhythmic motion as a single unified unit, expanding and contracting as one*
a. During the expansion phase, the whole body expands and widens away from the midline, as vitality rises up from the sacrum to the cranium
b. During the expansion phase, the head widens, flattens, and slightly shortens

Inhalation/exhalation

In the context of the primary respiratory system, Sutherland described the expansion phase as inhalation and the contraction phase as exhalation. These terms present obvious potential confusion with thoracic respiration, and so are not used in this book.

We can summarise the phases of motion with their corresponding expressions as follows:

Expansion phase
- expansion
- flexion
- external rotation
- inhalation.

Contraction phase
- contraction
- extension
- internal rotation
- exhalation.

Stability of rhythm

All three rhythms are relatively stable. Unlike heartbeat and respiration, which vary widely in response to exercise or even thought and emotion, cranio-sacral motion shows little change in this respect.

It is likely to fluctuate only slightly during everyday life – for instance whether you are awake or asleep. The characteristics of the cranio-sacral rhythm – its amplitude, strength, speed, fullness and other aspects of its nature – will also reflect aspects of the person's nature and circumstances.

- Someone with an open, expressive, outgoing nature is likely to express cranio-sacral motion in an open, expressive manner with a wider amplitude and greater variation.
- A person with a closed, contained, unexpressive nature is likely to manifest a closed narrow amplitude and a less expansive cranio-sacral motion.
- Someone high powered, highly active, busy and fast-living is likely to have a faster rhythm.
- Someone very calm, relaxed and peaceful is more likely to have a slower rhythm.

However, there are many factors which contribute to the picture, and such features cannot be interpreted quite so simply.

One factor which perhaps has the most significant effect on the rhythm is cranio-sacral treatment. Someone who has received a substantial amount of cranio-sacral treatment tends to have a slower calmer rhythm.

Changes in rate, in so far as they do occur, are also most noticeable during treatment. As the system settles, the rhythm is likely to become gradually slower, calmer and of greater amplitude. This is most noticeable following specific releases, whether at cranio-sacral rhythm or middle tide level, at which point, following the release of a restriction, the rhythmic motion is likely to settle into a slightly slower, more expansive motion.

During the build-up to a release, the amplitude of the rhythmic motion may gradually become smaller and smaller, until it reaches a point of stillness, where the rhythmic motion stops completely, before releasing and settling into an even, balanced rhythmic motion again, usually at a slightly slower rate than previously. This point of stillness is, for obvious reasons, known as a still point. These points of stillness are significant moments of healing and release.

Interaction of rhythms

When working therapeutically with the cranio-sacral system, clear distinctions between the rhythms are not always apparent. They may blend into each other; the system may shift seamlessly from one rhythm to another. The very existence of separate rhythms may be questionable, as the system settles steadily through a continuum of gradually lengthening phases of motion into deep dynamic stillness.

The perceived rhythmic motion is not an absolute objective rhythm. Like everything in the cranio-sacral process, and indeed everything in life as recognised in this quantum age, the rhythmic motion is the outcome of an interaction between patient and therapist, between observer and observed, and will therefore change in response to each therapist, and so will be perceived differently by different therapists.

This process is known as *entrainment* – the same phenomenon by which pendulum clocks synchronise – and it influences not just the rhythm, but the whole therapeutic interaction. Through entrainment, the presence of the therapist – their calmer, quieter rhythmic motion and their calmer, quieter state of being – can influence the patient's rhythm and overall state, bringing them into greater harmony. We will explore entrainment, along with other aspects of rhythmic motion and ways of enhancing engagement with the deeper tides, in Chapter 35.

Rhythmic motion is a reflection of the person, an expression of a whole state of being. Tuning in to these different expressions of rhythmic motion is not simply a matter of feeling or following movement; it is engaging with a state of being. Being in the middle tide, or the long tide indicates, not just tuning in to that particular rhythm, but engaging with the person on a particular level of depth, along with all the associations and implications that arise from that level of engagement.

Box 7.1 Rhythmic terminology

Terms vary from one source to another, with various terms being used for the same rhythms, the same terms being used to refer to different rhythms, and some sources using different terms altogether. For the purposes of this book, we will use the following terms:
- *Cranio-sacral motion*: indicating all the different levels of rhythmic motion expressed by the cranio-sacral system.
- *Rhythmic motion*: also indicating any or all of the different levels.

Within the all-encompassing term of cranio-sacral motion, there are three main rhythms:
- *Cranio-sacral rhythm*: indicating the fastest of the three commonly defined rhythms at 4–14 cycles per minute.
- *Middle tide*: indicating rhythmic motion at 2–2½ cycles per minute.
- *Long tide*: indicating rhythmic motion with a length of 100 seconds per complete cycle.

The term cranial rhythmic impulse is used by some to indicate the cranio-sacral rhythm and by others to refer to all cranio-sacral motion.

The terms potency tide and mid-tide are used by some in place of middle tide.

The term involuntary motion is used by some to refer to all cranio-sacral motion.

Primary respiration is the term originally used by Sutherland to describe the manifestation of the Breath of Life as rhythmic motion, expressed on various different levels as long tide, middle tide and cranio-sacral rhythm.

Box 7.2 Slime mould

In the 1950s William Seifriz, Professor of Botany at the University of Pensylvania, investigated one of the most primitive life forms, a slime mould (which can readily be found growing on tree stumps and rotten logs). Slime mould is so primitive that it doesn't even have a cellular structure. It is simply protoplasm, the basic material of all living things. Seifriz was able to show on film that even this primitive form of life expresses rhythmic motion (Seifriz 1954). His film shows a regular rhythmic cycle of 100 seconds (the same as the long tide) and also shows that the protoplasm is exhibiting multiple rhythms. He expressed the view that what he was witnessing was very close to identifying the source of life itself.

Chapter 8

Treatment
Fundamental Principles
– The Inherent Treatment Process

Lifelong accumulation
When the body is unhealthy, it is very seldom due to one injury or illness (even though there may be a predominant injury or an apparent trigger). We all have a lifelong history of accumulated injuries, tensions and traumas and these create disturbances throughout the body – in the muscles, the fascia, the membranes, the bones, the fluids, the organs, the psyche, the energy system, the matrix. We might identify some of these specifically as pains or tangible dysfunctions, others we might not acknowledge or recognise.

Tangled web
This accumulation steadily builds a complex tangled web of intertwined patterns of imbalance and restriction, transmitted from one part of the body to another, reflected in different areas and on different levels, resulting from an interaction of physical, structural, postural and emotional influences all interlinked, causing tensions, restrictions and dysfunction which may reflect to any part of the body or affect the whole balance and integrity of the body. Again, this might manifest as symptoms, or we might remain unaware of the underlying accumulation.

Depleted health
All of this depletes our health, sometimes gradually, sometimes suddenly, depending on the nature and severity of the injuries and illnesses. Initially we cope, we adapt, we compensate. Gradually, as our bodies labour under the weight of adaptation, we may become exhausted and function less and less effectively or start to display symptoms. The symptoms we experience may sometimes be attributable to one or other of these many injuries, but they are inevitably a consequence of everything that has gone before, everything that has accumulated up to that point.

Reintegration of the whole
When we treat through cranio-sacral integration, we are not looking to identify and 'fix' each little injury and illness individually; such a task would be impossible – there are hundreds of them in each individual history, and the effects of such an approach would inevitably be very limited. We are not looking to mobilise bones, release sutures, or stretch membranes. Instead we are looking for reintegration of the whole, and in order to enable this we are looking to the body's inner wisdom to disentangle the complex web of underlying injury and illness, knowing that it has the capacity to do so and that all it needs is a little help to enhance its potential, to help it to get back in touch with its inner forces of underlying vitality, and point it in the right direction. The inherent vitality can then do the rest, bringing about true healing and integration.

The essence
The essence of cranio-sacral integration is therefore *to enable the free expression of the body's fundamental vitality throughout the matrix*, through which it is able to maintain health, restore health and resolve ill-health.

In an irrigation system on a farm, you need a plentiful supply of water and you need a system of pipes to distribute that water and its nutrients to the various parts of the farm. If the water supply is inadequate or feeble, the whole farm may suffer. If individual pipes are broken or blocked, the affected areas of the farm may not receive adequate irrigation and the crops there will wither and die. The farmer needs to ensure a plentiful and powerful supply of water and ensure that all the pipes are functioning effectively. In the same way, a cranio-sacral therapist needs to ensure a potent underlying vitality and the removal of any obstacles to the free distribution of that vitality.

Influencing basic physiological processes

Release of restrictions within the cranio-sacral system – whether they may manifest as bony compressions, soft tissue tensions, fascial restrictions, energy blockages, shock effects, emotional tensions, depletion, or complex imbalances reflected throughout the body – is not only restoring the flow of vitality but also enabling the free flow of arterial blood, venous drainage, lymphatic drainage, energy flow, nerve supply and immune function, and thereby enabling proper functioning of all body tissues, organs and systems and enabling the body's own inherent healing mechanisms to combat infection, inflammation and disease, to restore homeostasis, and to restore and maintain health. Cranio-sacral integration is not merely addressing some abstract underlying life force. It is directly influencing the body's basic physiological processes to function more efficiently, as an integral part of restoring and maintaining health.

The process of cranio-sacral integration therefore involves two main elements:

- establishing a powerful fundamental underlying vitality
- identifying and enabling the release of any restrictions to the free expression of this vitality.

We enable this process by:
- *engaging* with the underlying vitality
- *allowing* it to express itself freely
- *enhancing* its inherent ability to identify and release restrictions to healthy function.

The whole process of cranio-sacral integration is biodynamic – in other words, it is allowing the inherent forces of nature expressed within the body to enable the healing process (rather than imposing forces onto the system). It involves engaging with the body's inner resources, knowing and trusting that the body has the inherent potential to bring about health and healing, balance and harmony.

You may ask, if the body has these inner resources and knows what to do, why does it need a therapist? The body, in its wisdom, knows what it needs to do in order to address dysfunction and resolve ill health. The underlying potential for health is always present in everyone. The natural forces of the universe generate the individual matrix – and this provides a blueprint for health.

But its *resources can be overwhelmed, depleted, or impeded*. This may be the result of severe trauma, persistent stress, an accumulation of injuries, exhaustion, or inadequate self-care. Consequently the body may need help, support and guidance in order to enable it to access its resources and make optimum use of its potential.

On the one hand we can appreciate the power and wisdom of the biodynamic forces within as the deepest and most powerful forces for healing and do everything we can to allow or enable these forces to operate fully. At the same time we can appreciate that the body may need assistance in accessing those forces. Injuries, illness, stresses and trauma create disorder. If we engage with the matrix, and allow those natural forces to be expressed freely, they can re-establish the original blueprint of health and restore a healthy state.

To a large extent, human beings are unaware of their inner resources, out of touch with their deeper needs, blocked off by injury and trauma, or imposing excessively demanding conditions of stress, overwork, busyness or overstimulation, and not allowing enough time and rest for healing, recuperation, and engagement with their inner healing potential. Consequently, many people are unable to engage with the body's inherent ability to heal and resolve.

Furthermore, a part of the body's wisdom is to protect itself in the short term, and these *protective defensive mechanisms* – aimed at coping or maintaining comfort in the present moment – may obstruct deeper resolution of injury.

When health does break down or become depleted, we therefore lack the resources to utilise our potential, and therefore need a therapist:

- to help us to get back in touch with those inner resources
- to enhance the natural healing potential within.

A fundamental function of the therapist is to provide a calm, quiet presence which can entrain with the patient's system, encouraging it to a greater degree of calmness and quietness and consequent engagement with its own resources.

Calm, quiet presence

The process of engagement with the subtle expression of the cranio-sacral system requires a correspondingly subtle sensitivity on the part of the practitioner. In order to enable such subtle engagement, it is therefore necessary first to develop your own calm, quiet presence. Through this calm, quiet presence you can establish an appropriate level of contact.

The ability to maintain a genuine calm, quiet presence does not necessarily come naturally to everyone. It is something which needs to be worked on, partly through day-to-day personal development, clearing out your own issues, traumas and tensions, clarifying your own system, and partly through developing the skills to take yourself into an appropriate state at any time, whatever the circumstances – a state of physical comfort, mental balance, emotional stability, spiritual equanimity. This process – both the underlying personal development and the establishment of the appropriate state in preparation for treatment – are sometimes referred to as *establishing practitioner fulcrums*.

Taking up contact
Butterflies and kittens

The process of treatment is entirely non-invasive, never imposing upon the body. The contact of the hands is exceptionally light, often described as a 'butterfly touch' – like a butterfly alighting upon the body.

The way in which you take up contact on the body can play a very significant part in everything that follows and in the whole evolution of the treatment process. If you simply place your hands on the body – suddenly, abruptly – the body's likely response will be to contract, defend itself and shut you out. If you come in very slowly, very softly, very calmly, then the body will not feel invaded; it will recognise that your touch is soft and safe, and is more likely to open up to your contact.

Imagine that you are walking down the street and you come across a kitten peeping out at you inquisitively. If you rush towards it eagerly (as an enthusiastic child might do) wanting to stroke it and cuddle it, the kitten will almost certainly run away and hide – however loving your intention might be. If you approach gently, without any sudden or abrupt movement, just reaching out your hand slowly and waiting for the kitten to come to you, it is more likely to approach.

In the same way, with the cranio-sacral system, if you come in too abruptly it will run away and hide. If you approach very softly and gently, and let it come to you in its own time, it is more likely to open up and reveal its innermost secrets to you and enable deeper engagement.

This applies not only to contacting the physical body, but also to the energy field around the body. The body will sense your approaching hands from some distance and will react or respond accordingly, whether or not the patient is conscious of their own internal reaction.

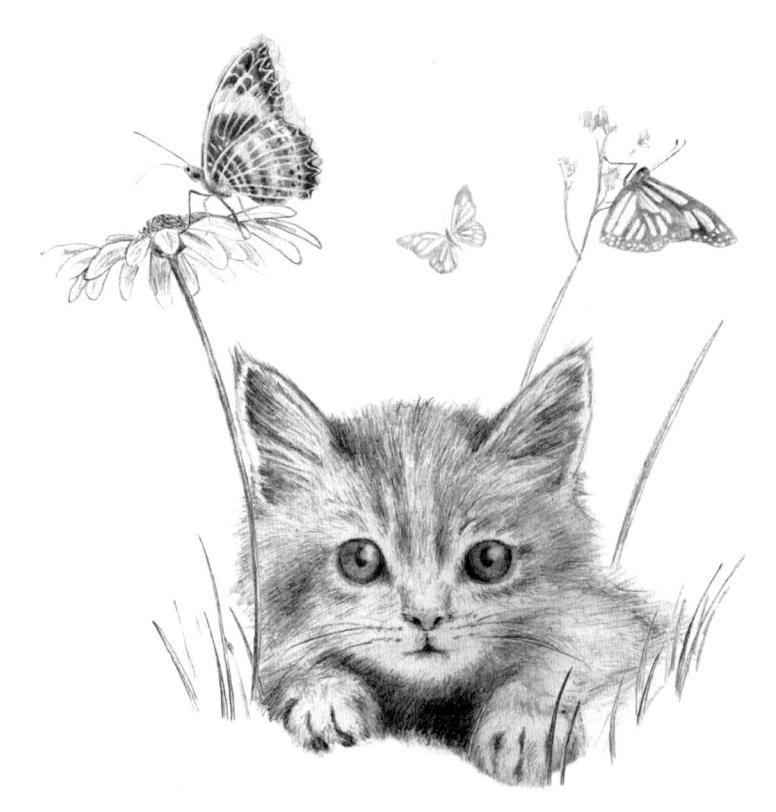

8.1 If you approach gently, this will enable closer connection and deeper engagement

Establishing appropriate levels

- Levels of physical contact.
- Levels of attention.
- Levels of tissue.

The first priority is to establish an appropriate *level of physical contact* in response to the demands of the body – always extremely light, not holding, not gripping, barely touching the body, simply being there. As you tune in through this soft gentle contact, you may feel an increasing sense of connection with the inherent vitality.

This might take various forms. You might feel a subtle vibration, a sense of magnetism, increasing warmth, a sense of aliveness, as if your hands were immersed in warm fluid which was gently washing over and through your hands, or as if you were holding a mouse or a small bird which was expressing tiny wriggling, twitching, fluttering movements.

The cranio-sacral system may demand more space, a lighter touch, or softer hands, perhaps pushing your hands off the body; or may invite a closer contact, drawing your hands into the body – but always completely soft and gentle.

Having established an appropriate level of physical contact, you can then establish an appropriate *level of attention* – relaxed, detached, open and receptive, a meditative state – not too intense or intent; focused and alert but not too concentrated – again allowing space for the free expression of the cranio-sacral system. An excessively intense focus of attention will restrict and limit the expression of vitality, perhaps even causing discomfort and disturbance. The appropriate level of attention is enabled by sitting back, waiting patiently, open and receptive to whatever arises – rather than looking hard or searching intently for something.

(To some readers, the fact that your level of attention, your thoughts, your intensity of concentration

could affect the patient may be an obvious fact. To others it might seem unlikely. In this quantum age, such an idea is now widely recognised. As you work with the cranio-sacral process, whatever your initial preconceptions, you will very soon experience for yourself and recognise the power of thought, the effects of your focused attention, the interaction between observer and observed.)

Having established appropriate levels of physical contact and attention, you can let your attention extend to an awareness of different *levels of tissue* within the body:

- bone, membrane, fluid, subtle energy
- solid, soft, fluid, cellular, energetic levels.

(We will explore how to do this subsequently).

Box 8.1 Therapeutic intention

Intricate, energetic interactions occur between nearby individuals, even if they are not in physical contact. Information can be transferred from one organism to another via energy fields, and living systems are very sensitive to them. Add therapeutic intention and touch to the equation, and whole new dimensions of subtle but measureable exchanges are brought into play. Intentions are not trivial, because they give rise to specific patterns of electrical and magnetic activity in the nervous system of the therapist that can spread through their body and into the body of a patient. (*Energy Medicine: The Scientific Basis.* Oschman 2000)

As you continue to tune in, you may increasingly become aware of different impressions arising through your gentle contact with this cranio-sacral system – *impressions of quality, symmetry and motion*. You may become aware of warmth, coolness, hardness, softness, tightness, looseness, activity, stillness, vibration, pulsation. You may observe differences between left and right, twists and turns, bulges, pulls and shifts, or myriad other possible impressions; and you may encounter subtle *rhythmic motion* of expansion and contraction.

All these impressions are indications of the beginnings of *engagement* with the cranio-sacral system – and recognition of rhythmic motion represents a true engagement with the cranio-sacral process and the establishment of a receptive neutral state through which the therapeutic process can evolve.

By *responding appropriately* to these impressions – mostly by simply being there, with your calm, quiet presence – you will find that the cranio-sacral system leads you, subtly but purposefully, through a journey of discovery, release and resolution, in which resistances and imbalances are identified, released, dissolved away – and the system gradually settles into a more balanced symmetrical state, in which the underlying vitality can be expressed more freely, and a state of improved health and function, harmony and integration is established.

This appropriate response is enabled by observing the development of the *inherent treatment process*, which is expressed through the evolution of certain *fundamental principles*.

THE INHERENT TREATMENT PROCESS: FUNDAMENTAL PRINCIPLES

The fundamental principles of cranio-sacral integration are:

1. Engagement.
2. Allowing the system to express itself.
3. Following the system wherever it may lead you.
4. Stillness – reaching points of stillness, points of balanced tension, fulcrums.
5. Release – softening, melting.
6. Reorganisation – settling to a balanced neutral state.

As mentioned previously, this is an *inherent treatment process*, a natural process which is happening within the body as a matter of course. But it can be enhanced through the therapist's specific attention.

1. Engagement

The secret of engagement is *simply being there*. Tuning in to the cranio-sacral system will very soon demonstrate that the process of simply being there, engaging with the cranio-sacral system, produces profound and widespread responses in the patient. These responses will vary from person to person according to their current state, their underlying condition, their nature and many other factors. These responses may occur in any part of the body or in the body as a whole, affecting and reflecting the physical, mental, emotional or spiritual state of the individual.

Recognise that your presence is in itself an influence on the therapeutic process. Be content simply to be there, not trying to do anything, or find anything. Continue to focus on your own *calm, quiet presence* – the most important factor in the whole process. The majority of your attention needs to be on yourself. Settle into deeper stillness, deeper softness, deeper spaciousness.

Lightness of touch in cranio-sacral therapy is fundamental. Lightness of touch precludes the need for the body to invoke any protective mechanisms of tension (which it might do in response to a more invasive touch). The absence of protective tension enables a deeper connection with the patient's system, direct to the core of the system. Any active input or firmer contact may prevent deeper contact and possibly prevent any connection or response at all.

Spaciousness of attention is also essential. As described above, if your attention is too concentrated, intense or invasive, the system will respond by closing you out. Again, simply being there establishing a connection – through your relaxed, spacious awareness, rather than by trying to do anything – will enable the most profound responses and connection with the cranio-sacral system.

Establish appropriate levels of physical contact. Establish appropriate levels of attention. Be aware of the different levels of tissues within the system:

- allowing your attention to shift from bone to membrane, to fluid, to energy
- observing in particular the molecular, subatomic, energetic levels
    - the sense of the body as a mass of subatomic particles
- engaging particularly with the energy matrix
    - the sense of the whole body as a coherent mass of vitality
    - the sense of the whole body softening and dissolving into a fluidic matrix, within which your hands can float.

Wait patiently in stillness and spaciousness – aware, alert, engaged, with full awareness of your own practitioner fulcrums – physical, mental, emotional and spiritual – but not trying to do anything or make anything happen, simply observing the response of your patient's cranio-sacral system as it revolves and evolves around the fulcrum of your light, non-invasive contact.

As you feel an increasing sense of interconnection or engagement with your patient, *be aware of any impressions* arising through this connection – quality, symmetry, motion. Observe gently, don't concentrate too intently. Remain spacious. Be aware of the whole person and impressions arising from the whole person, allowing your focus of attention to spread through the body to encompass the whole body.

2. Allowing the system to express itself

As you remain engaged with the patient and observe the evolution of the cranio-sacral process, you may encounter a wide variety of different responses. You may feel qualities of stillness, warmth and fluidity, or you might feel impressions of agitation, tightness and solidity. You might encounter twisting, turning, swirling, figure-of-eight patterns, bending, bulging, pulling, shifting, vibrating, pulsating, shaking, buzzing, rocking.

All these expressions of movement are the body's attempt to resolve disturbances. Your engagement with them enhances the body's ability to do so – simply by allowing their expression – leading to a more settled state through which you and the patient's cranio-sacral system can engage with deeper patterns of disturbance.

As you continue to observe the impressions that arise – simply being there – those impressions may change. Activity may become more settled. Hardness may soften. Tightness may loosen. Vibrations may diminish. Pulsations may come and go, building and fading. Allow the system to do whatever it wants – expand, contract, pull, twist, soften, harden, wriggle, shake.

Without any physical input or trying to do anything or achieve anything, you can observe these changes and allow them to happen, allowing your hands to allow them to happen, giving permission for this system to manifest whatever it wants, giving space for the expression of these various responses.

As you *allow these impressions to be expressed*, the system may gradually become more settled, softer, more balanced, more still, less busy, less solid. As the system settles, you may *feel the gradual emergence of rhythmic motion*, gently expanding and contracting. Continue to observe, allowing your hands to float on the surface of this fluidic medium, or to become more deeply absorbed into the soft, warm fluidity of the energy matrix.

3. Following the system wherever it may lead you

As you allow the system to express itself, you may notice further changes. As the system softens it may feel as if the head is expanding and your hands are being pushed away. Your hands can follow this tendency. Alternatively the system may draw you in as if the head is contracting. Again your hands can follow this tendency. Or the system may be twisting and turning, pulling and bulging. Again, your hands can follow these tendencies wherever they lead you – but always from a basis of stillness and ease within yourself.

Follow the system wherever it may lead you – but be absolutely clear that *following does not involve any input from you*. You are not initiating any movement, you are not encouraging any movement, you are not making any decisions, you are not moving your hands – they simply feel as if they are being moved by subtle fluidic forces.

Imagine your hands like fronds of seaweed washed to and fro by the currents, eddies and waves under the ocean. Fronds of seaweed don't make decisions, nor do they move of their own accord; they are simply washed this way and that by the sea. The movements you are feeling are a sense of fluidic energy moving like currents under the ocean. You don't need to do anything about them, just *allow your soft fluent hands to flow with the currents, eddies and tides.*

Take care that the emphasis on not initiating movement does not prompt you to hold your hands in any way rigid or immobile – simply allow them to be soft and fluidic.

The movements may feel very expansive, as if your hands are being drawn or pushed vast distances – but if you open your eyes, you will probably see that there is no visible movement at all. On the other hand, keeping your eyes closed will probably help you to engage with and become absorbed into the movements more deeply.

If the head seems to bulge to one side, allow your hands to be drawn into that bulge. If the system rocks, let your hands be rocked. If the system rolls, let your hands be rolled. If the system wants to rock and roll, let it rock and roll. If the system wriggles, let your hands be wriggled – all with the same soft sense of your hands floating within a fluidic medium.

Initially, you might feel that the system is drawing you all over the place (the superficial patterns and day-to-day tensions).

As the system settles, rhythmic motion may become clearer and clearer; and as you allow your hands to follow this rhythmic motion, you may find the system drawing you persistently into the extremes of rhythmic motion – extreme expansion, or extreme contraction.

As the system becomes increasingly settled, you may find that the movements settle into a more persistent pull in one direction (the more chronic, underlying patterns of tension and injury) as if your hands are being drawn consistently towards a particular point – like a continuous current under the ocean. Allow your hands to be drawn in that persistent direction – not pushing, not adding anything, not doing anything – just allowing yourself to be drawn by the inherent pulls within the system – floating with the tide, maintaining your soft, meditative, spacious level of consciousness, which enables you to remain connected with the subtleties of the cranio-sacral process and the subtleties of rhythmic motion.

4. Stillness – reaching points of stillness, points of balanced tension, fulcrums

As you follow the persistent pull of the system, whether into an extreme of rhythmic motion or into its specific chosen direction, you may eventually reach a point of stillness, a point of balanced tension, where the system doesn't seem to want to go any further, nor return – just stays there. It is not particularly encountering any barrier or resistance, but just seems to be floating freely.

As the system moves towards this point of stillness, you may feel a gradual build-up of tension or pressure in the system, and a gradual diminution or reduction in rhythmic motion, until the rhythmic motion ceases.

Wait patiently at this point of stillness. Observe the quality of the stillness. Feel the vibrant quality of balanced tension held in that stillness. Allow yourself to become immersed in the quality of stillness.

Within this stillness, you may feel a subtle vibration, pulsation, shaking, wriggling, rocking – as if something is trying to break free. Allow this to be expressed, while remaining in stillness, feeling the dynamism within the stillness.

The stillness may last a few seconds. It may last several minutes. Stay with this dynamic stillness. Stay with the point of balanced tension. Wait patiently at the point of stillness, within the stillness, not trying to do anything – simply being there.

5. Release – softening, melting

Eventually, as you wait patiently at the point of stillness, you may feel a sense of release.

When the release occurs, it is likely to feel like a sense of softening or melting, a change from tightness to looseness, from solidity to fluidity – in the tissues, in the energy matrix – as if the whole system has been holding its breath and has just let go. Allow this sense of softening, melting, releasing, without feeling the need to do anything, maintaining your calm, quiet presence.

6. Reorganisation – settling to a balanced neutral state

As the system releases, it is likely to go through a transitional period of reorganisation, as if it is milling around somewhat aimlessly, trying to find itself, reorientate itself, re-establishing its state of balance, settling back to the centre. *Feel the sense of this reorganisation spreading through the whole body, as the system rearranges itself around its new-found unrestricted state.*

Imagine, for example, that you have just released a long-standing injury in the patient's foot, which had led them to shift their weight on to the other leg with a corresponding adaptation in the pelvis, spine and right up through the body. As the foot releases, and the body returns to a more symmetrical state, the whole body will adjust to its new state of balance and adaptations and decompensations will spread through the ankle, knee, hip and pelvis, up the spine, into the neck and head, and throughout the body, with corresponding changes in all the muscles that have been maintaining the unbalanced state. In the same way, wherever a release occurs, reorganisation will spread through the body on all levels.

During this phase, continue simply to observe, and to allow the system to express itself in whatever way it wishes, remaining deeply engaged and absorbed. Gradually the system will settle back into a centred, balanced, *neutral* state – and rhythmic motion will be re-established. You will know that the process of reorganisation and settling is complete by:

- the quality of settled, balanced centredness
- the gradual re-emergence of rhythmic motion.

Neutral

The term *neutral* (in the context of cranio-sacral integration) refers to the state in which the cranio-sacral system is resting comfortably, balanced and receptive, with rhythmic motion being expressed freely and evenly, not drawing into any asymmetries or still points, rather like a car in neutral with the engine gently ticking over but not about to go anywhere. This neutral is most clearly experienced following release and reorganisation, when the system settles back to neutral. Generally, it is preferable for the system to settle back to neutral after every release.

Neutral – with those same characteristics of a settled state and gentle regular expression of rhythmic motion – is also experienced near the start of a treatment, as true engagement develops, with the initial wavelets and ripples subsiding and rhythmic motion emerging clearly – indicating that the system is ready to proceed into deeper treatment.

Recognising the neutral state is vital to recognising what stage the treatment process has reached, and to finding appropriate moments of completion, or places from which to move on, or places to move into deeper engagement.

The definitive characteristic of neutral is feeling a clear expression of even balanced rhythmic motion. Awareness of rhythmic motion is also a very valuable indicator that you are still engaged with the cranio-sacral system, not losing touch with the subtleties of the system through tensing your hands, or imposing on the system in any way.

(Different texts may use the word *neutral* to represent different concepts.)

When the system reaches neutral, be prepared to wait in that neutral state, simply being there, appreciating the sense of ease, peace, calmness, allowing the system to rest in that state. Within that neutral state, the system may choose:

- to rest there for a while
- to express further impressions of asymmetry and movement
- to move into another phase of evolving fundamental principles
- to settle into more profound expressions of subtle integration at a deeper level
- or it may just continue to express settled even rhythmic motion.

Continuation or completion

Once the system has settled into a balanced, neutral state, you may choose:

- to simply be there, settling into deeper stillness and deeper engagement
- to wait for the next pattern to arise
- to move to a different part of the body
- to finish the treatment there.

Reaching neutral is like reaching a plateau during a long mountain climb, a time to pause and take a breath before choosing whether to embark on the next phase of the journey, or to camp for the night, or simply to admire the view.

The neutral state that arises following release and reorganisation can represent an appropriate point at which to allow the treatment process to come to an end.

It can also be a time when the system can be very receptive to profound subtle integration, a good place to stay for a prolonged period, allowing that process of deeper integration.

Subtle integration

Once the system has settled into neutral, particularly as the treatment session progresses through several releases, it may settle into a state of *subtle integration*. If you stay there in deep stillness and observe more closely, you may notice subtle movements, little wrigglings, tiny adjustments, perhaps a multitude of them, perhaps just occasional adjustments, perhaps continuous, perhaps intermittent, perhaps feeling very quiet for a while and then going through a few microscopic movements, not particularly following into fundamental principles, not particularly drawing into any focal point or fulcrum, not particularly doing anything other than a gentle sense of subtle integration.

It might be easy to think that nothing much is happening and that the treatment is complete, but these can be the most significant times of therapeutic effectiveness, the clearest connection with deeper levels, so it is essential to *stay with the system through these times*. Everything that precedes this stage of the treatment may be leading towards this moment; and if you stop here, then you may only be addressing the superficial patterns and not really reaching to the depths. Be prepared to wait, be prepared to stay with this stage, be prepared to engage with these myriad miniscule movements, to engage with the process of subtle integration – *it may be the most profound aspect of the treatment.*

Therapeutic pulse

One of the movements most commonly felt during the cranio-sacral process is the *therapeutic pulse*. This is a pulsation very similar to the arterial pulse, except that it is transient and it varies both in intensity and in rate. It can arise at various times and in different forms, appearing out of nowhere, gradually speeding up or slowing down, building up and fading away.

Box 8.2 Unlatching

The process of following the cranio-sacral system to a point of balanced tension or stillness, and waiting at that point of stillness for release and reorganisation, is sometimes described as *unlatching*. This term provides an analogy which, while it may be inaccurate in actuality, is a useful concept through which to understand and therefore more readily recognise the process occurring.

You will no doubt have encountered at some time a gate or door on which the latch is difficult to lift, or the handle difficult to turn. By pressing the gate more firmly into the closed position, the latch can then more readily be lifted or turned, and the gate can then readily open. In the same way with the cranio-sacral system, by following into the persistent pattern (into the 'closed' position), a point is reached where the resistance can be released, the latch can be lifted and the system can then move more freely into an open, clear, balanced state.

Similarly, you could consider a fishing line or a kite string that has become caught in a branch. Pulling is likely only to tighten the knot and increase the resistance. By moving towards the restriction, the kite string will go slack and can then be more readily unhooked from its impediment; the kite can then fly freely wherever it wants to go. In the same way, by following the cranio-sacral system towards the site of resistance, the system goes slack and the restriction can be released; the system is then able to move freely wherever it may wish to go.

It is associated with the process of release, but may arise in the build-up to a release or in the aftermath of a release.

In the build-up to a release, as rhythmic motion diminishes and the system closes down to stillness, the therapeutic pulse may appear very faintly, gradually become stronger, increasing in intensity, slowing down as the system builds to a point of balanced tension (rather as cyclists slow down as they ascend a steep hill) perhaps stopping as a still point is reached.

As a release occurs, the therapeutic pulse may appear quite suddenly as a rapid pulsation which soon fades away as the release spreads through the body (as if a stream of butterflies had been let out of a box and were fluttering away into the surroundings).

A similar pulsation may also appear while waiting at a still point awaiting release, along with other subtle vibrations and rocking movements, at which point it is not to be mistaken for a release.

It also arises in a slightly different form within the process of an *energy drive* (see Chapter 54) and may appear at various other times.

Like all movements experienced during cranio-sacral integration, the therapeutic pulse can be acknowledged, observed, and allowed to express itself, appreciating it as a valuable part of the therapeutic process.

Variations in the treatment process

Levels of engagement

These fundamental principles apply at whatever level you are engaging, whether you are working with the cranio-sacral rhythm level, the middle tide, or with fascial unwinding. There will be subtle differences in the way that the inherent treatment process manifests and consequently subtle differences in application, which we will explore subsequently, but the principles remain essentially similar. The level at which you engage with the system is best determined by whatever arises spontaneously, by whatever the system chooses.

A common progression within a treatment session might be as follows:

- engaging with initial responses and superficial levels
- settling to cranio-sacral rhythm level
- deepening to middle tide levels
- further deepening to long tide levels
- further deepening to deep dynamic stillness.

Initial stages

In the early stages of treatment, particularly when working with initial responses and cranio-sacral rhythm levels, this process of allowing the unfolding of the inherent treatment process plays a vital role in *settling and grounding* the patient. This stage is *highly therapeutic in itself*, clearing patterns on certain levels, releasing physical discomforts and contained emotions, and addressing specific symptoms – aches, pains, agitation, emotional disturbances, emotional holding.

If emotional responses arise, this can be a valuable part of the therapeutic process and is no cause for concern – as long as the therapist is well-grounded and understands the process, and provides the patient with sufficient grounding and sufficient understanding of the process of therapeutic release. These responses can help the patient to feel better – more settled, more relaxed, more comfortable, more at ease – and this in turn helps the treatment to *progress more readily towards deeper engagement* and more effective treatment. This can also be assisted by giving attention to the patient's breathing, inviting them to breathe a little more deeply and particularly to let go throughout their whole body with each out-breath.

Deepening engagement

As the superficial layers settle and you engage with deeper patterns manifesting within the middle tide level, the same process can continue, but it is likely to be expressed more subtly, more slowly, more profoundly. This stage is addressing more deeply ingrained patterns of disturbance, which may take longer to resolve and may enable more profound therapeutic responses.

Progressing to deeper levels

As the system settles into an even deeper state, these fundamental principles may fade into the background, becoming less relevant; and as you settle into a deeper absorption and consequent deeper connection with the more subtle levels of the system, you may find that the process of fundamental principles is superseded by the process of subtle integration and you may experience the long tide.

Dynamic stillness

As you settle into even deeper connection, you may encounter deep dynamic stillness, where everything else becomes less relevant – the fundamental principles, the physical body, the tissues, the whole material world may seem to fade into the background and everything dissolves into a profound, fluidic, unified matrix as you settle into deep dynamic stillness.

Variations according to circumstances

The way in which the process progresses will vary from person to person. Sometimes the initial stages may need very little time and attention. The system may already be settled and clear and ready to proceed to deeper levels, or may settle readily. At other times, when the patient is more unsettled, these initial stages may need a greater degree of attention and much longer time and may become the predominant component of the treatment.

These fundamental principles, in various forms, are the principal and most common way in which the cranio-sacral process will unfold. But the way in which they are expressed can also be very variable, and a treatment session will not necessarily always follow a clear expression of the inherent treatment process. Depending on circumstances, the therapeutic process may involve parts or all of the fundamental principles, or may involve greater emphasis on certain aspects of the fundamental principles:

- A session might consist of simply being there allowing the system to settle, soften, melt, dissolve, allowing the subtle expression of the system through a series of tiny movements without specifically going through any recognisable expression of the fundamental principles.
- Another session might consist of a series of short still points and releases at the cranio-sacral rhythm level, each minor release bringing the system into a more balanced settled state.
- Another session might settle readily to middle tide level and consist of one or a few long processes of drawing into an extended still point at the middle tide level leading to profound release.
- Another session might involve progressing through a series of initial settling movements, a series of shorter still points and releases

in cranio-sacral rhythm, leading to a longer, deeper still point and release in middle tide motion.
- Another session might involve settling rapidly into a deep, settled neutral and simply being there allowing subtle integration of the whole system.
- Another session might go through many of the earlier variations and then settle into the long tide level, deep dynamic stillness and profound subtle integration.

These are just a few examples of endless possible variations. *The approach in cranio-sacral integration is to work without an agenda or expectations, simply allowing the spontaneous expression of the system in whatever way it wishes, according to individual circumstances, responding to the needs of the individual.*

Chapter 9

Stimulus

Within the context of the inherent treatment process and the fundamental principles of the cranio-sacral process, we can recognise and understand the value of various stimuli.

The basis of cranio-sacral integration is to allow the cranio-sacral system, in its own wisdom, to bring about healing in a biodynamic manner, without imposing on the system or trying to make anything happen. But there is no such thing as cranio-sacral therapy without stimulus. There can never be a complete absence of stimulus.

What constitutes a stimulus?

A stimulus is anything which might potentially elicit a response in the patient.

In other words, to give a few examples:

- the presence of the therapist
- the reputation of the therapist, even before the patient arrives
- the atmosphere and environment of the treatment space
- the manner and demeanour of the therapist
- any hand contact at all, however light, off-the-body, non-intentional
- the focus of attention by the therapist on the patient
- the words of the therapist
- the thoughts of the therapist
- the intentions of the therapist
- the focus of attention on particular anatomical structures or areas of the body
- the engagement with the patient's cranio-sacral system, on whatever level
- the depth of engagement.

The cranio-sacral process arises from the body's own inherent healing potential. Any inappropriate imposition on the system may restrict or block the process, invoking its protective mechanisms, leading it to shut down. Yet, by the very presence of the therapist, some degree of stimulus is inevitable. So the question is not whether or not to introduce a stimulus, but rather what degree of stimulus and what quality of stimulus is appropriate and therapeutic. This will vary according to circumstances and according to the level or depth at which you are engaged.

Within the cranio-sacral process:

- all stimuli are very subtle – offering, inviting, asking, responding – rather than doing anything
- all stimuli consist simply of *enhancing* the body's natural inherent tendencies.

For present purposes, the various stimuli listed above can be conveniently reduced to a shorter summary, in which the main stimuli can be summarised as:

- your presence
- your contact
- your thoughts
- enhancing the body's inherent tendencies
- following any propensities as required by the body.

(Remember, following doesn't involve doing anything – fronds of seaweed don't make decisions.)

Enhancement

Enhancement involves the recognition of a tendency within the cranio-sacral process, and responding appropriately by allowing and following that natural inherent tendency within the body to an appropriate point of resolution.

- This might involve recognising the body's natural tendency to draw into the extremes of rhythmic motion (expansion or contraction) to a point of stillness and release.
- It might involve recognising the body's natural tendency to draw into a twist or

pattern of asymmetry until it reaches a point of stillness, through which the imbalance releases and untwists.

- It might involve recognising a pattern of compression, deeply locked into the tissues, and enhancing the body's natural tendency to follow into that compression to a point of release.
- It might involve recognising the body's need to expand or stretch, and offering the thought of traction to see if the body takes up the invitation and gently stretches out on a subtle energetic level.

All of these responses will always be carried out from a basis of stillness and ease within yourself.

(The terms compression and traction within the cranio-sacral process involve no physical input, just the thought, just the offer, just the invitation, inviting the body to decide and to respond if it wishes. Any physical input will simply invoke the protective mechanisms of the body and make it close down or resist, or at least limit the effects of any input to a more gross, superficial level.)

(Remaining in touch with the rhythmic motion ensures that the therapist is engaged with the cranio-sacral process rather than imposing; and the level of rhythmic motion with which the therapist is engaged determines the depth at which the process is taking place – that depth being best determined by the body's own spontaneous expression. The appropriate level is the level which is relevant to that patient at that moment, within the context of that particular cranio-sacral interaction.)

Enhancement is an inherent part of cranio-sacral therapy. It may be particularly appropriate:

- when it is specifically invited by the system
- in response to extraneous movements that are not resolving
- on encountering a particularly resistant restriction which is not responding readily through its own inherent treatment process
- in order to encourage a further response from a system which is not responding
- in order to explore more deeply into the system once the superficial patterns have settled.

Still point induction

As we have seen, an inherent tendency within the cranio-sacral system is the tendency to go into points of stillness, leading to release and reorganisation. By interacting appropriately with the patient's system, the therapist can specifically enhance this natural tendency. This process is called *still point induction* and will be described in greater detail later.

Responding to extraneous movements

Any movements other than the fluent flow of expansion and contraction, represent imbalances or resistances that the body is trying to address. As we have seen, they can take many different forms, from vibrating or twisting to rocking from side to side or figure-of-eight patterns. (*These various movements are sometimes collectively described as* lateral fluctuations – *although they may not be lateral or fluctuating. This term is particularly appropriate for the common pattern of rocking from side to side and different variations of this pattern.*)

There are various ways of responding to these movements and the appropriate response can be established by allowing a natural sequence of possible options – all of which reflect the usual cranio-sacral process:

1. Simply engage with them, observing them and focusing your attention on them. Many of these movements will subside and dissolve away when you simply observe them with your calm, quiet presence.

2. As you observe them, these movements may tend to become more exaggerated and you can allow them to do so – for example, a rocking movement might gradually rock from side to side with increasing amplitude – until it seems to break free, resolve and settle.

3. If this doesn't happen spontaneously, you can ask the movements if they want to exaggerate, for instance enhancing the side to side movement from one extreme to the other through your focused attention, until it releases and resolves.

4. Particularly when the system is rocking from side to side and is not resolving, you can ask the system if it would like to move consistently towards one side or the other, following the sideways movement to the extreme until it resolves.
5. If it is not responding to any of the above, you can contain the movement, observing as the rocking gradually reduces in amplitude in response to your containment, until it reaches a still point at the centre of the movement, closing down, becoming still, and releasing.

Containment

Containment can be a valuable option to use at various times during a treatment, usually arising after initially allowing the system to express itself freely, for example:

- containing an unsettled system that is jumping around all over the place
- containing a system into a still point
- containing a system into a compression pattern
- containing a system that is unwinding aimlessly
- containing a system that is avoiding focal points
- containing a system that is rocking from side to side or expressing other repetitive movements
- containing as a way of bringing the system into focus
- containment as a stimulus to enable a more profound response.

Containment can be introduced purely with your focused attention, or may involve a subtle physical containment introduced very gradually until the system reaches a point of more specific engagement or reaches a point of stillness.

Presence

The 'presence' of the therapist is a deliberately ambiguous term: on the one hand, indicating that the very fact that the therapist is present has an influence on the patient – physically, mentally, emotionally, spiritually, energetically – but more significantly, indicating that the quality of the therapist's 'presence' plays a vital and fundamental role in the interaction of the therapeutic process, the progress of which will inevitably be profoundly influenced by:

- the ability of the therapist to maintain a calm, quiet presence
- the ability to be centred, grounded, and balanced in themselves
- the contribution which they bring to the interactive process through their presence
- their whole state of being
- their depth of presence.

All the qualities that they bring to the process are of significance to the interactive therapeutic cranio-sacral process. It is this, above all, that will determine the depth of engagement with the patient's system, and the degree and level of response in the patient.

The quality of presence in the practitioner is in turn dependent on the degree and level of development within the practitioner, which is in turn determined by:

- depth of personal development
- depth of awareness
- depth of spirituality
- depth of knowledge
- life experience
- current state of balance, centredness and groundedness.

The most fundamental factor in the whole cranio-sacral process and the most significant stimulus is your own *calm, quiet presence.*

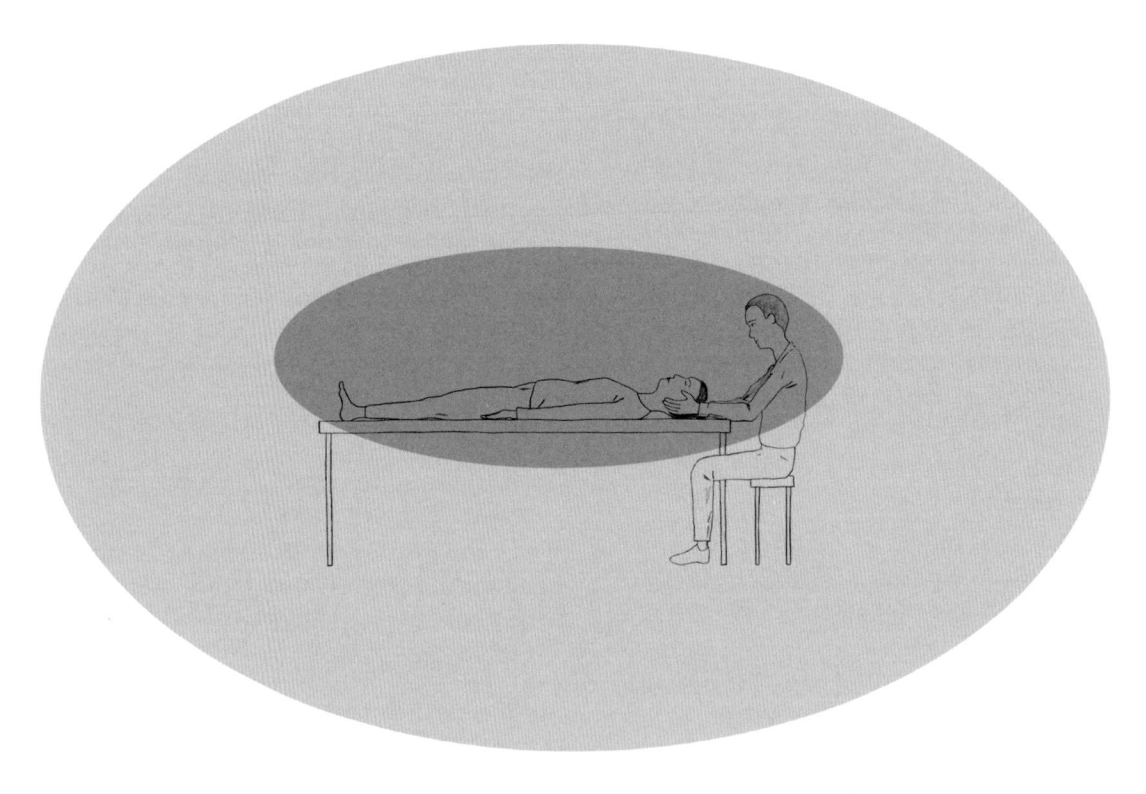

9.1 The therapist's calm, quiet presence can itself be the most profound and significant stimulus

Chapter 10

Responses to Treatment

Relax
The most common response to a cranio-sacral treatment is a profound sense of relaxation, often accompanied by various other associated sensations of softness, ease, comfort, contentment, a sense of being more at one with the world and with oneself.

Sleep
Each patient will experience this relaxation differently, some with a sense of lightness, some with a sense of heaviness. Some patients report sensations of floating. Many patients fall asleep during a treatment and, while they sometimes apologise, there is nothing at all wrong with that; it is a positive indication that they are relaxed – and the cranio-sacral system is usually very responsive during sleep, precisely because it is so relaxed.

Rumbling
Various other sensations may arise during a treatment – sensations of tingling, vibrating, pulsation, warmth or coolness. There may be muscle twitches, or the patient may feel subtle pulls and twists anywhere in the body. A particularly common response is a rumbling or gurgling tummy. This is a frequent source of embarrassment to patients, who will again often apologise, and sometimes tense up in embarrassment or in a vain attempt to stop the noises, so it is good to reassure them that it is very common, very understandable, and simply a sign of the digestive system relaxing.

Breathing
Changes in breathing are also very common, although not necessarily noticed by the patient. The most common is perhaps a long sigh or deep breath as a release occurs deep within the cranio-sacral system. There can be other changes in the breathing – holding the breath, breathing faster, taking a deep breath. For the most part, the general tendency is for the breathing to become gradually deeper and calmer as the session progresses.

All over the place
Patients may become aware of different parts of their body (assuming that they're not asleep). They may feel changes under the therapist's hands – warmth, buzzing, softening – or they may feel changes in areas of the body distant from the therapist's contact. This can often surprise patients, when you are sitting at their head and they feel things happening in their legs, or sacrum, or digestive system. It is of course an indication of the interconnectedness of the body, both in terms of injuries and imbalances transmitting their effects throughout the body, and in terms of all the tissues being connected.

Hot and cold
A predominant sensation is of the whole body softening, warming, sometimes glowing – but along with this apparent release of heat, it is common for patients to feel cold as the treatment progresses. This reflects changes in the autonomic nervous system as they relax, and it is advisable for the therapist to take it into account (especially if the therapist may feel quite warm and think that the room is quite warm). Many therapists will cover the patient with a blanket as a matter of course throughout the treatment, and it is at least necessary to have a blanket available and to offer it to the patient – bearing in mind that many patients are too polite to say that they are cold; they may lie there shivering until you ask them, and this is not helpful to their degree of

relaxation and therefore to the effectiveness of the treatment.

To pee or not to pee

Another common response, associated with the relaxation of the autonomic nervous system, is a need to pee. Many patients will find that after a cranio-sacral treatment they will need to pee, often copiously, but this may also arise during the session – something to be aware of, particularly with small children!

Pain

Pains will usually ease during treatment and tensions will generally soften, but it is not realistic to expect every long-standing ache and pain to disappear instantly. Many symptoms will fade gradually, or shift some days after the treatment, as the body adjusts and rebalances.

It is also possible for pains to *arise* during treatment. This will generally be due to old injuries rising to the surface – sometimes familiar old injuries, sometimes long-forgotten ones, sometimes aches and pains that can't readily be traced to any known incident. This can occasionally be a concern for patients who are not familiar with the concept of natural healing. It is therefore helpful to explain, where necessary, the process of release whereby old aches and pains which have been held under the surface perhaps for years, using the body's protective mechanisms of adaptation and compensation, tension and holding, will often come to the surface when allowed to do so in response to release and relaxation, in order to be cleared out and dissolved away. Such aches and pains can be welcomed.

If you have been sitting cross-legged on the floor, you might feel perfectly comfortable, until you try to get up and find that your leg has gone numb. Moving can be acutely painful, but that does not mean that you need to spend the rest of your life sitting cross-legged on the floor; you move the leg around, give it a little time to restore circulation and release pressure on the nerve, and then you are able to walk again. In the same way with old injuries, you can allow the transient discomfort to emerge, in order to move forward to a place of greater ease and comfort.

Therapeutic pain

The slight pains experienced at these times are sometimes described as *therapeutic pain*, and they often have particular qualities that distinguish them as therapeutic pain. It is not easy to describe them precisely, because they vary from person to person and according to the nature of the original injury, but those who have experienced therapeutic pain will generally recognise it. It will often be in an area of an old injury or former discomfort; it may be a sensation which feels familiar from the past, perhaps associated with a specific injury or incident; it often has a broad, expansive, open, alive, achy quality, as opposed to a sharp, intense, acute, contracted feeling (although in certain circumstances releases can occur with sharp pain). It is helpful for the patient to relax into the pain, to welcome it, and to allow it to be expressed – and definitely not helpful for them to contract against the pain, or worry about it. Helping the patient to breathe and relax into the pain can be very significant to the therapeutic outcome. Therapeutic pain is generally transient – seconds, minutes, sometimes hours – occasionally days if the body is adjusting to some very long-standing and deeply suppressed pattern.

Laughing – and crying

Just as old physical injuries may rise to the surface, in the same way emotions can arise. This can include all sorts of feelings: pleasant or unpleasant (laughter, smiles, sadness, tears); feelings relating to specific events in life (rejection, loneliness, loss); feelings reflecting deeply ingrained psycho-emotional patterns (depression, abandonment); abstract feelings of discontent that don't necessarily relate to anything specific. It tends to be uncomfortable feelings that will arise, because it is uncomfortable feelings that we suppress. We don't usually suppress feelings of joy and happiness and contentment. When laughter does come up, it is usually relating to nervous laughter, perhaps particularly in those who tend to respond to embarrassing or disturbing circumstances by laughing or giggling.

Such emotional feelings can be mild, almost unnoticed, or can be profound and dramatic. As with the physical sensations, the first priority is to ensure an appropriate understanding by the patient of such responses. Emotions can be harder to address and put into perspective than physical sensations, but the principles remain the same – acknowledging them, and understanding that they are simply rising to the surface to be released, that they are better out than in. Once again it is helpful for the patient to relax and let them out, welcome them, allow them to be expressed – talking about them if they wish, crying, or just feeling the feelings – so it is definitely not helpful to tighten up or suppress them, or push them back under the surface, where they continue to trouble the patient, depleting their resources and energy, and arise again at future, perhaps less appropriate, moments.

Memories are made of this

Along with both the physical and emotional sensations, a patient may often experience memories. As with the other sensations they can be happy or sad, pleasant or uncomfortable, they can relate to specific injuries, incidents or traumas. They can relate to recent situations or long-forgotten events, sometimes bringing back memories of situations that haven't been thought about for years, even decades. Once again they can also be abstract, sometimes puzzling, sometimes dream-like in their quality. Memories can arise at any time during a treatment, but they are most likely to occur as a particular focal point of restriction or injury releases, consciously or unconsciously. Sometimes this can be dramatic and very specific, as we shall see in various examples later. Sometimes these memories can be very insightful, helping a patient to understand their situation, to see where their tensions or pains have come from, and consequently helping them to address and release them more effectively.

Tissue memory

Memories arising in response to changes in the tissues are often known as *tissue memory*. The term tissue memory has two components or interpretations:

1. When tensions in the tissues release, memories associated with the incident which caused that tension may arise.

2. The tissues physically hold on to patterns imposed by injury or stress, maintaining and perpetuating the physical disturbance even though the original source has been removed. In other words, the memory of the pattern is imprinted in the tissues and remains there (unless released) perpetuating symptoms – pain, weakness, tension, twist – even though it has supposedly healed. Hence a sprained ankle may carry the memory of that injury for years afterwards, remaining weak, tense, susceptible to collapse, or with a tendency to twist repeatedly into its familiar pattern of injury – unless the tissue memory held in the tissues is addressed and released. This can apply to any tissues in the body, but is particularly noticeable in the fascia, so working with the fascia is particularly likely to bring up memories.

It may be surmised that memory actually resides in the tissues – after all, various experiments, particularly on rats, have demonstrated clearly that memory certainly doesn't reside in the brain.

Letting go

In the majority of cases, these responses are relatively mild, but any of them can occur in more dramatic form – depending on the circumstances. If a patient arrives for treatment in a highly charged emotional state, barely holding back their tears, then the treatment process – or simply giving them some attention or the opportunity to talk and let go – may lead to a flood of tears and emotion. This again can be welcomed as a positive release of tension. A good cry can be very therapeutic and can then lead to a more productive and profound treatment – far better than trying to work with a patient who is desperately trying to hold back their tears and their feelings, and holding onto a great deal of tension in order to do so.

Handling trauma

In patients with more severe trauma – rape, sexual abuse, post-traumatic stress disorder – any of these responses can be more exaggerated, and it is necessary to prepare the way and establish secure grounding and understanding of the process of trauma release before entering into any deep release of severe trauma. This is something which we will explore at a later stage. One advantage of the cranio-sacral process is that, as long as you are working gently and non-invasively, the system is only likely to bring up what the patient is ready to address.

Responses at the end of the treatment and after a treatment

Waking from a deep sleep

As mentioned at the start, the most common response to a cranio-sacral treatment is a profound sense of relaxation; at the end of the treatment the vast majority of patients will feel comfortable, relaxed and pleasant. As with any deep relaxation, this pleasant sensation and ease can sometimes be accompanied by feeling a bit vague, distant, detached. Patients may feel that they have been on a long journey deep inside themselves, and may need time to return to a fully conscious, fully awake, fully alert state – as if waking from a deep sleep.

As we have seen, many patients will actually fall asleep during a treatment and this may also leave them feeling a little light-headed or disorientated.

Light-headedness

Getting up after lying down for a long period under any circumstances can induce a brief sense of light-headedness or dizziness (particularly in elderly patients), and it is good to be prepared for this, encouraging patients to get up slowly, helping them off the couch and onto a chair. All such responses are perfectly understandable within the context of a deep state of relaxation, and are usually very transient, but it is also helpful to ensure that every patient feels settled and alert again before leaving the treatment room and returning to the outside world, particularly if they are planning on driving.

A few days later

Some therapeutic responses may arise some time after the treatment, hours or days later. These may include deep sleep (particularly if the patient has a backlog of tiredness after weeks, months, or even years of overstretching themselves and burning the candle at both ends). This is the body telling them that they need more rest in order to bring themselves into a more balanced state. In the same way, some patients may feel deeply tired. Babies and children will often sleep deeply soon after a treatment, or the night after a treatment – again, especially if they have not been sleeping much previously – and they will generally settle into a calmer, happier, more settled state.

Postural shift

Responses may also include vivid dreams, long-forgotten memories, or perhaps a shift in postural balance, as long-standing postural strains resulting from old injuries are released, allowing the body to adjust back to a more balanced, healthy position. The process of readjusting back to a more balanced state may bring on transient minor aches and pains, as muscles which have been out of use for some time come back into use – as happens when taking up exercise after prolonged lack of exercise.

Since responses may not arise until some time after the treatment, it is advisable to provide patients with a possible contact number, so that if any concerns arise they can be reassured.

Mostly minor, transient, therapeutic responses

Most of the responses described above are minor, transient, therapeutic, and either very pleasant or easily coped with. If cranio-sacral therapy is carried out in a well-integrated manner, then it is unlikely to have any significant adverse side-effects – other than those transient discomforts as the body adjusts to the newly balanced state. There are situations in which the responses can be more extended, more dramatic, and more significant, especially in cases of severe trauma, deeply embedded chronic patterns, and multiple complex injuries, and we will look at how to approach these situations later – but these are not the usual picture.

Remaining alert

Most of these therapeutic responses – tensions easing, old injuries rising to the surface – are the body adapting and adjusting to its newfound balance. Most will be transient. But the therapist should never be blasé or casual. While recognising that most responses are therapeutic, you always need to be alert for the occasional symptom that might not be – especially with a patient who you know to have a pathology or underlying condition, or with any sign that seems unusual or strange. As always in cranio-sacral therapy, the sensitive cranio-sacral therapist is likely to pick up on any unusual sensations. If in doubt, keep in touch with the patient after the treatment, and refer as necessary.

Pleasant and relaxed

Always be alert, always be observant, always be aware of any possibilities, in preparation for the very occasional adverse reaction. Always provide the necessary back-up and support – but for the most part, the response to cranio-sacral therapy will be a pleasant state of relaxation and well-being.

Chapter 11

To Treat or Not to Treat
Contra-Indications

The term *contra-indications* means situations in which treatment is not advisable. These can be described under two main categories:
- contra-indications for an experienced and sensitive cranio-sacral therapist
- contra-indications for beginners.

Contra-indications for an experienced and sensitive cranio-sacral therapist

As long as the therapist is genuinely sensitive to the needs of the patient and the subtlest responses within the system and is using cranio-sacral integration in an appropriately subtle, sensitive, gentle and non-invasive way, there need be no contra-indications for an experienced and sensitive cranio-sacral therapist. They can treat anyone, whatever their condition or circumstances. Cranio-sacral integration involves enhancing underlying vitality – and everyone can benefit from that.

Cranio-sacral integration (at least as presented here) does not involve doing anything to the patient. It does not involve exerting any pressure. It does not involve imposing on the body in any way. It involves allowing the system to do what the body, in its profound wisdom, needs to do. So long as the therapist is sensitive to the cranio-sacral system, listens to everything it says, and responds with due sensitivity and awareness, then it is not possible to cause any harm.

There may be times when the body says it doesn't want treatment, and that's fine so long as the therapist reads that message and responds accordingly. There will be treatment responses which may sometimes be uncomfortable – and these need to be evaluated and monitored carefully within the context of the therapeutic process and the patient's circumstances – but as long as the therapist has carried out treatment appropriately, then those responses will be a positive therapeutic response to sensitive and appropriate treatment.

It must be emphasised, however, that this applies to experienced cranio-sacral therapists, who have sufficient sensitivity to recognise and identify the body's subtlest needs accurately, and who can be absolutely confident in their ability to do so. It is not a licence for inexperienced therapists, or less sensitive therapists, or cranio-sacral therapists who practise in a more physically invasive way, to assume that they can do whatever they like without due care and consideration.

Contra-indications for beginners

A beginner may not have the sensitivity to read the system accurately and to recognise all the signs that may be put out by the system. A beginner may use too firm a contact, or apply inappropriate pressures.

Even in such cases it is difficult to do any harm. One of the advantages of the cranio-sacral process is that in order to engage with the system, the therapist needs sensitivity; and in order to engage with deeper levels of the system, the therapist needs profound sensitivity. Without such sensitivity the therapist is unlikely even to connect with the system. If they do have the sensitivity to connect, they are likely to have the sensitivity to read the system.

Another advantage is that if inappropriate pressures are imposed on the system, it will simply close down, put up barriers of protective tension and lock out the therapist. This might leave the patient with a transient feeling of being closed down or tight, but is unlikely to leave any long-term effects. So again it is difficult to do harm with a system that is self-protective.

Various texts describe possible contra-indications for cranio-sacral therapy, but all of these tend to assume a certain level of physical pressure or imposition on the system as a reason for the contra-indication, which when practising cranio-sacral integration appropriately is not the case. Nevertheless, it is sensible for beginners to err on the side of caution and to work with healthy stable practice partners until they gain sufficient experience.

It may therefore be advisable for the beginner to avoid practising initially on anyone with significant health problems, or significantly delicate circumstances. Standard advice to beginners might include the recommendation not to practise on:

- anyone with a significant health problem, or significant health history
- anyone with significant mental or emotional instability or volatility
- babies and children
- pregnant women.

Of course, it must be emphasised that these provisos are only for beginners. Treating babies and children is of course a major aspect of cranio-sacral integration. Treating women during pregnancy is a vital aspect of health care; and treating people with significant health problems, including mental and emotional instability, are the everyday process of cranio-sacral practice. So these are not to be regarded as danger areas, but simply as areas to be avoided by beginners.

Interlude 1

A Time for Reflection
Key Concepts in Cranio-Sacral Integration

Calm, quiet presence
- Your own calm, quiet presence is the most significant factor in the whole cranio-sacral process.
- Establish and maintain practitioner fulcrums.
- Simply being there.

Vitality
- At the heart of cranio-sacral integration is the acknowledgement of an underlying vitality which pervades every cell throughout the body.
- It is not primarily about bones, membranes, or fluids.
- It is about underlying vitality – expressed as rhythmic motion.

Engagement
- The essence of cranio-sacral integration is to engage with and enhance underlying vitality.
- Without engagement, it isn't cranio-sacral integration.

The matrix
- Maintain constant awareness of the cranio-sacral system as a fluidic matrix through which the fundamental forces of nature are flowing.

Establishing contact
- Establish appropriate levels of physical contact, levels of attention, tissue levels.
- Allow impressions of quality, symmetry, motion to arise.

The inherent treatment process
- Allow the evolution of fundamental principles.
- Engage with rhythmic motion – cranio-sacral rhythm, middle tide, long tide.
- Still point.
- Neutral.

Subtle integration

Dynamic stillness

Part II
Essential Concepts

Chapter 12

Pigs, Elephants and Snakes
The Concept of Quality

Quality – in the context of cranio-sacral integration – is the most valuable and powerful diagnostic tool that you can possess. It tells you everything there is to know – about the patient, about the process, about how things are progressing, about yourself. Understanding quality is an irreplaceable and invaluable gift.

Characteristics

When we talk about quality in cranio-sacral terms, we don't mean 'good' or 'bad', we are not assessing whether something is right or wrong, better or worse. Rather we are evaluating its *characteristics* – just as one might talk of the quality of a material or cloth – is it rough, is it smooth, is it silky, is it soft? Clearly wool feels different from cotton or silk – they have a different quality. Simply by feeling these materials, most people could distinguish them from each other. In the same way, every cranio-sacral system has its own distinctive qualities reflecting the nature of the individual.

Their whole life story is there for us to read

Quality in this context means the characteristics of something, and by learning to distinguish different characteristics – hundreds and thousands and millions of subtle distinctions in characteristics – we can establish a complete picture of the patient – their current state, their history, their physical injuries, diseases and pathologies, their emotional state, their psychological state, their spiritual state. Their whole life story is there for us to read – and quality is the secret to evaluating accurately and precisely everything about them.

Broken legs

If someone has broken one leg (and not the other leg) whether recently or a long time ago, and you rest your hands lightly on their feet, do you think that those two legs are going to feel exactly the same? Of course they're not. They will feel different. They will have a different quality. The leg that was broken will probably feel more solid, less mobile (partly due to the fracture and the scar tissue, partly because of the peripheral effects of the original injury on the leg as a whole). These are aspects of quality, and they enable you very readily to distinguish sites of injury.

Not only can you assess that the leg has been injured, but as you survey the legs, you will be able to identify different qualities at different parts of the leg. As you run your attention up the leg, you will feel changes in quality from place to place, you will feel the increasingly dense quality as you approach the site of an old fracture, and you can locate precisely the site of injury and all the effects on the surrounding tissues. (The very fact of taking your attention there will potentially instigate healing and change, but for the moment we are focusing on quality, so we will leave those aspects for now.)

People are different

When you rest your hands lightly on the shoulders of various patients, you will soon notice that each pair of shoulders feels different. Some are tight, some are relaxed, some feel agitated, some feel still. There are endless variations. These are not simply abstract words; they are telling you something about that patient. Has there been a shoulder injury, are they holding a lot of tension in their shoulders, is that agitation telling you that they are anxious about something?

This is still a very simple preliminary exploration of quality, but as you develop the concept, and refine your understanding of quality and gain experience of reading the quality of each and every situation, each and every part of the body, each and every patient, so you can extend your perception of quality to understand more and more about the patient.

The stillness that you felt in those shoulders – was it a stillness of being calm and at ease, or was it a stillness of being stuck and immobile? Learn to make that distinction through practice and experience and constant refinement of your skills in evaluating quality, and everything will become clear, so that you can distinguish the frozen shoulder, the fractured clavicle, the emotional tension held into the shoulder and all the other infinite variations that you might encounter, not just in the shoulders but also on every part of the body, and so gain a deep insight into your patient's state, situation and current circumstances on every level so that you can engage with their system more effectively.

Fear, anger, happiness

When someone is frightened, what do they tend to do? Contract, shrink. When someone is happy, what do they do? Relax, open up. When someone is angry, what do they do? Burn, boil, become fiery and tense.

So when you rest your hands lightly on the body, do you think the frightened person, the happy person and the angry person are all going to feel the same? Of course not – their whole body will reflect their emotional state; particular parts of the body might reflect certain emotions more specifically (something we will explore in greater depth later), but you will be able to read their emotional state as readily as their broken leg. And again as you refine your skills through practice and experience, you can read every detail – not just the immediate superficial emotions but also the more deeply held emotional patterns. You can distinguish the different levels – the current emotional state from the underlying emotional personality; you can feel the effects of the person who is suppressing their emotions – the tight holding quality on the surface, with the bubbling rumbling volcanic activity contained within.

You can feel emotion, not just as a general characteristic throughout the body, but also in key areas of emotional holding in the body – such as the emotional centres. You can feel agitation in the heart centre of someone who is anxious or stressed. You can also feel the deeply held tight quality in the solar plexus of someone who has been controlling their emotions and holding them in for years.

Judith was in her forties, suffering from various symptoms on her left side – tightness in her chest, pains and numbness down her left arm to her little finger. This had been developing for several years, gradually getting worse. The obvious immediate concern suggested by her symptoms was a possible heart condition. She had been to her doctor and undergone various tests which showed no cardiac pathology.

Tuning in to her system, there was certainly a distinctive quality around her heart and her pericardium – but not the qualities of a heart pathology, more the qualities of contraction, containment, holding on to something, holding on to sadness, holding on to grief. As I treated her, my hands resting gently around her heart and pericardium, I told her about the qualities that I was feeling and asked her if it meant anything to her.

She explained that a few years earlier her husband had died. She had two small children, so she had tried to be strong and supportive for them, and not upset them by showing her grief. She had tried to get on with life. As she talked, she began to cry. She continued to tell me her story and continued to cry gently as she spoke. She told me that she had never had a chance to express her grief, had never really cried about her husband's death, and how it was such a relief to be able to talk about it and cry about it now.

As she spoke, the quality around her heart and pericardium softened, loosened, relaxed, opened up. Her symptoms, both in her chest and down her left arm, disappeared instantly – those symptoms that were indeed indicative of the heart, but not as a heart pathology, not anything that a cardiac test could reveal, but grief held in her heart.

The whole picture

All of these – broken legs, shoulders, emotions, grief held in the heart – are just simple isolated examples. As you look at the whole picture, you can gain a vast overview of the whole person, with all these many details of qualities adding together to provide the broader picture:

- the qualities pervading the whole body
- the qualities in various different local areas
- the qualities reflecting physical injuries
- the qualities reflecting the emotional state
- the qualities on the surface
- the qualities under the surface
- the qualities at various levels of depth within
- and so on, ad infinitum.

A vast store of information is contained within their cranio-sacral system and is there for you to read and interpret – so long as you have the understanding of quality and the skills developed over years of practice and experience to read those qualities accurately.

Just a body?

Of course a casual observer, without any understanding of quality or any experience, might place their hands on a body and say 'I don't feel anything – just a body'. Beginners in cranio-sacral therapy often find the concept of quality quite elusive. But it is just a matter of practice and experience. Once you start exploring quality, defining quality, refining your definitions and building experience, so quality becomes clearer and more and more revealing and you too will come to recognise that it is the most valuable diagnostic tool available.

Identifying pathologies

Quality can also help you to recognise pathologies. If a patient has diabetes, it will affect the quality of their whole system and you can learn to recognise the distinctive qualities of a diabetic. Of course you will need to feel many diabetic patients before you can recognise those qualities. Describing the features theoretically is not enough; it might help, but ultimately *feeling* the quality, taking it into your subconscious memory bank of qualities, is what will enable you to recognise the next diabetic – perhaps developing the ability to recognise an incipient diabetes before it has been identified and diagnosed. This is of course a speciality, and one would not expect every cranio-sacral therapist to have the specific clinical experience to enable that specific diagnosis.

Lilian came to me with pain in her abdomen. She was a forthright woman in her fifties who knew what she wanted – and she wanted to be rid of this pain. She paid careful attention to her health, ate a very healthy diet, and looked after herself, as she had done for many years. She didn't like going to doctors, because she said they didn't listen, and were dismissive, and they didn't share her interest in natural health care.

I treated her and her pain eased, but something about the quality of her system concerned me. I said to her that, despite her misgivings about doctors, it would be a good idea to see her doctor and have these pains investigated. I saw her a week later and she hadn't contacted her doctor and didn't want to. I treated her again, her pain was again relieved, again I was concerned by the qualities I felt in her system. I didn't want to alarm her by saying too much of what I felt, but this time I insisted that I would not continue to treat her unless she went to her doctor and underwent investigations.

The following week, she reported that she had (reluctantly) seen her doctor, he had been dismissive as usual, had told that there was nothing wrong with her, that she was being neurotic and had sent her away – without any investigations.

This time I insisted that she must see another doctor and that I wouldn't treat her until proper investigations had been carried out. This was difficult because her own doctor wouldn't refer her for investigations and she didn't know where she could find another doctor. I said if necessary she would need to go into the accident and emergency department of the local hospital.

A few days later she phoned me from her hospital bed. She had been to the hospital, they had taken her in immediately, operated the next day for bowel cancer, and she was now recuperating in hospital.

Quality can make the difference between life and death.

Doing drugs

Similarly, one might feel the effects of drugs. Various medications will have their effects on the system and recognising that these are the result of medication, rather than emotional qualities or part of the patient's underlying physical condition, may be helpful in understanding your patient and helping them appropriately.

Recreational drugs also have their effect. When a patient comes in after a few drinks, you will soon recognise the effects (even when they've done their best to cover up the smell of their breath) by the slippery, slidy quality of their cranio-sacral system. Heroin, cocaine, cannabis, skunk, ecstasy will all have their distinctive effects on the system, and no doubt a cranio-sacral therapist specialising in treating drug addicts would gain the necessary experience to make those distinctions.

Meningitis

The chronic effects of meningitis have a very clearly distinguishable effect. Meningitis causes sclerosis (hardening) of the meningeal membranes, so not surprisingly, when you tune in to the system, you can feel that quality of intense contraction in the membranes.

Timothy was just 15 months old when he was brought to me. He had been crying, screaming, waking every hour through the night, and constantly hyperactive for over a year, since contracting meningitis at the age of three months. The meningitis had of course been treated medically, but Timothy was not the same child. The family doctor insisted that his symptoms were nothing to do with his meningitis, that there was nothing wrong with him, that he was just a 'crying' baby. His parents knew perfectly well that he had been a perfectly happy peaceful baby before the meningitis, and they were deeply concerned about him. Their life of endless sleepless nights with Timothy waking up screaming every hour was deeply disturbing – but the doctor wouldn't refer them for further investigations.

Eventually they encountered the Meningitis Trust, who referred them to me. His whole head felt so contracted and tight, it was as if it had shrivelled like a dried fruit. It was immediately recognisable as the classic effects of meningitis. Appropriate identification of the cause of his condition – through its quality – enabled appropriate cranio-sacral treatment, and within a few sessions he was a peaceful, calm, contented, happy little boy again.

Every meningitis patient I have ever felt (and there have been a great many of them, because I have found cranio-sacral therapy to be exceptionally effective in addressing the often-misdiagnosed chronic effects of meningitis) has had that same quality of intense contraction in the membranes. Often the same qualities can be felt in patients who have not been diagnosed with meningitis, but who have clearly suffered a milder inflammation of the meninges (known as meningism) in response to some infection, whether a serious ear infection or a severe flu that has spread to their meninges.

Healthy and unhealthy tissues

Quality is not just valuable for identifying and diagnosing pathologies and injuries. It is an inherent aspect of every moment of the cranio-sacral process. Quality enables you to distinguish between different tissues – bone (a hard solid quality), membrane (pliable, malleable), fluid (fluctuating, flowing), energy (floating, buzzing, vibrating) – although each of these can of course vary according to the current state of the tissues. Chronically sclerosed membrane feels very different from healthy mobile membrane; energy varies enormously in its different expressions and manifold manifestations (and after all, in the final analysis, all matter is energy in different degrees of density). Quality enables you to distinguish healthy tissues from unhealthy tissues and so to identify sites of injury and disease and the underlying source of ill health. You can also distinguish muscle from tendon or ligament, and the presence of inflammation or other damage to these tissues, and you can explore the viscera and the qualities within them – distinguishing a liver with cirrhosis from one with hepatitis or suppressed anger.

What would be the qualities of acute inflammation? Heat, swelling, immunological activity. These characteristics might be visible for anyone to see on the external surface in some circumstances. But as a cranio-sacral therapist with a clear concept of quality, you can feel these characteristics expressed more subtly, and internally – even when there are no visible signs.

The quality of time

Inflammation is a response to an acute condition. It therefore tends to feel hot, active, dynamic. As time goes by, the body deals with the injury as best it can – forms scar tissue where appropriate, contains the injury where necessary – and gradually the tissues tend to harden. So when you feel a quality of undue hardness in tissues, this may tell you that there is an old injury there. Hardness develops gradually, so after a short space of time you might feel a slight degree of hardness; with an injury that's been deeply embedded for many years, you might feel a far more solidified degree of hardness. So you can distinguish recent injuries from older injuries from even older injuries; and with practice and experience you can refine your assessment of time – 'this injury feels approximately five years old, that one approximately twenty years old' – and perhaps further refine your skills until you are able to put a more specific time to the injury – 'this feels like an injury from three years ago, that one from seventeen years ago; this feels like a pattern from childhood around the age of seven; this feels like a birth pattern'. So you can distinguish how a patient's history has developed from some primary original injury through a number of compensatory patterns that have developed; you can identify the original source of their condition; you can explain why certain symptoms or aspects of their condition might respond more readily and others more slowly; you can predict how their situation might respond to treatment, depending on its chronicity.

(Again, the very fact of identifying the relevant time will influence the therapeutic response, but again we are exploring quality here, so we will leave that for now.)

Monitoring the progress of the cranio-sacral process – through quality

Quality enables you to follow the cranio-sacral process from moment to moment – feeling the quality of an easeful gentle neutral state, the quality of a build-up of pressure in the system, the quality of a point of balanced tension, the quality of holding or floating at a point of stillness, the quality of dynamic vibration that may precede a release, the quality of softening and melting as a release occurs, the quality of abstract meandering during reorganisation, the quality of ease and calm as the system settles back into neutral.

Quality will enable you to know to what extent you are engaged with the system; it will tell you when it wants to push your hands away to a more spacious contact, or draw your hands in. All of these qualities enable you to follow the process more accurately, to be more deeply engaged with the system at all times, to identify the precise details as they happen within the system, and therefore to be more effective in your therapeutic response.

The focus of your attention is a crucial aspect of the therapeutic process. When your attention is specifically focused on a particular tissue restriction (identifiable by its quality) that restriction will respond. If you can accurately identify the time of life when that injury occurred (by its quality) and focus your attention on that restriction within the context of that moment in time, then it will respond more readily and more fully. Sometimes the whole picture of the incident, the injury, the position of the patient at the time of injury, the age of the patient at the time, will all come vividly to mind as your attention rests on a particular focal point of restriction, and release occurs. The more accurately your attention is focused on every detail (each detail identified by its quality) the more profoundly and effectively you will enable the therapeutic process to progress.

As your attention spreads through the whole body, different qualities will become apparent in different areas, thereby identifying focal points of restriction, areas of injury, tension or disease. If you project your attention down through the spine, you can feel changes in quality as you move from one vertebral level to another – tightness, agitation, stuckness, turmoil – reflecting restricted vertebral joints, facilitated segments, neurological input (perhaps due to visceral disturbances or sympathetic inflow). As you project down the spine, your attention might seem to be flowing smoothly through certain areas, then the quality might change and you encounter choppy waters, a stormy sea, or a sense of a boat rocking from side to side – as you reach the fourth thoracic segment associated with the heart centre, or the ninth to twelfth thoracic segments associated with the solar plexus – the quality indicating the emotional turmoil which the patient is holding at those areas.

Plumbing the depths

Qualities also reflect different levels of depth within the patient. You can feel the changes in quality as the treatment process deepens, feeling the system shifting from one level to another, or gradually settling into a deeper softer quality. You can feel the quality of the rhythmic motion (as distinct from its rate or its amplitude) as a gentle easeful motion, a turbulent or agitated motion, a smooth settled motion, a dynamic forceful motion. Cranio-sacral rhythm, middle tide and long tide are not just different rhythms; they are different levels of being and have vastly different qualities – the middle tide level has a very different quality from the cranio-sacral rhythm level, and the long tide level a very different quality again.

Quality enables you to evaluate the overall quality of a patient's *vitality* – dynamic, potent, vibrant and strong, or weak, emaciated, feeble and lacking vitality – partly through the expression of rhythmic motion, but primarily through the quality of the vitality itself, indicating their level of underlying resources, all of which will again guide your treatment approach.

Your perception of different levels will depend partly on the demands of the system, partly on the practitioner's choice, and partly on the progress of the treatment. Sometimes a particular level will draw your attention – you could rest your hands on a patient's feet and feel superficial agitation crying out for your attention, or engage immediately with the long tide, or be drawn to some profound pull that seems to lead you deeply into the depths of the system. You might choose to explore the superficial levels, or look deeper into the system – some practitioners will automatically tune in to certain levels, whether superficial or deep, as a matter of course – although mostly it is preferable not to impose any agenda on the patient and rather be guided by the system as to which level it wants to engage. Also, as a treatment progresses, so the superficial levels are likely to become more settled, and access to deeper levels more readily accessible and more appropriate. It is always helpful to keep track of all levels, and you may choose to take your attention through different levels – superficial, deeper, deeper still – not just in terms of tissues – skin, muscle, bone, viscera, and so on – but in terms of levels of energetic depth, emotional depth, personality depth, cranio-sacral depth.

You can feel changes in quality throughout the treatment process, enabling you to recognise the evolution of the treatment process, the progress from moment to moment, the changes from start to finish, and the appropriate moment at which to allow a treatment to come to an end – when the quality feels suitably settled and complete.

Putting on a brave face

Everyone presents some degree of external face to the world, whether it be a polite pleasant manner hiding a shy inner self, a calm outer display masking a troubled inner being, an open happy clowning exterior disguising a traumatised soul, a controlled performance belying a confused nature, a confident air disguising a fearful underlying nature.

The external face is often very convincing; most observers will probably take the person at face value and believe them to be what they seem. Even close friends and family may not be aware of deeper feelings and true underlying personality. But the cranio-sacral system can never be fooled, the cranio-sacral system never lies. The cranio-sacral system reflects every aspect of the person, on all levels. Quality is the means of recognising all these characteristics, these hidden depths and the whole complexity of the person's nature. The cranio-sacral system will reflect everything about the person exactly as it is – the controlled quality on the surface, with a tortured quality inside, the apparently open relaxed superficial qualities covering a solid hard core that is not prepared to open up, and so on. Not that everyone (or anyone) is merely two-dimensional or two-levelled. On the contrary, everyone is multidimensional and multilayered. And the qualities in the cranio-sacral system can reveal all the many layers of the personality in their infinite complexity – so long as you have the skills to read them.

Teresa was in intense pain every moment of her life. She was barely able to cope, life was unbearable; she often felt suicidal. Tuning in to her system, the quality was beautifully soft, open and responsive; everything felt fluent and mobile; the whole system felt balanced and settled. So why was she in pain? Staying with her system, the level of engagement gradually deepened. Still everything felt soft and fluent, open and easeful. What was the explanation for her pain?

Taking my attention ever deeper, we reached very profound levels of her being; and there at the very core of her being there was a very intense quality of hardness and immobility, like a steel rod down the centre of her being, a hardness that was deeply held, intensely guarded and unresponsive.

Teresa had been in pain for a long time. She had been working on herself and her personal development in many ways. She had received huge amounts of therapy of various kinds – medical treatment, acupuncture, osteopathy, homeopathy, psychotherapy, cranio-sacral therapy, medication, meditation, and a huge amount besides – her whole life had been orientated around trying to address and resolve this overwhelming pain.

All this treatment and self-development had been beneficial; this is why her system felt so soft and open and balanced; a great deal of good therapeutic work had been done and her system reflected that. But nothing had penetrated to reach that deeply embedded, intensely guarded level at the core of her being.

Teresa's pain arose from deeply embedded childhood trauma – severe trauma that, even though she genuinely wanted to address it, she was unable to face and deal with. Everything she did helped her in various ways, but despite her conscious desire to address it, on an unconscious level she had never been able to let go of the protection, and engage with that deep pain from childhood.

The quality of her system, although apparently surprising and contradictory at first, reflected everything about her with absolute accuracy – as always – and led the way clearly to the appropriate treatment approach.

Practitioner quality

Quality also applies to the practitioner. The quality of your own presence is crucial to the interaction of the cranio-sacral process. Developing your own inner qualities, your grounding, your practitioner fulcrums, through treatment and personal development, maintaining awareness of your own qualities, monitoring your own state and ensuring that you maintain appropriate qualities of calmness, stillness, openness, and caring, is vital.

Pigs, elephants and snakes

When you first start exploring quality, you may want to start with some kind of framework, some possible examples that you could explore: hot or cold, hard or soft, solid or fluid, tight or loose, warm or cool, active or passive, busy or still, tense or relaxed, agitated or calm, dynamic or lethargic, powerful or weak.

But this is just the beginning. Qualities are not limited to these words, or to any particular words. They could include any word that comes to mind and which seems to convey the sense of what you are feeling. They are not limited to adjectives; they might include images – a boat floating on water, a stream, a waterfall, a lake, a cloud, cotton wool, candy floss, a heavy vehicle lumbering along a track. They might include more abstract concepts – colours, images, impressions. The words might not always seem to make immediate sense or have obvious meaning, but often the significance of the images will become clear in due course – as a vivid representation of the nature of the person – and it is helpful to keep in mind every impression or image that arises, rather than dismissing images as irrelevant or too abstract or meaningless.

You might experience impressions of a bright sunny day, a dark forest, a storm, a fire, or a roller coaster. The impression might be of a small furry animal, and in due course you may find that this fits the nature of the person perfectly. On the other hand, you might get a sense of a pig, or an elephant, or a fish, or a snake. Everything has its significance.

Jumping to conclusions

It is of course possible to project your own imagination into your perceptions, and it is therefore helpful not to jump to conclusions, not to believe that every word or image that leaps into your mind must be a definitive reflection of your patient, not to be dogmatic in your interpretation of quality. Trust your impressions, explore their validity, seek substantiation for your perception, and investigate for confirmation or otherwise of your findings. Find the right balance between being open to the valuable information potentially provided by your perceptions of quality received through the cranio-sacral system, and a healthy desire to find further confirmation of your impressions rather than imposing them dogmatically on your patients.

Defining and refining

Defining your perceptions is vital. It is easy to feel an abstract sensation and acknowledge it and tell yourself that you know what it is. But if you don't put it into words, it may remain abstract and elusive and certainly harder to remember or recall. Putting words to your perceptions is essential; it clarifies what you are feeling, it enables you to be more specific, it identifies characteristics more clearly, it makes the qualities more memorable – and gives you something identifiable to record in your case notes, so that you can monitor changes in quality over the course of several sessions. Words come more readily to some people than to others. If you have difficulty defining what you are feeling, make the effort to discover the right words. It enhances your perception enormously and is essential. Make a point of defining your perceptions as clearly as possible.

As you look for precise words to describe what you are feeling, this inevitably leads you to look more closely in order to find the exact words, noticing that some are not accurate enough or don't quite convey what you are feeling. As you continue you can refine your definitions, which will lead you to an increasing accuracy and clarity in your perception of your patient.

Refinement of your perception of quality enables deeper and more accurate understanding of every situation. Take stillness, for example. You could feel stillness that is peaceful and contented, stillness that is stuck and immobile, you could feel stillness that is dynamic, you could feel stillness that indicates a point of balanced tension building up to a release. All of these would have different interpretations and significance. We will explore this further in Chapter 16.

You might feel solidity, but you can refine that definition: does it feel solid like steel, like rock, or like wood? If it feels like wood, is it a hard wood like oak or a soft wood like pine, or even a very soft wood like balsa? If it feels soft, is it soft like a pillow, like a balloon, like a marshmallow, or as soft as a cloud? If it feels fluidic, is it a thin watery fluid or a thick viscous fluid like honey? These distinctions might seem arbitrary and meaningless at first, but by exploring these refinements of definition, you will be developing your ability to distinguish bone from membrane from fluid from energy, muscle from tendon from ligament from fascia, diabetes from multiple sclerosis from rheumatoid arthritis, and a multitude of other different qualities.

Nothing

You might say that you feel nothing – but what sort of nothingness? Do you mean that there is no movement, in other words a quality of immobility. Or do you mean a sense of nothing there, in other words a quality of emptiness. These distinctions can have far reaching implications. It is easy to think, when you feel nothing, that you are not feeling anything; in fact, you may be feeling a very definite and meaningful quality of nothingness. It is easier to recognise activity and movement than absence of movement, but within the cranio-sacral process, it is most often the areas of lack of mobility, the areas of immobility, of inertia, that are most significant, so identifying the qualities of apparent nothingness can be crucial.

You can also refine your definitions of the quality of movement and activity. You might identify a system as dynamic, but is it a positive, potent, vital dynamism, or an aggressive, scattered, overbearing, destructive dynamism? You might experience impressions of rocking, turbulence, choppy waves, stormy seas – and find that they exactly reflect the way the patient is feeling. Countless times I have described to patients qualities such as these which I am feeling in their systems and they have replied that my description describes exactly what is happening in their life and how they are feeling.

You might ask

You might ask, what do these various conditions feel like, why don't we describe them for you in detail – every disease, every circumstance, every emotion – so that you can recognise them?

- Words can never describe the details of quality sufficiently; it is the experience of quality that enables you to recognise and understand quality; the human mind, conscious and unconscious, can identify, recognise and differentiate millions of qualities more accurately than any words could ever describe.

- It would take countless volumes to describe just a small portion of the millions of qualities and combinations of qualities that you will encounter in practice.
- Every patient is different and is a complex mixture of vast numbers of individual qualities and variations of qualities. It is not a matter of reading, learning and diagnosing by rote; it is a matter of feeling and experiencing and relating to the qualities you feel in each patient.
- Every experience is individual, so you can't work from a textbook.
- The individual relationship that you create through your perception of qualities is an integral part of the integrated therapeutic process.
- It is through experience, practice and application that you gain an understanding of quality, not by reading about it – words are just to get you started, to introduce the concept, so that you have some basis from which to operate and develop your own perception of quality.

Summary

Everyone is an individual, with a multitude of different characteristics. These characteristics are reflected in the cranio-sacral system as qualities. The quality of a patient is the combination of all their various characteristics.

There will be qualities which reflect the whole person, qualities which reflect specific parts or areas, qualities reflecting physical, emotional, psychological or spiritual characteristics, qualities reflecting current circumstances and qualities reflecting past events.

Their whole life story is there for us to read – and quality is the secret to reading accurately and precisely everything about them.

Chapter 13

Fluid Analogies

In cranio-sacral integration, analogies with fluids are often drawn. We tend to talk in terms of waves, tides, currents, fluctuations, letting your hands sink into the warm fluidity of the system. This is understandable and useful because what we are feeling is very fluidic. The overall progress of a treatment, from first tuning in through to the deepest levels of engagement can evocatively be described in terms of fluid analogies.

The fluidic progression of a treatment

Wavelets and ripples
When you first tune in, the initial impressions you encounter are often experienced as a multitude of minor movements, like the wavelets, ripples and other minor perturbances that you might find on the surface of the sea. These reflect the superficial day-to-day disturbances affecting the patient on the surface.

Currents
As the superficial activity subsides, you may encounter pulls drawing this way and that, like currents under the sea. These are the patterns of relatively superficial injury and tension that are more readily accessible.

Waves
As these patterns release you may feel the increasing emergence of rhythmic wave-like motion, like waves rising onto a beach and ebbing away. This is the cranio-sacral rhythm.

Deeper currents
At this point, you may encounter more persistent and resistant pulls drawing consistently in certain directions, like deeper, stronger currents under the ocean. These are the deeper patterns of resistance within the system, the more severe injuries, the more chronic deeply ingrained levels of trauma and disease.

Oceanic waves
Within the context of these deeper patterns, you may feel the increasing emergence of a slower rhythmic motion, like oceanic waves rolling across the ocean. These are the middle tide, reflecting deeper levels of health and being.

Tides
In due course as you settle into deeper and deeper engagement, you may feel a long slow movement like the rise and fall of the ocean tide. This is the long tide. The ocean tides are of course a reflection of the gravitational pull of the moon influencing the whole planet, just as our own long tide is a reflection of the natural forces of the universe.

Stillness
As you settle into the deepest levels of engagement, you may reach dynamic stillness, like the stillness at the very depths of the ocean where everything is quiet and still.

The value of fluid analogies
Using fluid analogies helps to move our attention beyond the more mechanical structures of bones, membranes and tissues. If we talk of forces, force fields, potency, vitality and energy, many people may not necessarily have a sense of what that might feel like, or how such forces move, so fluid analogies help to convey that sense. We can see fluids in everyday life and see how they ebb and flow and swirl, so they provide a useful, visible, recognisable analogy for describing something that is not so readily recognisable.

Fluid analogies are also used to describe more general concepts. Sutherland talked of 'the fluid within the fluid' as a way of describing the potency, energy or vitality spreading through the system carried by the cerebrospinal fluid. The term 'fluid body' is sometimes used to describe the force field which extends beyond the physical body as the individual matrix. Cranio-sacral therapists sometimes talk of 'working with the fluids' as a means of describing engagement with levels beyond bones, membranes and tissues. This can often be interpreted as working with the subtle forces and energies within the matrix – forces that feel fluidic and respond in fluidic ways.

Using fluid analogies helps us to describe the way the matrix feels. When you truly engage with the cranio-sacral system, it can feel as if the whole body has dissolved into fluidity and your hands are floating on the surface of this matrix or are deeply immersed within this fluidity.

As cranio-sacral therapists, we are of course working with actual fluids in the body, not only cerebrospinal fluid but also arterial blood, venous blood, lymphatics, extracellular fluids, intracellular fluids, and others – and we certainly want to tune in to these as well, just as we tune in to other tissues of the body. But these fluids are not what we are primarily concerned with. We are primarily working with forces transmitted through the matrix, forces which transcend the fluids, which move through all the tissues, which extend beyond the perimeter of the body – forces which feel fluidic and which can perhaps be more readily recognised and identified through analogies with fluid, but which are not in fact fluids.

The tides which move the oceans are not fluids, they are forces within the fluid. The same applies to currents, eddies and waves. They are not fluids, but powerful forces within the fluids.

Beyond fluids

Analogies with fluid are useful, but they can also be misleading. 'Working with the fluids' doesn't really describe what we are doing. Talking of 'the fluid within the fluid' is evocative but it is not really an accurate description. Using a term such as 'the fluid body' to describe a force field outside the body which clearly isn't fluid doesn't altogether make sense.

This was understandable in Sutherland's day when terms such as energy and force fields were less acceptable. But these days when there is a much wider understanding of natural forces, biofields, quantum science and energy medicine, it may be clearer to express these concepts for what they actually are – energy, force fields, matrices. Instead of expressing such concepts somewhat misleadingly as if they were fluids, we can think beyond fluids.

Treatment

Stormy seas

During treatment, if the sea is stormy and there are many waves on the surface, then the priority is to settle the surface. Otherwise it may not be advisable to swim or go out to sea, let alone to dive deep. It may be difficult even to see what lies under the surface.

Once the sea is calmer, after addressing the waves and settling the turmoil, and opening up the system, then you can not only see more clearly under the surface – like looking into a clear calm azure Mediterranean sea – but also swim more safely, dive underneath, go to greater depths, and explore what lies therein. Under appropriate conditions of fair weather and calmness, it may be safe to dive right down to the depths without fear of losing connection with your mothership.

Working only on superficial wavelets will tend only to settle the surface. This may be what's appropriate.

Working with deeper currents will help to resolve deeper, more intransigent, deeply ingrained issues.

Working with the deepest tides and dynamic stillness helps to integrate the underlying natural forces and therefore the underlying state of health within the whole person.

Appropriate levels

Addressing the wavelets and superficial storms through engagement with the superficial movements and opening up the system is vital to enable grounding and stability.

Addressing the medium-depth currents, pulls and patterns is also vital. If you try to go under the ocean without taking into account strong currents, you might get into trouble. So we need to address these medium-depth currents before settling into the deepest levels.

Trying to work with deeper levels when the surface is stormy, you may find that the deeper levels are not accessible or that trying to work with them may be turbulent.

So with every treatment it is advisable to ensure that the surface is settled, taking whatever time is needed to settle as necessary through initial engagement, through attending to wavelets and ripples, addressing the surface levels, opening up the system, so that you can then gain access to deeper levels, and address them comfortably.

Every treatment is likely to involve some sort of evolving process like this – proceeding purposefully from superficial to deep. The starting point will of course vary from person to person depending on the weather and the climatic conditions within and around their system – whether it is stormy, inundated by waves, or calm, peaceful, halcyon days; and the rate of progress will also vary depending on the degree of strong currents under the surface. But the overall pattern of gradual deepening is likely to be a consistent and recognisable theme.

Forces and fields

In summary, fluid analogies are useful but fluids are not our principal concern. We are primarily concerned with forces – forces which feel fluidic but are not in fact fluids. They are the forces of nature expressed throughout the matrix.

Chapter 14

Fulcrums

A fulcrum is a pivotal point around which a system operates – whether it be a simple mechanical lever, or a more complex system:
- A see-saw has a central fulcrum around which the two ends move.
- The hinges of a door act as fulcrums around which the door can open and close.

and the occipit-atlas joint. Within the vertebral column there are also various key pivotal areas such as the fourth thoracic vertebra, the ninth thoracic vertebra, or the thoraco-lumbar junction. Awareness of these fulcrums enables a deeper understanding of the way the body operates and of the therapeutic process.

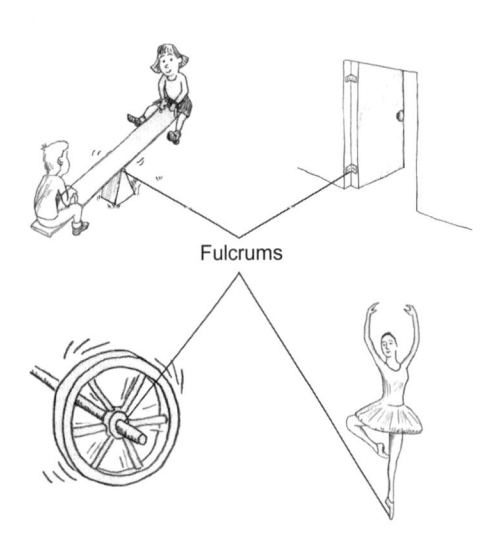

14.1 Fulcrums

As a cranio-sacral therapist it is helpful to take into account many different types of fulcrum – fulcrums within the patient, fulcrums within the practitioner, fulcrums within the mechanics of the physical body, fulcrums within the cranio-sacral system, and fulcrums on other levels.

Mechanical pivots

Within the body structure there are countless fulcrums. Every joint – vertebral joint, knee joint, finger joint, any joint – acts as a fulcrum in relation to localised activity. The body also operates as an integrated unit, with certain pivotal areas acting as fulcrums for the body as a whole. Significant pivotal areas are the lumbo-sacral joint

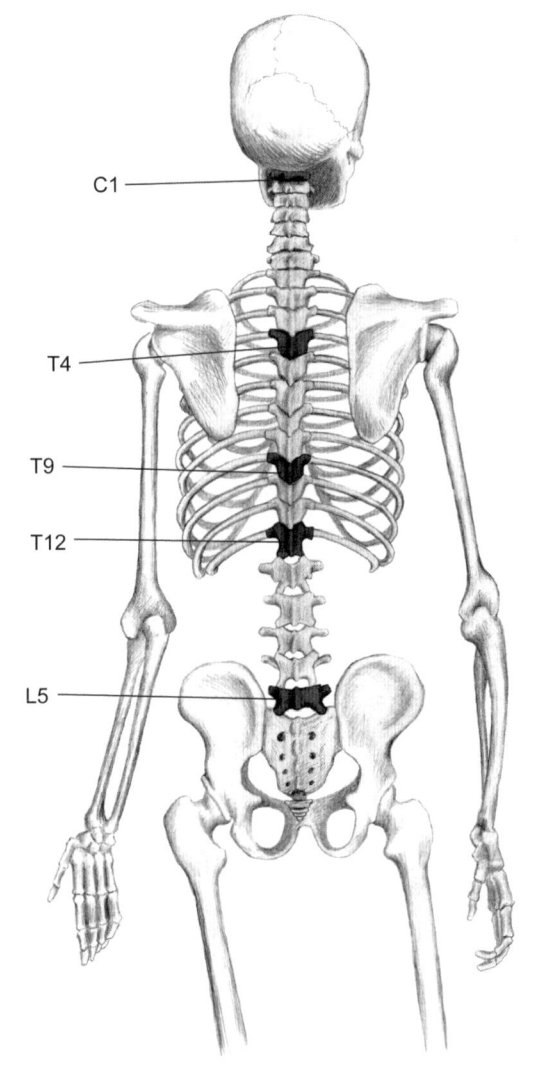

14.2 Within the vertebral column there are various significant fulcrums

Cranio-sacral fulcrums

Within the cranio-sacral system, certain pivotal areas can also be identified as significant fulcrums:

- In relation to the bones of the cranio-sacral system, the *spheno-basilar synchondrosis* is regarded as the fulcrum around which the bony structures operate.

- In relation to the membrane system, the *straight sinus* – where the falx cerebri, falx cerebelli and tentorium cerebelli meet – is seen as the fulcrum around which the whole membrane system operates. The significance of this fulcrum was identified by William Sutherland and is consequently known as Sutherland's fulcrum.

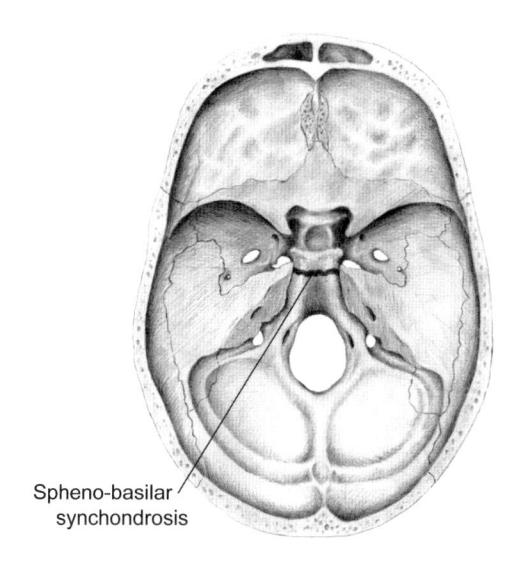

14.3 The spheno-basilar synchondrosis is the fulcrum around which the bony structures operate

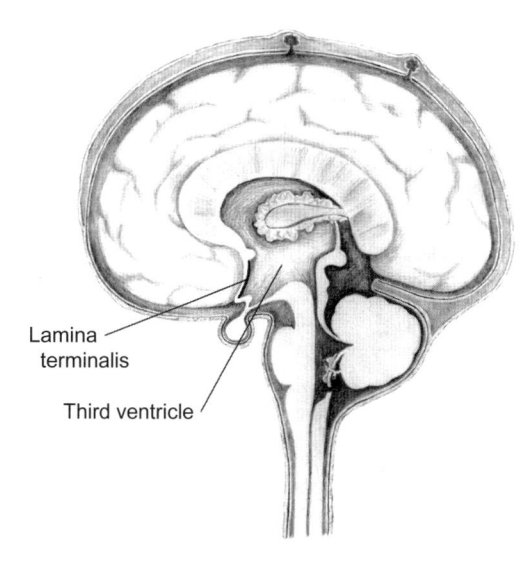

14.5 The central nervous system moves around a fulcrum at the lamina terminalis, which forms the anterior wall of the third ventricle

- The central nervous system moves around a fulcrum at the *lamina terminalis*, which forms the anterior wall of the third ventricle.

Mental fulcrums

The concept of fulcrums can also be extended to the mental level. Certain concepts, ideas or beliefs may be fundamental to our whole way of thinking. Certain thoughts and ideas inevitably influence our response to every situation we encounter, creating prejudices and preconceptions, which may in turn determine our attitudes and behaviour. Establishing balanced mental fulcrums can be fundamental to our progress and development in life.

Mental fulcrums can provide a very positive focal point around which to determine your life, or can also become a barrier which limits

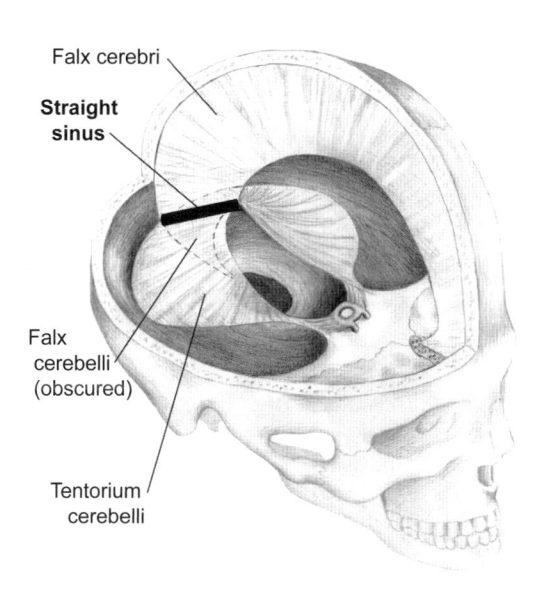

14.4 The straight sinus is the fulcrum for the membrane system

your thinking and your ability to respond to circumstances in a positive, flexible, fluent way. A religious belief, for example, can be a very strong motivating force for a positive purposeful life, but can equally become a dogmatic prejudice which is unable to respond to circumstances in an appropriately flexible manner.

Clear mental fulcrums can provide stability and clarity. A particular philosophy or way of thinking can provide a secure foundation from which to respond to the world with a flexible and broad-minded perspective. However, rigid attachment to a particular idea or way of thinking can become restrictive, limiting your ability to respond positively to circumstances, whereas a willingness to alter that way of thinking, or see things differently, can open up new vistas which can enable life to progress more positively and freely.

Such limiting views could include negative thoughts about yourself and your own abilities, pessimistic views regarding your health, excessive attachment to job security preventing you from exploring new opportunities, inability to throw off unhelpful viewpoints imposed on you by your upbringing.

As a therapist, it can be helpful to recognise when a patient's health, progress and whole being is being blocked by a particular mental fulcrum, and thereby to help them to acknowledge, recognise and re-examine their viewpoint and move forward in their life.

Emotional fulcrums

Just as mental fulcrums are inevitably determined by our experience of life, so in the same way emotional fulcrums are created. Emotional events in our life – whether positive or traumatic – may influence our response to every subsequent event, potentially influencing our whole direction in life. Day-to-day emotional events and changes influence our responses and well-being. On a therapeutic level, identifying emotional fulcrums in a patient which may be creating emotional resistance, may play a significant part in the therapeutic process.

Emotional fulcrums are everywhere; they are present in all of us; our personalities and our whole lives are moulded by a continuous succession of emotional events which determine our subsequent behaviour and our subsequent response to everything around us – our relationships, our friendships, our work, our overall direction in life.

Patterns set up in childhood by our parents and our upbringing, starting school, changing school, specific triumphs or traumas at school, bullying, academic success, a charismatic teacher, an overbearing teacher, happy relationships, broken relationships, births, deaths, marriages, break-ups and countless other events in our lives create pivotal moments – some of great magnitude, some relatively minor – which determine the way in which we respond to subsequent events – most of it entirely unconscious, of course.

Recognising these pivotal moments, understanding how our behaviour may have been determined by specific events, can be a key to unlocking the door to a more balanced and appropriate response to life and circumstances, thereby leading us to greater harmony and fulfilment. An example is the case of Judith (described in Chapter 12) whose unexpressed grief over her husband's death had adversely affected her life and health – until it was resolved.

In some cases there may be a very specifically identifiable event, but emotional fulcrums are often less clearly recognisable. Daughters growing up with a violent father may repeatedly choose violent partners or husbands, apparently locked into a pattern of behaviour imprinted at an early age, a habit which they subconsciously feel the need to perpetuate, even though it is unsatisfactory and destructive for them. Emotional fulcrums can also be imprinted by the nature of one's birth, or during intrauterine life. (Research following the 9/11 bombings in New York demonstrated that babies born to mothers involved in the attack showed higher than average levels of stress hormones.)

Much of what we do is determined by the multitude of emotional fulcrums established in our unconscious consciousness throughout our lives.

Time fulcrums

We can all identify particular moments or events in our lives which were fundamental in determining our direction and our very nature, whether they be happy events – marriages, new relationships – or difficult circumstances, such as traumas, accidents, illnesses, times of stress, childhood incidents or birth. Identifying these key moments in our lives can be helpful, both in identifying positive influences in our lives, and in changing negative patterns created at that time, whether on physical, mental or emotional levels.

When a patient becomes aware of such patterns, recognising the fulcrums around which they revolve and the events which initiated them, then simply becoming conscious of them and talking about them can instigate changes – changes in perception, changes in action, changes in circumstance.

However, working cranio-sacrally with time fulcrums is not just a matter of identifying the event (as in the emotional fulcrums above). A much more profound process of release and reorganisation of past patterns can be enabled through a deep connection with a specific moment in time, engaging with the physical, emotional and energetic changes that occurred in association with a particular incident. This may or may not involve conscious acknowledgement of the event. Conscious recognition of the event may arise only after an initial cranio-sacral engagement with the time fulcrum, with vivid memories of long-forgotten events arising apparently out of nowhere – images, feelings, even smells reminiscent of the incident – accompanied by physical changes, emotional changes, and significant therapeutic releases. Connecting with these time fulcrums on a cranio-sacral level can contribute greatly to the therapeutic process. We will explore how to do that shortly.

Natural fulcrums and unnatural fulcrums

Many fulcrums exist as standard pivots around which one expects the body or the system to operate. These can be regarded as natural fulcrums – such as the mechanical pivots within the spine, or the fulcrums mentioned above in relation to the cranio-sacral system – the spheno-basilar synchondrosis, the lamina terminalis, and Sutherland's fulcrum.

Unnatural fulcrums, where a fulcrum is displaced or where a new unbalanced fulcrum appears, may arise in the body as a result of trauma, tension, injury or disease creating a pivotal point, which pulls the body out of alignment causing strains and tensions in the body and consequently leading to pain, discomfort or other symptoms.

A fall in the snow might lead to a restricted sacro-iliac joint, which becomes a fulcrum around which the whole body pivots in an unbalanced way, creating strains and tensions throughout the body, resulting in back pain, neck pain, headaches or a multitude of other symptoms. Identifying that unnatural fulcrum at the sacro-iliac joint is vital to the restoration of health.

Similarly, a sprained ankle might lead to a patient habitually shifting their weight onto the opposite leg, so that once again the ankle becomes a fulcrum around which the whole body pivots in an unbalanced way. A car accident or fall might leave a multitude of mechanical pivots throughout the body out of alignment. An operation scar might pull the body tissues towards a specific fulcrum of restricted scar tissue. Poor posture may create postural tensions. Releasing these unnatural fulcrums enables the body to return to a healthy balanced state around its natural fulcrums and therefore to function more freely, comfortably and effectively.

Unnatural fulcrums can be identified not only on these obvious physical levels but also in relation to cranio-sacral fulcrums, mental fulcrums, and emotional fulcrums.

Fulcrums as the main focal points of the cranio-sacral process

All the fulcrums described above represent an essential grounding in the understanding of fulcrums. But the fulcrums with which we are most concerned during the cranio-sacral process are those which are the main focal points within the cranio-sacral process – the points of balanced tension, the points of stillness, the points to which the cranio-sacral system draws as we allow the evolution of fundamental principles.

These fulcrums are of course unnatural fulcrums, brought about by injury, trauma or tension, resulting in focal points of resistance where there is restriction of cranio-sacral movement, restriction of rhythmic motion, restriction of vitality, of energy flow. They are sometimes known as inertial fulcrums – inertia meaning lack of movement.

They are points of resistance which can be anywhere; they can be physical, mental, emotional; they can be anywhere in the body – a bony fracture, a joint restriction, a muscular strain, an emotional tension, a visceral contraction, a fascial sprain; they can be outside the body in the energy field, they can be felt in more abstract ways, not apparently relating to any physical tissues, but palpable in the surrounding matrix. They can be the result of injury, trauma, tension, birth.

Identifying these fulcrums within the context of the fundamental principles of the therapeutic process, allowing the system to draw to points of stillness and release around such fulcrums, is an essential part of the cranio-sacral process.

Practitioner fulcrums

Fulcrums are significant not only in relation to an understanding of patients and restoring a patient's system to a more balanced state, but are also significant in relation to the practitioner. A practitioner will operate more effectively when working from a clear and balanced perspective. It is therefore vital for every practitioner to be aware of his or her own practitioner fulcrums on all levels.

Physical awareness

As a practitioner, you need to be aware of the way that you sit, move and use your own body in order to avoid undue strain. Strain in your own body creates tension, reduces your sensitivity, projects into the patient, and interferes with the interaction of the cranio-sacral process. Maintaining this awareness throughout the cranio-sacral process will enhance your interaction with the patient. For this purpose, constant consistent awareness of your own body and your own breathing contribute considerably to your effectiveness.

Within this overall mechanical balance, you can also be aware of more specific points of balance or fulcrums within the way that you are operating. Your elbows, resting on the couch, will act as fulcrums for your forearms, enabling your forearms to operate more freely, enabling subtle responses to the cranio-sacral process. If you lean too heavily on your elbows, you will create tension in your own arms and shoulders and restrict mobility and sensitivity. If you hold your arms up in mid-air, without support, you may again create tension in your arms and shoulders.

The contact of your hands on the patient's body will also act as a fulcrum around which the interaction between the two systems – the patient's system and your own system – will revolve and evolve. Subtle change in these fulcrums in response to the cranio-sacral process can be profoundly significant – for instance, leaning forward very slightly into your elbows, leaning back from your elbows, allowing your hands to soften away from the contact or to sink into the contact. A fundamental aspect of the cranio-sacral process is the observation of the patient's cranio-sacral system revolving and evolving around the fulcrum of your contact.

As a practitioner, you need to be aware of your own fulcrums on all levels – the physical and mechanical fulcrums within your body, and your own cranio-sacral fulcrums at the spheno-basilar synchondrosis, Sutherland's fulcrum and the lamina terminalis (primarily addressed through receiving good cranio-sacral treatment for yourself).

Mental fulcrums

You also need to establish appropriate mental fulcrums, establishing a clear and uncluttered mental state, free of prejudices and preconceptions instilled by your own past experiences, and an ability to maintain this clear and uncluttered mental state despite the distractions of everyday life. You want to be able to view each patient with unconditional love – not the remote impersonal detachment of a clinical psychologist, but the warm empathetic sympathetic understanding of an open-hearted but well-centred and grounded human being. This is something which can be developed through constant and continuous personal development.

As a therapist you need to be free of prejudice, whether racial, religious, or any other kind. This means not just observing the letter of the law, but being genuinely unprejudiced – the cranio-sacral system is never fooled by a superficial facade –

and able to respond to anyone, from an iconic idol to a murderer, without losing your fulcrums. Whatever the circumstances, you need to be able to maintain your own grounding, balance, centredness, and equanimity.

Self-awareness: no one is perfect

Of course, no one is perfect and you don't need to be perfect in order to become a therapist. You need to be aware of your fulcrums, work assiduously on them, be aware when your own underlying patterns are being triggered, and have the means to address this appropriately without being thrown off balance. Developing these abilities is all part of the training and development in cranio-sacral integration.

Emotional balance

You also need to establish an appropriate level of emotional balance, both on the macroscopic level of clearing your own underlying emotional patterns (perhaps the result of past emotional traumas, childhood influences, deeply ingrained emotional patterns) and also in dealing with the transient emotional distractions that arise from day to day. Both levels require a continuous process of personal development and self-awareness in order to establish a more clear and balanced perspective, and so to operate more effectively – both in response to patients and in our lives generally.

If a practitioner has, for example, suffered a miscarriage some time ago and has not fully acknowledged, addressed and processed the grief and upset which she experienced at the time, then when a patient comes to her having recently suffered a miscarriage, that practitioner may find her own unresolved grief and memories arising and interfering with her ability to help the patient from a calm, grounded, balanced perspective. On the other hand, if the practitioner has fully addressed and processed her reactions to her own miscarriage, this not only will help her to maintain her practitioner fulcrums, but also may help her in providing specific insight and empathy for the patient who is now going through a similar experience.

Suppression is not the solution

In some quarters, it might be thought that you should simply put your own problems behind you and get on with the job. This is not generally a good idea as it would tend to lead to the practitioner holding down a lot of suppressed feelings, emotions and issues, perhaps becoming irritable, impatient and ill-tempered despite their best intentions, inevitably projecting their own unresolved inner tensions onto their patients and those around them. Within the cranio-sacral process it is generally recognised that suppression is not the solution, that these inner tensions will inevitably be reflected into the process anyway – if not on a conscious level, then at least on an energetic level – and that the practitioner can operate far more effectively from a more grounded, centred, balanced perspective if they have genuinely acknowledged and addressed their own issues rather than merely suppressing them.

Establishing appropriate fulcrums

Establishing appropriate practitioner fulcrums is essential to establishing the calm, quiet presence which is fundamental to profoundly effective practice, something which every practitioner needs to address from the start, and also something which every practitioner can continue to develop throughout life.

It has two main elements:

1. Clearing the long-established, deeply ingrained patterns that have arisen within your own system throughout your life – birth patterns, childhood patterns, traumas, tensions, prejudices, beliefs – something which can be worked on steadily through cranio-sacral treatment, self-awareness, personal development and continuing self-exploration.

2. Developing the skill to ground yourself on a day-to-day basis, in the present moment, maintaining the ability to remain centred, balanced, open and grounded for your patients whatever is going on within you or around you – the ability to maintain your calm, quiet presence, even when you're having a difficult day, when events

in your life are not progressing smoothly, when you receive unhappy news, or when circumstances are not ideal. A well-grounded practitioner can operate effectively in the middle of Oxford Circus, amid the hustle and bustle of Varanasi, at a rock festival, in the midst of a war. You might not specifically choose those circumstances in which to set up your regular practice, but it's good to be able to operate under any conditions.

This is a skill which develops through extensive practice and application, and through the deeper clearing of your own patterns. The degree to which you can implement the second element is largely dependent on the degree to which you have addressed the first, but also involves the development of specific skills for this purpose.

Balance of spaciousness and grounding

Another aspect of establishing practitioner fulcrums is maintaining a balance between spaciousness and grounding – developing a wide perspective through which you can be aware of the space around you, open to the subtle forces and impressions arising within that space, while at the same time remaining well-grounded in your physical body and the material world.

One way of enabling this can be to keep part of your attention at a point somewhere above you, part of your attention at your seat comfortably settled into your chair, and part of your attention at the soles of your feet firmly grounded on the floor, maintaining awareness of all these fulcrums (and more) simultaneously.

Attention to practitioner fulcrums is fundamental

The cranio-sacral process is an interactive process. The establishment of a clear and balanced perspective from which to operate is essential for every practitioner in order to enable the most profound therapeutic effectiveness. Attention to practitioner fulcrums is therefore fundamental.

Box 14.1 Time fulcrums revisited: working with time fulcrums in practice

Arising spontaneously

There are various ways in which time fulcrums can operate within the cranio-sacral process. Often they will arise spontaneously. As you work with the cranio-sacral system, or as a particular inertial fulcrum releases, *the patient may suddenly remember* a long-forgotten incident from years ago. They may remember it vividly or vaguely; they may remember very specific details – sounds, smells, sensations, the taste of an anaesthetic, feelings experienced at the time – or just a brief flashback to that moment. This will often be accompanied by a physical change in the tissues, as the tissue tensions which were imprinted into the body at the time of the incident release along with the emergence of the memories. As has been mentioned earlier, this is sometimes described as tissue memory.

Tissue memory

Tissue memory, as described previously, has two main components:
- The physical patterns of tension and restriction imprinted into the tissues are remembered and held by the body as tissue memory. In other words the tissues themselves 'remember' the patterns of injury imposed on them at the time and are held in that state of tension by those tissue memories.
- The conscious memories of the incident are also held in the tissues in association with the physical tensions, and are therefore released into consciousness when the physical tensions in the tissues are released.

Similarly, as you work with a patient's system, and you encounter a specific resistance or fulcrum, *you may be spontaneously drawn* to a particular time in their life. This could be partly because you can feel from the quality of the restriction that it dates back a long time, but it can often arise much more specifically – a specific age may spontaneously come to mind as you engage with that particular restriction. As you acknowledge that age, the tissues may then release. On asking the patient if anything happened at that age, you will often find that something very relevant occurred then – and the patient may be very surprised at your perception.

Deliberate access to time fulcrums

Time fulcrums can also be used more deliberately, in several ways, as discussed below.

TRACING BACK THROUGH TIME

On encountering an area of resistance within the cranio-sacral system (an inertial fulcrum) which is not responding or releasing readily, you can run your attention back through time, starting from the patient's current approximate age, thinking back year by year. As you take your attention back in time, you may feel changes in the tissues – changes in quality, symmetry and motion – as you reach the relevant age at which the tissue tensions were imprinted. In this way, you can not only identify the age at which the incident occurred, but also facilitate a response from the tissues.

This is a significant aspect of the cranio-sacral process. As we have seen previously, your informed attention can have a profound influence on the cranio-sacral process – whether in identifying a specific location in the body (such as when projecting your attention up through the legs or down through the spine, vertebra by vertebra) or in identifying specific patterns of asymmetry (such as when exploring spheno-basilar patterns) or in facilitating the release of an inertial fulcrum simply by virtue of focusing your attention on it. When your attention identifies a specific moment in time that is relevant to a particular tissue tension, then the physical patterns in the body are more likely to change in response to your focus of informed attention.

Sometimes you (the therapist) may experience a vivid image of the whole incident (even though the patient has not told you about it, and may not even remember it themselves). This could be a detailed impression of a car accident, or a clear image of a birth process. It can involve specific directions of impact or pressure, images of other people involved or the surrounding environment – or you might not experience any of that, just a physical change in the system as your attention reaches a specific age or a particular year in the patient's life – thereby knowing that whatever it was that happened at that time has now released and evaporated away.

CONSCIOUS RECALL – WITH EQUANIMITY

Time fulcrums can also be used in a more specific conscious way. When you and your patient are aware of a specific incident or time in life that was traumatic or stressful, you can deliberately look back at that time. The patient – in an appropriately settled, grounded and supported environment – can think back to that time and to the events that occurred. The therapist can also think back to that time and picture the events as described by the patient, at the same time observing the changes that arise in the cranio-sacral system. This can be helped by maintaining a dialogue during the treatment process, the patient describing the events as they remember them and the feelings they are experiencing as they think back to those events. Once again, the process of release is helped by the focused attention of the patient and therapist – so long as the attention is appropriately calm, settled and grounded.

This process can also be used very effectively in treating birth trauma, whether in babies or adults, with the therapist taking their attention back to the birth process, envisaging the patient as a baby as they were being born and feeling the changes in the body that arise as a result and the patterns of tension and trauma that become apparent and release accordingly. (When working with birth trauma, you would not of course expect the patient to remember the process or describe it verbally – especially with babies! – although it is interesting to observe how many patients do describe experiences that feel very much like birth.)

Surveying back through time

Even without engaging with a particular inertial fulcrum, you can take your attention back through time year by year, in order to identify and engage with times of particular significance in a patient's life, observing how the patient's system responds as a whole to the focus of attention on particular ages by observing changes in quality, symmetry and motion. It can be fascinating to observe how the quality can change very specifically – tightening up as you reach a time of greater tension in the patient's life, becoming turbulent as you reach a time of emotional turmoil, easing and softening as you reach times of greater ease and comfort, reflecting sudden shock as you reach a time of a major accident, reflecting debilitation at a time of prolonged illness such as glandular fever or ME, reflecting the patient's birth process, sometimes in highly accurate detail as you reach the time of birth.

INFORMED AWARENESS IS A KEY FACTOR IN THE THERAPEUTIC RESPONSE
These are not merely points of interest, nor merely diagnostic. Your informed awareness engaging with these responses is a key factor in enabling the therapeutic response and release of deeply held patterns.

NOT NECESSARILY READILY ACCESSIBLE
These images and impressions can sometimes be very vivid and clear. However, they are not always so readily accessible and cannot necessarily be brought to mind as a matter of course. The patient's circumstances can be complex, the patterns may be intricately intermingled and obscured by layers of subsequent traumas and tensions or by current more demanding circumstances. Some cranio-sacral therapists will engage with the images and impressions more readily than others. Some patients' systems will reveal this information more readily. Different circumstances will render the patterns more or less accessible. Above all, matters will arise in their own time – the time has to be right. So it is not something that can always be turned on at will by every therapist. On the other hand, when circumstances are right and these impressions do arise clearly, it can be remarkably accurate and vivid.

DAY-TO-DAY USE OF TIME FULCRUMS
In day-to-day practice, the more common application of time fulcrums is perhaps simply reflecting back through time as you encounter and address specific inertial fulcrums, and experiencing the changes in quality, symmetry and motion as releases occur in response to your focus of attention – without necessarily experiencing any vivid imagery or dramatic memories.

Chapter 15

Calm Quiet Presence
The State of the Practitioner

The whole therapeutic interaction evolves and revolves around the state of the practitioner. Consequently the ability to maintain your own calm, quiet presence is the most fundamental factor in the whole cranio-sacral process.

Entunement and entrainment

Entunement with the forces of nature

Why is the state of the practitioner so significant? Primarily because it is through developing and maintaining your own peaceful and receptive presence that you are able to *get in touch with the natural forces* that are the principal element in the therapeutic process of cranio-sacral integration – the external forces within the wider universal matrix, and the expression of those forces within the individual matrix – both within the body and in its surrounding energy field, both within your patient and within yourself, thereby enabling you to engage with the interaction of those forces between you, your patient and the surrounding matrix. Without such engagement, the cranio-sacral process will not occur.

An interactive process

Cranio-sacral integration is an interactive process. In fact, in this quantum age, it is well recognised that everything in life is an interactive process, but this is not generally taken into account in most aspects of our daily lives, even within medical and therapeutic interactions. Recognition of this quantum scientific fact is valuable to any interaction, but it becomes all the more essential in the field of cranio-sacral integration where we are working more specifically with quantum levels of being. *Everything about you contributes to this interaction.*

Quality of presence

The beneficial influences of cranio-sacral integration arise partly as a result of specific engagement with the cranio-sacral process – tuning in to rhythmic motion and allowing the inherent treatment process to lead towards points of stillness and release – and this in itself is dependent on your state, but this is not the only factor.

Even in day-to-day life, being in the presence of someone who is calm, who can keep their head when everyone else is losing theirs, tends to be a beneficial influence. Similarly, this beneficial influence also arises in the therapeutic process through the *quality of your presence* as it envelops and interacts with your patient's matrix – your stillness, your peacefulness, your grounding, your thoughts, your intentions, your focus of attention. If your system is calm, this tends to encourage calmness in the patient. If your system is clear and balanced and integrated, this tends to bring clarity, balance and integration to your patient's system; and there are also other influences – including the biomagnetic fields radiating from your heart and brain, the extremely low frequency (ELF) radiation emanating from your hands, or the many other *measurable forms of energetic radiation*, all of which are dependent on your own inner state (see Figure 15.1). All of these influences will contribute to the *entrainment* of your two systems, with a tendency to bring both systems into harmony around the more settled balanced system.

Entrainment

Entrainment was first recognised in 1685 by Christiaan Huygens (1629–1695), a Dutch mathematician, astronomer and physicist, who noticed that the pendulums of grandfather clocks within the same room gradually start to swing in time with each other, all the clocks gradually synchronising with the heaviest pendulum. The same phenomenon can be observed throughout nature, as crickets and cicadas start to chirp in unison, women's menstrual cycles coordinate when living in close proximity, and the cardiac cells of the heart beat in time.

The concept of entrainment was originally conceived in relation to rhythms, and as such it is a significant factor in the perception of the rhythmic motion of the cranio-sacral system. But the concept of entrainment goes beyond rhythms and also reflects the wider influence of all aspects of systems on each other. When any two people are in the same room, their systems will entrain and influence each other in measurable ways (see Figure 15.2).

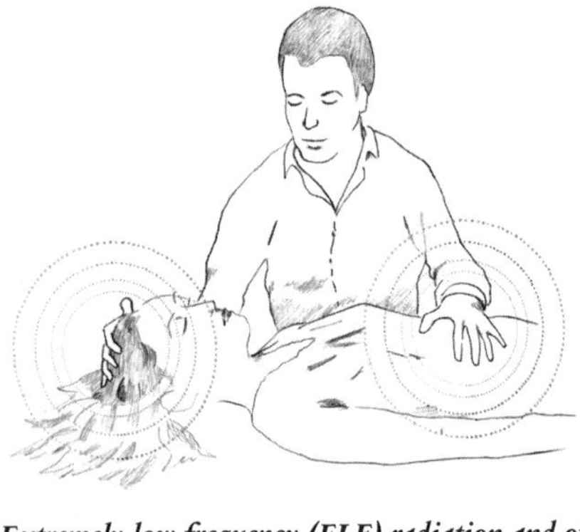

In the therapeutic process, the patient's and therapist's systems entrain. Just as clocks gravitate towards the heaviest pendulum, so the cranio-sacral systems gravitate towards the more settled calm cranio-sacral system, so the patient's system tends to harmonise increasingly with the therapist's more settled, steady system.

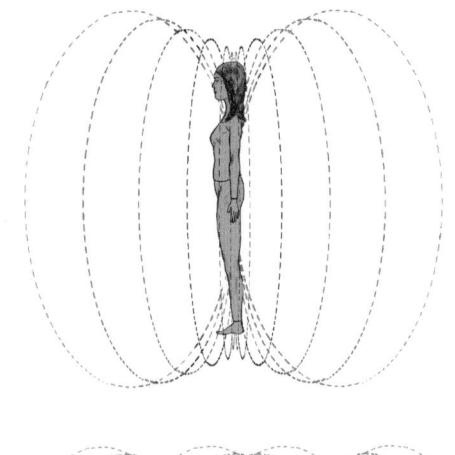

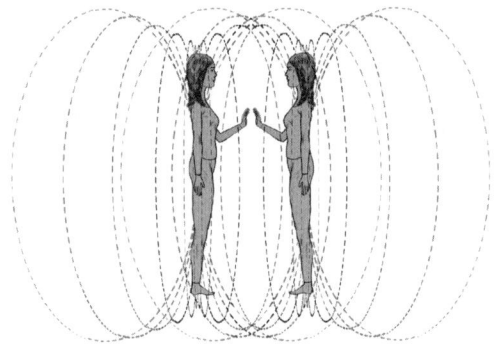

15.1 Extremely low frequency (ELF) radiation and other measurable forms of energetic radiation emanate from the hands of practitioners

15.2 Around each individual there exists a measurable biomagnetic field, which interacts with the fields of those around them

Box 15.1 Biomagnetic fields in modern medicine

Modern physicians may prescribe an energy healing method called Pulsed Electromagnetic Field Therapy (PEMF). The prescription is for a small, battery-powered pulse generator connected to a coil that you will place next to your injury for 8–10 hours per day. Clinical tests have proved that PEMF therapy will jump-start bone repair. Medical research has revealed that magnetic fields can convert a stalled healing process into active repair, even in patients unhealed for as long as 40 years. To be effective, PEMF pulses must be of low energy and extremely low frequency. Recent research shows that comparable fields emanate from the hands of practitioners of therapeutic touch and related methods.

Superconducting Quantum Interference Device (SQUID) detectors have been used to detect a large biomagnetic field, emanating from a practitioner's hand. The therapeutic touch signal from the practitioner's hands pulsed at a variable frequency, ranging from 0.3 to 30Hz, with most of the activity in the range of 7–8Hz. In studies, non-practitioners were unable to produce the biomagnetic pulses.

The heart produces the strongest electrical and magnetic activity of any tissue in the body. The biomagnetic field of the heart extends indefinitely into space, its strength diminishing with distance, until it becomes undetectable in the noise produced by other fields in the environment. Quantum physics has led to the development of instruments that can map the energy fields of the human body. There are devices that can pick up the field of the heart 15 feet away from the body. (*Energy Medicine: The Scientific Basis.* Oschman 2000)

Box 15.2 Balancing energy fields can reverse disease processes

The living matrix extends into every nook and cranny of the body, forming a systemic, energetic continuum. Coherent vibrations in living systems are as fundamental as chemical bonds. The energy fields projected from the hands of bodyworkers are in the range of intensity and frequency that can influence regulatory processes within the body of another person.

Harold Saxton-Burr, Professor of Anatomy at the University of Yale School of Medicine, implemented a series of studies on energy fields between 1932 and 1956. He obtained evidence that abnormal fields show up before serious pathology sets in, and that balancing or restoring the field can reverse disease processes. (*Energy Medicine: The Scientific Basis.* Oschman 2000)

Box 15.3 Therapeutic energy fields emanate from the hands of practitioners

Disease and disorder alter the electromagnetic properties of molecules, cells, tissues and organs. When a particular molecule is deficient, or altered, or in excess because of a disease or disorder, normal functioning can sometimes be restored with a drug. This is the basis of pharmacology. Vibrational medicines such as homeopathy demonstrate that similar or even better results can be obtained by providing the electromagnetic fingerprint or signature of a natural substance. In bodywork, the emanations from a therapist's own tissues can provide electromagnetic information that opens or augments vital communications in a patient's tissues.

Electromagnetic fields, at the frequencies and intensities emitted from the hands of the therapist, are capable of producing biological effects. The low frequencies emitted from the hands of therapists, and from pulsing electromagnetic field therapy devices, in the range of 2–30Hz are beneficial. (*Energy Medicine: The Scientific Basis.* Oschman 2000)

Further benefits of an appropriate presence

Sensitivity, perception, depth, grounding

Your calm, quiet presence also contributes to your:

- sensitivity to the cranio-sacral process
- clarity of perception
- ability to engage with deeper levels
- ability to remain grounded and centred at any time of disruption, or in working with a patient who is upset, disturbed or experiencing difficult circumstances.

A steadying influence

If a baby is screaming in pain or if a patient is unhappy, crying, angry or telling you the story of their severe trauma, injury, rape or abuse, it is a natural human response to feel upset for them or with them; anyone might be affected. However, as a therapist you need to be able to listen not only with compassion but also with grounding – not impersonal, uncaring detachment, but sympathetic, well-centred empathy.

If you can provide a settled and yet sympathetic responsive environment and connection through your own clear, balanced cranio-sacral system, then the patient's state and their cranio-sacral system will tend to become more settled and balanced.

Adverse effects

Conversely, if you don't have that well-grounded presence, your own disturbed or unsettled state can be projected into the interactive process – your own inner tensions, anxieties, lack of clarity; your mood, emotions, beliefs, prejudices and preconceptions – any of these may adversely affect the interaction.

Also, your own unresolved issues may be brought to the surface by the interaction, not only disrupting your state of being, your focus, and consequently your level of engagement, but also potentially leaving you unsettled or disturbed.

So once again it is necessary to maintain a clear balanced state of being – a state which can cope with the vagaries of life and the imbalances of others, through being well-grounded in calmness and stability – just as an oak tree can cope with the vagaries of the weather, its branches adapting flexibly to the wind, the rain and the storms that arise from time to time, while remaining steady and stable with its roots well-grounded in the earth.

Your own system is only likely to be disturbed if you have unresolved issues lurking under the surface waiting to be stirred up. The more you clear your own system the less you are likely to react. So long as you have the fundamental grounding, the skills and the awareness, then you can recognise and address any potential disturbances as they appear, allow them to arise, to flow through you, and to evaporate away, while maintaining your own grounding – like the oak tree. The more you have worked on your own *personal development*, the more clear and settled you will be.

Perfection

Obviously you don't have to be perfect in order to be a cranio-sacral therapist – but you do need to understand the significance of your own state and to address your own issues and your own process of personal development as far as possible, so that you can maintain a true inner state of balance despite your imperfections, rather than being ruled by them.

You certainly don't need to think that you have to be perfect before you embark on becoming a cranio-sacral therapist. Many prospective cranio-sacral therapists may be attracted to cranio-sacral therapy precisely because they aspire to a greater degree of stillness and calmness in their lives. It is something which you develop during a training in cranio-sacral integration, and this helps you not only in your development as a cranio-sacral therapist, but also in every aspect of your life – personal relationships, work relationships, your whole relationship with the world around you – often transforming life.

The cranio-sacral system is never fooled

It is not enough simply to maintain a superficial impression of calmness and equanimity. You might present a very professional appearance by wearing a white coat and behaving in a correct, controlled, impersonal manner. That might impress some patients, but it won't impress the cranio-sacral system.

You might be extremely knowledgeable, well versed in anatomy, physiology and pathology, science and technique. All of that is useful, but it is not what really counts and may come to nothing if your underlying state is not clear and balanced.

You might be very caring and loving, deeply concerned for your patients, eager to help them, determined to heal them. This is worthy and admirable, but it is not necessarily helpful to the process if it is emanating from a state of imbalance and unresolved needs within you. Your eagerness can be overwhelming, too intense, imposing on the system, and may therefore obstruct the easeful flow of the cranio-sacral process. By all means be caring and loving and want to help your patients – but these good intentions need to come from a balanced perspective, recognising that it is not your eagerness and determination that will help the patient, but the ability to allow the fluent evolution of the cranio-sacral process from a well-grounded, settled and peaceful state.

This is fundamental to the cranio-sacral process. Trust in that realisation of simply allowing the cranio-sacral process to take its course. Don't try too hard. Let the process flow. What is needed is to be truly stable and grounded – from deep within. The cranio-sacral process is at its most profound when there is minimal interference from the therapist. All you need to do is be there with your calm, quiet presence, engaging with the natural flow of life within your patient and within yourself, not feeling the need to do anything, trusting the process to take its course, understanding that life goes on within you and without you.

Enhancing the development of cranio-sacral skills

Developing your own presence also assists in the development of various other skills essential to the cranio-sacral process. By settling into a quieter, calmer state:

- you can develop a greater degree of spaciousness, a *wider perception*, a greater ability to see the whole picture

- you can create the ability to get in touch more readily with your *intuition* and deeper insight
- you can develop the ability to let your *attention be in several places* at the same time
- you can enhance your ability to *project* your attention through the body.

Divided attention

Developing the ability to have your *attention in more than one place* simultaneously enables you to take a broader and more comprehensive view of the whole picture – like an artist standing back from her painting to gain an overview of the whole picture, seeing how the detail of her artistry fits within the overall perspective. It might include taking your attention to a point somewhere above you, as if looking down from above:

- aware of the space around you and of your patient and yourself within that space
- while at the same time making you aware of specific impressions and responses at your hands
- increasingly aware of several things at once your patient, yourself, the whole interaction, a sense of spaciousness around you
- increasingly, within that wider perception, able to see the whole patient and the detail within the patient the whole body and the specific fulcrums, restrictions and asymmetries within the wider picture.

Projection

Developing the ability to *project* through the body is an invaluable skill, which enables you to identify what is going on throughout the body, wherever you may be, identifying focal points of tension or restriction, identifying fulcrums, imbalances and asymmetries, reading whole body patterns. It is an essential component of diagnosis, but it is much more than that. The very fact of identifying fulcrums and patterns enables therapeutic responses within the cranio-sacral process, as they change and release in response to your specific focus of attention. Projecting your attention through the body is an inherent part of every moment of the cranio-sacral process.

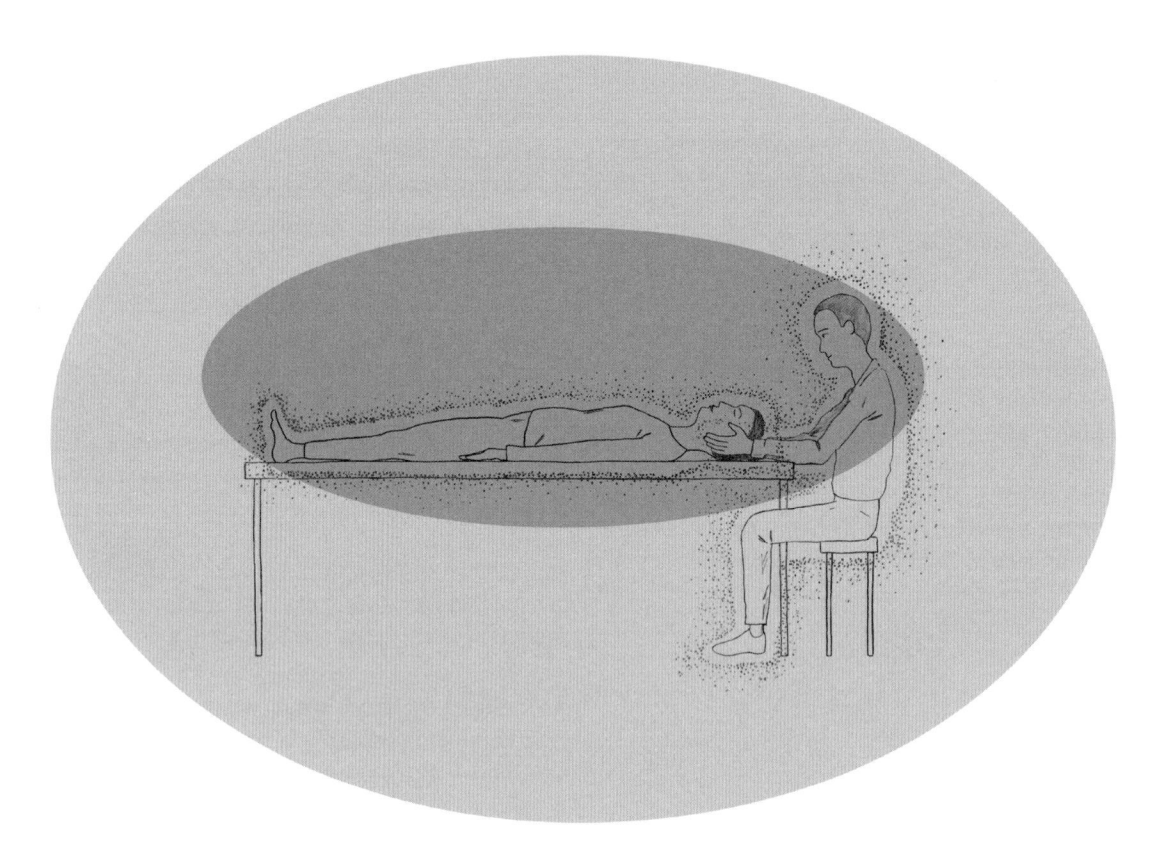

15.3 Allow your attention to expand into the space around you, and be aware of yourself and your patient within that space

PRACTICAL EXERCISE

Initially you might develop your projection skills by practising projecting from different parts of the body.

With a practice partner lying supine (on their back) on the couch, gently take up contact at the feet, resting your hands softly on the dorsum (upper surface) of the feet. Settle into a calm quiet state, aware of your own practitioner fulcrums, and feel the gradual development of engagement with your partner's system. Once you feel truly engaged, project your attention gradually up through the ankles, shins, knees, thighs, hips, pelvis, trunk, to the shoulders, neck and head, noticing any changes in quality, symmetry or motion as your attention moves from one place to another.

In the same way, you can practise projecting:

- from the shoulders down through the body
- from the head down through the body
- from the occiput down through the spine
- from the sacrum up through the spine
- from the sacrum up through the trunk, spine, viscera, muscles
- increasingly viewing the whole body with all its fulcrums and patterns
- increasingly describing the overall patterns in greater detail.

In due course you can develop your skills to project:

- from anywhere to anywhere
- through the tissues
- through the fluids
- through the energy system
- through the energy field
- through the whole matrix and beyond
- viewing the whole person and everything about them on all levels.

Don't expect to be able to do all this instantly. It may seem impossible at first, but all it takes is time and practice.

Establishing an appropriate presence

There are two principal aspects to establishing an appropriate therapeutic presence:

- Developing an *underlying state* of clarity and equanimity through receiving treatment and therapy, a supportive lifestyle, and through *personal development*.
- Developing the ability to bring yourself into an appropriate state of grounding and calmness *in the moment*, whatever may be going on within you or around you, through *specific grounding skills*.

There are no universal rules on how to go about this. The process will be different for each individual. But there are various possible initial guidelines:

- Establish a *lifestyle* that provides you with space and time for yourself.
- Avoid an *excessive bombardment* of input and stimulation from the world around you.
- Address your *underlying patterns* of tension and trauma, through treatment and therapy.
- Incorporate *adequate times of quietness* and peacefulness into your day-to-day life.
- Give attention to your *breathing*.

Breathing

Breathing is a very valuable asset, always with you wherever you go, and inevitably reflecting your state with unerring accuracy. Through your breathing, you can both monitor and influence the state that you are in. Establish habits of breathing in a deeper, more relaxed way, particularly letting go with each out-breath. This is something that you can work on constantly 24 hours a day – while walking, sitting, travelling, while drifting off to sleep, on waking up in the morning, while working, or while playing – until it becomes so natural that you can maintain it unconsciously as a matter of course, awake or asleep, so that whenever necessary, you can readily re-establish easy breathing, and thereby encourage a calmer quieter state. (We will explore breathing further in Chapter 37.)

Reflective practice

Set aside time each day for reflecting on the events of the day, your responses to those events, how you might have managed them differently, how you can learn from your reflections and gain deeper insight into yourself and the way that you are living your life.

Daily practice

Maintain a daily practice – of reflection, of meditation, of breathing, of awareness of your own fulcrums, your state of physical comfort, your mental balance, your emotional tranquillity, your spiritual equanimity. Allow yourself to settle into deeper stillness, calmness, peacefulness and consequent contentment.

The pursuit of personal development in all its many aspects doesn't have to be ascetic, strenuous or unpleasant; it can be enjoyable, rewarding and satisfying, and it will help you in all aspects of your life.

Regular and consistent daily practice will enable you all the more easily to ground yourself and settle yourself whenever you need to – at the start of a day in clinical practice, at the start of each treatment session, throughout each moment of therapeutic interaction, throughout life.

Your presence is the most important factor in the therapeutic process – more important than knowledge, technique or skills. The cranio-sacral process will proceed most effectively simply through your appropriate presence. Be content just to be there, trusting in your calm, quiet presence.

Summary

At the start of this chapter, we asked: why is the state of the practitioner so significant?

- Because it is through developing and maintaining your calm, quiet presence that you are able to get in touch with the forces of nature that are the principal element

in the therapeutic process of cranio-sacral integration.
- In order to ensure that your contribution to the interaction is a positive influence of calmness and centredness.
- Because it enables greater development of your own sensitivity and receptivity.
- It enables the development of many other skills necessary for effective cranio-sacral therapy – spacious perception, projection, levels of attention.
- Because it enables deeper levels of engagement.
- So that you can respond most positively and helpfully to your patient.
- So that you don't find your own state of balance disturbed by whatever may come up.
- Because it enhances your ability to remain grounded and centred.

Most significantly, because your own calm, quiet presence is the most significant factor in the whole cranio-sacral process.

Chapter 16

Stillness

Stillness is one of the most essential components of the cranio-sacral process. It arises in many different forms, most of which are quintessentially vital:
- stillness in the patient
- stillness in the practitioner
- stillness in the environment
- stillness in the therapeutic process
- points of stillness
- dynamic stillness
- stillness of movement
- stillness of motion
- qualities of stillness
- outer stillness
- inner stillness
- all pervading stillness.

Environmental awareness

Stillness starts with the therapeutic environment. For the most part we tend to create a calm, peaceful environment, undisturbed by noisesome distractions. This is preferable and often helpful for patients in enabling them to settle into deeper relaxation – but it is not essential. A well-grounded practitioner can operate under any conditions – in the middle of Piccadilly Circus, Times Square, or a Mumbai market. The key is not so much in the environment but rather in the therapist.

True inner stillness

Stillness in the practitioner is essential. As we have seen, it is the most fundamental factor in determining the fluent progress of all other aspects of the cranio-sacral process, the most vital factor in the healing process. When a therapist is well-grounded and can maintain a calm, quiet presence, healing will occur. Without that, it is less likely. Most significantly, it is not just a matter of maintaining a veneer of stillness. It is not enough to be sitting still, to be holding yourself firmly and determinedly in stillness. It is a true inner stillness – a stillness that comes from deep within and from dedicated application to your own personal development in order to be able to maintain that true inner stillness, whatever is going on within you or around you.

Patient stillness

Stillness in the patient is, like stillness in the environment, something that is preferable but not essential. In most cases, we tend to work with the patient lying still and peaceful; and the more they can settle into deep relaxation, the more their system will respond and the inherent healing process can take effect. But there is no way we can expect every baby to stay still; some of them are screaming in pain and wriggling in agony – or just having fun. When it comes to treating children it is very likely that we will be treating them while playing and singing and maintaining a juggling act of keeping them happily entertained while at the same time focusing on the deepest levels of the treatment process. And when it comes to hyperactive toddlers, you may well be treating them as they run manically around the room. So stillness in the patient is relative – desirable, but not something you can always insist upon. It's no good being over-concerned about having complete stillness. Sometimes it happens, sometimes you just have to accept that it is not to be. Don't worry, be happy just to be there, absorbed in your own profound inner stillness amidst the surrounding activity.

Shake, rattle and roll

When you first start to engage with a patient's system, there will often be a multitude of extraneous movements – buzzing, vibrating, wriggling, pulsating, rocking, rolling, shaking, twisting, turning and many others – reflecting the initial state of the patient. As you tune in, the stillness of the environment and above all, your own inner stillness, will start to pervade the patient and encourage an increasing level of stillness. Simply by being there, allowing these movements to be expressed and maintaining your own calm, quiet presence, these movements will start to subside into stillness, a stillness within which there is less movement, a stillness which can then reveal the underlying rhythmic motion more clearly.

There is a distinction to be made between stillness of movement (the multitude of extraneous movements) and stillness of motion (rhythmic motion), for, ironically, it is through stillness of movement that we are able to feel motion more clearly, and we find motion within the stillness of movement.

Still points

The next level of stillness is within the rhythmic motion. As we have seen, as the treatment process proceeds, the rhythmic motion will in due course draw into points of stillness, gradually closing down to a still point – where rhythmic motion has ceased – perhaps around a specific fulcrum, perhaps simply within the rhythmic motion itself. These are the essential moments of the therapeutic process. It is primarily at these points of stillness that healing occurs.

Dynamic stillness – part 1

Within these points of stillness, you may feel one form of *dynamic stillness*, where the rhythmic motion has become still and yet there is a dynamism within the stillness, a sense of vibration, wriggling, underlying activity, a sense that something is about to happen, a sense of building up to something. These qualities within the still point are indications that you are truly engaged with a point of stillness, that the therapeutic process is in process. The dynamism within the stillness helps you to recognise that you are in the right place, that it is not just a stoppage, and so helps you to maintain your engagement at that vital point of stillness for as long as it takes to move on to release and reorganisation. These subtle dynamics are the indications that the system is building towards a release and the healing that ensues from such a release.

These still points can take many forms and can occur at many different levels. They can release in milliseconds before you have even acknowledged them; they can last several seconds, they can last several minutes, or longer. They can occur in cranio-sacral rhythm, in middle tide, or in fascial unwinding. They may release into a slower expression of rhythmic motion, or they can represent a transition from cranio-sacral rhythm to middle tide, or from middle tide to long tide. Some still points will be felt in the local tissues, some will seem to spread through the whole body. Others may pervade the whole patient, the practitioner and the whole room with a deep sense of stillness.

A summer's day – qualities of stillness

As the treatment process proceeds, perhaps through a series of still points, the system may increasingly take on an overall quality of stillness. A quality of stillness is different from a still point or point of stillness. It is an overriding quality that expresses the overall characteristics of the system with a sense of calmness and ease – which may or may not include movement and motion.

It is like a tranquil summer's day, peaceful and quiet; bees are still buzzing, birds are still singing, life still goes on, so there is movement around – but there is a quality of stillness which pervades the atmosphere. This may be an indication of the state or quality of the patient – calm, quiet, relaxed and at ease – or it may be an indication of the progress of the process, perhaps having reached a point of conclusion where it would be appropriate to bring the treatment to an end, or a plateau where it wants to rest for a while before moving on along its journey.

There will be other qualities which may also reflect stillness, but different forms of stillness – such as stuckness – which may feel very still, but is not an easeful, peaceful, calm stillness, but rather a more solid, obdurate block of hard stillness, perhaps indicating an old injury or a deeply held tension. Distinguishing these different qualities of stillness will have significant implications for the treatment process.

When first taking up contact, you might also feel an initial quality of nothing happening, which you might interpret as a type of stillness. This could simply indicate lack of engagement, or a solid stuck quality, or a frozen locked quality of being in shock. You will need to differentiate the different qualities of stillness and differentiate the stillness due to lack of movement from other aspects of stillness. They are readily identifiable – by their quality.

The deepest healing occurs in the deepest stillness: dynamic stillness – part 2

As the treatment proceeds through a series of longer still points and ever deepening qualities of stillness through levels of long tide motion, you may eventually encounter a deeper level of stillness, a profound level of dynamic stillness: where the stillness seems to pervade everything – the patient, the practitioner, the room, the whole surrounding matrix; where rhythmic motion ceases to be apparent – not because it has reached a still point, but because it has simply ceased to be noticeable or relevant; where the surrounding environment seems to fade into the background; where the whole physical universe seems to disappear into oblivion; where patient, therapist, awareness, consciousness and everything have dissolved into spaciousness; where there is nothing but a profound sense of deep dynamic stillness.

These are the moments when the most profound healing occurs.

Part III

A Framework for Integrated Treatment

BASIC SKILLS

Chapter 17

Integrated Treatment

Introduction
Every cranio-sacral treatment is individual. There are, however, certain elements of the treatment process which are particularly significant in enabling effective integrated treatment:

- engagement
- settling and grounding the patient
- deeper engagement with more profound levels
- appropriate completion.

So it can be useful to keep in mind the concept of *A Framework for Integrated Treatment*, which will enable all these factors and others to be catered for, ensuring that each treatment session has a cohesive wholeness and that each treatment is concerned with overall integration of the patient.

This is not a rigid protocol to be followed at all times, nor a standardised treatment system to be applied mechanically – but a broad framework within which to respond individually to each patient's needs. As we have seen, cranio-sacral integration is not about applying techniques. It is about simply being there, engaging with the inherent healing forces, allowing the system to express itself, observing and allowing the responses within the system. So while this section will describe various contacts, hand positions, and stimuli that may be used at various times during a treatment, all of these need to be understood within the context of the treatment approach outlined earlier, rather than with the idea of doing anything to the patient.

Infinitely variable
Since it is just a framework, the way in which each treatment starts, evolves, continues and finishes will vary substantially. The format outlined below provides a useful starting point – for beginners, for new patients, for any treatment session. Even for experienced therapists, the principles within the framework provide a valuable foundation for every treatment, but the form of the treatment around those principles will change from session to session. Some practitioners may choose to maintain a fairly recognisable structure to their treatments, especially with new patients. Others may apply the principles of the framework, without necessarily using an obviously recognisable format. Particularly as you get to know a patient, you will readily realise which elements of the framework are significant for that individual and adapt your sessions accordingly. With increasing experience, the practitioner can identify the patient's needs more readily, and again adapt the format appropriately.

Four stages
This broad framework consists of four stages:

1. Engagement (tuning in).
2. Opening up the system (settling and grounding).
3. Core treatment.
4. Completion.

1. Engagement (tuning in)
Engagement with the cranio-sacral system is fundamental to all cranio-sacral integration. Without engagement, it is not cranio-sacral integration. Engagement doesn't necessarily happen instantly or automatically. Appropriate conditions need to be established – both in the patient and in the practitioner. Only when true engagement has been established can the cranio-sacral process proceed. This is essential to each and every treatment session.

2. Opening up the system (settling and grounding)

When patients arrive for treatment, they have generally come in from the outside world, perhaps in a suitable state to manage the outside world, but not necessarily in the most appropriate state for deep therapeutic interaction. Opening up the system is an essential part of settling and grounding the patient, bringing them to a more appropriate responsive state, relaxed and at ease, ready to gain the most benefit from their treatment.

Failure to give attention to opening up the system where appropriate may lead to lack of engagement, lack of progress, unwanted side-effects and treatment reactions, or the patient's time being wasted with little or no progress being made.

The degree to which each patient needs settling and grounding will vary substantially, so the form it takes and the length of time it takes will similarly be adapted to their needs. In some patients who are significantly unsettled, particularly when they first start receiving cranio-sacral integration, settling and grounding may occupy the majority of the treatment session, or be the principal focus for several sessions. In others it may barely be necessary at all. As always there is no premeditated protocol or format – simply an appropriate response to individual circumstances.

3. Core treatment

On the whole, core treatment, as its name suggests, will be the deepest, most significant stage of the treatment (although, as just mentioned, there is no premeditated protocol, and if a patient needs the whole session devoted to settling and grounding, then there is no requirement to enter into core treatment where it is not appropriate or where the patient is not ready). It may therefore be the stage which is most variable according to the needs of the patient or circumstances. It involves deeper connection with the very core of the system, and is likely to involve the most profound healing.

4. Completion

Every treatment needs to reach a suitable state of completion, in order to ensure that the patient leaves in a suitably balanced and settled state – not left in limbo, or incomplete.

If someone goes into hospital for an operation, they are not ejected out onto the street immediately after the operation with their wound open. The incision is sewn up, and adequate time for recovery and recuperation are allowed (one would hope).

In the same way, with a cranio-sacral treatment, having opened up the system and penetrated to the depths of a patient's being, it is essential to bring the process to a satisfactory conclusion, with the patient settled and ready to go out into the world again.

With most treatments, this is likely to occur spontaneously as the treatment process comes to a natural conclusion, but the therapist always needs to be observant and aware, alert to any unresolved or unfinished activity, and to check that the system feels balanced and complete before bringing a treatment to an end.

Chapter 18

Tuning In – 1

This chapter introduces the first stage in the four-stage integrated treatment framework:

1. *Engagement (tuning in).*
2. Opening up the system (settling and grounding).
3. Core treatment.
4. Completion.

Engagement

In order to work effectively with the cranio-sacral system, you will first need to establish a connection. This does not mean merely resting your hands on the body or on the head. It doesn't mean simply palpating skin or bone or muscles. It means establishing a connection with the underlying vitality, with the subtle expressions of quality, symmetry and motion within the energy matrix of the body. It means genuine engagement.

In order to clarify this, we will here describe a practical process of tuning in to a patient at the shoulders and at the head. It is of course possible to tune in and engage anywhere in the body and the same principles would apply wherever you tune in.

A practical process of tuning in
Allow approximately 40 minutes.

Stillness
Stillness, as we have seen, is an essential characteristic of the cranio-sacral process. Initially you will find it helpful for your patient to be still and relaxed in order for you to identify the subtle expressions of the cranio-sacral system and for them to receive maximum benefit from the cranio-sacral process.

Self-awareness
The continuing development and maintenance of an inner stillness within yourself throughout the treatment process is also essential:

- in order to maximise your own sensitivity
- in order that your own qualities of stillness and calmness can contribute positively to this subtle interaction between you and your patient
- ultimately, because your own calm, quiet presence is the most significant factor in the whole cranio-sacral process.

Most of your attention (90%) needs to be on yourself.

Patient preparation
Invite your patient to lie supine (lying on their back, face up) on the treatment couch, with the top of their head approximately 4 inches (10 cm) from the end of the couch. (This position of the head is helpful, as it enables the therapist to establish a comfortable position sitting at the head, with enough room to rest their forearms on the couch if necessary, without feeling cramped or squashed when they take up contact on the patient's head – and the comfort of the therapist is vital to the cranio-sacral process, since any discomfort may reduce their sensitivity and awareness.)

Invite the patient to take a deep breath, to let go completely – physically and mentally – and to continue to breathe easily.

Self-preparation
Sit comfortably and symmetrically at the head of the couch. Before you take up any contact with your patient, take time to focus on yourself, to bring yourself into an appropriate state of quiet, calm, relaxed sensitivity – to become aware of your own 'practitioner fulcrums' – physically, mentally, emotionally.

Sit comfortably in your seat, your body balanced and relaxed, the soles of your feet comfortably grounded on the floor – grounding you posturally and grounding you energetically.

Take a deep breath or two, letting go physically and mentally with each out-breath (taking care not to breathe into your patient's face), then settle into easy, relaxed, natural breathing.

Maintain a consistent awareness of your breathing. As you continue to let go with each out-breath, run your attention through your body from the top of your head to the soles of your feet, feeling your chest open, your shoulders drop, your arms hanging loosely, your back relaxing, your pelvis settling into your seat, your legs letting go, your feet grounded on the floor.

Continue to be aware of your easeful, relaxed breathing. Maintain this awareness of your breathing throughout the treatment process, coming back to it again and again, a thousand times and more.

Let go mentally – settling into a relaxed, detached, open and receptive, meditative quality of mind. Allow your attention to expand out into the space around you – the space above you, the space below you, the space in front of you, the space behind you, the space on each side of you.

You may become aware of sounds around you – voices, bird song, traffic. Allow the sounds to come and go – not trying to block them out, nor giving them attention, not being disturbed or irritated by them, just letting them be there, simply letting them come and go.

Similarly, you may be aware of thoughts arising. In the same way, allow the thoughts to come and go – not trying to block them out, nor giving them attention, not being disturbed or irritated by them, just letting them be there, simply letting them come and go, gently putting them aside and bringing your attention back, again and again, to letting go of each out-breath.

This part of the process is likely to take several minutes. When you feel completely settled and at ease, you are ready to consider making your first direct contact with your patient.

Continue to maintain your awareness of your breathing and your awareness of your own practitioner fulcrums throughout the process.

Initial contact – on the shoulders

Inevitably some parts of the body are more sensitive than others. A patient's system will be more comfortable with an initial contact on a less sensitive area – such as the shoulders – taking a few minutes to tune in and connect with the system through this less delicate area.

The body has many protective mechanisms. The body's natural response to any physical contact is to defend itself from potential intrusion. In order to minimise these defence mechanisms and connect more deeply with the core of the system, it is essential that your initial contact

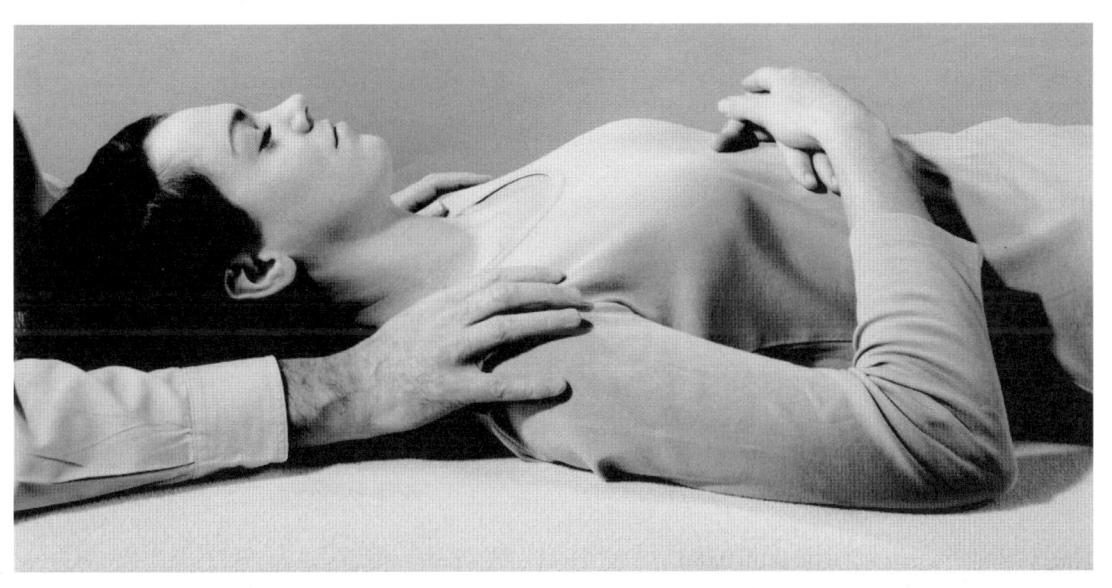

18.1 Gradually, almost imperceptibly, allow your hands to sink down through the energy field, until they come to rest very lightly onto the shoulders

should be extremely light – like a butterfly alighting on the body – reassuring the patient's subconscious awareness that your touch is gentle, non-threatening and safe.

The body will feel and react to your approaching hands – even before you have made contact – through the sensitive energy field which surrounds the body.

Not only will your contact need to be extremely light, but also you will need to approach the body very slowly since any sudden or abrupt movement or contact will immediately alert the body and arouse its protective mechanisms. Again, this will apply long before you make actual contact with the body, as your hands move softly through the energy field.

So, when you are ready to take up contact, don't rush into it, and don't abandon the gentle, settled spaciousness that you have been developing for the previous few minutes. Move slowly, carefully, gently, reflecting on what you are going to do before you do it, so that you can move fluently.

Maintaining your awareness of yourself, move slowly to place your forearms or elbows so that they are resting gently on the end of the couch, in such a position that your hands can hover, soft and relaxed, a few inches above your patient's shoulders.

See if you can feel the warmth of the body – energy is radiating off all parts of the body in the form of heat; see to what extent you can feel this heat energy. Then gradually, almost imperceptibly, allow your hands to sink down, millimetre by millimetre, through the energy field – noticing at what point you begin to feel the warmth of the body, or perhaps how the warmth intensifies as you come closer – until eventually your hands come to rest very lightly onto the shoulders.

Maintain self-awareness

As your hands settle onto the shoulders, allow them to sink softly and gradually into the body, gently allowing your hands to relax completely as they sink into the body, until you are no longer holding on to any tension in your arms and hands.

Come back into yourself. Maintain awareness of your own practitioner fulcrums and your own breathing. Let go in your heart. Let go in your solar plexus. Run your attention down through your head, neck and shoulders, down through your arms, forearms and hands – softening and letting go completely. Feel your hands so soft and relaxed that they seem to melt into the shoulders, the shoulders melting into your hands.

Feel the increasing sense of interconnection between your two systems – your patient and yourself.

Quality, symmetry, motion

Through this connection, gradually become aware of the various characteristics of this patient's system:

- Do these shoulders feel warm or cool – what does this tell you about the patient?
- Do the shoulders feel tight or loose? What does this tell you about the patient, about the degree of tension they may be holding in their body, or about a possible site of injury and restriction?
- Do these shoulders feel agitated or calm? Again, what does this tell you about the patient?

In the same way, you can evaluate everything that comes to your attention:

- The distinctive *qualities* – softness, hardness, warmth, coolness, tightness, looseness, activity, stillness, vitality, or whatever other qualities or characteristics may come to mind.
- Any disturbances to *symmetry* – differences in the perceived position of the two shoulders – whether one is higher or lower than the other, pulling up towards the neck, down into the body, across into the midline – or differences in quality between the two shoulders – one tighter or looser than the other, more active, more still, more stuck – perhaps revealing some site of injury or restriction.
- Any sense of movement or *motion* – vibration, pulsation, swirling, shaking, twisting, turning, rocking, pulling.
- Any sense of *vitality* – are there any indications that this patient is alive – warmth, movement, activity, a sense of dynamism? Is there a powerful sense of vitality, or a weak feeble vitality?

Each and every one of these characteristics reflects the nature of the person you are connecting with – their physical state, their mental state, their emotional state, their spiritual state, physical injuries, emotional tensions, their personality, their very nature.

With practice and experience, you will be able to identify and interpret every subtle reflection of the person's being – to assess their physical health and well-being and to gain a subtle and profound understanding of their situation – simply through this gentle but infinitely perceptive touch.

Allow the system to express itself. Take several minutes to observe whatever arises, content to 'simply be there'.

Allow your attention to expand to encompass the whole body, projecting beyond your contact at the shoulders to encompass the whole person, perhaps drawn by a specific asymmetry, perhaps simply opening up your attention to a wider perspective. Allow your attention to expand to encompass the whole fluidic matrix – within and around the body (see Figure 18.2).

Observe whatever impressions you encounter, putting them into words in order to define them more clearly, summarising your findings and making a mental note of your impressions. The more specifically you define your findings, the more accurately you will understand your patient.

Taking up contact on the cranium

When this process feels complete, *after several minutes*, once you have a clear sense of connection, and a clear assessment of qualities, asymmetries and movements, still maintaining your self-awareness, prepare yourself to move very slowly and sensitively in order to make a gradual transition to the sides of the head.

Before you move, reflect again on the need to respect the sensitivity of the system, the need to avoid any sudden abrupt movements that will arouse the body's protective mechanisms. Plan your moves so that you can move smoothly and fluently, and when you are ready, allow your hands very gradually to float away from the shoulders, so softly that your patient may not even be aware that your hands have moved away.

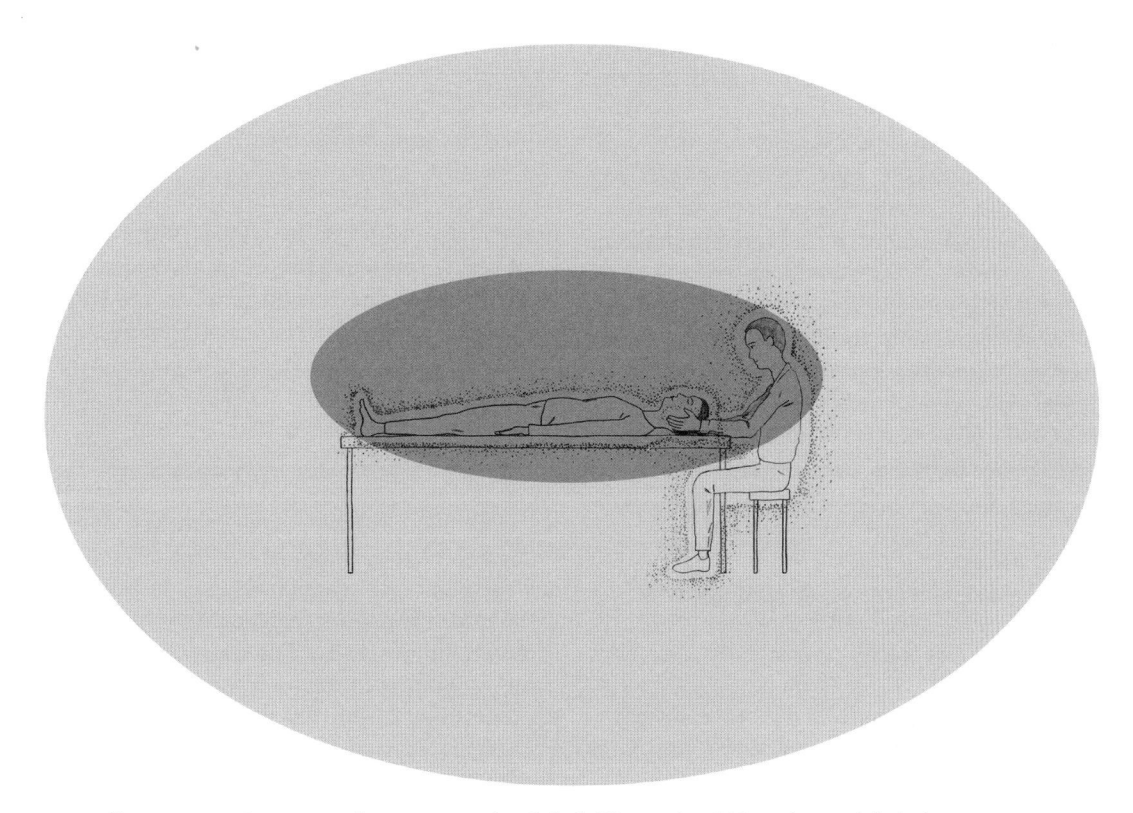

18.2 Allow your attention to expand to encompass the whole fluidic matrix within and around the body

Still moving slowly and softly, adjust your forearms on the couch so that your hands can come to rest about 2 inches (5 cm) away from the sides of the head.

Again, see if you can feel the warmth of the body. Again, approach slowly, almost imperceptibly, letting your hands sink in millimetre by millimetre, feeling the gradual intensification of warmth as you come closer, respecting and experiencing the energy field – perhaps feeling it as a layer of warmth or a cushion of energy around the body.

Again, sink though the energy field, to settle very lightly with the same butterfly touch onto the sides of the head.

Let your hands be completely soft and relaxed, not holding the head, not gripping, just being there with a soft light contact, your hands or forearms supported by the couch or head-cushion so that they can relax completely.

Maintain self-awareness as before, aware of your breathing, aware of your practitioner fulcrums, letting go in your heart and solar plexus, running your attention down through your head, neck and shoulders, arms, forearms, wrists, hands, fingers, thumbs, and palms of your hands.

Let your arms and hands be so soft and relaxed that your hands seem to melt into the head, the head melt into your hands, as if to become one continuous structure.

Feel the increasing sense of interconnection.

Observe the quality, symmetry and motion of the system as expressed through the cranium, just as you did at the shoulders, putting your observations into words for greater definition and clarity, defining your findings as specifically as possible for greater precision and understanding. Evaluate the level of vitality or potency within the system, defining it and making a mental note of what you encounter.

Allow the system to express itself.

Take *several minutes* to observe whatever arises, content to 'simply be there'.

Make a mental note of your impressions.

Fluidity

Observe the fluidic nature of the process.

Initially, you are likely to encounter the more superficial aspects of the system (the day-to-day tensions and activities) which often manifest as the kind of movements one might find on the surface of a lake or sea – wavelets, ripples, turbulence. This is the beginning of engagement.

As these impressions subside and settle in response to the stillness that you bring to the interaction of the cranio-sacral process, you may encounter deeper aspects of the system (the persistent effects of injuries, illness and emotional tensions) manifesting as the kind of movement one might find under the surface of the sea – swirling, shifting, eddies and currents – together with a gentle wave-like motion, like waves ebbing and flowing on a beach. This is true engagement.

As these movements subside and settle, you may encounter aspects of the system that are deeper still (the underlying personality and nature of the person) manifesting as the kind of movement one might find deep within the ocean – the deep tides that rise and fall at the very depths of the ocean. This is profound engagement.

Rhythmic motion

Maintain your sense of interconnection with the system. After several minutes simply being there, observing and noting the various impressions, while still engaging with the system through the contact of your hands on the head, see if you can feel the *arterial pulse*. The arterial pulse is transmitted from the heart through every artery of the body, including the arteries of the head. It is, of course, more readily felt at the radial pulse at the wrist or the carotid pulse in the throat, but it is also present, albeit less obviously, in the arteries of the head. See if you can feel it – maybe you can, maybe you can't. Don't be concerned either way. Keep focused on your own sense of ease and calmness.

If you don't readily feel these subtle features, the most likely reason is your own lack of ease, softness and relaxation. The more relaxed you are, the more sensitive you will become. Anxiety and concern about not feeling anything can only obstruct and get in the way. Don't try too hard. Focus on your own fulcrums, on your breathing, on letting go physically and mentally, on just being there, on your own calm, quiet presence, on being soft and relaxed. Keep the majority of your attention on yourself. Let the impressions come to you in their own time – like the kitten.

Keeping your eyes closed, see now if you can feel your patient's *breathing*. As the lungs expand and contract, subtle pulls are transmitted up through the body tissues, from the lungs and thorax to the head. See if you can feel these subtle movements. Maybe you can, maybe you can't. Don't worry, be content just to be there.

If you think you can feel your patient's breathing, open your eyes slightly to observe the rise and fall of your patient's abdomen. Does the rise and fall of the abdomen match what you are feeling in the head? Don't try to make it match, simply acknowledge whatever you are experiencing.

Having acknowledged the breathing, close your eyes again and see if you can feel another rhythmic motion, similar to breathing but perhaps a little slower and a bit more even – and also more subtle – as if the head were a balloon, being slightly blown up a little and slightly let down a little. If you can feel this movement, then you are tuning in to the *cranio-sacral rhythm* – gently expanding and contracting at a rate of around 4–14 cycles per minute (each complete cycle lasting approximately 5–10 seconds) – as if the whole body were breathing independently of the respiration of the lungs. Again, you may feel it or you may not. Don't worry, be happy with whatever you experience (or don't experience). Continue to focus on your own sense of ease and relaxation, recognising that trying too hard will only limit your sensitivity, trusting that with time and practice and softness and spaciousness, the various impressions will come to you more clearly.

If you are very still and sensitive and if your patient is very still and relaxed, you may also identify a further rhythmic motion, a similar expansion and contraction but at a much slower rate of around 2½ cycles per minute (each complete cycle lasting approximately 25 seconds). This rhythm is even more subtle. It is likely to take time and practice before you experience it, but if you feel it, then you are tuning in to the *middle tide*.

Eventually, with experience, and in conducive circumstances of profound stillness and subtlety, you may encounter an even deeper rhythmic motion, with a cycle of 100 seconds. This is the *long tide* – expanding and contracting slowly and deeply throughout the whole of our being.

Completion

Having penetrated to the deepest levels of your patient's being, bring your awareness gradually back to the surface, to the physical realities of the room that you are in, to the present moment.

Make a mental note of your impressions, putting them into words, evaluating what they might signify, what they might tell you about this patient, again defining your findings as clearly and precisely as possible, refining your definitions, summarising the whole interaction.

When it feels appropriate, gently allow your hands to soften away from the head, floating away so softly that your patient may not know your hands have come away, taking care not to move too suddenly, or to create any disturbance or shock to this subtle sensitive system with which you have been connecting, and allow the process to come to completion.

(This tuning in process has been described at length and in detail, and for a beginner, practising the process in this way, taking 30 or 40 minutes, will be a valuable way to develop the skills of tuning in to the cranio-sacral system. As you develop those skills and become experienced, you will be able to tune in instantly or almost instantly to the cranio-sacral system, absorbing everything that has been described here instinctively, so that this whole 30–40 minute process may take just a few minutes or even just seconds.)

Chapter 19

Tuning In – 2

In this chapter we will be deepening engagement by exploring how the process of tuning in can be affected by different levels of connection – different levels of physical contact, different levels of attention, different tissue levels.

Exploring different levels of physical contact

The level of contact appropriate for craniosacral integration is perhaps hard to imagine for practitioners who have not yet experienced it. In most aspects of day-to-day life, we are accustomed to 'doing' rather than 'being'. If we want to achieve something, we do something about it, rather than simply being there waiting for it to happen. Consequently, with beginners (including highly experienced practitioners used to working with more physical therapies) the level of contact they use – even when they think they are being extremely light – is often more like an elephant than a butterfly.

Lightness

The first point to make about the level of contact is the extreme lightness of touch – not holding, not gripping, not exerting any pressure at all, not trying to feel anything, not trying to find anything – but simply being there, your hands completely relaxed, in calm, quiet stillness, open and receptive to whatever may arise.

Softness

The second point is that together with lightness of touch – more fundamental and significant than lightness – is the quality of *softness* in the hands. It will soon become apparent that, *even when the hands are very light, even off the body, even several inches away from the body* – if the hands are tight, tense, or hard, then the patient may experience that tightness and hardness, and may find it disturbing, invasive or uncomfortable; and it will also block off the practitioner's sensitivity to the impressions arising within the patient's craniosacral system.

Conversely, even when the hands are in close contact with the head, if they are truly soft, the patient may be unaware of their presence, or experience them as a warm soft fluidity, through which the hands may seem to melt into the head in a way that is completely soft and comfortable.

This softness is not simply in the hands. It can only come from your whole being. So you need to soften in your heart, soften in your solar plexus, soften in your whole body, feel that softness spreading down through your head, neck, shoulders, upper arms, elbows, forearms, wrists, hands, fingers, thumbs, and palms. Feel your hands soften further with each out-breath, as if breathing out through your hands. Let your hands become so soft that you feel a sense of your hands melting into the head, the head melting into your hands – not so much you feeling the patient's head, as the head and your hands seeming to become one continuous structure, a sense of continuity, of interconnection, of melting into each other, a sense of your hands being immersed in a warm fluidic medium. When you feel that deep sense of melting into the matrix without separation between hands and head, then you are reaching an appropriate level of softness and a truer sense of engagement with the craniosacral system.

Exploring different levels of attention

Equally important is your level of attention. If your attention is excessively concentrated, intent, or intense, your patient may feel this, consciously or unconsciously, whether as an intensity, or as a discomfort – even if your hands are off the body, or some distance from the body.

Partly, this intensity may be conveyed through your hands. But partly, the intensity of thought itself will affect the patient through its effect on the matrix. So once again the therapist needs to develop the ability to maintain a less intense concentration, letting the attention expand out to a more relaxed, detached, open and receptive, spacious, meditative quality of mind. This does not of course mean losing connection with your patient, but rather finding the right balance of attention. In order to do this, you will need to develop the ability to keep your attention in two places at the same time, or in fact in more than two places at the same time.

This is a skill which may not come readily to every practitioner at first, but which can easily be developed over a few weeks or months of practice, enabling you to be:

- aware of yourself and of the patient simultaneously
- aware of the whole body at the same time as being aware of specific focal points within the body
- aware of the wider picture at the same time as details within that wider picture
- aware of the space around you and of yourself and the patient within that space, developing the ability to keep a part of your attention somewhere in the space above you – as if looking down from above, open and spacious – while at the same time aware of impressions arising within your patient's cranio-sacral system, and at the same time aware of yourself.

Exploring different tissue levels

Once you have developed the appropriate levels of physical contact and the appropriate levels of attention, you can use these skills to help in exploring different levels of tissues and energy within the body.

In order to develop all these skills, we will here present another practical tuning in process, similar to the one in Chapter 18, but with a specific emphasis on these three aspects of the process:

- levels of physical contact
- levels of attention
- levels of tissues within the body.

A second practical process of tuning in

Allow approximately 45 minutes

Start by entering into the same tuning in process as in Chapter 18, settling into position with the patient on the couch and the practitioner sitting at the head. As before, establish the appropriate state of the patient – encouraging

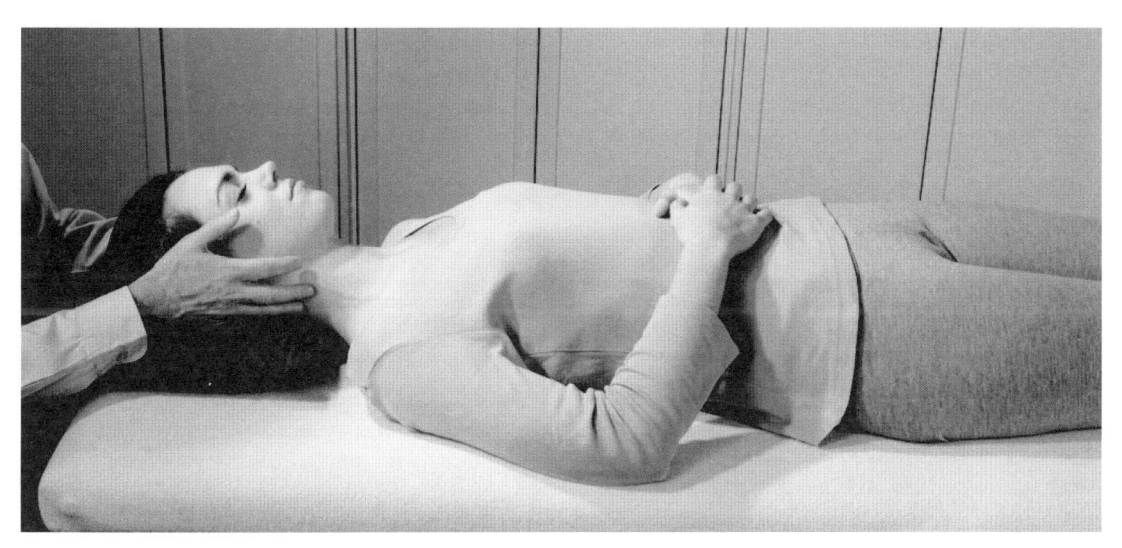

19.1 Let your hands be completely soft and relaxed, not holding the head, not gripping, just being there with a soft light contact

the patient to take a deep breath, relax and settle into an easeful state. As before, establish the appropriate state of the practitioner – giving attention to your own practitioner fulcrums, breathing easily (taking care not to breathe into your patient's face), sweeping your attention through your body, settling into a comfortable state of ease and relaxation.

Gently, slowly, carefully take up contact on the shoulders as before, engaging with the system through the shoulders over a period of 5–10 minutes.

When you are ready, make a gentle, careful transition to the sides of the head, engaging with the system through this contact on the head as before, being open to impressions of quality, symmetry and motion, observing whatever impressions arise.

After a further 5–10 minutes, having established this sense of engagement with the patient's system, maintain a constant awareness of the impressions that arise, and changes in those impressions, as you explore different levels of physical contact.

Exploring different levels of physical contact

Maintaining a constant awareness of any impressions that arise – quality, symmetry and motion – as you settle in, allow your hands to soften and relax as much as possible. Soften from your heart, soften from your solar plexus, soften through your head, neck and shoulders, your upper arms, elbows, forearms, wrists, hands, fingers, thumbs, and palms.

When you think that you have softened as much as possible, soften even more, feeling your hands soften further with each out-breath, as if breathing out through your hands. Soften so deeply that your hands seem to melt into the head.

Observe any changes in the impressions that you are perceiving.

Maintaining this constant and complete sense of softening, allow your contact to become a little lighter, so that your hands are barely touching the head (not a sudden deliberate movement, but a gentle, subtle sense of your hands softening away from the head).

Observe any impressions, and any changes in impressions.

Maintaining this constant and complete sense of softening throughout the process, allow your hands to become even lighter, so that you are barely touching the hair.

How does this affect what you are perceiving? Do you still feel connected to your patient's system? Do you feel more connected, or less connected?

Allow your contact to lighten even further so that your hands are no longer in contact with the head or the hair (again, not a sudden deliberate movement, but a gentle, subtle sense of your hands softening away from the head).

Do you feel impressions more clearly, more strongly, or less clearly, less strongly, or perhaps different impressions? Do you feel that the system is able to express more expansive movements and impressions?

Allow your contact to lighten even further, so that your hands are an inch or two (3–5 cm) from the head.

Do you still feel connected to your patient's system? Do you feel more connected, or less connected?

Move gradually back and forth through these different levels of physical contact, observing the different impressions that you experience at each different level.

Notice at which level you observe impressions most clearly, and how different impressions may be apparent through different levels of contact.

Observe that the system may seem to be pushing your hands away, or drawing them in, or inviting different responses on each side of the head – pushing one hand away, drawing the other hand in.

Notice that at certain levels you may feel a stronger connection, interaction, or sense of engagement with the system. Observe at which level you feel the strongest sense of engagement and allow your hands to settle into that level of contact.

Observe that the appropriate level may change from moment to moment in response to changes in your patient's system – perhaps expanding continuously for some time, then reaching a point of stillness and release, whereupon your hands may feel able to sink in towards the head again.

Gently let your hands explore and experiment, flowing seamlessly from one level of contact to another, guided by the responses within your patient's cranio-sacral system. Explore through the various levels, moving in from off the body to on the body, feeling where the system wants you to settle, where you feel the strongest sense of interconnection. Find the most appropriate level of physical contact for this particular patient at this particular moment within this particular interaction.

This description has taken several minutes to read. This is an appropriate length of time to spend tuning in as an exercise for a beginner. With time and experience, you will tune in more rapidly, sometimes instantly, sometimes within seconds, sometimes over several minutes according to circumstances.

Every time you tune in to a cranio-sacral system, explore different levels of physical contact to establish the most appropriate level for that interaction at that moment. Practise this repeatedly until it becomes instinctive and instant with every contact that you make.

Observe that the more space you allow, the more the cranio-sacral system can express itself and the more you are likely to feel. Observe that you may pick up different impressions at different levels of contact.

Throughout every cranio-sacral process, be aware of changes throughout the process, requiring lighter or deeper contacts according to the needs of the moment.

Be aware that the level of contact may vary from moment to moment within a treatment session, as patterns change, as releases occur, pushing your hands away, drawing your hands in, expanding, contracting, twisting turning, building up, becoming still, releasing, reorganising. So don't become attached to one particular level of contact (whether off the body or on the body) as being the best, or better than others, or your preferred option. Remain flexible to each situation, each patient, each treatment session, each moment within each session.

Exploring different levels of attention

Having established an appropriate level of physical contact, still maintaining your engagement with the system, you can now explore different levels of attention. The initial tendency is for the attention to be concentrated on the patient and on the impressions arising in the patient's system. So allow your attention to soften away from your patient.

Bring your attention away from your patient, back and up to the centre of your own forehead – your third eye. Observe how this affects your perception. Can you still maintain awareness of your patient's system while bringing your attention to your own forehead? Do you notice a difference in what you are feeling?

Take your attention deep inside the centre of your head – around your pituitary gland, your pineal gland, into the spaciousness of your third ventricle. Do you feel a sense of wider perception, a broader perspective? Does the system express itself more expansively, more clearly within that wider perspective? See what impressions arise as you continue to move your attention back away from your patient.

Take your attention to the back of your head, finding a comfortable place to rest your attention, around your straight sinus, just inside your occiput, or just outside your occiput, behind the back of your head, wherever it feels comfortable for your attention to rest.

Take your attention to the top of your head, letting your attention rest for a while on the crown of your head.

Let your attention float up from the top of your head to a point somewhere above your head – two or three feet above, a metre or so, wherever it feels comfortable for your attention to rest. Feel the greater sense of spaciousness, as you look down from above – like the artist standing back from her canvas to gain a broader perspective on her painting. Keep part of your attention somewhere up above you, while at the same time keeping another part of your attention on your patient, the impressions arising through your contact, the whole patient, the specific details within that wider picture. At the same time keep a part of your attention on yourself, aware of your own breathing, your own sense of ease and spaciousness, your own grounding, your own fulcrums and presence.

Allow your attention to float up through the ceiling, through the roof, as if looking down from somewhere above the building that you're in. Feel the greater sense of spaciousness. Observe how your patient's system responds to this greater spaciousness. Feel the lessening of intensity, the greater sense of ease, the broader perspective and the patient's greater responsiveness to this sense of ease and spaciousness.

Allow your attention to float up through the sky, out into space, as if looking down from a distant planet. Feel the vast sense of spaciousness and the infinitely broad perspective. Do you still feel connected to your patient? Do you still feel grounded in yourself? Can you still maintain a combined awareness of the patient, yourself and the vast spaciousness?

Observe that the more space you allow, the more your patient's system can express itself. Observe that at certain levels you may feel a stronger interconnection and interaction with the system. At other levels, whether close or far, you may feel less connection. Observe that the appropriate level may change from moment to moment in response to changes within your patient's system.

Explore different levels of attention, letting your attention shift seamlessly, from the distant planet, through the sky, to a point somewhere above your head, to inside your head – even right in to your patient's body, noting how this may perhaps feel too intense and invasive – sweeping gently in and out, to and fro, between the different perspectives. Establish the most appropriate level of attention for this particular interaction, with this particular patient, at this particular moment – bearing in mind that this may change from moment to moment, according to the responses within your patient's system.

Throughout every cranio-sacral process, be aware of the ever-changing needs of the moment, adapting your level of attention to the needs of the moment, allowing as much space as the cranio-sacral system needs to express itself fully. Practise this repeatedly throughout every treatment, until it becomes instinctive and instantaneous.

Develop the ability to see the whole picture – as if looking down from above – while at the same time observing minute detail within the process, without losing the whole picture. Develop the ability to be open, detached, spacious and meditative, while at the same time grounded, focused, alert and aware. Develop the ability to be both distant and present. Develop the ability to be aware simultaneously of yourself, your patient, your immediate environment, and the universe around you.

Exploring different tissue levels

Having established appropriate levels of physical contact and appropriate levels of attention, we can now explore different tissue levels.

Maintaining your engagement with your patient's system, your awareness of impressions arising from moment to moment, and your overview of the whole picture, be aware of the contact you are making with your patient's hair – feel the quality and characteristics of the hair. As you do so, you may notice not only the hair, but also impressions relating to the energy field that surrounds the body, perhaps experiencing it as heat, perhaps feeling it as a cushion of energy. (If patients have very little hair, let your attention rest where their hair would be if they had any – the intention here is actually to tune in to the energy field around the head, rather than the hair itself.)

In due course, be aware that on one level, this head is composed of a bony cranium. Experience the head as a solid bony cranium. Let your attention rest gently on the *bones* of the cranium, be aware of the whole cranium – observe the qualities and characteristics that you feel, the sense of hardness, the sense of solidity.

In due course, be aware that within this cranium, there is a soft membranous lining. Allow your attention to penetrate deeper to the *membranes* lining the cranium. Experience the cranium as a soft membranous balloon. See how this affects what you feel, perhaps feeling that the head seems to become softer, more pliable, more malleable. Allow that malleability to be expressed, feeling the head softly moving – bulging, twisting, expanding, contracting.

In due course, be aware that these membranes contain fluid. Allow your attention to penetrate deeper to the *fluids* contained within the membrane system. Observe any changes in your impressions. Experience this cranio-sacral system as a fluid-filled balloon, fluent, flowing and fluctuating. Feel the fluidic motion. Allow that fluidic motion to be expressed freely – rippling, swirling, ebbing, flowing. Allow your hands to become absorbed into this warm fluidic motion.

Let your hands be washed this way and that by the gently fluctuating fluidic movements.

In due course, be aware that at a deeper level this head is composed of cells, of molecules, of subatomic particles, of elementary particles, a mass of vibrating particles in constant motion and with infinite potential for changing shape (like a swarm of bees, each individual bee busily buzzing, while the whole swarm continuously shifts in shape). Allow your attention to penetrate to a deeper and more subtle level, a quantum level. Experience this cranio-sacral system as a ball of *energy* – a mass of elementary particles – perpetually vibrating and with infinite malleability, a coherent energetic matrix. Feel the movement of the vital forces within, gently shifting this way and that. Let your hands melt into this ball of energy to be moulded by this malleable mass.

Explore the different levels. Let your attention shift seamlessly from one level to another. See how your attention can be drawn to specific structures – bony, membranous, fluid or energetic – and how it can also be aware of the whole integrated mass, the whole matrix. See how you can choose to explore solid bony structures, pliable membranous tissues, fluent fluidic fluctuations, or the malleable mass of the molecular matrix. See how you might identify individual bones that feel free or restricted, areas of membrane that feel tight or loose, areas of fluid that may feel more or less fluent, areas of energy that might feel blocked.

Throughout every cranio-sacral interaction, be aware of all levels simultaneously, allowing your attention to shift to different levels according to the needs of the moment.

As you come towards the end of the session, let your attention return more specifically to the rhythmic motion, observing the even balanced flow of rhythmic motion, whether at the cranio-sacral rhythm level or the middle tide level. If you are feeling cranio-sacral rhythm, allow your attention to deepen and open into greater spaciousness to see if you might encounter the middle tide motion.

As before, as you come to the end of the session, let your attention rise to the surface, summarise everything you have felt throughout this process, defining every quality, asymmetry and movement as precisely as you can, every change, every response to different levels of perception. Refine your definitions to give them greater clarity and significance. Gently, softly, let the process come to a settled completion and conclusion. Allow your hands to float away from the head, so softly that your patient may not be aware that they have come away.

Chapter 20

Opening Up the System
Settling and Grounding

This chapter covers the second stage in the four-stage integrated treatment framework:
1. Engagement (tuning in).
2. *Opening up the system (settling and grounding).*
3. Core treatment.
4. Completion.

The emotional centres

As we go about our day-to-day lives, we need to maintain appropriate boundaries between the outside world and our inner selves. It is neither practical nor sensible to expose our deepest sensitivities to the potentially invasive vagaries of day-to-day life.

Inevitably we all wear a protective cloak – physically, mentally, emotionally and spiritually – and this is reflected in our physical bodies and consequently in our cranio-sacral systems.

This defensive shield is present to some extent throughout our bodies. Tension can be held anywhere and everywhere in the body. Each individual may hold particular protective tensions in particular areas. There are certain areas of the body, however, which are universally common areas of holding – physical holding and emotional holding – reflecting into the body as tissue tension and restricting access to deeper levels of the person's being. There are clear physiological reasons for this.

Four such areas are of particular significance:
- the *heart centre* – in the upper thoracic region
- the *solar plexus centre* – in the abdominal region
- the *pelvic centre* – in the pelvic region
- the *suboccipital centre* – in the suboccipital region.

The tensions held in these four centres are reflected in the quality, symmetry and motion of the area – the quality perhaps feeling tight, tense or agitated, the symmetry drawing in to focal points of tightness, and the motion restricted so that rhythmic motion is not being expressed freely. These tensions restrict blood flow, nerve supply and the free expression of vitality and therefore predispose to malfunction, dysfunction and disease within the surrounding tissues, organs, and muscles, with repercussions of restricted motion, vitality and energy flow throughout the body.

Crucial benefits

The release of restrictions, agitation and disturbances in these areas provides several crucial benefits. It is *therapeutic in itself*. It also *opens up the system, enabling access to deeper levels* of the cranio-sacral system, and consequently a more effective response to the cranio-sacral process. It therefore serves as a valuable preparatory release in the initial stages of every treatment, adapted as always according to the needs of the patient. Releasing these emotional centres is also a crucial component in *settling and grounding* the patient in preparation for subsequent treatment.

Failure to release these areas, especially where it is particularly needed, is likely to block progress, leading to reduced access to deeper levels of the system, decreased response and therefore less effective treatment. Failure to address these areas may also lead to adverse reactions and discomfort, stirring up the tensions held in these areas by trying to access deeper levels without first preparing the way and establishing a settled stable environment within which to explore deeper patterns.

Underlying reasons

The reasons why these four areas are particularly significant can be recognised on many different levels, reflecting different body systems.

Throughout the body, certain key areas can be seen to be of greater significance than others on many different levels; and the arrangement of different levels of structure can be seen to be reflecting each other – gross structures reflecting more delicate structures, reflecting more subtle levels of being. An obvious example is the spine, with the bony vertebral column, lined with the softer structure of the membranes, in turn containing the subtler level of the cerebrospinal fluid, in turn enveloping the delicate and vital spinal cord, and also reflecting the deeper subtlety of the midline energetic core of the body.

Similarly, in these four emotional centres, we can again see several different levels of structure, or different systems, gathered together in specific regions, reflecting the relevance of those specific areas.

Sympathetic nerve plexi

All fours areas are focal points of sympathetic nerve plexi. The sympathetic nervous system (which we will look at in greater detail later) is the part of our nervous system which processes emotional responses to our environment. The particular sympathetic plexi involved at these emotional centres are:

- the cardiac plexus – in the thoracic region
- the solar plexus – in the abdominal region
- the pelvic plexus – in the pelvic region
- the superior cervical sympathetic ganglia – in the suboccipital region.

Chakras

Within the context of the oriental system of chakras, these regions are focal points as chakras or energy centres:

- the heart chakra – in the thorax
- the solar plexus chakra – in the abdomen
- the root chakra – in the pelvis
- the throat chakra – in the suboccipital region.

Both of the above systems provide ample explanation for why emotional tensions are particularly held in these areas.

Endocrine glands

Furthermore, there are focal areas within the endocrine system:

- the thymus gland – in the thoracic region
- the adrenal glands – in the abdominal region
- the gonads – in the pelvic region
- the thyroid and parathyroid glands – in the cervical region.

Fascia (the transverse diaphragms)

From a structural point of view, these regions are also significant, since they are all *transverse diaphragms* – areas where the body tissues are more transversely orientated as compared with the longitudinal orientation of tissues through most of the body. This specifically involves the fascia in these regions – since fascia envelops every structure in the body, including these transversely orientated structures.

- The *thoracic inlet*, in the upper thoracic region, is the area where the rib cage closes in to form a narrow inlet through which the oesophagus, trachea, jugular veins and vagus nerves enter the upper thorax, as well as an outlet for the carotid arteries and sympathetic nerve supply exiting from the thorax and passing up into the head.
- The *thoracic diaphragm* forms the division between the thorax above and the abdomen below, consisting of a transversely orientated muscle (the diaphragm), which like all muscles is enveloped in fascia.
- The *pelvic diaphragm* consists of two muscles – levator ani and coccygeus – forming a muscular hammock across the pelvic floor; again like all muscles this hammock is enveloped in fascia.
- In the *suboccipital region*, the base of the cranium closes in to form the foramen magnum where the cranium sits on top of the cervical spine with many surrounding suboccipital muscles and consequently many layers of enveloping fascia.

Each of these systems has components elsewhere in the body, but these four regions represent particular aggregations of significant structures on the various levels.

Emotional centres

Above all, these areas can be regarded as emotional centres, where significant levels of emotion are felt, expressed, suppressed and held in most people. This is perhaps most clearly evident in the solar plexus, where most people will have experienced 'butterflies in the tummy' while awaiting an exam, an interview, or a public performance, or other stressful events which stimulate the sympathetic nervous system (along with reactions in the organs supplied through these areas). These sensations of fluttering or agitation reflect the neurological activity occurring in the synapses of the coeliac ganglia in that area. The common response to such sensations is to suppress them, to control them, to hold them in, to tighten up in that area; hence, persistent stress or emotional suppression leads to a chronic, deeply ingrained tension in these emotional centres (with corresponding disturbance and disease in related organs).

All of these systems – plexi, chakras, glands, fascia, emotional centres – are significant; all of them will reflect the emotional tensions held into these areas and it is helpful to be aware of all of these factors as we allow the unfolding of cranio-sacral principles in each of these areas, enabling the release of blockage and restriction, enabling the settling of agitation and emotional disturbance, enabling the free expression of vitality, enabling easier access to deeper levels of the patient's being.

In order to address these emotional centres, we will, for each of the areas, first establish a comfortable and appropriate hand contact, then allow the unfolding of the usual fundamental principles of the inherent treatment process – engage, allow, follow, to points of stillness, release, and reorganisation – or whatever variations of them may arise.

The heart centre

The heart centre (thoracic inlet) is in the upper thoracic region. It is not a specific anatomical structure. It is an area of emotional holding, as reflected in the various systems described above. Engaging with the heart centre involves an awareness of:

- the heart centre
- the cardiac and pulmonary plexi
- the heart chakra
- the heart, the lungs
- the upper thoracic spine
- the sympathetic nerve supply emanating from the upper thoracic vertebral levels and supplying the heart and lungs and other local structures
- the thoracic inlet and the structures passing through this area
- the fascia enveloping the various structures in this area
- the emotional factors that contribute to stimulation of this area, with consequent tensions and activation of the organs and structures and energy field in this area
- the whole matrix
- how all of these various factors interact and influence each other.

It involves feeling the emotional holding in that area, with an understanding of the underlying factors that might be held there, together with the tensions in the tissues, the organs and the energy field that result from that and which may contribute to disturbances ranging from tension, discomfort, pain, palpitations or anxiety to asthma or cardiac pathology.

The term heart centre reflects all of these elements and the interactions between them. Working with the heart centre involves engaging with all of these elements, feeling the qualities, symmetries and movements that they express, and responding to them within the usual cranio-sacral framework in order to bring greater integration of the local area and of the whole person.

The process

With your patient lying supine on the treatment couch (see Figure 20.1), take up a position sitting to one side of them, above the level of the shoulder, at the corner of the couch. Invite your patient to arch their upper back so that you can slide your hand under the upper thorax between the top of the shoulder blades (using the hand nearest to your patient's head). This hand is vertically orientated, with the fingers pointing more or less straight down towards the sacrum, the fingers fitting snugly between the shoulder blades for greater comfort of both patient and practitioner.

The palm of your hand will be around the cervico-thoracic junction, with the spinous process of the seventh cervical vertebra (the 'vertebra prominens' or most prominent vertebra) sitting roughly into the centre of your palm.

Invite your patient to settle back down, resting onto your hand and relaxing completely.

Check with your patient that this hand position is comfortable. Ensure that you and your hand are also comfortable, adjusting your sitting position as necessary in order to enable maximum comfort. *(In order to work most effectively as a craniosacral therapist, it is essential that you ensure your own comfort and balance at all times.)*

Once you are settled, bring your other hand slowly and gently to rest on to the upper thorax, approaching slowly, respecting the energy field, coming in lightly with a butterfly touch, gently allowing the weight of your hand to settle onto the body. This hand is transversely orientated across the front of the upper chest. The most appropriate position for your hand is just below the bony prominences which form the medial ends of the clavicles. Take care that your hand and thumb do not rest above this level onto the throat, causing discomfort and tension. Allow your forearm to relax completely, sinking down gradually, until it comes to rest gently but comfortably onto your patient's shoulder. Be sure to relax your own shoulder and arm, not holding on to any unnecessary tension.

As you settle into the contact, come back into yourself, breathing easily, letting go physically and mentally, and settling your own practitioner fulcrums. Maintain a relaxed detached state of

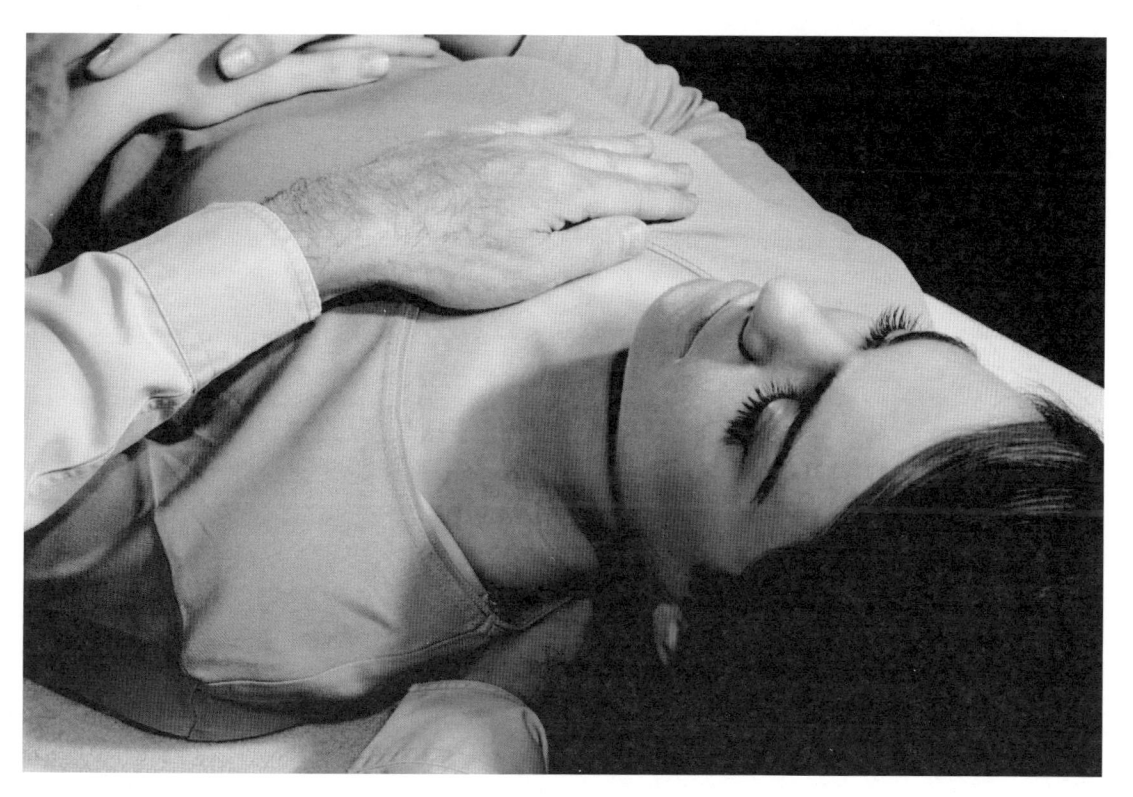

20.1 Contact for the heart centre

mind, open and receptive, alert and attentive, maintaining an overview as if looking down from above while at the same time observing the detailed impressions arising between your hands. Maintain a consistent awareness of yourself and your own fulcrums. Feel the increasing sense of interconnection between the patient's system and your hands. Feel the space between your hands, feel the quality of that space, the spaciousness of that space. Feel an increasing awareness of the patient's whole body, as well as the local area between your hands. Observe the various impressions emerging from this interconnection.

Observe impressions of *quality* – tightness, looseness, softness, hardness, warmth, coolness, activity, stillness, calmness, agitation. What do these impressions tell you about the nature of this person and about what is going on in this particular region? Is the patient tense, held, contained; soft, open, warm; agitated, anxious, restless, settled, still? If there is stillness, is it the stillness of a peaceful calmness, or the stillness of tightly held contained stuckness? Observe the changes in quality as the process evolves.

Observe impressions of *symmetry*. Is there a greater tightness on one side or another – increased activity, stillness or restriction or resistance on one side, or in one area or another? Do the body tissues seem to be pulling in any particular direction? Do your hands feel drawn towards one shoulder – perhaps with one hand, perhaps with both – towards the shoulder blade, towards an old fracture of the clavicle, towards the heart, towards one of the lungs, down towards the diaphragm, up into the neck, or pulling medially into the thoracic spine, into the rhomboid muscles, or towards a particular vertebral level? What do these impressions of symmetry or asymmetry tell you about this patient, and about focal points of physical tension or injury within this region of the body?

(Recognise that while movement and activity are more readily felt in the body, it is restriction of mobility, or lack of movement, that is more significant from a cranio-sacral perspective since this represents blockage of cranio-sacral motion, restriction to the free expression of vitality, and represents the focal point or source of a dysfunction.)

Observe impressions of *motion* – vibration, pulsation, swirling, squirming, twisting, turning, pulling, shifting, or whatever movements or combination of movements you may encounter. What do these tell you about the patient? Is there agitation or anxiety (vibration, fluttering) in the heart centre? Is the heart centre tightly held and closed (contracted, immobile)? Is there active emotional turmoil (swirling)? Is it peaceful, open and calm (soft stillness)? Or are there persistent pulls drawing you towards specific structures, organs, muscles, bones, reflecting injury or disease, recent or in the distant past.

Observe the combination of quality, symmetry and motion. See what it tells you about this person and this region of the body.

Allow the system to express itself, observing any subtle changes and movements. Follow any pulls, twists and turns to points of stillness – not doing anything, just letting your hands be washed this way and that by the subtle fluidic movements. Points of stillness may occur in milliseconds (so quickly that they've released almost before you notice them, or even without you noticing them consciously); they may occur in a few seconds, or over several minutes. Stay with each point of stillness until it softens, dissolves and releases. Allow the system to reorganise and reorientate – settling into a more balanced and freely mobile state.

As the process continues, feel the changes in quality as the system becomes more settled; feel the greater degree of symmetry as resistances and pulls release; and feel the greater fluency of motion as the release of resistances allows a freer flow of energy through the area and reflecting through the whole body.

As the superficial restrictions release and the system becomes more settled, you may encounter deeper, more persistent resistances. Allow these patterns to be expressed in the same way, as directed by the subtle movements within the body, drawing your hands this way and that, encountering points of stillness and staying with the points of balanced tension or stillness until the resistance softens. For more deeply embedded resistances and chronic restrictions, be prepared to stay longer in the stillness (perhaps several minutes, perhaps longer) waiting for it to soften.

Superficial resistances will release readily. Deeper, more chronic resistances will take longer. Not every resistance will resolve completely in one session, so for the deeper more chronic resistances you may need to be content with partial releases. Chronic resistance may release through a series of partial releases, opening up layer by layer. Resistances may also be maintained by other restrictions elsewhere in the body in a complex interaction of pulls and compensations, so by working through the body and then returning to a resistance, you may find a greater response in that specific area once other restrictions have released.

When the system feels settled following a release, or a series of releases, and the quality, symmetry and motion are such that the process feels complete, then you can allow the process to come to an end. Release your attention from the area. Let your upper hand float away from the body gently and slowly, taking care not to introduce any sudden, abrupt movements that might disturb or create shock in the body. Slide your lower hand out from under the thorax and prepare to move on.

The solar plexus centre

The solar plexus centre (thoracic diaphragm) is in the abdominal region. Like the heart centre, working with the solar plexus centre involves an awareness of various structures:

- the solar plexus
- the coeliac ganglia
- the superior mesenteric plexus
- the lower thoracic spine
- the sympathetic outflow from the lower thoracic and thoraco-lumbar spine
- the thoracic diaphragm
- the surrounding organs – the stomach, the liver, the adrenal glands and other local organs
- the fascia enveloping all of these.

It also involves an understanding of the emotions and stresses held there and the underlying factors that might contribute to those emotional and physical tensions and the consequences, discomforts, or pathologies – including digestive disorders, duodenal ulcers, irritable bowel syndrome and many others – that might arise from the interaction between the emotions, the sympathetic nervous system, the organs, and the fascia – just as in the heart centre.

The process

Sitting at the side of the patient, a little below waist level, your chair angled to face towards your patient's opposite shoulder, invite your patient to arch their back so that you can slide your hand transversely under the back around the thoraco-lumbar vertebral level (using the hand nearest your patient's head).

Allow the vertebral column to rest comfortably into the palm of your hand with your fingers extending to the erector spinae muscles on the far side of the spine, the heel of your hand resting under the erector spinae muscles on the near side of the spine.

Check with your patient that this hand position is comfortable. Adjust as necessary. Ensure that you are comfortable in your hand position, your arm and your shoulder. Ensure that your body is not unduly twisted or under any postural strain or tension. Adjust your sitting position as necessary to ensure maximum comfort.

Ensure that your patient allows their back to relax down completely onto your hand. (Some patients are very considerate and concerned for the welfare of your hand, and will hold their back up in order to avoid squashing it. This is not helpful to them or to you or to the therapeutic process, so encourage them to relax down onto the couch.) Invite them to take another deep breath and to let go completely.

Once you are settled, bring your other hand gently and slowly to rest onto your patient's abdomen, vertically orientated with the fingers pointing up towards the head, the heel of the hand resting into the soft abdominal area between the two halves of the rib cage, the fingers spreading out across the rib cage to gain a wider perspective.

Bring your contact in slowly and gently, respecting the energy field and coming to rest lightly with a butterfly touch onto the body. Gradually allow the weight of your hand to settle onto the body, relaxing your hand completely, allowing your forearm and elbow to rest gently onto your patient's ilium or hip region, relaxing your shoulder.

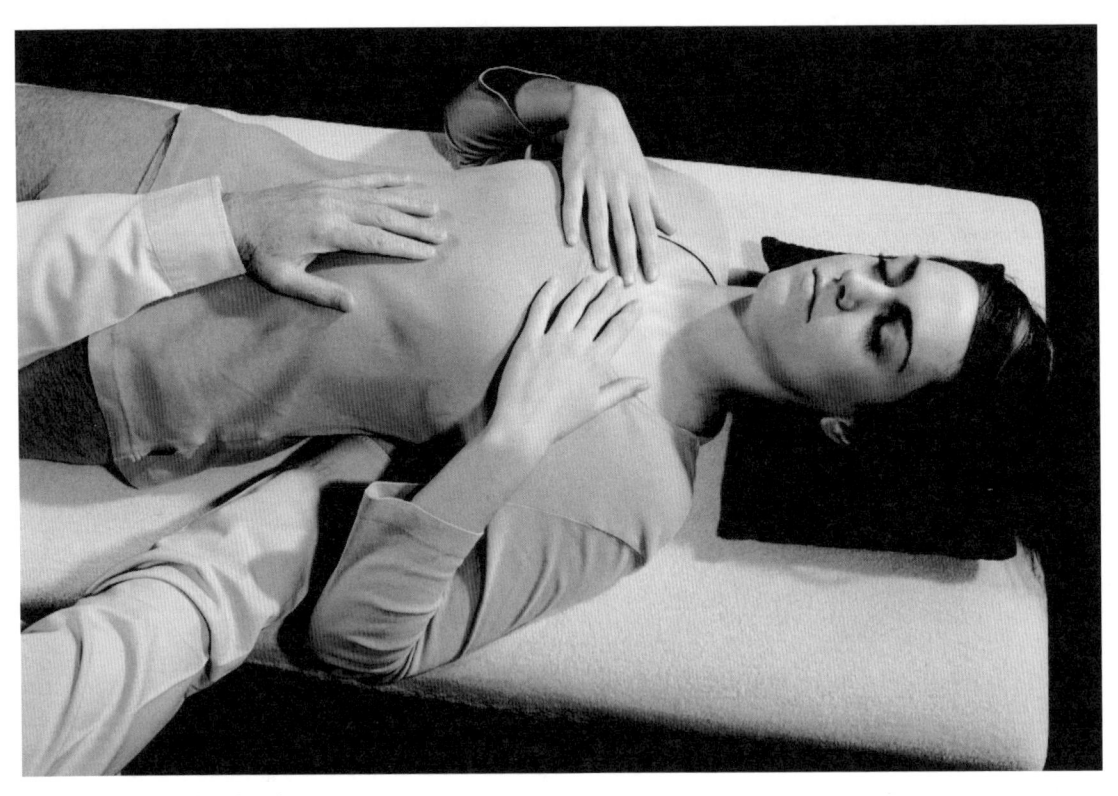

20.2 Contact for the solar plexus centre

Come back into yourself, breathing easily and re-establishing your own practitioner fulcrums. As you settle into the contact, follow the same principles as outlined above for the heart centre.

Feel the space between your hands. Feel the quality of that space, the fluidity of that space, and any movement within that space. Observe the various impressions of quality, symmetry and motion that arise from this interconnection. What do they tell you about the patient? Is there a mass of tension held in the solar plexus (from many years of suppressed, contained emotion) or is it soft and open? Is there agitation or turmoil, current or longstanding, or is it calm and peaceful? If there is stillness, is it a stillness of being stuck and tightly held, or a stillness of being at ease? Is your attention drawn up into the diaphragm? Is the diaphragm tight, held, breathing only shallowly? Are you drawn towards the stomach on the left, or the liver on the right, or the gall bladder, or the kidneys, or the adrenal glands, or to muscular, fascial, and other soft tissue pulls, or into the spine at a particular vertebral segment.

How does the solar plexus area feel relative to the heart centre? Are they similar, or different? Do they reflect each other, or contrast with each other? Do they feel connected (the control of the solar plexus keeping the emotions of the heart at bay)? Do you feel drawn up towards the heart centre, perhaps on one side more than the other, or down towards the pelvis? Is there a consistent pattern of tightness or restriction down one side of the body, and where is its most significant focal point within that broader pattern of tension?

Allow the system to express itself, observing any subtle changes and movements. Identify the focal points of resistance, the fulcrums within the matrix, the points of resistance towards which the tissues, the movements, and your hands seem to be drawn. Define these focal points more specifically – the gall bladder, an adrenal gland, the solar plexus, a particular vertebral segment or muscle – identifying the relevant structures in detail, while at the same time maintaining an overview of the wider perspective of the whole person, the combination of the detail and the wider perspective providing you with the foundation for your overall diagnosis of the patient and their situation.

Stay with the points of stillness until they soften, dissolve and release. Allow the system to reorganise and reorientate – settling into a more balanced and freely mobile state. Feel the changes in quality, symmetry and motion throughout the body as the system becomes more integrated.

When the process is complete, release your attention from the area. Gently release your upper hand. Invite your patient to arch their back so that you can slide your other hand out from under the spine and prepare to move on.

The pelvic centre

Working with the pelvic centre (pelvic diaphragm) involves an awareness of:

- the pelvic plexus, also known as the inferior hypogastric plexus
- the pelvic diaphragm
- the root chakra
- the sacrum
- the sympathetic and parasympathetic neurological associations in the area
- the various pelvic organs – uterus, ovaries, bladder, prostate, colon
- the emotional and physical tensions held in those structures
- the whole matrix of the body, and the interaction of all these various components with their possible repercussions – including menstrual disorders, cystitis, genital dysfunction and others – just as in the heart centre and solar plexus.

The process

Sit at the side of your patient, a little below the level of the pelvis, again with your chair angled up to face your patient's opposite shoulder. Invite your patient to bend their knees up, with the soles of their feet on the couch. Ask them to place their feet well apart and knees together for greater stability. Invite your patient to raise their pelvis so you can take up contact with your fingers under the sacrum (using the hand nearest your patient's feet). Your hand is best placed vertically orientated, fingers pointing up towards the head, the curve of the sacrum sitting comfortably into your fingers. The sacrum is resting on your fingers rather than weighing heavily onto your hand, your fingers slightly separated to accommodate

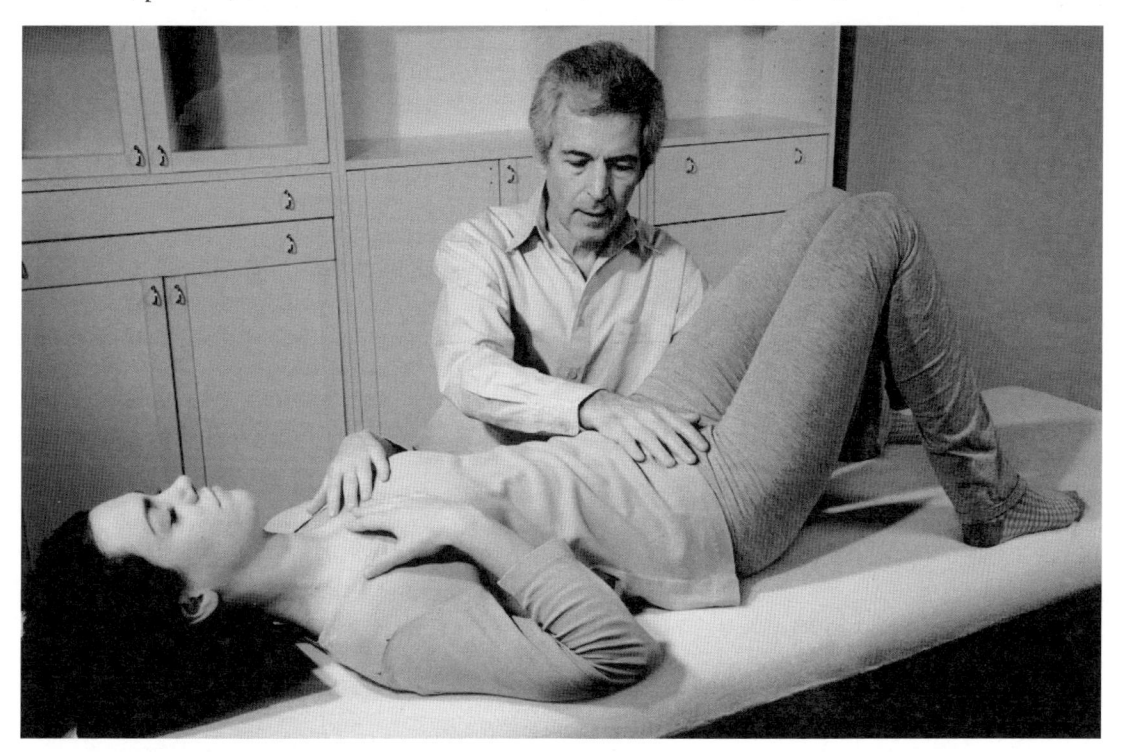

20.3 Contact for the pelvic centre – oblique view

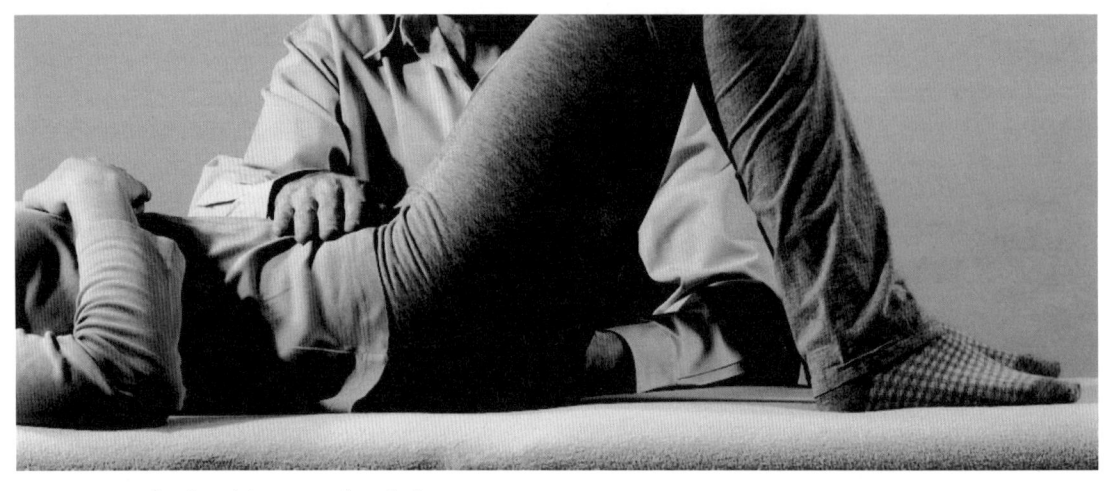

20.4 Contact for the pelvic centre – lateral view

the spinous processes of the sacrum, so that they don't dig into your fingers or hand. Invite the patient to let the weight of their pelvis sink down into the couch, ensuring that they relax and let go completely.

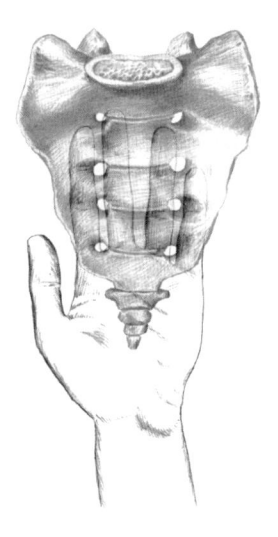

20.5 Contact for the sacrum – the sacrum is resting on your fingers rather than weighing heavily onto your hand, your fingers slightly separated to accommodate the spinous processes of the sacrum

Check with your patient that this hand position is comfortable. Ensure that your hand is also comfortable, and that it is symmetrically balanced and centred. If necessary, ask your patient to raise their pelvis again so that you can adjust your hand position. (It is vital to establish a comfortable balanced position. You won't be able to operate most effectively if you are making do with a position that does not feel satisfactory, whether for you or for your patient. A common tendency is to place the hand too far up under the sacrum, with the weight of the body weighing heavily onto it, with the result that your hand becomes numb, thereby reducing your sensitivity; this is not helpful or necessary; taking up a contact with just your fingers, rather than your hand, under the sacrum is far more comfortable and effective.)

Relax through your hand, arm and shoulder. Ensure that you are comfortable throughout your body, adjusting your sitting position as necessary. Once you are comfortable and settled, bring your other hand slowly and gently to rest onto the body over the front of the pelvis. Your hand can be placed transversely orientated across the body just above the pubic area. As your hand comes to rest with a butterfly touch, gradually allow the weight of your hand to sink down onto the body, letting your elbow and forearm come to rest onto your patient's ilium. Relax your shoulder and arm.

Come back into yourself, breathing easily and settling your own practitioner fulcrums.

As you feel an increasing sense of interconnection between your two systems, follow the principles outlined above. Feel the space between your hands. See how this pelvic area feels relative to the heart centre and solar plexus. How does the quality of each area compare or differ? Is there a consistent quality throughout the body, or variations from place to place? What do these variations tell you? Is there a greater degree of tightness, tension or restriction on one side or the other? Is this pattern of tightness reflected consistently up through one side of the body, or twisting across to the opposite side of the body?

Are you drawn to any specific focal points of resistance – a sacro-iliac joint on one side or the other, the bladder, an ovary? Does the sacrum seem to be twisting to one side, or pulling up one side – and if so, where is it pulling to, and how does this relate to what you have felt previously at the heart and solar plexus?

As always, identify the specific focal points of resistance towards which you are drawn, within the perspective of the whole person, thereby building up your overall picture and diagnosis of the patient. In the meantime, allow the system to express itself, follow to points of stillness and release. Feel the quality becoming softer and looser, the symmetry becoming more balanced, the motion becoming more settled and freely expressed. Feel the whole system settling into a more balanced, integrated state.

As you do so, the patient is likely to feel an increasing sense of ease, calmness and well-being as their body (and mind) come into greater balance and harmony. They may experience this physically, they may experience it mentally, or emotionally. They may feel the release of specific tensions. Most of all, they are likely to feel a more abstract overall sense of greater ease and well-being physically, mentally, emotionally and spiritually – even though at this stage we are only opening up the system.

When the process is complete, release your attention from the area. Gently release your upper hand. Invite your patient to lift their pelvis so that you can slide your other hand out from under the sacrum and prepare to move on.

The suboccipital area

The suboccipital area is a little different from the other emotional centres, and so deserves a chapter of its own.

Chapter 21

The Suboccipital Region

The significance of the suboccipital region

The suboccipital region, where the occipital bone at the base of the cranium meets the upper cervical spine, is an area of particular significance. It is a focal point around which many issues tend to accumulate. Restriction here not only is particularly common, but also can have particularly far-reaching consequences on health and function.

There are many reasons for this – and these reasons can be divided broadly into two categories:

- *It is an area where many crucial structures are located and through which many vital pathways pass.*
- *It is an area that is particularly susceptible to trauma, injury and tension.*

Structures in the suboccipital area

There are a great many crucial structures located in, and passing through, the suboccipital region – connecting brain to body and body to brain – with essential functions of blood supply to the brain and overall control of vital functions throughout the body. Restrictions here can therefore be particularly debilitating.

Vertebral arteries

The *vertebral arteries* are one of the main providers of arterial supply to the brain, and yet they follow a tortuous, right-angled, S-bend route over the atlas vertebra and in through the foramen magnum, a pathway which renders them liable to be squashed between the occiput and atlas. This can be a major contributory factor in reducing oxygen distribution to the brain and may be relevant to anyone who has suffered a head or neck injury or who holds significant levels of tension in this area. It is perhaps most noticeable in elderly people, where it can lead to dizziness, vagueness and fainting. But compression of this vital arterial pathway may be of greatest significance in babies and children, whether through compression during birth or due to falls and head injuries, restricting the blood supply to the brain and potentially limiting brain development with consequent ramifications throughout life.

Carotid arteries

The *carotid arteries* are the other major providers of arterial supply to the brain. They pass up through the carotid canal, immediately in front of the suboccipital joints with the atlas vertebra. They again follow a right-angled, S-bend route, but in this case are a little less vulnerable.

These two paired arteries between them (the vertebral and carotid arteries) provide the total blood supply and therefore oxygen supply to the brain, and so constriction of these vessels – whether from birth or from subsequent injuries and tensions – can have significant repercussions on brain function.

Internal jugular veins

The *internal jugular veins* provide the channels of drainage for virtually all venous blood from the cranium. They pass through the jugular foramen on each side of the suboccipital region. Restriction of these major veins may lead to venous congestion within the cranium, and stagnation of all fluids, including arterial blood and cerebrospinal fluid, around the brain.

Vagus nerves

The principal function of the *vagus nerves* is the regulation of parasympathetic supply to most of the viscera – including the heart, lungs, stomach, spleen, liver, gall bladder, small intestine and large intestine. They therefore play a major part in the regulation of cardiac, pulmonary and digestive function. They are very often one of the factors involved in infant colic. They also pass through the jugular foramina. The vagus also serves various other functions relating to swallowing, taste and receiving sensory information from the viscera.

Accessory nerves

The *accessory nerves* supply the trapezius and sterno-mastoid muscles, and also pass through the jugular foramina. Vicious cycles of mutual interaction between the jugular foramina, the accessory nerves and these muscles are a common source of problems. They are almost invariably involved in cases of torticollis – whether infant or adult, particularly arising from birth trauma – as well as other neck imbalances and shoulder tension.

The accessory nerves also assist the vagus with its functions in the throat.

Glossopharyngeal nerves

The *glossopharyngeal nerves* receive sensation from the pharynx, larynx and palate, and also work in close conjunction with the vagus nerve in relation to swallowing. They are also concerned (through their parasympathetic component) with the secretion of saliva from the parotid glands. They also pass through the jugular foramina.

Carotid nerves

The *carotid nerves* are the sympathetic nerve supply to the head. This sympathetic supply arises from the upper thoracic spine, passing up through the neck, synapsing at the superior cervical sympathetic ganglia on each side of the suboccipital region. It then continues as the carotid nerves, entering the cranium through the carotid canal on each side along with the carotid arteries. Compression of the sympathetic supply to the head anywhere along its pathway can have significant implications for the eyes and for the innervation of the meninges and the blood vessels within the cranium. They are particularly susceptible to compressions and tensions in the suboccipital region.

Superior cervical sympathetic ganglia

The *superior cervical sympathetic ganglia*, located on each side of the vertebral bodies of the upper cervical vertebrae, are the crucial points of synapse for sympathetic nerve supply to the cranium, again with vital functions including pupil dilation and regulation of blood vessel constriction within the cranium. They are located on either side of the upper cervical vertebrae in the suboccipital region, and overstimulation due to injury, tension or restriction here may readily influence not only these specific functions but also engender repercussions throughout the sympathetic nervous system as a whole.

Nuclei of the vagus

The *nuclei of the vagus* contain the cell bodies of sensory neurons carrying sensation from the viscera. They are also located within and around the jugular foramen on each side.

Suboccipital muscles

There is a particular accumulation of small *suboccipital muscles* congregated around the base of the cranium and upper cervical spine, whose role is to maintain balance and equilibrium in this crucial area and around these many vital structures, together with other larger surrounding muscles.

One of these muscles is of particular significance. The *rectus capitis posterior minor* attaches bilaterally from the atlas vertebra to the occiput, but it has a bridge of fibrous soft tissue extending from the muscle, passing between the atlas and occiput, to attach to the dural membrane. The function of this bridge is not clear, perhaps to draw any slack membrane out of the way in order to avoid compression of the dura during backward bending of the neck. It can be of substantial clinical significance, since tension, restriction or imbalance in this muscle – perhaps due to a whiplash or other neck injury – can have direct restrictive effects on the dura locally, and consequently on the whole reciprocal tension membrane system and on cerebrospinal fluid flow;

this can be a significant but often unrecognised factor in maintaining a debilitated state of health, particularly severe chronic head and neck pain.

With so many crucial structures present in such a specific localised area, it is clear that any injury, trauma or tension here could have widespread repercussions; and yet this is the area of the body most susceptible to trauma and tension, perhaps more than anywhere else in the body.

From the very beginning of life in the outside world, starting with the birth process, the suboccipital region is the area most susceptible to the compressive forces and the shock effects of *birth trauma*, as the head is pushed back into backward bending and compressed down into the spine. This can leave patterns of restriction which may have lifelong effects if not addressed.

Head and neck injuries from falls, accidents, whiplash effects and sports injuries – from childhood through adulthood – will all tend to gravitate towards this focal point, as the pivotal area around which the cranium sits on the upper cervical spine, and as the many small suboccipital muscles struggle to maintain balance and equilibrium.

Structural imbalances throughout the body due to injuries, accidents or tensions – in the pelvis, the legs, the spine or anywhere else in the body – tend to put strain on the suboccipital area. The body adapts its position and posture to compensate for any imbalances. One of the principal priorities of the body is to keep the eyes level. Consequently much of this adaptation and compensation will occur at the subocciput, again mediated by adaptations and tension in the subocciptal muscles.

Postural imbalances readily result in strain and tension here for the same reasons. The habitual postural patterns of modern society, from sitting (perhaps reluctantly, bored and collapsed) at school desks for hours on end, and subsequently at office desks and in car seats, along with many other common positions of postural collapse prevalent in everyday life, further contribute to the strain and tension imposed on the suboccipital area.

The suboccipital region is one of the most common sites for the holding of *emotional tension*. The instinctive reaction of any mammal under threat or pressure is to contract in the suboccipital region, pulling its head protectively down into its neck. Consider, for example, a cat reacting to a sudden loud noise. Similarly, humans under persistent stress tend to contract and tighten in this area as a matter of habit. Day-to-day tensions will readily accumulate here, but most significantly, chronic patterns of tension and pressure will create deeply ingrained patterns of restriction and blockage in this crucial region – as is reflected by its inclusion as one of the four principal emotional centres.

The combination of all the above factors means that this suboccipital region is very commonly restricted and therefore very commonly in need of attention to release the potentially debilitating effects of blockage here – and yet it is an area that is often neglected.

Consequences
Ranging from colic to poor brain development

In babies, the consequences can be particularly significant, not only in terms of their immediate symptoms, but also in terms of their long-term development. As mentioned above, compression of this area is particularly common during the birth process. The effects on the sympathetic and parasympathetic nerve structures travelling through the area can be associated with the symptoms experienced by so many babies – colic, poor sleep, restlessness – often developing into longer term consequences of hyperactivity, inability to settle at school, and poor learning, the pattern evolving from a restless baby, through the hyperactive child, to an overactive, overworking or disturbed adult. Similarly in the long term, the effects on arterial supply and venous drainage may lead to reduced blood flow to and from the brain, leading to poor growth and development of the brain, with a range of possible repercussions from low ability, through learning difficulties, to brain damage.

Vertebro-basilar insufficiency

In adults, whose growth and development are already more advanced, the brain is already developed but function can still be affected.

The effects of suboccipital restrictions, whether due to head injury, tension or postural collapse, may lead to poor memory, poor concentration, vagueness, lack of clarity and less efficient brain function. This, as mentioned above, is particularly noticeable in elderly people – where postural collapse often leads to vertebro-basilar insufficiency, with increased pressure and compression in the suboccipital region.

Irritability, aggression and depression

Irritability, intensity, aggression, persistent feelings of constant overstimulation, pressure, stress and a persistent drive to be active, hyperactive, moving, or working can all arise from restrictions in this same area. Depression is also a particularly significant consequence.

Headaches and migraine

Headaches and migraine are other potential effects of the disturbed vascular and neurological supply to the head, with headaches often arising from stress and tension held in the neck. There are many factors which contribute to migraine, but a susceptibility to migraine is often the result of a significant head injury or due to birth trauma, often combined with or aggravated by emotional tensions held in that same area, and excessive sympathetic stimulation.

Asthma and heart conditions

The effects on the vagus nerve can also have widespread effects, contributing to respiratory disorders including asthma, and also to heart conditions, and digestive dysfunction.

The association of so many specific conditions and symptoms associated with a particular area should not distract attention from the overall perspective. No symptom or condition exists in isolation. No part of the body exists in isolation. We are all complete integrated beings, integrated within ourselves and integrated into our environment and surroundings. Any patient needs to be assessed and understood within that overall perspective. Every treatment is a complete integrated treatment, perceiving and taking into account every aspect of the situation. The specific factors and associations mentioned above are valid and relevant, but they are of course only a part of the overall picture.

The whole cranio-sacral system blocked

Apart from these more specifically identifiable factors, restriction in the suboccipital region can also have profound effects on the system as a whole, with the entire cranio-sacral system potentially blocked, restricted in its motion, and unable to manifest free expression of vitality – again with widespread repercussions for the health and well-being of the whole person, the function of all their systems, and on their very nature and personality.

Blockages here, perhaps more so than in any other area in the body, can have far-reaching obstructive effects on the whole treatment process. The cranio-sacral system as a whole may become very unresponsive to treatment, making engagement and diagnosis more difficult, and treatment less effective – or even ineffective.

Restriction in the suboccipital area can also block access to higher levels of consciousness, so release of the subocciput can help to open the doors of perception.

The significance of suboccipital release

Release of the subocciput will therefore not only in itself improve the patient's condition considerably, due to the release of restriction to the many crucial structures in the area, but also enable the whole system to respond, opening up the system, enabling easier and more profound engagement, clearer diagnosis, and more effective cranio-sacral treatment.

Conversely, working on the rest of the cranium without releasing the subocciput (when it is restricted) is one of the factors most likely to cause discomfort and unpleasant side-effects in a patient – most commonly headaches, feelings of congestion, vagueness and nausea, but potentially more debilitating symptoms.

The suboccipital region needs to be assessed with every patient and released where necessary. It is one area, above all, which you can't afford to neglect – and yet it is far too often neglected.

SUBOCCIPITAL RELEASE

Like all cranio-sacral processes, the suboccipital release involves the usual fundamental principles of engaging with the system, allowing it to express itself, following to points of release and reorganisation, always within the context of the whole person and the overall circumstances.

Like the previously described processes for release of the heart centre, solar plexus centre and pelvic centre, it plays an important part in the process of opening up the system and settling and grounding the patient. But it also has many distinctive features.

It is clearly not practical to take up contact on the suboccipital region in the same way as with the other emotional centres (with a hand under the back and a hand at the front) since the anatomy of the body in this area is not conducive to a comfortable and effective contact of that nature.

Also, the specific area of effective application within the suboccipital region is very precise – high up under the occiput, deep within the curve of the neck – and for optimum effectiveness the contact needs to be equally precise.

One can of course access any area from anywhere in the body, through the focus of attention on that area. One can engage with the subocciput from the feet, from the sacrum, from the cranium, or from anywhere else on or off the body. But there are specific benefits from taking up particular precise contacts and working specifically with particular processes, which are not readily obtained by other means or other contacts.

With most cranio-sacral contacts, the exact hand position is not highly significant. But there is no adequate substitute in this case. More than any other cranio-sacral process, this contact benefits from precise positioning of the hands and fingers. This is not always easily mastered and requires attention, diligence and persistence. It is a contact and an area often inadequately addressed.

Suboccipital release – the process

Sitting at the head, bring your hands in softly through the energy field to make a gentle connection onto the sides of your patient's head.

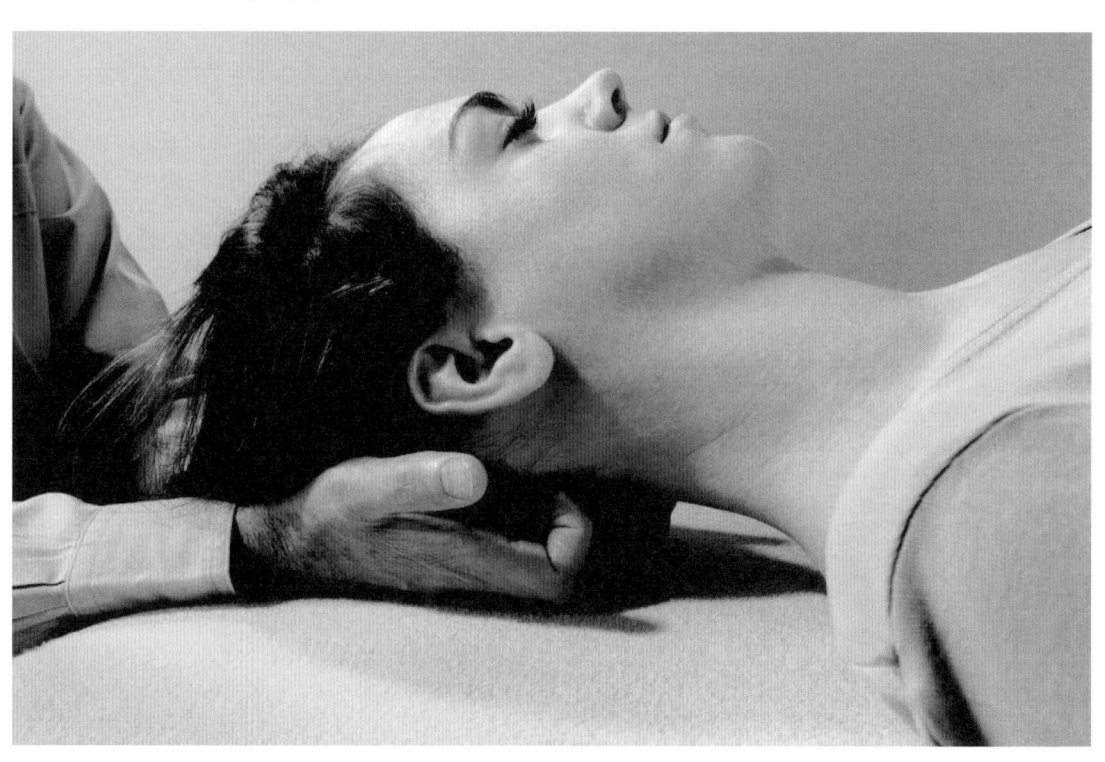

21.1 Contact for suboccipital release – keep your fingers and hands very soft

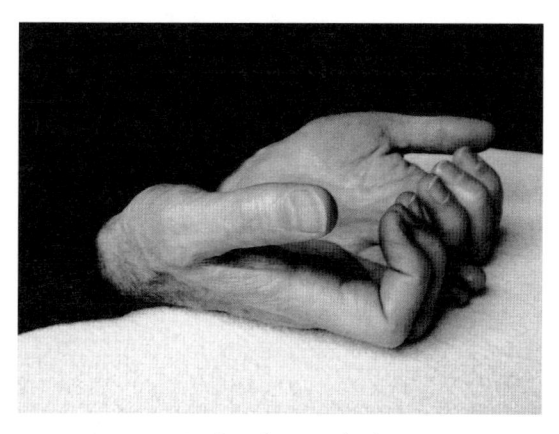

21.2 Finger position for suboccipital release

Once settled, rolling the head as necessary, lift the head gently in order to take up contact with the heels of your hands under the occiput, your hands well down towards the neck (just above the level of the tops of the ears) in such a position that your fingers can curl up into the suboccipital area. Keep the heels of your hands close together, thereby raising the head to create enough space for your curled fingers. Keep the heels of your hands soft, taking care not to squeeze or compress the occiput at all.

Curl your fingers into a C-shape, so that the tips of your fingers are pointing towards your own face, the ring fingers close together at the midline. With the fingers just brushing lightly against the skin at the back of the neck, establish the appropriate position for your fingers in the groove between the occiput and atlas. The contact is with the ring and middle fingers of each hand; the other fingers play no part and can rest wherever they feel comfortable. The appropriate point of contact between your fingers and the suboccipital tissues is right on the tips of your nails. Keep your fingers soft and springy, each interphalangeal joint slightly curved, not pushing up into the tissues at all.

Allow the heels of your hands to soften further. Gradually, almost imperceptibly, allow your wrists to drop, allowing the occiput to sink down towards the couch. As you do so, the subocciput will gradually, almost imperceptibly, sink down onto your fingertips and you can allow your fingers to sink deeper into the tissues as appropriate. Keep your fingers soft and springy as the contact deepens.

Feel the quality of the area, observing differences between left and right, greater softness on one side, greater tightness on the other, observing subtle pulls, twists and turns. Where the tissues are soft, allow your fingers to sink deeper; where there is tension, wait patiently at the surface, waiting for softening and release which gradually allows your fingers to sink deeper. Let your attention focus on the area of greater tension or restriction.

As always, allow your attention to trace any pulls down through the body, maintaining awareness of whole body patterns and relationships between the subocciput and other areas. You can also survey in detail the different structures in the area, the various suboccipital muscles, and particularly the *rectus capitis posterior minor* with its direct fibrous attachment to the dura.

Allow the system to express itself. Allow the unfolding of the usual fundamental principles. Allow the whole process to progress deeper and deeper, layer by layer, as the tissues soften through a series of releases until you reach an appropriate moment of completion.

Attention to detail

As mentioned above, this contact needs precision, and there are various factors to consider in order to enable this process to be most effective:

- *The heels of the hands need to be far enough down* towards the neck (just above the level of the tops of the ears – depending on relative size of head and hands) since otherwise the fingers are unable to reach an appropriate position – and this undermines the whole process.
- *The heels of the hands need to be close together*, particularly at the start, so that the head is sufficiently raised to create enough space for a very light contact of the fingers.
- *The fingers need to be sufficiently curled*, so that the tips of the nails are in the groove between the atlas and occiput.
  - Contact with the nails sounds potentially invasive, but will not be uncomfortable so long as the fingers are soft and light. Check with your patient for reassurance

that the contact of the nails and fingertips is not uncomfortable. Your nails do need to be short.

- It is of course possible to establish a perfectly comfortable contact with the fingers flatter and the fingertips contacting the cervical spine, but this would not be a suboccipital release and would not enable the same responses and effects.

- It is also possible to curl your fingers too much, presenting the flat surface of the distal phalanges. This will not enable effective engagement into the appropriate position within the groove.

- If your fingers don't have enough space to curl into the appropriate degree of curve, it is probably because the heels of your hands are not far enough down towards the neck.

- *The fingers need to remain in a soft springy curve, not rigid or upright*, not pressing into the suboccipital tissues, but simply letting the subocciput rest lightly on the tips of the nails.

- *The heels of the hands and the fingers need to remain soft* throughout the process. This is perhaps the most demanding aspect of this contact, at least for beginners. The position of the hands and fingers may not be immediately conducive to maintaining complete softness and relaxation. The precise attention to detail can also distract from softening. It is therefore necessary to keep reminding yourself again and again to soften your hands and fingers. As always this softening needs to come from deep within, from your heart, solar plexus, head, neck, shoulders, arms, hands, fingers and palms. Ideally you may reach a stage where the patient is completely unaware of your hands or fingers.

In the absence of adequate softening, this contact may initially seem too firm, potentially invasive and ineffective. If you don't address sufficiently the need for softening, then it may remain too firm and consequently ineffective, possibly even uncomfortable – both for patient and therapist – which is perhaps why some practitioners abandon this process having never managed to master it properly. It may take weeks – even months – to gain adequate mastery, but it is worth persisting because when you do master it, it is a most vital, essential, powerful, indispensable and irreplaceable process.

The procedure – further detail

In taking up this contact, one of the first actions after connecting with your patient's system is to *lift the head*. This needs to be done in an appropriately gentle and sensitive manner. Lifting the head is a physical, mechanical action, but it still needs to be carried out with the same softness and sensitivity as any other cranio-sacral contact in order to reassure the patient's system of your non-invasive gentleness. Anything too rough or abrupt will induce tension and resistance – tensions which may then leave the system apprehensive and unable to relax completely, and may therefore block progress for the rest of the treatment.

Initially, the head is supported by the heels of your hands, enabling your *finger contact to be extremely light*, just brushing against the skin.

The exact degree of curl in your fingers is vital – gauged by the position of the tips of the fingernails into the groove between the atlas and occiput.

Observe any difference between the two sides. *Observe any movements* – pulsation, vibration, twisting, turning, pulling. Acknowledge any pulls, noticing their direction, extent and location. Identify any focal points that become apparent, whether locally within the suboccipital region, or drawing you elsewhere to other parts of the body – down into the neck, thorax or pelvis, on one side or another, or up into the head, *maintaining awareness of whole body patterns*.

In this area, there is often a mass of accumulated tensions. You may often experience a multitude of tiny wriggling movements as the tensions release, along with various pulsations, vibrations, twists, turns and pulls. Allow the system to express itself, letting your fingers be alive to the subtle activity – not doing anything, but feeling your fingertips *responding to the myriad micro-movements*, as if being moved by tiny bubbling swirling movements under the ocean, letting your fingers become a part of the process –

involved and yet always observing from a position of quiet calm stillness. As the activity settles, and the system gradually subsides into deeper softness and stillness, observe any persistent patterns drawing you to more persistent focal points. Allow the system to settle into stillness around those fulcrums, and wait patiently for release and reorganisation.

As you allow your fingers to sink into the suboccipital tissues in response to the continuing softening, allow your wrists to drop, allowing the occiput to sink down towards the couch, so that *your fingers can gradually sink in deeper as appropriate.* At this stage, *your hands may gradually, unconsciously, start to move slightly apart,* to accommodate the head sinking down into them; however, you don't need to specifically initiate this – simply allow it to happen spontaneously.

If the tissues are soft on one side, then your fingers may seem to sink in readily through the softness to deeper fulcrums. If the tissues are tight, then your fingers can wait patiently at the surface, until softening occurs, allowing your fingers gradually to sink in, layer by layer, to deeper layers. There are many layers of small suboccipital muscles and enveloping fascia in this region, with a mass of complex pulls and twists reflecting the complex of muscles as they struggle to maintain equilibrium in this crucial area. *Allow these many patterns of movement to unravel of their own accord, step by step, layer by layer, spontaneously releasing every little twist, turn and tension in response to your light touch,* steadily penetrating to deeper and deeper layers, gradually, through a long chain of releases, bringing the whole suboccipital region into a more settled, balanced, freely moving state of equilibrium and free-flowing vitality.

Each individual will of course be different. There will be those in whom the subocciput is relatively free and responsive. In the majority of patients, the suboccipital region is significantly restricted and needs attention. The process of suboccipital release may require a considerable length of time, and may need to be repeated over several sessions, as well as addressing any new tensions that may arise in this area from week to week with each new session. Not every subocciput will release completely in one session. You may reach various different stages of progress. As with all cranio-sacral processes, there will be releases and reorganisation. At any of these stages you may consider it appropriate to bring the treatment process to an end, or to continue to deeper layers.

In some cases you may reach more specific stages of release. If the suboccipital tissues have released substantially, you may reach the stage where *the atlas disengages from the occiput.* The condyles of the atlas fit into a wedge shape within the condyles of the occiput, a stable arrangement in which they may be firmly held by the suboccipital muscles. As the suboccipital tissues release, the bony joints between the occiput and atlas may become free to move and the atlas vertebra may seem to float anteriorly (with your patient lying supine – this means up towards the ceiling) as the occiput drops posteriorly. This stage can feel significantly profound in its degree of release, with a powerful sense of floatiness, and is a good indication of a freely mobile suboccipital region. However, it is not the sole objective of this process, and will be experienced only when the subocciput is particularly free, not as a matter of course.

Whatever stage of release is attained, following an appropriate degree of release and reorganisation, the treatment process can be allowed to come to an end, the fingers gently softening away from the suboccipital tissues, the hands flattening out, and the head gently rolled to one side to remove the hands, taking great care not to pull the hair, jolt the head, or introduce any abrupt or sudden movement. You can then move on to the next part of your complete integrated treatment.

Subtle integration

Following the more specific application of a suboccipital release, it can often be appropriate to settle into a more abstract subtle integration of the suboccipital area, allowing the contact to become less specific, with the fingers gently resting on the sides of the atlas, the axis, the occiput and the surrounding tissues, the hands melting away from under the occiput, observing the tiny adjustments and engaging with the microscopic activity of subtle integration. The initial suboccipital release is helpful, often essential, in clearing the more substantial gross restriction, enabling the deeper process of subtle integration to be expressed more effectively. This can be a particularly profound aspect of the therapeutic process.

Reluctance to release

If the subocciput is reluctant to release, there are various factors to take into account in exploring the reasons for this and how to address the situation:

- current emotional tension – holding the subocciput tight
- tension in the heart centre, solar plexus centre, or pelvic centre reciprocally maintaining and perpetuating corresponding tensions in the subocciput
- shock, trauma or psycho-emotional tension held throughout the system
- compression or restriction in the lumbo-sacral joint and spheno-basilar joint, reciprocally maintaining and perpetuating corresponding restriction in the subocciput (these three areas of reciprocal compression are sometimes described as the triad of compression)
- deeply ingrained muscular and fascial patterns in the soft tissues of the neck
- meningeal restriction in the falx cerebelli, the dura encircling the foramen magnum, or the dura of the upper cervical spine – perhaps due to previous meningitis or meningism
- a very chronic deeply held pattern of restriction (perhaps arising from birth trauma or a severe head injury or a deeply ingrained emotional or postural habit pattern) which will require consistent persistent treatment to enable permanent release.

Appropriate approaches to assisting the release of such persistent resistances may consequently include:

- release of the heart centre, solar plexus centre and pelvic centre
- release of the lumbo-sacral joints and spheno-basilar synchondrosis
- falx release
- fascial unwinding of the neck
- addressing major shock, trauma and emotional patterning in the patient
- addressing underlying patterns – such as birth trauma, postural tension, habit patterns – in their entirety – as one would inevitably do in any cranio-sacral process.

In other words, the complete process of cranio-sacral integration.

Chapter 22

Core Treatment
Overall Approach

Within the context of our four-stage treatment framework, having tuned in and opened up the system, we are now, with the patient suitably settled and grounded, ready to progress to the third stage – core treatment:

1. Engagement (tuning in).
2. Opening up the system (settling and grounding).
3. *Core treatment.*
4. Completion.

The core of any structure is generally the innermost centre or heart of the matter – the core containing the seeds at the centre of an apple, the engine throbbing away at the heart of a machine – and as such is generally the most vital part.

Within the context of cranio-sacral integration, when we talk about the core, we are similarly referring to the vital structures at the centre of the system, at the midline, and these comprise:

- the membrane system, enveloping and containing the central nervous system
- the bones attaching to the membrane system – the bones of the cranium, and the sacrum and coccyx
- the cerebrospinal fluid, contained within the membrane system.

As we have seen already, cranio-sacral integration involves the whole person, working with an integrated approach, always maintaining a constant awareness of the whole. But in order to understand how the whole system works, we need to understand the individual parts.

A car engine can only operate effectively as an integrated unit, but in order to understand or repair a car engine, we need to understand the individual parts which make up that engine.

So in this section we will explore the different individual parts which make up the core of the cranio-sacral system so that we can gain a better understanding of the integrated system as a whole.

We will look at the individual anatomy, specific hand contacts and different technical aspects of each area, so that we can see more clearly how it all fits together and operates as a unit.

Pianists may practise scales and arpeggios, study technical aspects of a piece and practise difficult passages over and over again – in order that they can then go out onto the concert

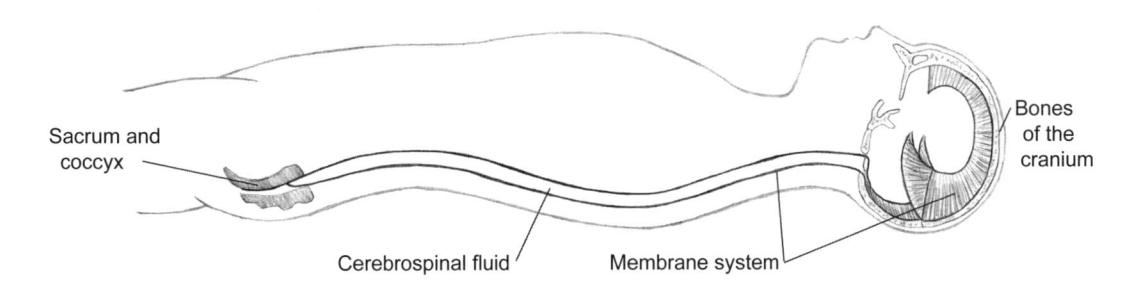

22.1 The core consists of the membrane system, the bones attaching to the membrane system and the cerebrospinal fluid contained within the membrane system

platform able to flow with the integrated unity of the music, the technical aspects safely absorbed into their fingers so that they don't need to think about them as they lose themselves in the flow of the music.

Similarly, as cranio-sacral therapists, we can study the technical aspects of the cranio-sacral system in detail, practise different hand contacts and processes, in order that that we can go into a treatment with all those technical aspects securely at our fingertips, so that we don't need to think about them as we lose ourselves in the flow of the integrated treatment process.

As we explore each area, we will see how we can allow the unfolding of the usual treatment principles in each area, and we can identify the individual characteristics and peculiarities of each area, so that when we are deeply absorbed in a treatment, we can respond appropriately to the system without needing to think – our response profoundly guided by our *informed awareness* – awareness of the evolving cranio-sacral process within the context of the well-grounded base of knowledge and understanding that we have absorbed.

These are not techniques to be applied; they are processes into which to become absorbed. As we look at each section, and particularly as you practise each process, it is vital to remember that with every contact, we are tuning in to the whole cranio-sacral system, as reflected through that particular window. We are not looking to 'fix' any specific structure; we are looking to allow the whole system to reintegrate and resolve around the fulcrum of our contact.

As we look at each section, we will tend to organise our description around the bony structures – being the most evident structural components of the body. But at all times we are engaging, not only with bone, but also with membrane, fluid, fascia, muscle, other soft tissues, blood supply, nerve supply, movement, physiological activity, cellular activity, molecular activity, subatomic activity, psycho-emotional activity, energy, vitality, potency, life force – the totality of the cranio-sacral process.

Prerequisites

Before we embark on the first of these core contacts, it may be useful here to summarise briefly and reflect on the various elements that constitute our overall approach to the cranio-sacral system – the prerequisites to effective engagement – all of which need to become an instinctive, inevitable part of the treatment process with every contact and every change of contact.

Interlude 2

Key Elements in the Overall Approach to Cranio-Sacral Integration

- Establish your own *practitioner fulcrums*.
- Take up each *contact slowly, gently, gradually*.
- Establish an appropriate level of *physical contact*.
- Establish an appropriate level of *attention*.
- Establish an awareness of the various different *tissue levels*.
- Establish an awareness of the *whole person*.
- Feel the increasing sense of *interconnection*.
- Allow a growing awareness of *quality, symmetry* and *motion* – including *rhythmic motion*.
- Be content to *'simply be there'*.
- Feel the gradual *deepening* of the process.
- Observe the sense of *shifting* from one level to another.
- Observe the natural evolution of the *inherent treatment process* through *fundamental principles*.
- Stay with the *neutral* state.
- Allow *subtle integration*.
- *Enhance* the inherent responses as appropriate.
- Settle into *deep dynamic stillness*.

Chapter 23

Core Treatment
Individual Processes

Contacts to be covered under core treatement are:
- the occiput and spine
- the sacrum and spine
- the sphenoid
- the temporal area
- the frontal area
- the parietal area
- the falx contact.

Like the car engine, taking these individual contacts apart can be useful in order to understand them fully, but it is not the way they are intended to be used. Unlike the car engine, each of these contacts *can* be applied separately, and certainly specific contacts may be of particular relevance to specific individuals and situations. But primarily, they are intended as part of an integrated treatment process.

Not every contact will be used with every patient. A treatment might not involve any of these contacts, might involve one or two, or several. They can be combined together to form a cohesive treatment – something which is particularly useful for beginners in establishing a clear sense of a complete integrated treatment.

Integrated unit

The body works as an integrated unit. Forces and stimuli are transmitted from one place to another throughout this integrated unit. Symptoms, conditions, disease and ill health may arise anywhere in the body as a result. Whether these forces are transmitted through fascia, membrane, bone, fluid, etheric body, energy field, nervous system, perineural system, the molecular web, or a combination of these and many others, proper understanding of disease requires acknowledgement of the totally integrated nature of the body.

In describing each contact, there tends to be a focus on bones, partly because they provide the most visible tangible framework for describing hand positions, landmarks, identification and location, partly because the whole cranial concept has derived from bony osteopathic origins, and also because the bones are an integral part of the process – but only a part. If you limit your perception to a mechanical view of the visible tangible structures, you will see only one part of the picture and it may be difficult to understand how forces can be transmitted by other more subtle, intangible, invisible means and to understand the many complex and unpredictable ways in which the body operates.

Disentangling the web

The layers and levels of complexity are infinite, far beyond the limited understanding of the human brain. But we don't need to work out every detail. We can simply let the body disentangle the web, which it is much better at doing that any human mind or therapist.

So with each contact that we explore, all we need to do is engage and simply be there. Every contact is a window into the whole system. So while we may take up various different contacts, with each contact that we take up, and at every stage of every treatment, it is simply a matter of tuning in, allowing the therapeutic process to evolve around the fulcrum of our contact, allowing the system to identify the relevant forces that it needs to address at that point in order to bring itself back into balance and harmony, enhancing its ability to do so.

Engaging the whole system – at all times

So as we look at each part of the core of the system, we want to understand the individual parts, but not get caught up or distracted into treating parts in isolation. Awareness of specific mechanical and other restrictions may play a part in the process, but is not the principal focus of what we are doing. Each process is valuable and useful in its way and through familiarity with all these various processes the therapist can maintain a subconscious memory bank of contacts and connections which can be introduced, in order to respond appropriately to each patient according to their needs.

Even as we identify and describe specific contacts and stimuli revolving around particular bony or membranous structures, we are inevitably engaging the whole system and offering our stimulus to the system as a whole rather than trying to release a specific structure. Every contact is a process – not just a technique that you apply, but a process into which you become fully absorbed – a process of interaction with the body's underlying healing potential to integrate itself.

Chapter 24
The Spine

C1 (Atlas)
C2 (Axis)

Cervical spine
C1-C7

C7 (Vertebra prominens)

T1

Cervico-thoracic junction

T4

Thoracic spine
T1-T12

T9

T12
L1

Thoraco-lumbar junction

Lumbar spine
L1-L5

L5

Lumbo-sacral junction

Sacrum

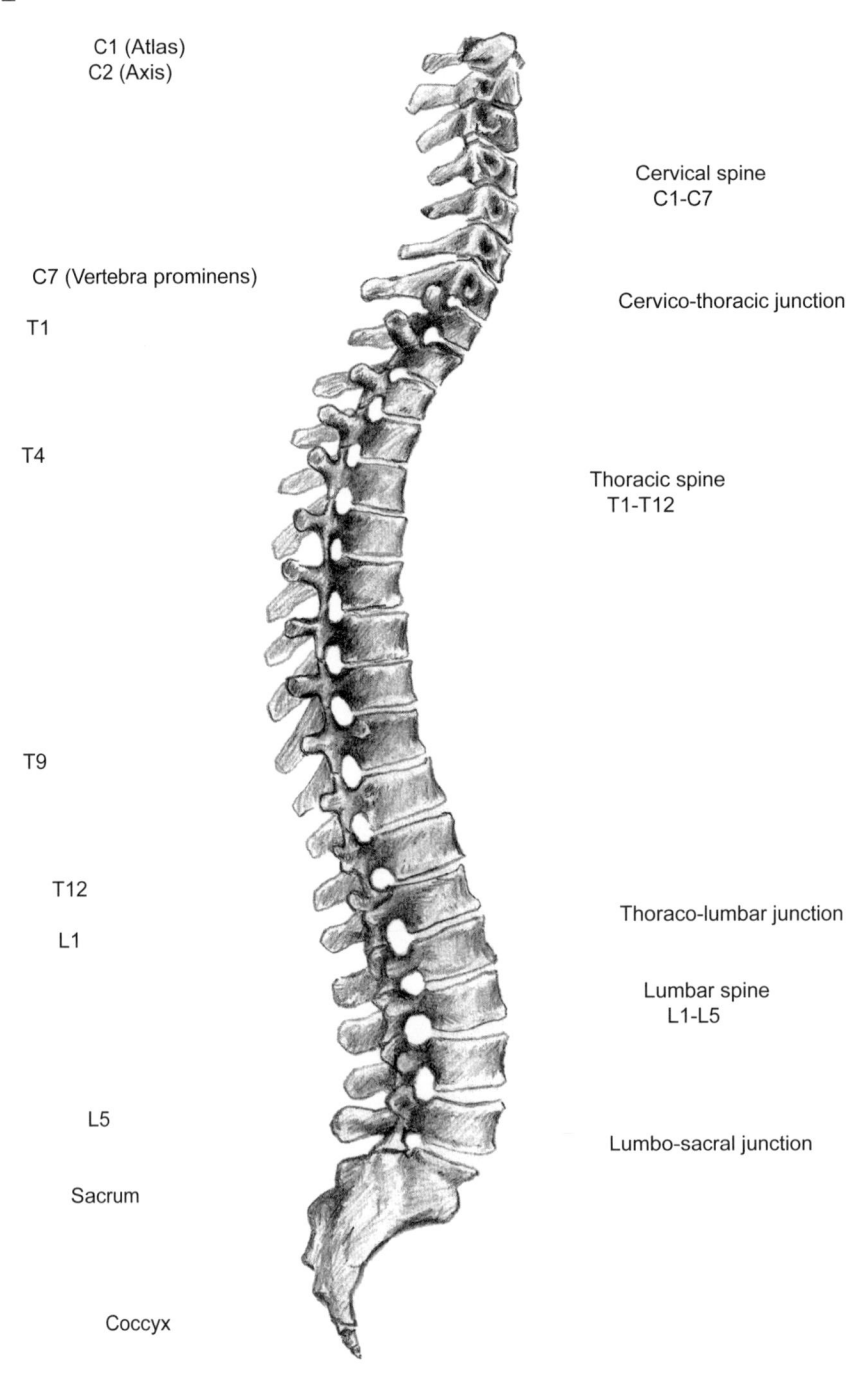

Coccyx

24.1   The vertebral column – lateral view

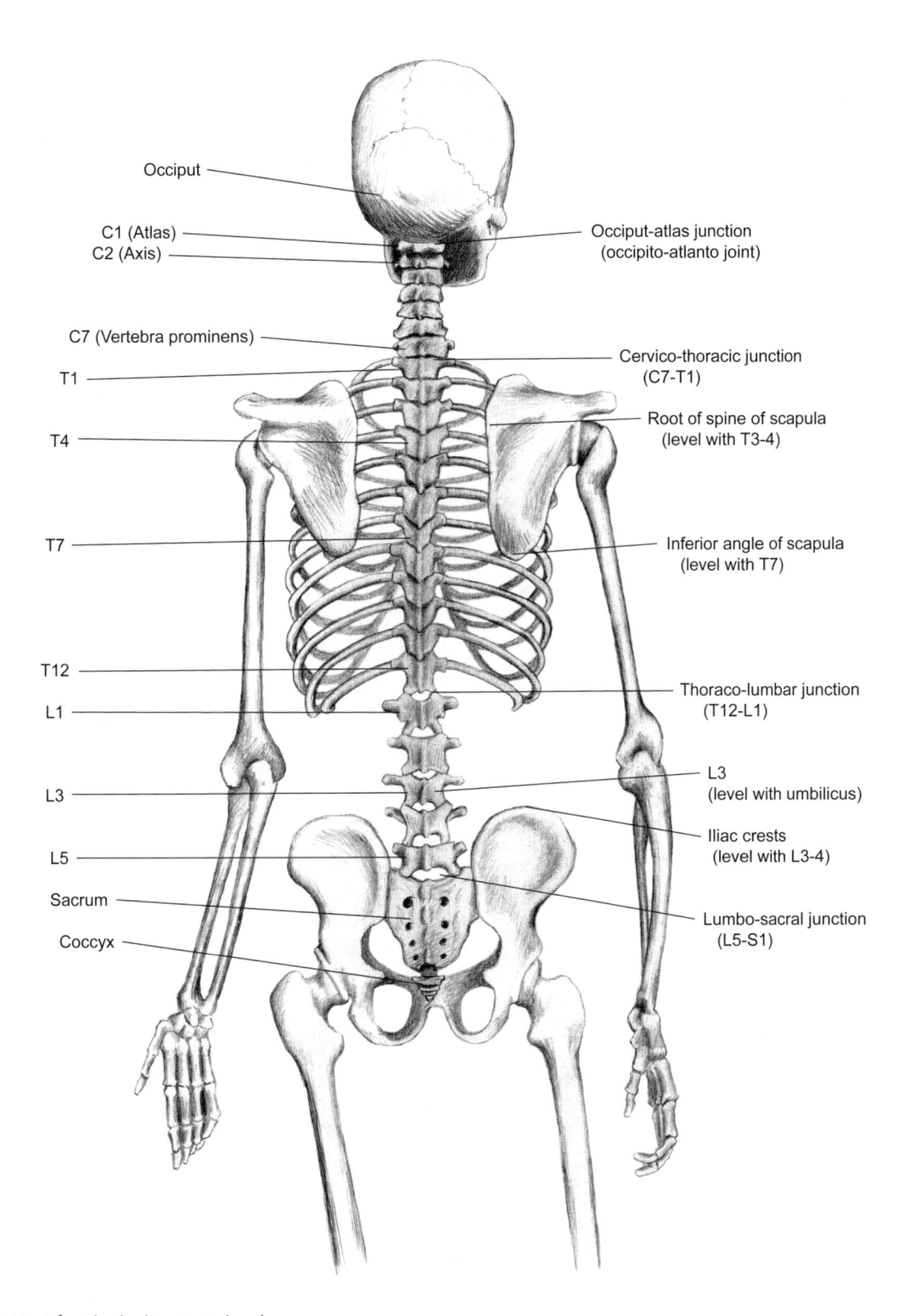

24.2 The spine in situ – posterior view

As we have seen earlier, significant areas of the body often have their significance reflected in different layers and levels, key areas in subtle energetic terms being reflected in and protected by significant areas on a structural level – and the spine is typical in this respect – with its bony structure, protecting the vital spinal cord and the deeper inner core of the energetic midline.

The spine (see Figures 24.1 and 24.2) consists of:

- a bony vertebral column
- lined with three layers of membrane (dura, arachnoid, pia)
- with cerebrospinal fluid contained within the subarachnoid space between the arachnoid and pia
- the spinal cord enveloped within these membranes
- with a central canal also containing cerebrospinal fluid
- with nerve roots entering and emerging from the spinal cord, the motor and sensory roots combining to form spinal nerves, which penetrate the membranes and exit through the intervertebral foramina between the vertebrae to travel to and provide innervation to all parts of the body.

The spine is therefore the source of neurological supply, motor and sensory, to most structures throughout the body – muscles, organs, fascia, blood vessels and many other structures.

Spinal membranes

The spinal membranes (dura, arachnoid and pia; see Figure 24.3) form a tube of membrane lining the vertebral canal and enveloping the spinal cord. As in the cranium, the dura is divided into two layers – the endosteal layer lining the bony vertebral column, and the meningeal layer forming a lining within a lining.

The meningeal dura passes from its firm attachment around the foramen magnum of the occiput, to its lower attachments within the sacral canal at the second sacral segment and via the filum terminale to the coccyx. It has a small but significant attachment to the second

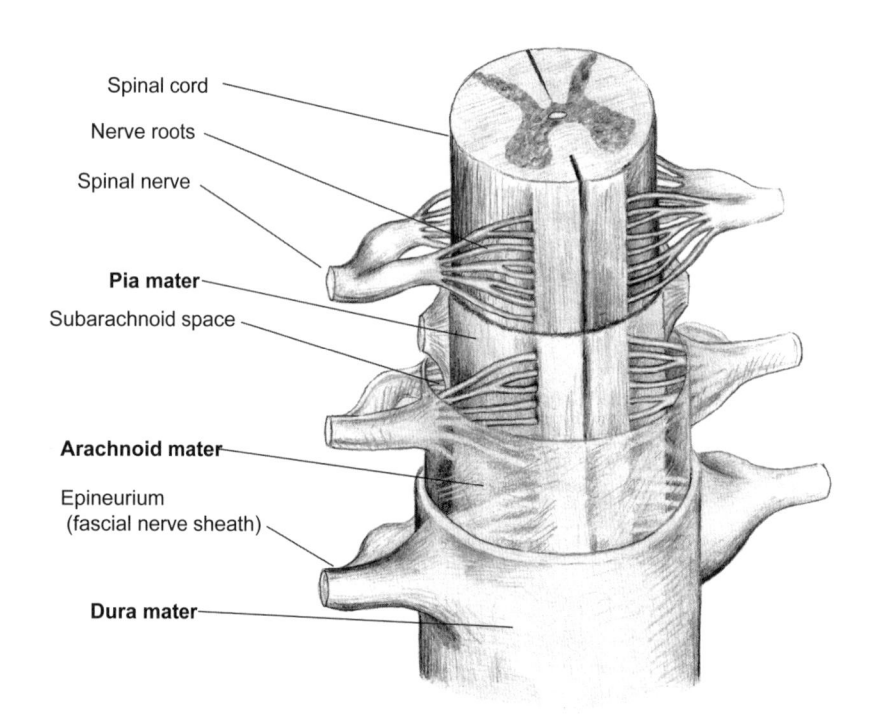

24.3 The spinal membranes (dura, arachnoid and pia) form a tube of membrane lining the vertebral canal and enveloping the spinal cord

and third cervical segments. It is otherwise free to float within the vertebral canal, although partly tethered by the nerve roots emanating from each side of the spinal cord and also by the denticulate ligaments passing between the dura and pia, particularly in the lower part of the spine.

There is also a small bridge of connective tissue from the rectus capitis posterior minor muscle to the dura at the level of the occiput-atlas junction.

The arachnoid terminates with the dura at the second sacral segment. The pia, closely enveloping the spinal cord, terminates with the spinal cord at the level of the second lumbar vertebra (in an adult).

Neurological irritation

Membranous restrictions readily impinge upon the nerve roots, activating the efferent (motor) nerves, with potential consequences throughout nerve pathways to organs, muscles and other structures, not only around the spine but throughout the body (see Figures 24.4a and b).

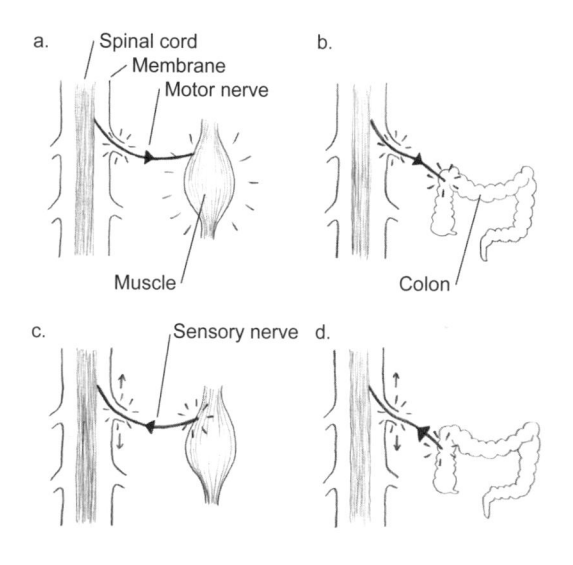

24.4 *Neurological irritation in the spine may induce:*
a. muscle spasm
b. disturbance in the viscera (organs)
Similarly, irritation in the spinal membranes and surrounding segmental structures may be induced by
c. muscle tension or injury
d. visceral disturbance
with ramifications throughout the system via the membranes and other communication channels

Conversely, afferent (sensory) neurological stimulation or irritation arising in the organs and peripheral structures and entering the spine can disturb the membrane and the surrounding vertebral segment, with ramifications both locally and to other parts of the spine and to the whole reciprocal tension membrane system, stirring up weak spots (facilitated segments) and potentially causing symptoms anywhere in the body (see Figures 24.4c and d).

Restrictions and imbalances anywhere in the body may have repercussions on the spinal membranes and consequently on the nerves and their areas of distribution. Restrictions within the occiput and sacrum are likely to be particularly relevant due to their direct attachment to the spinal dura.

Flow of vitality (fluid drive, potency)

The spine is also the principal pathway for the flow of vitality rising up from the sacrum through the midline core of the system to the cranium. Vitality rises up from the sacrum towards the cranium during the expansion phase of rhythmic motion and ebbs down from cranium to sacrum during the contraction phase. (This rhythmic flow up and down the spine is sometimes described as longitudinal fluctuation.) The potency of this flow through the midline of the body, the power, the dynamism within the flow of energy through the spine (sometimes known as the fluid drive) is a reflection of the underlying vitality and therefore the overall health of the individual.

Ensuring a healthy, balanced, freely mobile, well-integrated spine is fundamental to health.

The spine is also particularly vulnerable to injury, as evidenced by the prevalence of back pain and the many disturbances to health arising from spinal disturbances, so integration of the spine plays a significant role in the integration of the system as a whole.

Accessing the spine

Within the context of a cranio-sacral treatment, the spine, its membranous lining, its nerve roots, and its inner core of vitality are most readily accessed from its two ends – the occiput and the sacrum (see Figure 24.2).

At the top of the spine, the cranium sits on top of the atlas vertebra – the first cervical vertebra – the condyles of the occiput at the base of the skull sitting on to the condyles of the atlas, held by several pairs of small suboccipital muscles and other pairs of larger surrounding muscles. As we have seen previously, this is a particularly crucial and vulnerable area.

At the base of the spine, the fifth lumbar vertebra sits on to the first segment of the sacrum, forming the lumbo-sacral joint – another very vulnerable area of the body.

Free mobility of the occiput and sacrum is therefore vital to healthy function of the spine, and to the integrated function of the body as a whole. Establishing free mobility of the occiput and sacrum is therefore fundamental to enabling healthy integration of the system as a whole, and an essential precursor to working through the spine.

Chapter 25

The Occiput and Spine

Location

The occiput forms the back and base of the cranium. It is composed of four parts, surrounding and forming the foramen magnum (through which the spinal cord connects with the brainstem and brain). These four components are:

- *Squamous portion* – posterior to the foramen magnum – the curved plate of bone at the back of the head.
- *Two condylar portions* – lateral to the foramen magnum – including the two occipital condyles which sit on to the condyles of the atlas vertebra (the first cervical vertebra).
- *Basilar portion* – anterior to the foramen magnum – at the base of the skull.

In the neonate (newborn) cranium, these four portions are still distinct bones separated by cartilage, not fusing fully until the age of six years (see Figure 25.3).

Articulations

The occiput articulates with the *parietal bones* superiorly (at the lamdoid suture).

Laterally, it articulates with the mastoid portions of the *temporal bones* (at the occipito-mastoid sutures) and the petrous portions of the temporal bones (at the petro-condylar sutures).

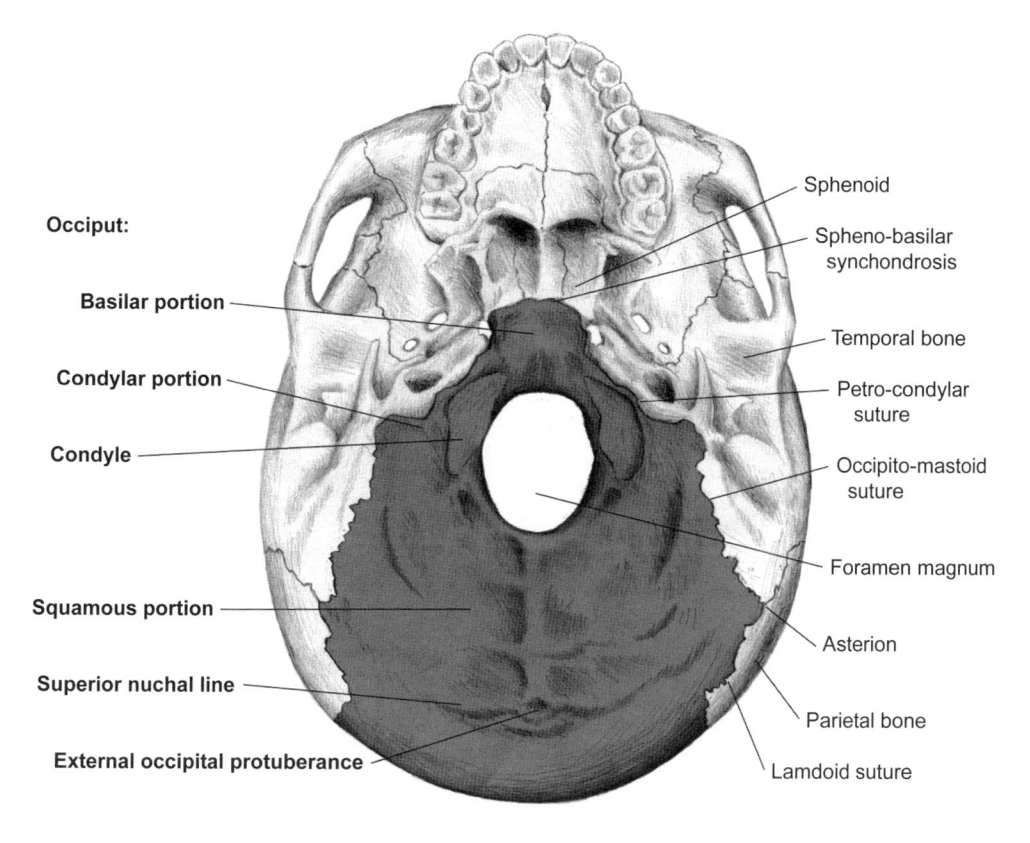

25.1 The occiput in situ – inferior view

155

25.2 The occiput in situ – superior view

Anteriorly, the basilar portion articulates with the body of the *sphenoid* (at the spheno-basilar synchondrosis).

Features

On the external surface of the occiput, there is a protrusion of bone (which you can usually feel on yourself) called the *external occipital protuberance* (also known as the *inion*). On the internal surface, there is a corresponding *internal occipital protuberance*. Ridges of bone emanate both horizontally and vertically from the internal occipital protuberance, marking the attachments of the various infoldings of membrane – the tentorium cerebelli, the falx cerebri, and the falx cerebelli – as well as the pathways of the venous sinuses which follow the contours of these membranes, coming together at the internal occipital protuberance to form the confluence of sinuses.

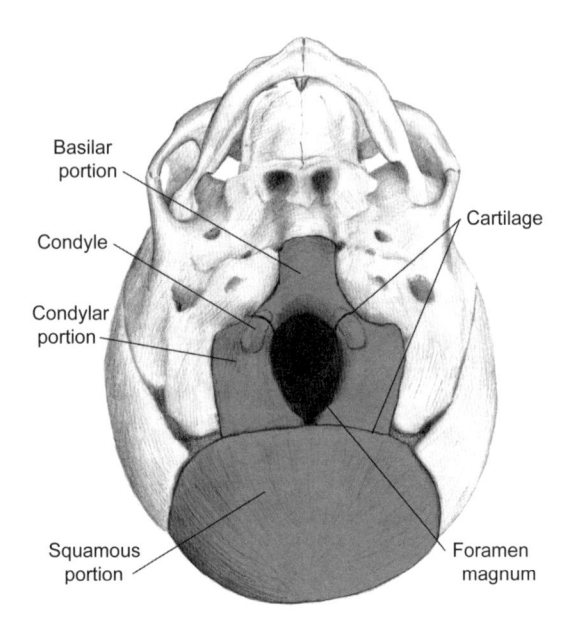

25.3 The neonate occiput is in four separate parts divided by cartilage

Membranous attachments

Like all cranial bones, the occiput is lined with membrane. It also receives attachment for several of the membranous infoldings. The *tentorium cerebelli* passes almost horizontally across the back of the cranium, (forming a tent or roof over the cerebellum). The *falx cerebri* passes down from above, along the midline of the upper part of the occiput as far as the confluence of sinuses. The *falx cerebelli* passes down from the confluence of sinuses along the midline of the occiput, blending into the membrane around the foramen magnum.

There is a more firmly attached thickening of membrane around the *foramen magnum*. The membrane then continues down through the foramen magnum, continuing as the spinal membranes enveloping the spinal cord, penetrated by spinal nerves at each vertebral segment, and extending down to the sacrum and coccyx.

Preparatory suboccipital release

The most common site of restriction for the occiput is at the suboccipital region, where the occiput meets the atlas vertebra and is held by many pairs of small suboccipital muscles, together with various larger pairs of surrounding muscles. As we have seen in Chapter 21, this is a particularly significant area due not only to the many vital structures that pass through the area, but also due to its particular susceptibility to trauma and tension.

In order to enable a freely mobile occiput, the first priority is therefore to release the suboccipital region. The suboccipital release has been described previously, but it needs to be emphasised that any work with the occiput needs to be preceded by checking the suboccipital region and addressing any restrictions there as necessary, otherwise effectiveness may be limited (see Figure 25.4).

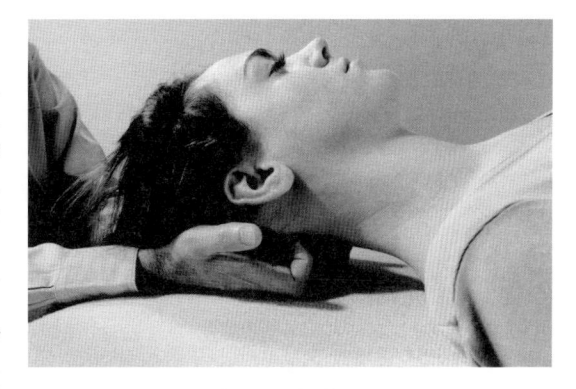

25.4 Preparatory suboccipital release

Occipital contact

Following a suboccipital release, you can settle into contact with the occiput, allowing your hands to relax into a soft receptive curve, adjusting the position of your hands to enable maximum comfort both for patient and practitioner. The curve of the occiput can rest comfortably into the curve of your fingers and hands, the two hands close together at the midline, your fingers extending just below the occiput into the upper neck (see Figures 25.5 and 25.6).

As you settle into this contact, re-establish your own fulcrums, settling into stillness, settling into spaciousness. Expand your attention to be aware of the whole body, as well as your local connection within that broader perspective. Allow the system to express itself, following any pulls and twists to points of stillness and release, gradually feeling the occiput (and the system as a whole) settling into a quieter state, through which you may find cranio-sacral motion emerging more clearly, whether at cranio-sacral rhythm level or middle tide level. The time taken for this process to reach a point of resolution and settle into an easeful neutral state will vary according to the degree of restriction in this area. It may settle very readily or it may take several minutes.

158 \ Cranio-Sacral Integration

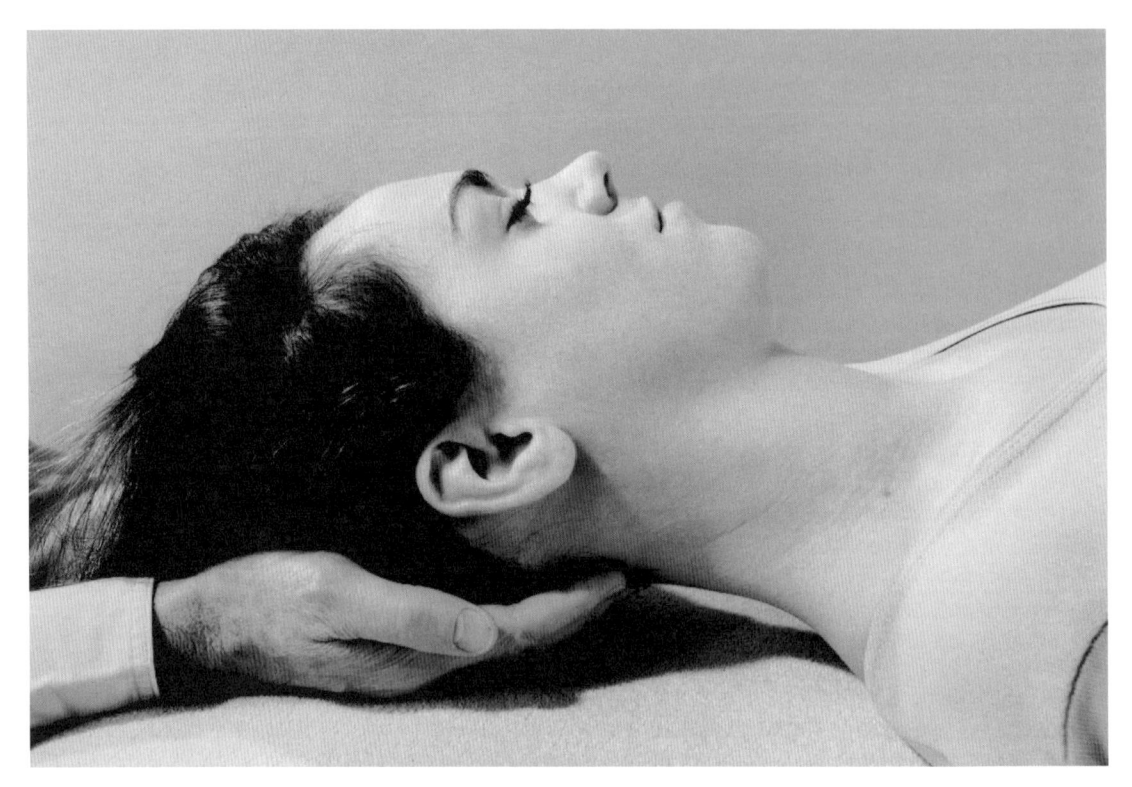

25.5 Occipital contact – allow your hands to relax into a soft receptive curve

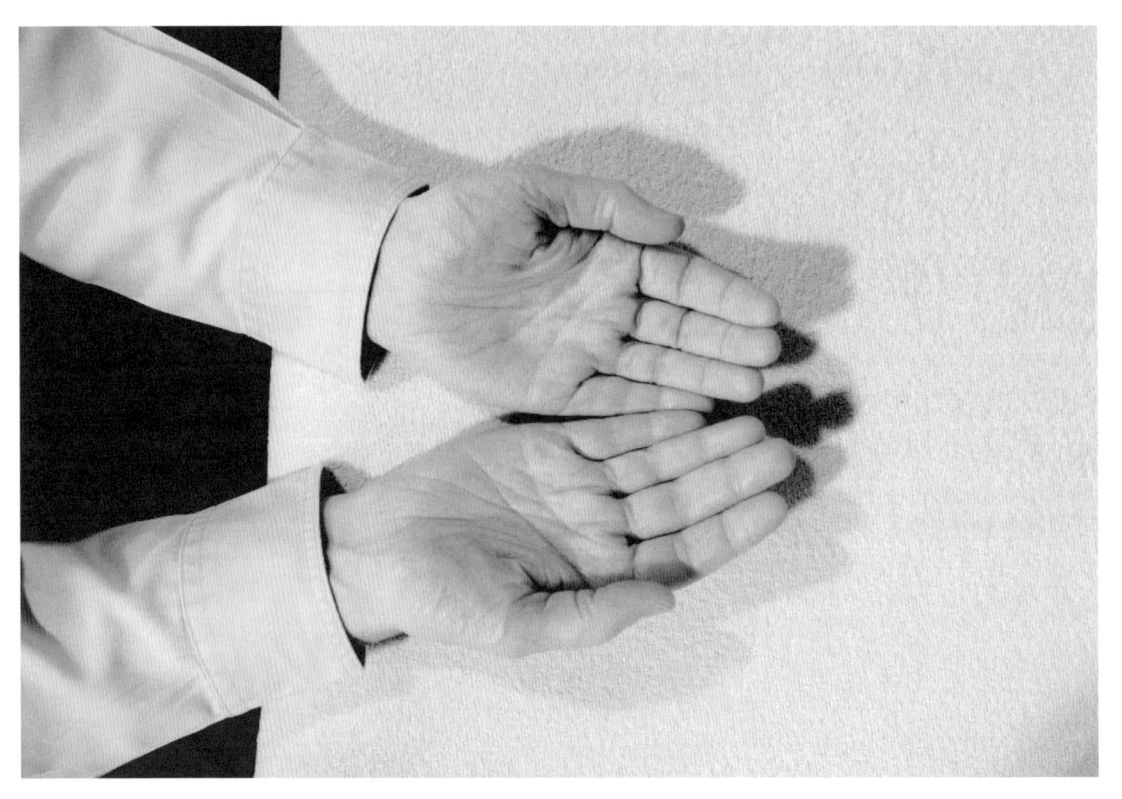

25.6 Hand position for occipital contact

Cranio-sacral motion

Rhythmic motion is expressed through the occipital region in two ways, longitudinally and laterally:

- *Longitudinal motion*: during the expansion phase, the occiput tucks under towards the neck, the basilar portion moving anteriorly and superiorly (as the spheno-basilar joint moves into flexion). During the contraction phase, it comes back and up.
- *Lateral motion*: during the expansion phase, as the cranium expands laterally, the occipital region also flares or widens around the midline, widening more expansively at the squamous portion than at the more solid basilar portion.

Integration of the spine through the occiput

When the occiput is restricted or imbalanced locally, these local restrictions and imbalances are likely to draw the therapist's attention, masking any imbalances arising from elsewhere in the body, or at least rendering them less clear. As the occiput settles, and local imbalances resolve, so any imbalances from elsewhere may become more clearly apparent, including imbalances arising from the spine – such as a restricted vertebral segment transmitting a pull up through the membrane to the occiput.

These imbalances might arise spontaneously, or they may become apparent when you explore more closely to see what impressions present themselves:

- *Spontaneously* – for an experienced therapist, it is, on the whole, preferable to allow the impressions to arise spontaneously – as long as you have a sufficiently spacious and perceptive informed awareness.
- *Surveying* through the spine is also effective and is a valuable means of developing this perception. The more you practise surveying through the spine and through the body, the more readily you will find impressions arising spontaneously.

Either way, once the occiput is settled and clear, you will soon find that any restrictions, imbalances, injuries, scolioses, tensions or other characteristics anywhere in the spine will – as your attention reaches the affected area – be reflected as changes in quality, symmetry or motion through the occiput in your hands.

Spontaneous imbalances

You might, for example, feel a pull drawing the occiput down on one side of the neck. Explore this pull with your attention to see how far it goes, where it seems to be coming from. As you follow it down through the body, keep monitoring any changes in quality, symmetry or motion in your hands under the occiput. Perhaps the pattern of asymmetry may become more exaggerated as your attention moves closer to the source. Perhaps the rhythmic motion will gradually reduce. Perhaps the quality will gradually intensify, until you reach a point of stillness – which will eventually release, releasing the source of the restriction in the spine, allowing the occiput and neck to settle into a more balanced position, with a looser quality and a more expansive rhythmic motion. Feel that sense of release and rebalancing spreading through the whole spine and the whole body, as the whole system adapts to that change.

Surveying the spine

Whether or not you feel any imbalances, you can survey the whole spine – whether as a unit, or section by section, or segment by segment. You can sweep your attention up and down the spine, observing any general tendencies to imbalance. You can let your attention rest broadly on different sections of the spine, observing how the quality may vary between the cervical, upper thoracic, lower thoracic, or lumbar sections, or how characteristics in certain key areas – the thoraco-lumbar junction or the cervico-thoracic junction, for example – may draw your attention.

More specifically you can *project your attention down, vertebra by vertebra*, segment by segment, observing any changes in quality, symmetry or motion that arise in your hands under the occiput as your attention moves from segment to segment. It may be enough simply to project your attention down the spine. Or you may prefer to think in terms of introducing *a subtle thought of traction*, as if your fingers were gently inviting the occiput to stretch away from the spine, as if you were gently stretching the spinal membranes. Of course there will be no actual physical input, just the thought.

Segment by segment

Let your attention pass down from the occiput to the atlas, from the atlas to the axis (the second cervical vertebra) and on through the third, fourth, fifth, sixth, and seventh cervical segments, observing any changes in quality, symmetry or motion as you project down, and continuing down through the twelve thoracic segments and five lumbar segments.

Perhaps initially you might feel resistance. Wait patiently at each segment for it to soften. Don't be tempted to try to make anything happen, to introduce any force, or any physical input. In due course, you might feel a sense of softening, as if the spinal dura were stretching out towards you, perhaps more readily on one side than the other. Allow that sense of stretch; follow into any imbalance.

Perhaps as you reach a certain segment, C7 for instance, you might feel a twist to one side, reflecting a rotation of the spine at that vertebral level. Allow the system to express that twist. Follow it wherever it takes you, to stillness, release and reorganisation. Perhaps as your attention reaches T4 you might feel the quality tightening, reflecting a tightness at that vertebral level, or in the associated heart centre. Wait with your attention focused at that point, understanding its significance in relation to the patient, until the tightness softens. Perhaps you might feel a section of several vertebral segments that are resistant. Wait patiently for them to soften. Perhaps you might feel other areas where it seems you can flow through more easily.

As you work your way down the spine, you may feel a multitude of twists, pulls, resistances, or contractions at various levels – all reflecting the state of the patient's spine, much of which in turn reflects sensory input into the spine from all over the body. Some of these resistances will release readily. At other points you may encounter more persistent resistances. Simply wait. Be prepared to be patient. However, resistances can often be interrelated, and maintained from elsewhere, so rather than wait indefinitely, move on, acknowledging the resistance or imbalance and continuing on through the spine, and you may find that as another resistance releases further down the spine, so the original resistance disappears of its own accord. Or if it doesn't, you can always come back to it later, and perhaps it will be more responsive once the system as a whole is clearer.

Perhaps as your attention reaches T9 you might feel some shaking or wriggling, perhaps indicating some injury or strain at that level, or reflecting some anxiety or agitation in the solar plexus. As always wait for it to subside, understanding its significance in relation to the patient, then move on.

In this way you can work your way down through the whole spine, allowing the system to release any restrictions, imbalances or tensions, gradually integrating the whole spine, down to the sacrum and coccyx. As restrictions dissolve, the whole spinal dura may appear to take on a looser quality, as if it can stretch out indefinitely. Allow that sense of stretch. You can in fact continue your projection through the whole body – pelvis, legs, feet, viscera, anywhere in the body – but for the moment we are concerned with the spine, so we will content ourselves with that.

Ramifications to the viscera and periphery

In working through the spine in this way, you are not only releasing restrictions in the spine but also contributing to the integration of the whole system – the viscera and the peripheral structures neurologically supplied from the spine, and consequently the overall balance of the body.

Through this approach you can address any vertebral restriction, or facilitated segment, just as manipulative therapy might do. And you are not simply releasing the tissues, but releasing the underlying forces which are maintaining those tissue restrictions.

Jane was in her mid-forties, crippled with back pain. She was on crutches, and even with the crutches every step was intensely painful. She had been in pain for many years, unable to do anything much – which was a severe burden, since she was by nature a very active woman.

She had seen several osteopaths, and one manipulation had severely aggravated her condition, leaving her very fearful of further treatment. She had undergone two operations and an injection to deaden the nerve. Nothing had helped. She was very wary of seeing any more practitioners or receiving any further treatment, due to her previous unsatisfactory experiences, so she was very reluctant to come and see me despite reassurances from her friends that I was extremely gentle and would not be manipulating her back at all.

Eventually she was persuaded. She hobbled in on her crutches, every step making her wince with pain. Getting onto the treatment couch was difficult, but at least once she was there lying on her back with her knees up, the pain was slightly reduced. Her back was so painful that I could not put a hand under it, or under her sacrum, or anywhere near her back. Any movement or contact was intensely painful. The only place I could contact her was her head. So I sat at her head, engaging with her cranio-sacral system. As I projected down through her spine, I could feel the various blockages and imbalances, and the effects of the various manipulations and injections, and the severe restriction around the site of the pain – and the cranio-sacral process doing its work. Gradually, the process of integration proceeded.

At the end of that first treatment, she got up and was able to walk. She no longer needed her crutches. Within a few treatments she was back to her former active self again – completely free of back pain, as busy as ever.

Chapter 26

The Sacrum and Spine

The sacrum (as the name cranio-sacral therapy suggests) is *fundamental* to cranio-sacral work. It is a powerhouse of cranio-sacral energy. The free mobility of the sacrum is therefore essential to the fluent expression of inherent vitality and consequently to the health and well-being of the individual.

The sacrum is also (like the occiput) particularly *susceptible* to injury, partly because of its position, carrying the weight of the body above and receiving a great deal of physical trauma from falls on the buttocks, sports injuries, the pressures and strains of giving birth, and many day-to-day activities. Many of these injuries are compressive – compressing the sacrum up into the spine, but may also cause other distortions – twists, side-bending, side-shifting, displacement, joint restrictions.

Injuries to the sacrum can be responsible for many of the *common symptoms* of low back pain and sciatica, together with various other pelvic disorders (particularly following childbirth) and conditions involving the pelvic organs and genitalia, including menstrual disorders, cystitis and sexual dysfunction. This can be attributed in part to pressures and strains on the sacral nerves which emerge from the foramina within the sacrum to supply those various organs and structures.

Disturbances to the sacrum can also be associated with symptoms *anywhere in the body* – headache, neck pain, digestive disorders – as a result of imbalances at this crucial area reflected through the rest of the body. (Just as a house may develop cracks in the walls right up to the top floor if the foundations are unstable, so the body may develop symptoms anywhere right up to the head if the structural foundation of the pelvis is disturbed or unstable.)

But perhaps *most significant* are the effects of sacral restriction and imbalance on the system as a whole, on the flow of inherent vitality – which in turn undermines the patient's ability to resolve the underlying causes of any and all symptoms and conditions.

Our primary concern is, as always, the quality and potency of the underlying vitality, so while we will of course address the symptoms of low back pain and sciatica and any other symptoms through whatever means may be appropriate, at the heart of the treatment process is the need to restore underlying vitality, so that the healing process can be not merely symptomatic, but long lasting and more profoundly far-reaching. Restoration of free mobility of the sacrum is fundamental to this.

The sacrum

The sacrum is an upside-down triangle, or perhaps more precisely an upside-down pyramid, with its base at the top and its apex at the bottom. It is an extension of the lower end of the spine, formed through the fusion of five vertebrae, the vertebral structure still clearly apparent through the fused vertebral bodies, the fused transverse processes, the spinous processes projecting posteriorly, and the five pairs of foramina – anterior and posterior – through which sacral nerves emerge to be distributed to their various destinations (see Figure 26.1).

Articulations

The sacrum articulates superiorly with the *fifth lumbar vertebra* at the lumbo-sacral joint at the base of the spine, the body of the fifth lumbar vertebra sitting on to the body of the first sacral segment, separated by a cartilaginous intervertebral disc. There is further articulation with the fifth lumbar vertebra through the two articular processes which project up from the sacrum to articulate with the two articular processes projecting down from the fifth lumbar vertebra, forming two synovial joints (see Figure 26.1a).

The Sacrum and Spine / 163

a. Anterior view

- Joint surface for articulation with L5
- Superior articular processes
- Base of sacrum
- Alae (wings)
- Anterior sacral foramina
- Apex of sacrum
- Coccyx

b. Posterior view

- Joint surface for sacro-iliac joint
- Posterior sacral foramina
- Coccyx

c. Superior view (transverse section through S2)

- Spinous process
- Sacral canal
- Ala (wing)
- Sacral foramina (anterior and posterior)

d. Lateral view

- Superior articular processes
- Spinous processes
- Joint surface for sacro-iliac joint
- Coccyx

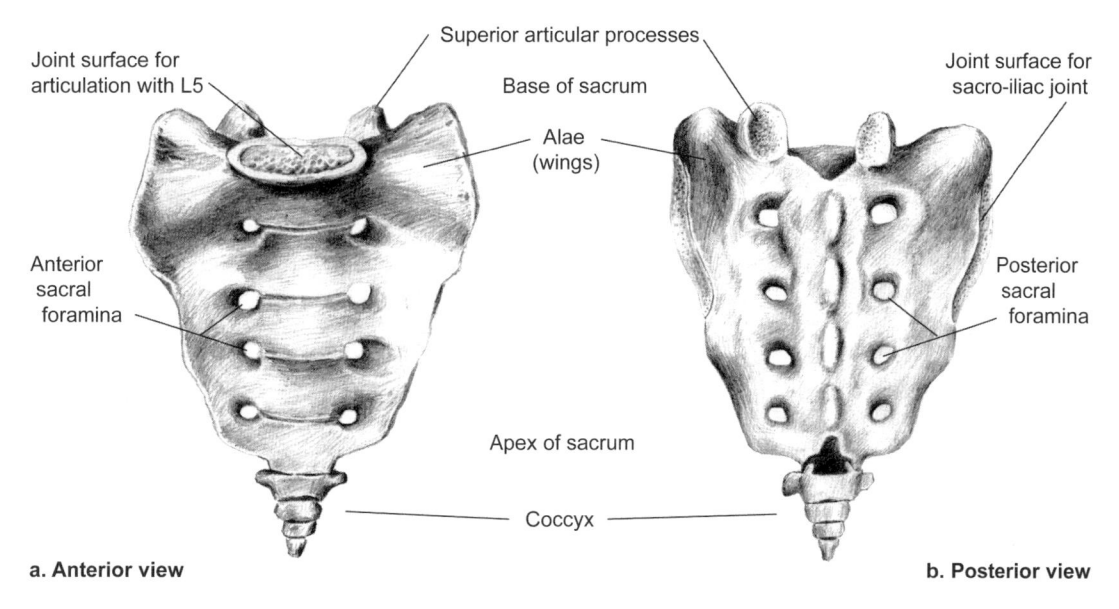

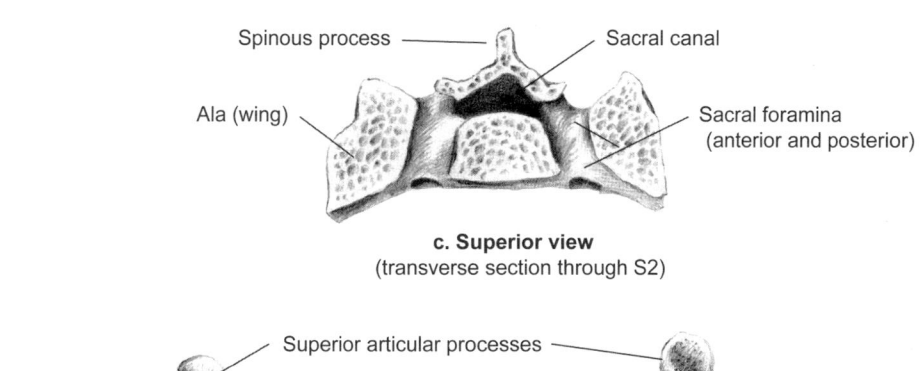

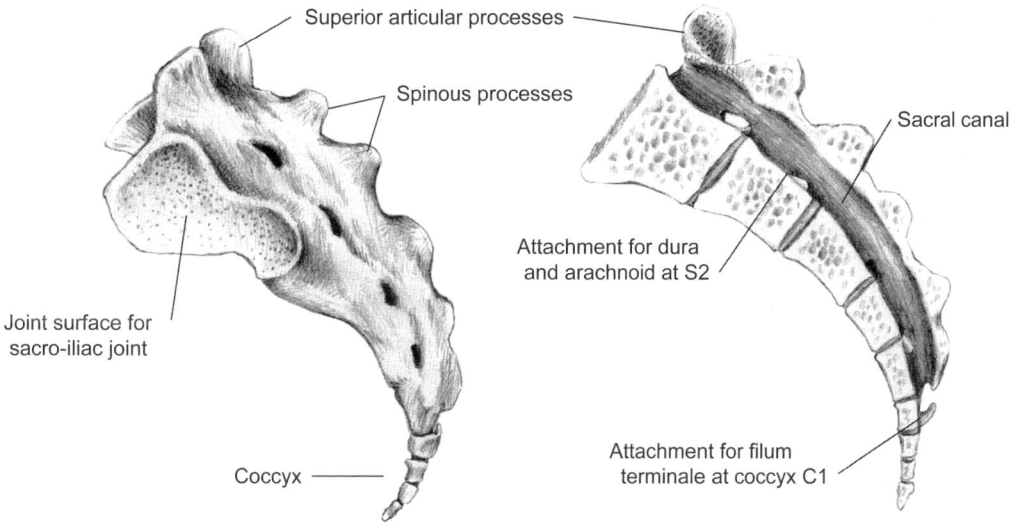

e. Mid-sagittal section

- Sacral canal
- Attachment for dura and arachnoid at S2
- Attachment for filum terminale at coccyx C1

26.1 The sacrum and coccyx

Laterally, the alae (wings) of the sacrum articulate on each side with the iliac bones of the pelvis, forming the two *sacro-iliac joints*. These are substantial joints, with large articular surfaces, firmly bound by ligaments which maintain the stability of these important joints (see Figure 26.1a, b, c and d).

Inferiorly, the sacrum articulates with the *coccyx*. The coccyx is also formed from fused vertebrae, four in this case, the first coccygeal segment articulating superiorly with the apex of the sacrum (see Figure 26.1a, b, d and e).

Membranous attachments

The spinal membranes lining the vertebral canal continue down into the sacral canal, which is an extension of the vertebral canal. The dura mater and arachnoid mater terminate within the sacral canal, where they attach to the *anterior wall of the second sacral segment*. However, the pia mater, which closely envelopes the central nervous system, terminates at the tip of the spinal cord – which extends down the vertebral canal only as far as the second lumbar vertebra – giving off a thin thread of membrane, the *filum terminale*. This continues down through the centre of the vertebral canal, penetrating the dura and arachnoid at their termination at S2, and continuing down (invested in dura and arachnoid) to attach to the coccyx, on the *posterior surface of the first coccygeal segment* (see Figure 26.1e).

Sites of restriction

The sacrum is highly susceptible to restriction, *particularly at the sacro-iliac joints*. The sacro-iliac joints are large joints which contribute substantially to the firm foundation provided by the pelvis for the stability of the structure of the body above. Conventional anatomy books often describe the sacro-iliac joints as having no motion. The many strong surrounding ligaments and associated muscles (although no muscles attach directly between the sacrum and the ilia) ensure that mobility is limited and that the pelvis is stable, but movement is certainly possible in healthy sacro-iliac joints and is, in fact, essential even to healthy everyday physical movement, let alone for the free expression of cranio-sacral motion.

Restriction of mobility will have extensive repercussions on the structure and balance of the whole body above and below, exerting extra strain on other joints throughout the body. It may also contribute to progressive osteoarthritis. And yet, restriction to the mobility of the sacro-iliac joints is very common and widespread, arising from a variety of different causes including falls, chronic tension in the pelvis, postural imbalances, and prolonged immobility through a sedentary lifestyle.

The sacrum is also prone to restriction at the *lumbo-sacral joint*, whether unilaterally or bilaterally, often in conjunction with sacro-iliac restriction – a common pattern being restriction of the sacro-iliac joint on one side combined with compensatory restriction of the lumbo-sacral joint on the opposite side – or due to bilateral compression of the lumbo-sacral joints through falls on the buttocks and other compressive injuries.

The whole cranio-sacral system may be *firmly tethered* or excessively anchored by a restricted sacrum. A fundamental priority in the treatment of any patient is therefore to assess the state of the sacrum and to ensure its free mobility.

ENGAGING WITH THE CRANIO-SACRAL SYSTEM THROUGH THE SACRUM – THE PROCESS

Initial contact

In preparation for taking up contact on the sacrum, invite your patient to bend their knees up, with the soles of their feet on the couch, as described previously (Chapter 20). For greater stability and comfort, invite your patient to place their feet apart and their knees together. If a patient has difficulty maintaining this position, it may be helpful to place a pillow, cushion or rolled blanket under their knees.

Sitting beside your patient, a little below the level of the pelvis, your chair angled to face towards the patient's opposite shoulder, ask your patient to lift their pelvis so that you can place a hand under the sacrum. Using the hand that is nearest to your patient's feet, take up contact under the sacrum with your hand vertically

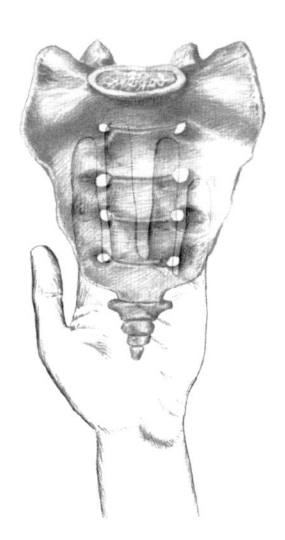

26.2 Contact under the sacrum – the curve of the sacrum sitting comfortably onto your fingers

orientated, fingers pointing up the spine towards the head, with the curve of the sacrum sitting comfortably onto your fingers, the fingers slightly separated to accommodate the spinous processes of the sacrum (see Figure 26.2).

It is not necessary to place your whole hand under the sacrum (as is sometimes described and depicted) since this results in excessive pressure on the practitioner's hand, and discomfort for both patient and practitioner, as well as reducing sensitivity. The sacrum only needs to be resting on the fingers, creating less pressure on the hand, and a lighter, softer contact.

Having established the position of your hand under the sacrum, ask your patient to lower their pelvis down to the couch again. Check that they let their full weight sink down and that they relax completely. If you find the sacrum weighing too heavily on your hand, you can position your hand slightly further inferiorly so that the sacrum is resting more on your fingers and even less on the palm of your hand.

Check that your hand position is central and symmetrical. Ensure that your own hand is comfortable. Check that the patient is comfortable. If your hand is not completely comfortable, ask your patient to raise their pelvis again, so that you can adjust as necessary. Make as many adjustments as necessary in order to establish a comfortable contact. It is not a good idea to try to make do with any contact that does not feel comfortable or balanced, since this will compromise your own sensitivity and focus, and therefore reduce the effectiveness of the treatment.

Initial impressions

As you settle into this initial contact under the sacrum, re-establish your own practitioner fulcrums, settling into stillness, settling into spaciousness, settling into increasing engagement. Adjust your sitting position if you feel overstretched, twisted, unbalanced or uncomfortable in any way. Allow any impressions to emerge through your contact with the sacrum.

Be aware of the *quality* of the sacrum. Does it feel mobile or stuck, tight or loose, hard or soft, tense or relaxed, or any of an infinite number of other possible qualitative impressions? Define your impressions precisely, in order to clarify them, to see what they may be telling you about your patient, their physical state, their nature, the state of their sacrum and pelvis, their whole being.

At the same time, allow impressions of *symmetry* or asymmetry to emerge. Does the sacrum feel well balanced between the two ilia and symmetrically aligned with the vertebral column? Does it feel *sidebent*, with the base of the sacrum pulling towards the sacro-iliac joint on one side? Does it feel *torsioned*, with the sacrum twisting posteriorly to left or right? Does it feel *sideshifted*, as if the whole sacrum has been shunted to one side (see Figure 26.3)? Does it feel particularly drawn into *flexion* (with the apex moving anteriorly) or into *extension* (with the apex drawn posteriorly)? Or do you feel any other asymmetries or complex combinations of asymmetries within the sacrum?

At the same time, be aware of any movements or *motion* expressed by the sacrum. Is it wriggling around, rocking from side to side, vibrating, shaking, pulsating, or expressing rhythmic motion? Is that rhythmic motion slow, fluent and of wide amplitude, or fast, restricted and of small amplitude? Is it even or uneven? Is it manifesting cranio-sacral rhythm or middle tide motion? Is it exhibiting a powerful vitality?

a. Sidebending - left

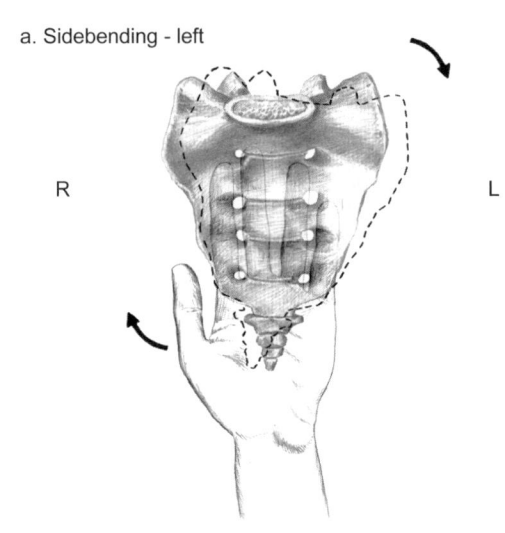

R   L

b. Torsion - posterior left

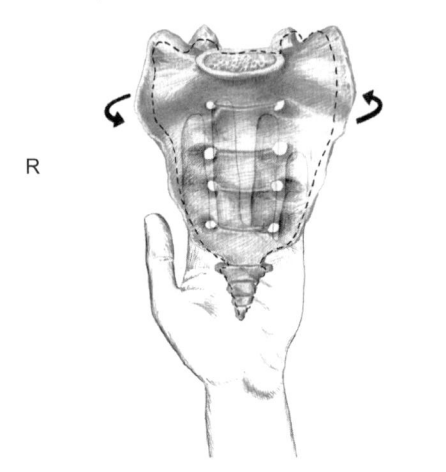

R   L

c. Sideshift - left

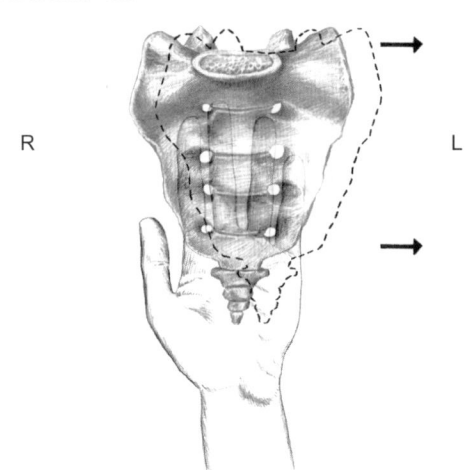

R   L

26.3 Asymmetries of the sacrum – sidebending, torsion, sideshift

Cranio-sacral motion

The sacrum, being a single midline structure, responds to the expansion and contraction of rhythmic motion by rocking forward and back into flexion (during the expansion phase) and extension (during the contraction phase).

a. Balanced position

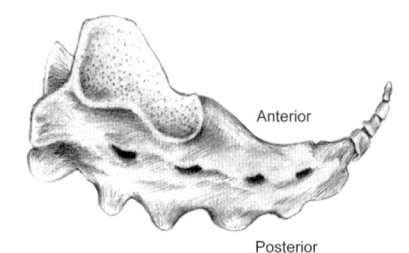

Anterior

Posterior

b. Flexion

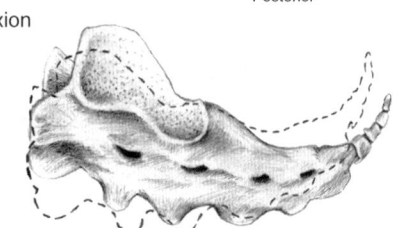

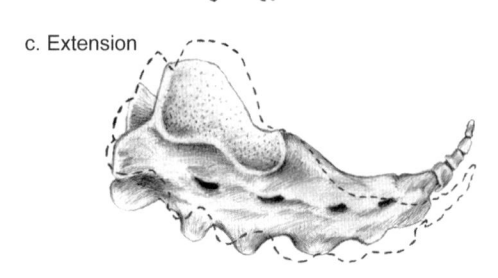

c. Extension

26.4 Cranio-sacral motion of the sacrum – the sacrum rocks forward and back into flexion and extension during the expansion and contraction phases of rhythmic motion

In cranio-sacral terms:

- flexion indicates that the apex of the sacrum is moving anteriorly
- extension indicates that the apex is moving posteriorly,

the movement of the sacrum revolving around the poles of attachment at the sacro-iliac joints.

Response to impressions

Does the sacrum feel solid and immobile? Is this solidity local in the sacrum, or is it characteristic of the whole body? Is this immobility due to the inherent nature or physical build of the patient (a rugby player's sacrum may feel very different from a ballet dancer's sacrum) or is it the result of a specific compressive injury, or is it chronic psycho-emotional tension held in the pelvis? Alternatively, does the sacrum feel soft, light, fluent, mobile? What does this tell you about the patient? Is it jumping around all over the place? Is it drawn strongly into flexion? Is it pulling towards one side, the base drawn towards one sacro-iliac joint, indicating a restriction in the sacro-iliac joint on that side? Or is it pulling up on one side, perhaps towards a lumbo-sacral restriction, or a pull from further up the spine, perhaps transmitted through the membranes.

As always, be content just to be there, allowing the gradual evolution of the inherent treatment process, allowing the system to express its various initial movements, gradually settling, and increasingly drawing into points of stillness and release. Observe the superficial patterns releasing more readily. Stay longer with the more chronic underlying patterns which emerge as the system settles and your connection deepens.

As you allow the various patterns to emerge, you may feel a build-up of pressure and tension within the system, as the movements and rhythmic motion close down towards a point of stillness. As you rest at the edge of that point of balanced tension, you may feel the whole system taking on a quality of stillness, a sense of focus, a feeling of floating. You may feel pulsation, vibration or other minor wriggling movements. Allow them, stay with them, observe them; don't feel that you have to do anything about them – except allow your attention and your hand to flow with them. As you continue to wait at the edge of that stillness, you may feel the eventual release of the sacrum as any resistance gives way, the tensions and tightness soften and dissolve, and the sacrum settles into a more balanced and symmetrical state with a softer, looser quality and an increased amplitude of cranio-sacral motion.

Points of stillness and release may occur at cranio-sacral rhythm level or at middle tide level. Middle tide motion may be clearly apparent from the start. If the system is expressing cranio-sacral rhythm initially, then with each release, rhythmic motion is likely to become increasingly evident, with increased amplitude and a slightly slower rate, gradually settling into clearer expression of middle tide motion.

Shifting to deeper levels

As the system becomes more settled, you may access deeper levels. This will be reflected both in the quality of what you are feeling, and also in the slower rate of rhythmic motion, particularly as middle tide motion becomes more apparent. As you connect with these deeper levels, allow your awareness also to become deeper and more subtle.

At various points, perhaps following a significant release, the whole system may seem to shift to a deeper level. Everything will seem to settle into a slower quieter deeper state – the rhythmic motion, the gentle pulls, the quality – and your responses will therefore become correspondingly more subtle, blending into the system more deeply, becoming absorbed into the system more deeply, as if you were sinking deeper under the ocean to a world of greater stillness and slow motion. Focal points of stillness may still appear, the system may still draw towards fulcrums, but the whole process will happen more slowly, more gradually, more subtly.

Addressing specific restrictions of the sacrum

Not yet ready

But perhaps the body isn't ready to settle into those deeper levels yet. Perhaps there are more superficial disturbances which are more relevant to the patient at this moment, which are blocking sacral mobility, or which are blocking access to deeper levels, or which are crying out to be heard and addressed.

Restrictions at the sacro-iliac joints and lumbo-sacral joints are not only very common, but often very deeply ingrained over many years; and since the mobility of the sacrum is so fundamental to cranio-sacral mobility and to health, it is helpful to assess and address such restrictions more specifically through more specific contacts, first in order to address the system's needs at that level, and second to enable more ready access to deeper levels.

As you work with the sacrum, you may encounter a very common pattern in which the base of the sacrum is pulling towards the sacro-iliac joint on one side (creating a pattern of distortion throughout the body). You may have allowed it to express itself, followed the inherent treatment process, and yet still that deeply ingrained, solidified sacro-iliac restriction is not responding, not releasing. You could continue to wait patiently, you could maintain your focus of attention on that area and on the patterns throughout the body that may be contributing to it and perpetuating it – or you could enhance the body's ability to release that sacro-iliac joint through the introduction of a gentle stimulus.

Release of the sacrum between the ilia

With one hand remaining under the sacrum, take up contact with the forearm across the front of the pelvis, so that the forearm, just below the elbow, is resting on the anterior superior iliac spine on the near side of the body, and the tips of the fingers are hooking round the anterior superior iliac spine on the opposite side of the body (see Figures 26.5 and 26.6). It is helpful to keep the wrist arched to create a position of mechanical advantage, as if to draw the two anterior superior iliac spines together. Maintain an equal degree of light contact on each side.

As you introduce this contact across the ilia, maintain a keen awareness of the responses within the sacrum, allowing the sacrum to express any responses to this contact – perhaps drawing into flexion, perhaps pulling to one side, perhaps following to points of stillness and release. Once any initial responses have resolved or subsided, or if there is no significant initial response, you can introduce a very slight further stimulus to the cranio-sacral system by envisaging that you are drawing the two ilia together between your elbow and your fingers. As the system responds, allow and follow any pulls, twists, turns, movements, resistances and releases that may occur, letting your attention be drawn to any focal points of stillness within the movements, allowing both hands – the hand under the sacrum and the arm across the ilia – to float with the subtle movements towards the fulcrum of stillness, and waiting there for release and reorganisation. As release occurs, observe how the sacrum settles into a more freely mobile, balanced and symmetrical state. Feel the sense of softening and release spreading up through the spine and throughout the body.

If you feel that the sacro-iliac region on one side is more specifically restricted, *you might choose to alter your contact in order to address that particular side*, so that the hand on the front of the body is resting specifically over the affected ilium (instead of resting the forearm across the front of the pelvis). With this contact, your attention may be more specifically focused on the area of restriction – but always within the context of the person as a whole (see Figure 26.7).

As the sacrum settles into increasing freedom of movement, re-evaluate quality, symmetry and motion, observing the softer looser quality, the more balanced symmetry, and the more expansive rhythmic motion, steadily taking on a wider amplitude and a slower rhythm. Note the difference with each release and the contrast in comparison to its original state. Feel the ramifications of the release spreading through the whole body as the body adapts to its new-found freedom of movement.

It is common for a sacro-iliac restriction on one side to be accompanied by a compensatory restriction in the lumbo-sacral joint on the opposite side. It is therefore often relevant to follow the sacro-iliac release with a lumbo-sacral release. Or you may in the course of a treatment identify a restriction in the lumbo–sacral area, irrespective of any sacro-iliac restriction. Either way you have the option of introducing, where appropriate, a lumbo-sacral release.

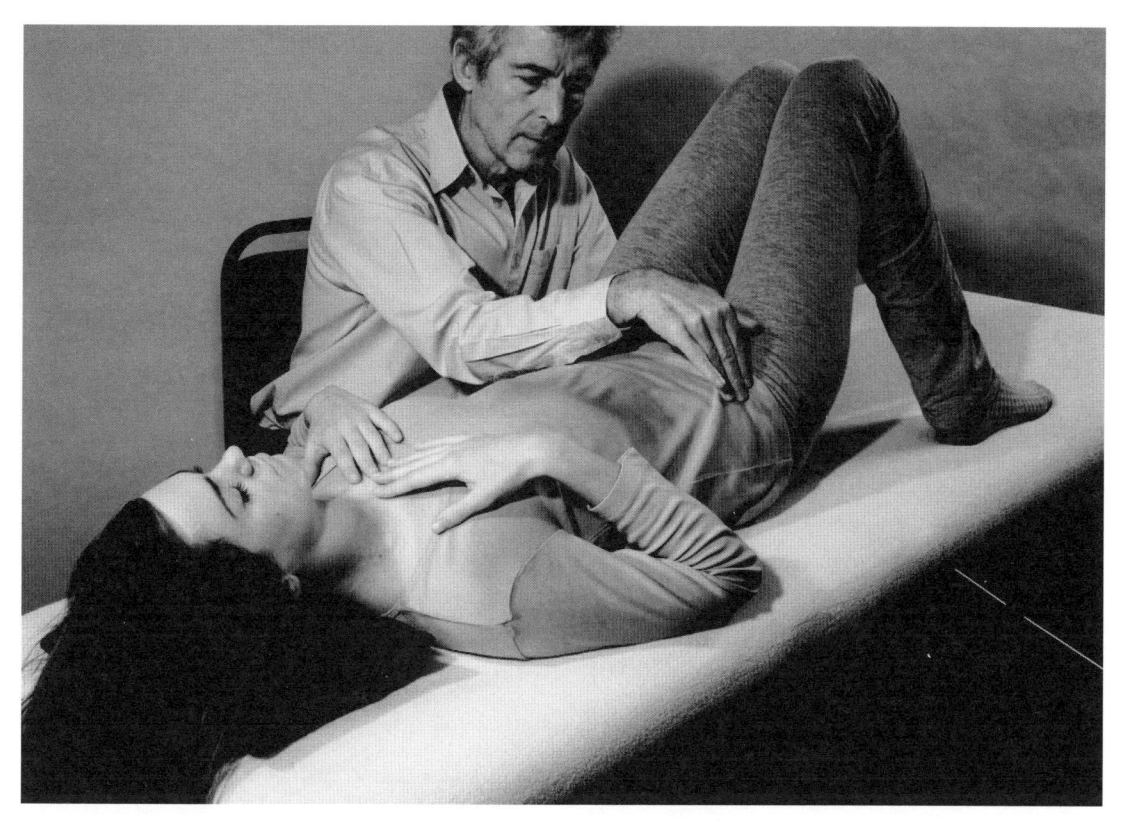

26.5 Contact for release of the sacro-iliac joints and their associated structures

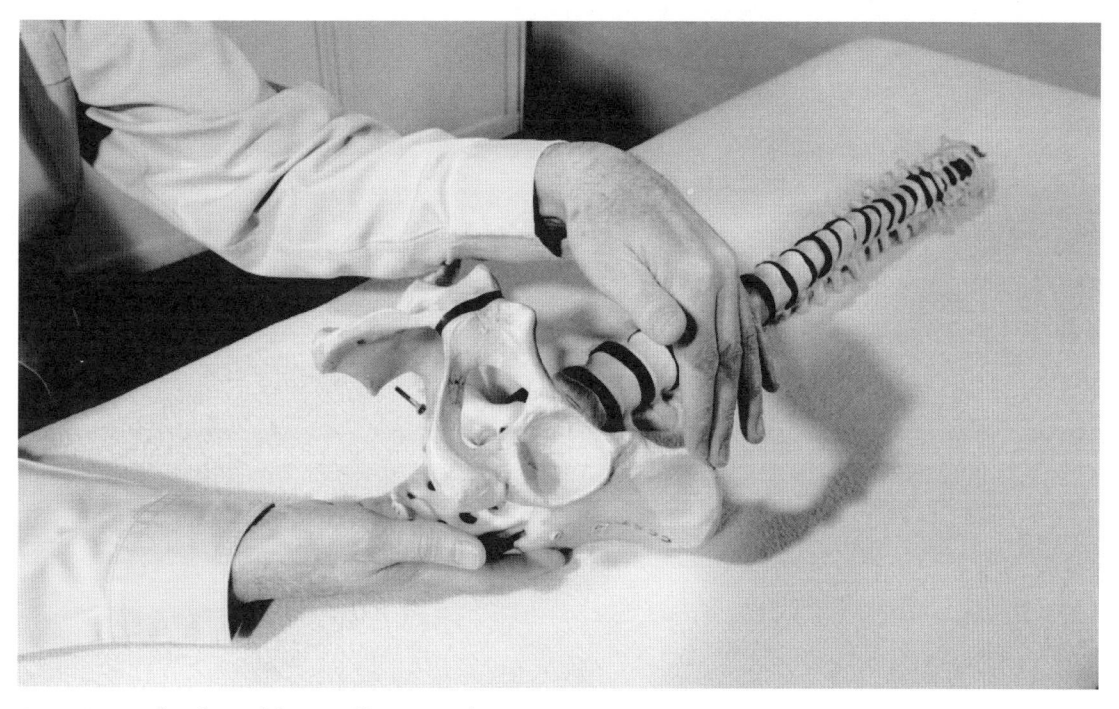

26.6 Contact for release of the sacro-iliac joints – bony perspective

170 \ Cranio-Sacral Integration

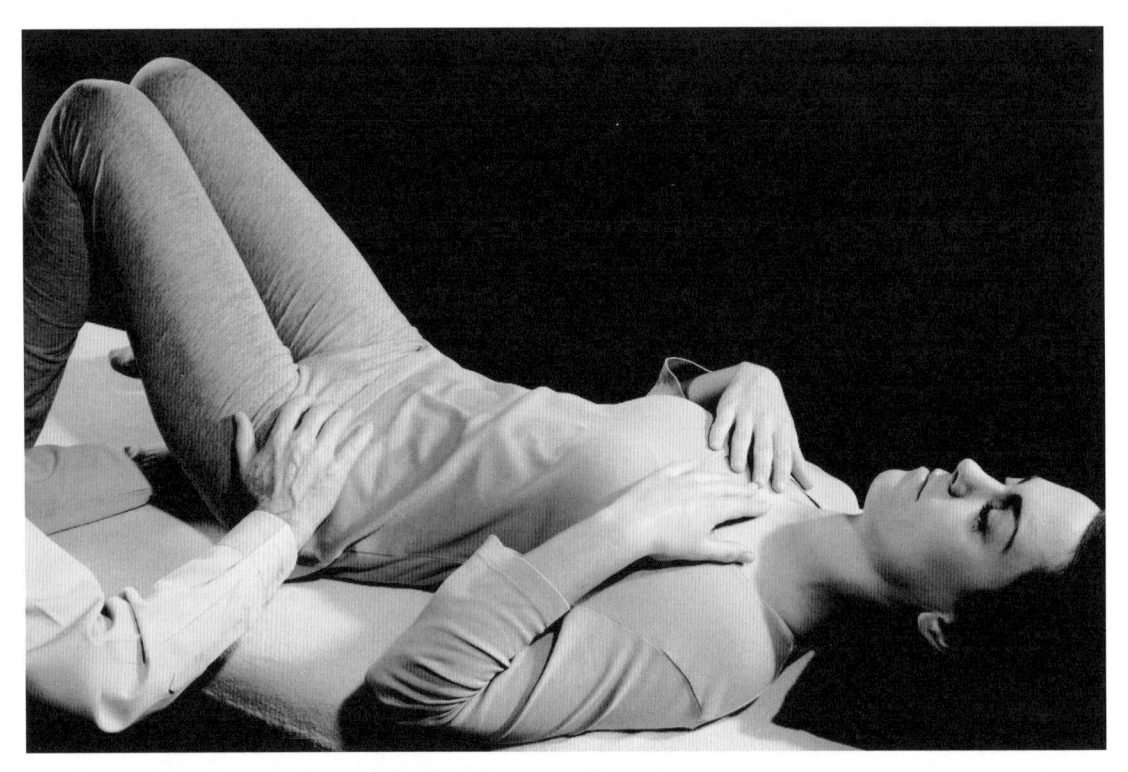

26.7 Contact for more specific focus on the release of one sacro-iliac region

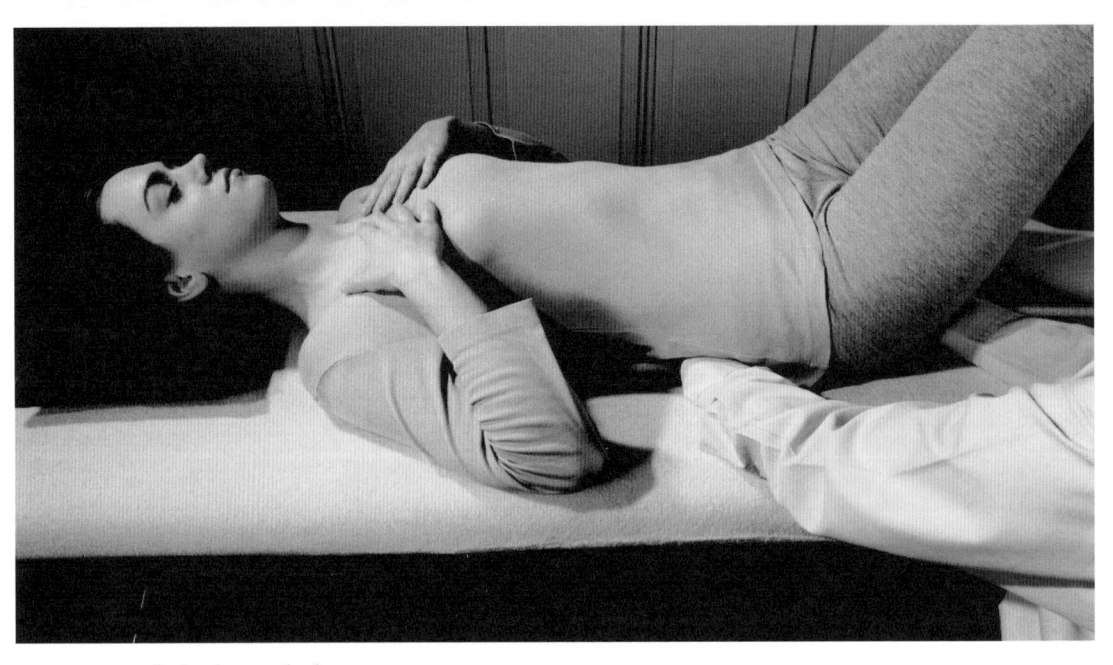

26.8 Contact for lumbo-sacral release

Lumbo-sacral release

With one hand remaining under the sacrum, ask your patient to arch their lower back slightly, so that you can slide your other hand under the lower lumbar spine, transversely under the back, close to the sacrum (see Figures 26.8 and 26.9). The edge of the second hand rests close to the tips of the fingers of the hand under the sacrum. The spine sits into the palm of your hand. Ensure that the patient relaxes down into the contact, inviting them to take a deep breath and let go completely.

As you settle into this new contact, re-establish your own fulcrums, and feel the gradual re-engagement with the system. Observe how quality, symmetry and motion are being expressed here, noticing any differences expressed through this new contact as compared to the previous impressions. Allow the sacrum and lumbar spine to respond to this new contact, allowing any spontaneous expression, following to points of stillness and release, until the system feels settled.

Compression

The lumbo-sacral area is particularly prone to compression, whether directly up the spine or at various oblique angles. Falls on the buttocks are very common in childhood and in adulthood, whether in sport, or falls in the snow and ice, or having a chair pulled from under you in the classroom. Particular sports such as horse-riding may leave more persistently ingrained effects. The prolonged sedentary lifestyles of modern life also contribute substantially to persistent compressive forces in the lumbo-sacral area. Compression is therefore an endemic condition in a substantial proportion of the population, partly contributing to the prevalence of low back pain and sciatica and many other health difficulties both locally and throughout the body. Assessing the degree of compression within this area, and offering the body the opportunity to release that compression is therefore a very valuable part of any treatment, with widespread benefits.

The sense of *compression may be immediately evident* as soon as you take up contact, the system drawing your two hands towards each other, in which case you can allow this spontaneous expression of compression – the sacral hand drawing towards the lumbar hand, the lumbar hand towards the sacrum – until it reaches a point of stillness and eventual release.

At other times, the *compression may be deeply buried* or not immediately apparent for various reasons, in which case you can explore for the presence of compression. Once the system has finished responding spontaneously and has settled into a balanced neutral state, ask the system if there is an underlying need to draw into compression, asking yourself whether your sacral hand feels drawn up towards the lumbar spine, your lumbar hand drawn down towards the sacrum, in order to engage with and release any underlying compressive pattern.

This may occur on a more forceful physical level, releasing the kinetic forces locked into the tissues by the compressive forces, or on a more subtle level, releasing the energetic forces held in the more subtle levels of the matrix. Either

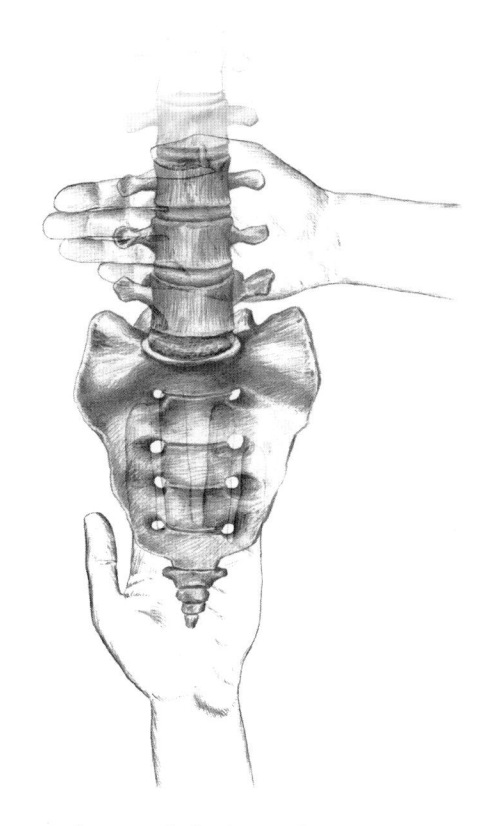

26.9 Hand position for lumbo-sacral contact

level may be relevant, depending on the needs of the patient, and working with both levels where appropriate may provide a more complete treatment process.

This process can be compared to *releasing a stuck drawer in an old chest of drawers*. If a drawer is stuck and is not pulling out easily, no amount of pulling will release it. But if you push the drawer in, then the drawer breaks free, straightens, and will then slide smoothly out from the chest of drawers. Of course we are not going to push or pull with any physical force, but on a subtle level, the same process can occur within the cranio-sacral system, as *we invite the system to take up the offer of subtle compression, until it releases or unlatches, and can then ease out freely from its compressed state*.

As you invite your hands to draw towards each other, see how the system responds. Does it welcome the offer with open arms, eagerly drawing into compression? Does it show no particular interest? Do your two hands feel readily drawn towards each other? Does the lower back seem to draw into a side-bending pattern, compressing more readily on one side than the other, reflecting a compressive injury up that side of the body, or a fall on that particular buttock?

As always, allow the system to express itself in response to this offer of compression, following to a point of stillness and eventual release. Feel the sense of softening, as the compressive forces held into the back are released and the whole area seems to open up into a softer, looser quality. Feel that softness spreading through the whole body, as the body adapts to the profound change, perhaps having released compressive forces that have been locked into the body for decades, and allowing the whole body to let go of compensatory patterns of restriction throughout the body, which may have been causing headaches, menstrual pain or personality changes. Feel the system settling into a balanced neutral state. Feel the re-emergence of rhythmic motion, more expansive than before. Follow the system through a few cycles of settled rhythmic motion.

Decompression

Having explored the possibility of compressive forces locked into the system, it is helpful to follow that with an invitation to decompression.

An invitation to decompression allows the system to *make the most of its new found freedom* to open out through the lumbo-sacral region, with consequent ramifications throughout the body. It also helps the body to release the *chronic compensations and adaptations which may have become deeply ingrained into the tissues* as a result of the long-term holding into compression. Decompression also invites the system to respond in a different way and to *address different forces* held in the system.

Once the system has settled into a balanced neutral state, invite your sacral hand away from the lumbar spine, your lumbar hand away from the sacrum, as if your two hands were drawing apart (as always, no physical force, just the thought).

Allow any responses, following any twists and turns. Continue until the system has decompressed as far as it wishes, sometimes seeming to float out endlessly. When it feels complete, gradually reduce any invitation to decompression, allow the system to settle back into a balanced neutral state. Re-evaluate quality, symmetry and motion.

Integration of the spine through the sacrum

With the sacrum released from any restrictions in the sacro-iliac and lumbo-sacral areas, the *vitality of the system is likely to be profoundly enhanced* – assuming that restrictions were encountered and addressed. This in itself will be of great benefit to the health of the patient.

It also provides us with *a sacrum through which we can more clearly and accurately access patterns of restriction emanating from the spine*. With the sacrum released from its local bony and soft tissue relations, the influence of pulls on the sacrum from elsewhere can be felt more clearly and the freely mobile sacrum can be more readily used to engage with these patterns.

Just as we have done from the occiput (as described in Chapter 25) we can project our attention up through the spine, segment by segment, allowing the system to respond, following the responses to points of stillness and release, releasing vertebral restrictions and facilitated segments, integrating the whole spine, and thereby enhancing the balance and integration of the whole system.

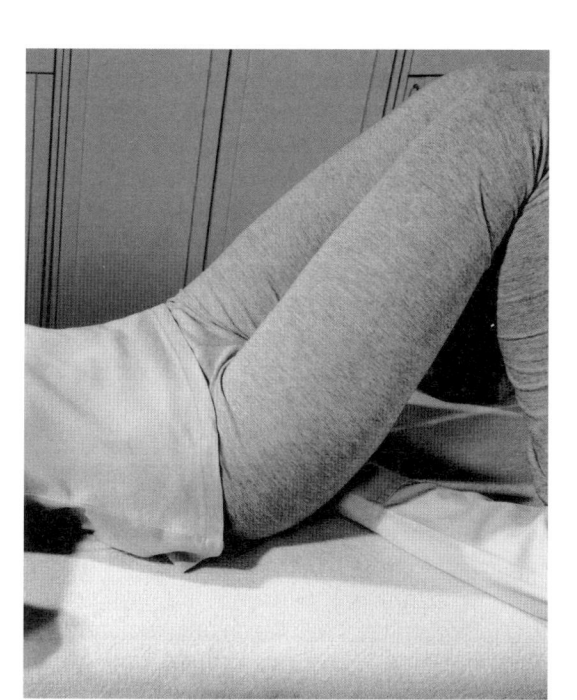

26.10 Contact for the sacrum

Keeping your hand under the sacrum, maintaining continuity of the connection that you have established previously, gently slide your other hand out from under the lumbar spine. Settle into the new contact, re-establish your practitioner fulcrums, re-engage with the cranio-sacral system, monitoring quality, symmetry and motion and settling into a balanced neutral engagement with the sacrum (see Figure 26.10).

Project your attention up through the spine, segment by segment, from sacrum to L5, up through the lumbar spine from L5 to L1, the thoracic spine from T12 to T1, the cervical spine from C7 to C1, all the time feeling the responses in your hand under the sacrum, noticing the changes in quality, symmetry and motion as your attention moves from segment to segment. These responses may be the result of vertebral restrictions, facilitated segments, adhesions or neurological input at these segments. Allow the sacrum to respond, following into any patterns of asymmetry to points of stillness and release.

As you continue your journey up through the spine, evaluate the overall state of the spine together with any ramifications relating to other parts of the body – understanding the relationship between particular vertebral levels and the specific organs or parts of the body neurologically supplied from those levels. Respond to any impressions that arise, allowing any twists and turns, waiting at any points of resistance for the resistance to soften, allowing any agitation to settle, identifying any areas of

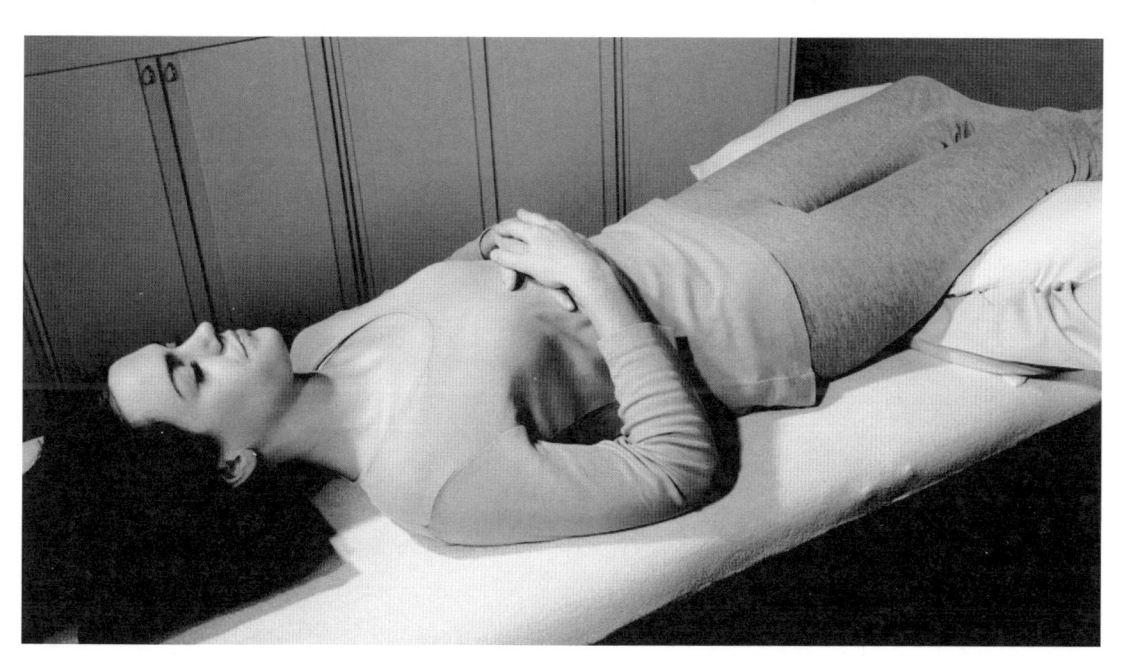

26.11 Sacral contact with a pillow under the knees

more persistent resistant restriction – reflecting more chronic patterns of injury or trauma, feeling the gradual release of each segment and the integration of the whole spine.

As before, you could continue up into the cranium, or project out to any other part of the body, but for the moment we will content ourselves with the spine. As before, you might wish to conceptualise a very slight thought of traction as you project up the spine, as if you were gently stretching the dural membrane, easing out any tensions and restrictions.

Once you have completed your journey up the spine and the whole spine feels integrated, release any thought of projecting up through the spine. Re-evaluate the quality, symmetry and motion at the sacrum. Feel the calmer quality as the system settles increasingly into a balanced neutral state. Feel the increasingly expansive rhythmic motion. Follow the rhythmic motion through a few cycles of even motion, allowing the process to come to completion.

Subtle integration

As the system settles following these releases, you may find the system spontaneously shifting to deeper levels and deeper tides, no longer needing to pull towards imbalances and fulcrums, settling into a more fluent expansive expression of middle tide motion, perhaps sinking deeper into long tide motion and dynamic stillness. Be content to stay there with this deeper engagement, not feeling the need to do anything, not feeling that the lack of pulls and twists means that nothing is happening, allowing the more subtle integration that is continuing at this level, allowing yourself to become deeply absorbed into the surrounding matrix and appreciating the deeper level of healing that emerges from this level of engagement. This stage of the process, when nothing much seems to be happening, but therapeutic responses are occurring on a deeper more subtle level, can be a very significant part of the treatment, so be prepared to stay there at length.

Chapter 27

The Sphenoid

The *sphenoid* is an *exceptionally beautiful* bone, beautiful in its complexity, beautiful in its delicacy. It has often been compared to a butterfly, or moth – with its body centrally, its two greater wings, its two lesser wings, and its pterygoid processes hanging down like the legs of a moth (see Figures 27.1 and 27.2).

The sphenoid is also a *central*, *pivotal* component of the cranio-sacral system, located centrally within the base of the cranium, articulating with every other bone of the cranium and also with several facial bones. Together with the occiput, it forms the spheno-basilar synchondrosis, the pivotal fulcrum around which the whole bony cranio-sacral system revolves (see Figure 27.3).

Most parts of the sphenoid are located internally, *deep inside the cranium*, not palpable on the external surface. The only parts of the bone which do emerge to the surface are the tips of the greater wings, emerging at the pterions, or temples, just behind the lateral corners of the eyes (see Figure 27.4). This deeply enclosed location

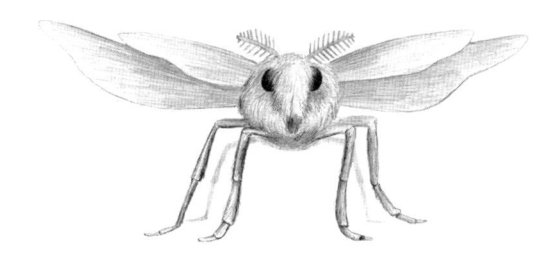

27.1 The sphenoid has often been compared to a butterfly or a moth

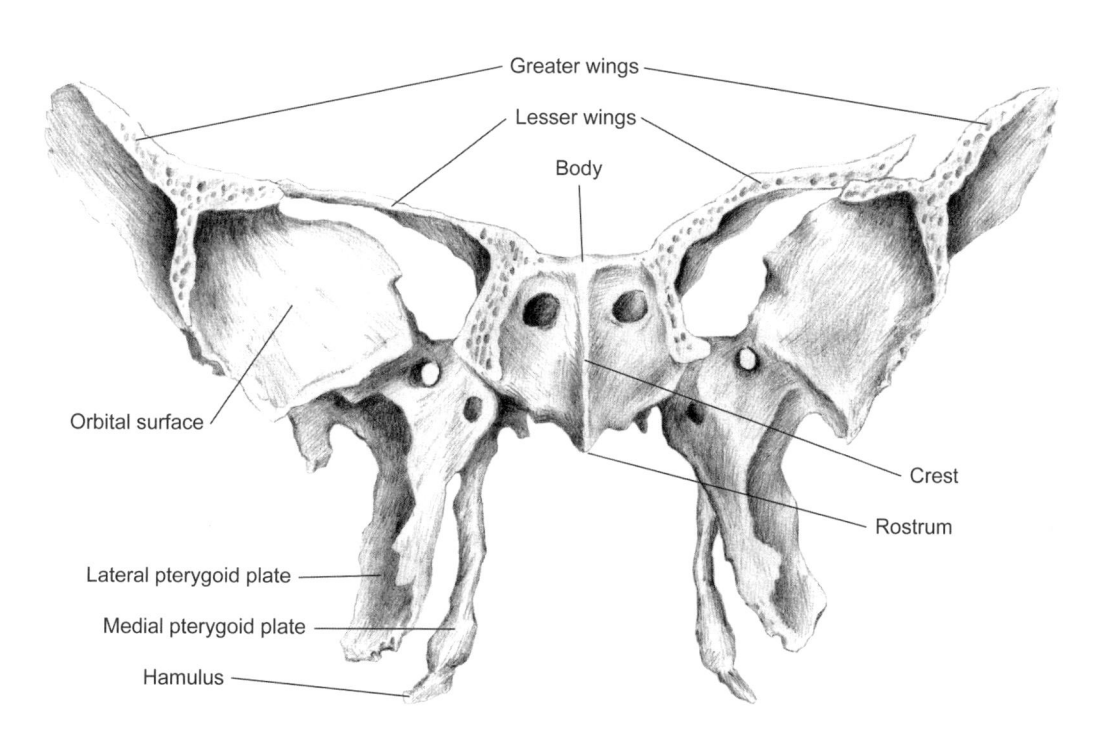

27.2 The sphenoid is an exceptionally beautiful bone – beautiful in its complexity, beautiful in its delicacy (anterior view)

is reflected in the fact that the sphenoid provides access to particularly profound levels of the patient's being.

In view of its pivotal nature, the sphenoid also readily reflects imbalances and tensions from all over the system. Restoring balance, mobility and symmetry around the sphenoid reflects the restoration of balance and integrity to the system as a whole at a deep level, perhaps more than anywhere else in the body.

Location

The sphenoid is located at the very centre of the base of the cranium, with its *body* at the midline just in front of the basi-occiput, its two *greater wings* spreading out on each side to form part of the floor of the middle cranial fossa, the two *lesser wings* – smaller thinner wings – emerging from the top of the front of the body to run along the posterior edge of the anterior cranial fossa (see Figure 27.3). The two *pterygoid processes* (the legs of the moth) project down (inferiorly) from the body, each process dividing into a *medial pterygoid plate* and a *lateral pterygoid plate*, terminating just behind the nasal cavity and palate (see Figure 27.3).

The superior surface of the *body of the sphenoid* is intricately shaped to form the *sella turcica* (Turkish saddle) so-called because the early anatomists, with their imaginative imagery, perceived that this structure resembles the ornate saddles used by Turkish horsemen, with two pommels at the front and two pommels at the back holding the rider securely in his saddle. In the case of the sphenoid, the sella turcica has two *anterior clinoid processes* projecting from the front and two *posterior clinoid processes* projecting at the back. Instead of a Turkish horseman sitting in the middle of your head, you have a *pituitary gland* (the 'master gland' of the endocrine system – again reflecting the pivotal significance of this area).

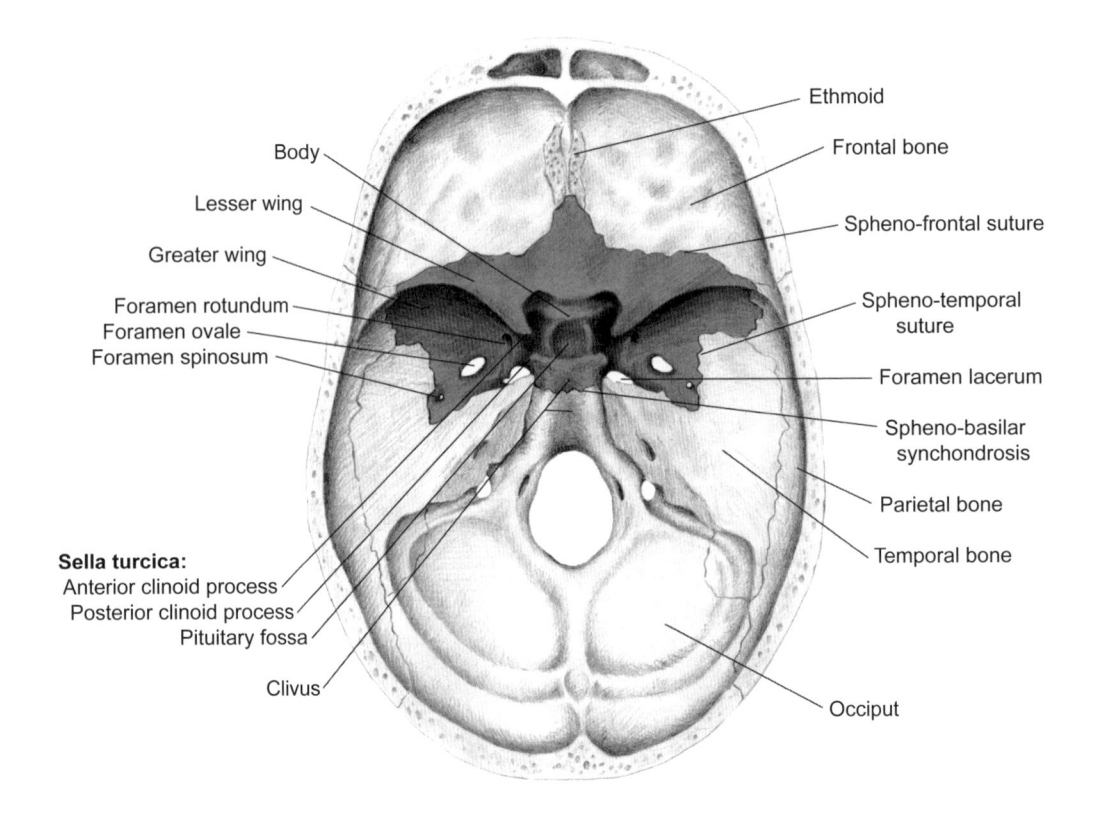

27.3 The sphenoid in situ – superior view of the cranial base

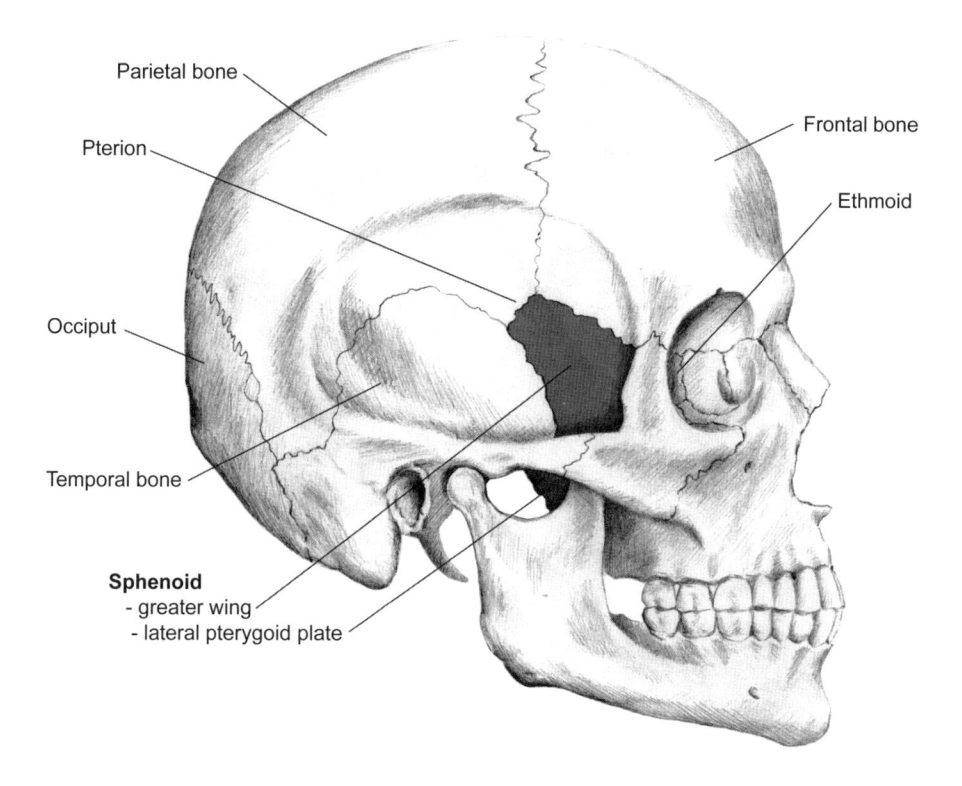

27.4 The sphenoid in situ – lateral view

Articulations

The sphenoid articulates with every other cranial bone – as well as several bones of the face (see Figures 27.3 and 27.4).

Anteriorly, the lesser wings articulate with the *frontal bone* (at the spheno-frontal suture). At the centre of this articulation, where the frontal bone opens out into a notch (the ethmoid notch) to accommodate the ethmoid bone, the sphenoid body meets with the *ethmoid* (the hollow sphenoidal sinuses within the body of the sphenoid opening into the ethmoid sinuses).

The tips of the *greater wings of the sphenoid* form a small articulation with the *parietal bones* on each side of the head, at the *pterions*.

The posterior edges of the greater wings articulate with the anterior edges of the *temporal bones* (at the spheno-temporal sutures).

(The word sphenoid derives from the Greek word for a wedge, since the sphenoid is wedged between the frontal and temporal bones. However, as we shall see shortly, the term wedge is actually more applicable to the temporal bones.)

The posterior portion of the body of the sphenoid meets the anterior portion of the basi-occiput to form the spheno-basilar synchondrosis.

Spheno-basilar synchondrosis

This joint is a synchondrosis (not a suture) because, unlike most joints in the skull, it is a cartilaginous joint (whereas sutures are fibrous joints). A synchondrosis is a primary cartilaginous joint, which means that it starts life as cartilage, and gradually ossifies to become solid bone (in this case ossification is considered to be complete by the age of 25). This distinction means that the spheno-basilar joint behaves differently from the sutures, a difference which we will explore in more detail later.

The spheno-basilar synchondrosis is also the central pivotal fulcrum around which the whole bony structure of the cranio-sacral system revolves; it is also the joint around which Sutherland established the terms flexion and extension to describe the rhythmic movement within certain structures of the cranio-sacral system, since flexion (the closing of an angle) and extension (the opening of an angle) are occurring at the inferior surface of the spheno-basilar joint during the expansion and contraction phases of rhythmic motion.

Membranous attachments

The sphenoid is lined with membrane. It also receives attachment of the *tentorium cerebelli*. As the tentorium projects forward, it forms four strands of membrane: two from the upper leaf of the tentorium attaching onto the anterior clinoid processes, two from the lower leaf of the tentorium attaching onto the posterior clinoid processes (see Figure 27.5).

The sella turcica is also covered by a roof of membrane, the diaphragma sellae (the diaphragm over the saddle; see Figure 27.6), a small membranous sheet which stretches across the four clinoid processes like a canopy over a four poster bed, and passes down the sides of the sphenoid body (like the curtains around the four poster bed). On first sight the diaphragma sellae appears to cover the pituitary gland, enclosing it within the sella. However, the diaphragm is actually invaginated by the pituitary, wrapping around the whole pituitary gland and stalk as they project down into the sella below, thereby enveloping and protecting the pituitary gland, and also ensuring that the pituitary gland is within the subarachnoid

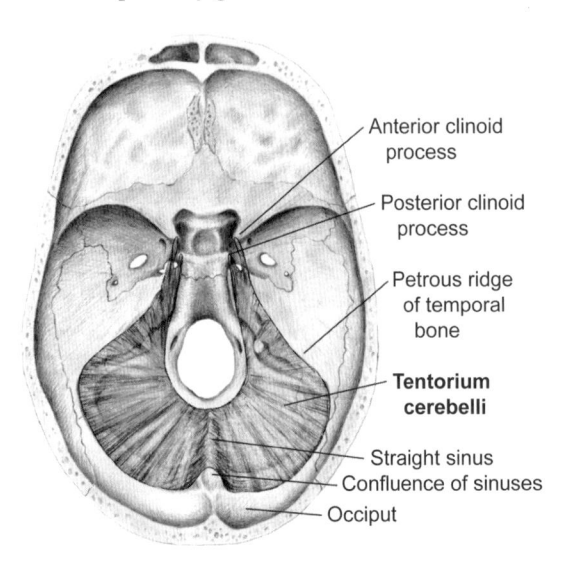

27.5 *Membranous relations of the sphenoid – the tentorium cerebelli*

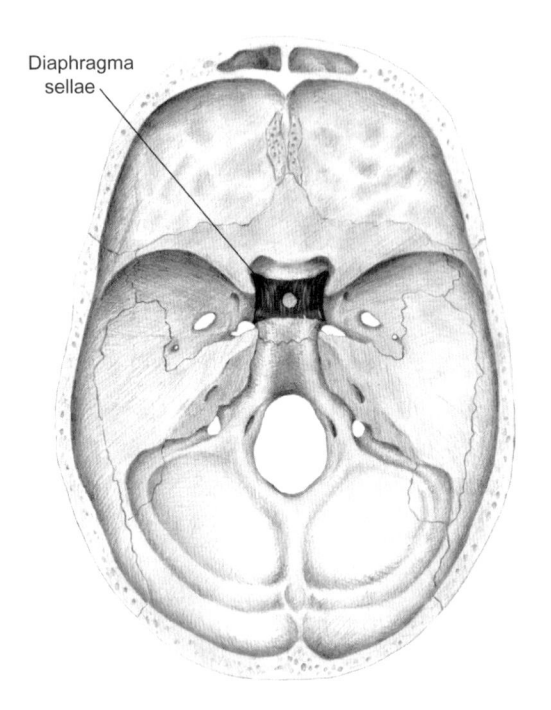

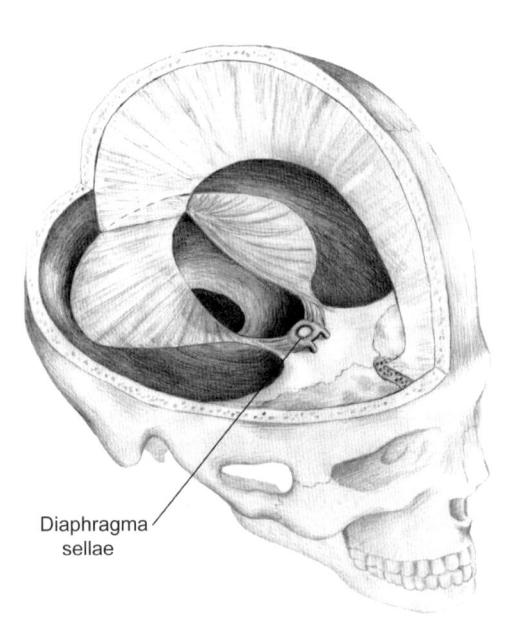

27.6 *The diaphragma sellae is a small membranous sheet forming a roof over the sella turcica*
  a. *Superior view*
  b. *Oblique view*

space and therefore continuously immersed in and washed by cerebrospinal fluid. The diaphragma sellae, like all the membranous infoldings, is not a separate piece of membrane, but blends into the surrounding membranes, as part of the continuous membranous meningeal sheath.

Cranio-sacral motion

During rhythmic motion, the sphenoid moves with the front part of the cranium, arcing forward and down (together with the frontal bone) during the expansion phase, coming back and up during the contraction phase, hingeing around the spheno-basilar synchondrosis (see Figure 27.7). This has been compared to a large bird, hunching forward as if to take flight, starting to lift its wings – and then changing its mind and settling back onto its perch.

This forward and down movement is the opposite of the movement at the occiput and back of the head, thereby creating the flexion/extension movement at the inferior surface of the spheno-basilar synchondrosis. This combined motion of sphenoid and occiput can most readily be felt through the sphenoid contact.

ENGAGEMENT THROUGH THE SPHENOID – THE PROCESS

Contact

In order to access the cranio-sacral system through the sphenoid, let your hands come in very softly through the energy field towards the sides of the head until the *pads* of your thumbs come to rest very lightly on the tips of the greater wings, where they emerge to the surface of the cranium at the pterions, just behind the lateral corners of the eyes. (It is preferable to use the pads rather than the tips of your thumbs, as this provides a softer, more relaxed and less intrusive thumb contact.)

If you take up contact on your own sphenoid, you will no doubt notice that this is a soft, sensitive area. All cranio-sacral contacts are extremely light, but here in particular, you want to ensure that your thumb contact is exceptionally light, establishing as always the appropriate level of physical contact in response to the system's demands – whether on the body or off the body.

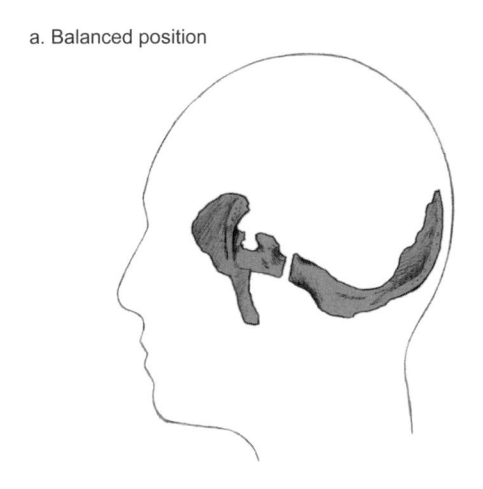

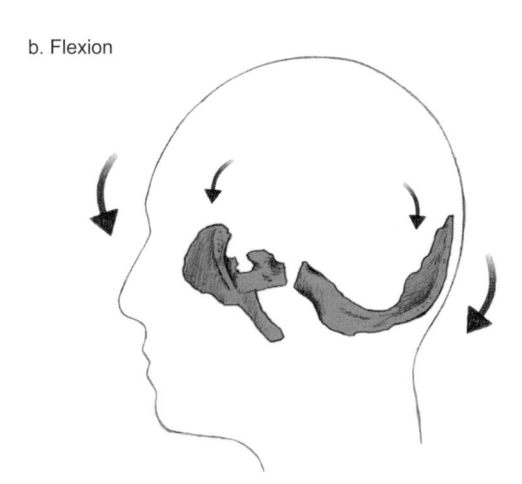

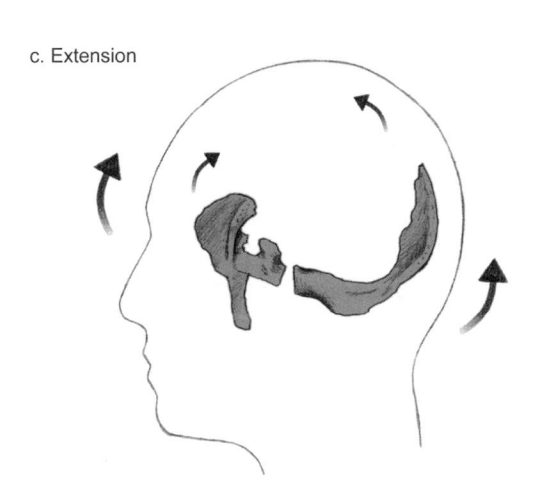

a. Balanced position

b. Flexion

c. Extension

27.7 Cranio-sacral motion of the sphenoid – during rhythmic motion, the sphenoid arcs forward and down during the expansion phase, coming back and up during the contraction phase, hingeing around the spheno-basilar synchondrosis

Having settled into the contact, with your thumbs appropriately positioned, allow your fingers and hands to settle gently onto the sides of the cranium, the little fingers extending round towards the occiput in whatever position is comfortable – without losing the contact of the thumbs at the sphenoid. Keep your hands relaxed, not stretching or straining in any way. Most significantly, take particular care to ensure that your thumbs, fingers, hands, arms and your whole being remain extremely soft.

Engagement

As you settle into the contact, establish the usual prerequisites for effective engagement with the cranio-sacral system – settling your own *practitioner fulcrums*, settling into the relaxed, detached, floating, meditative state of mind which will enable you to be at your most sensitive and receptive. Establish the appropriate *level of physical contact* in response to your patient's system, whether on the body or off the body. Establish the appropriate *level of attention* – allowing a sense of spaciousness and a wider perspective. Connect with the different *tissue levels*, feeling the malleability and pliability within this soft, membranous balloon, allowing your hands to become immersed in the fluidity of the system, experiencing this cranium as a ball of energy, a mass of vibrating subatomic particles in constant motion, a fluidic matrix, with infinite potential for movement, change and flexibility.

Impressions

As your hands dissolve into the fluidity of your patient's system and your patient's system melts into your hands, and you feel the increasing sense of interconnection between your two systems, allow your attention to become increasingly aware of any *impressions* that may come to you – without losing the sense of your own ease and detachment – as if looking down on the whole spacious picture from above, while at the same time being aware of impressions arising at your hands.

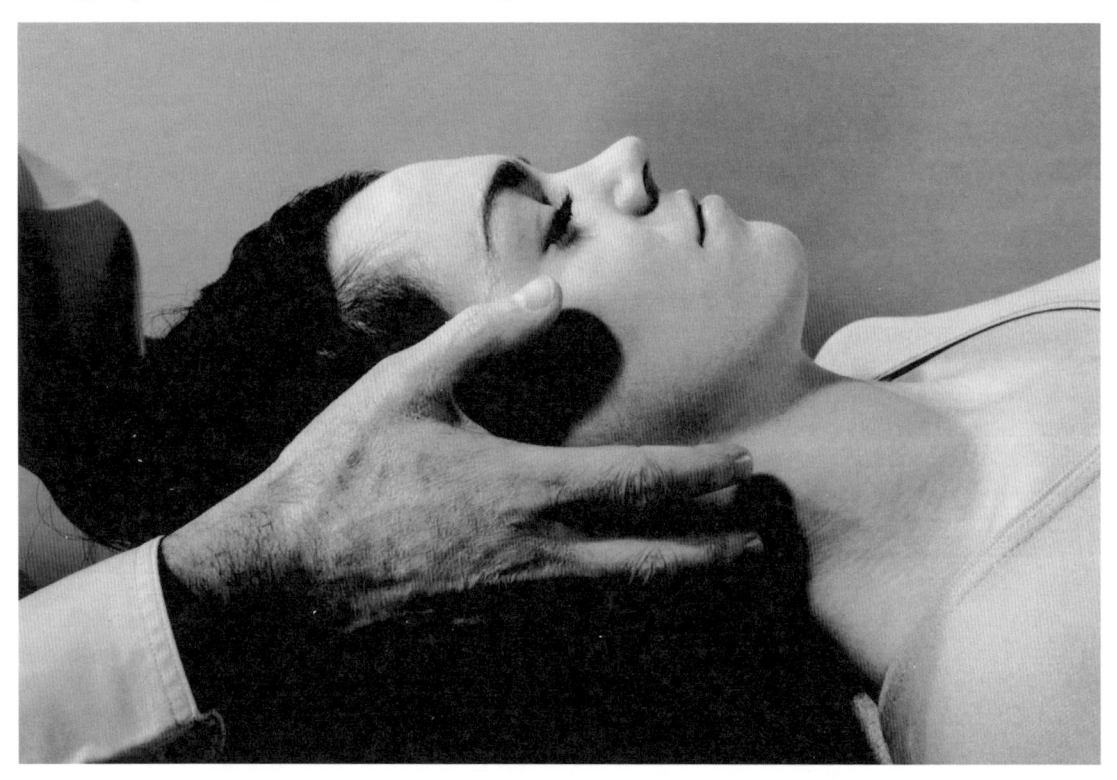

27.8 Contact for the sphenoid – lateral view – let your hands come in very softly towards the sides of the head until the pads of your thumbs come to rest very lightly on the tips of the greater wings, where they emerge to the surface of the cranium at the pterions, just behind the lateral corners of the eyes

The Sphenoid / 181

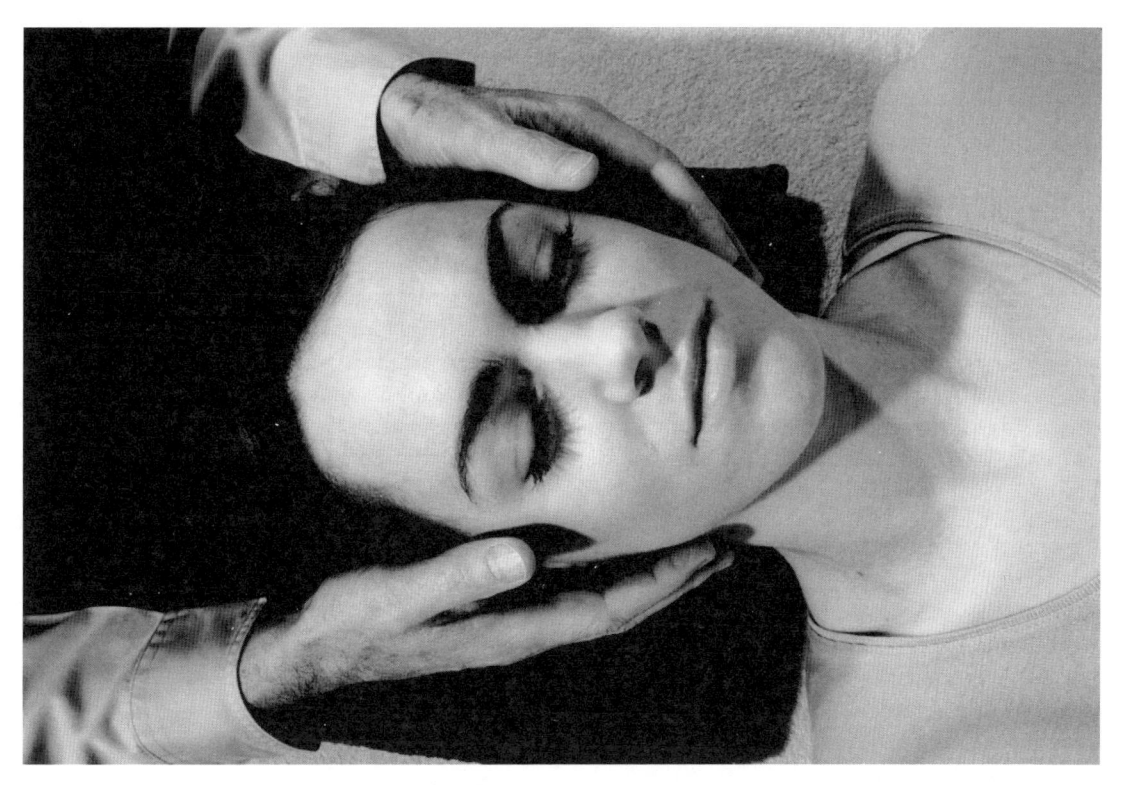

27.9 Contact for the sphenoid – anterior view

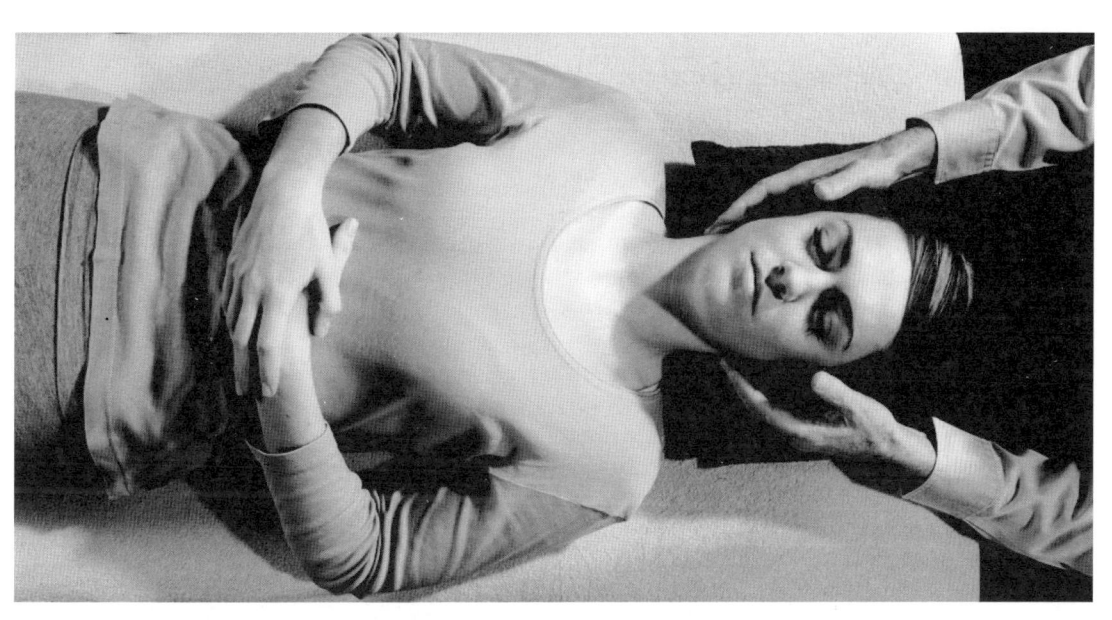

27.10 Contact for the sphenoid – wider perspective

Be aware of impressions of *quality* – the quality of the system as a whole, local qualities and differences in quality from one area to another.

Be aware of impressions of *symmetry* or asymmetry – any overall sense of asymmetry, any difference between the two sides, any bulging, twisting, pulling, any sense of greater contraction or expansion on one side or the other, any sense of greater restriction or stuckness on one side or the other, differences of solidity and fluidity, of activity and stillness.

Be aware of impressions of *motion* – subtle, generalised movements of vibration and pulsation, swirling, rocking, agitation, dancing, twisting or pulling – or the increasing emergence of *rhythmic motion*.

Allowing

Allow the system to express itself, allowing the different movements to arise, allowing your hands to float freely with the subtle movements, allowing your hands to become immersed in the fluidity, allowing your hands to be washed this way and that by the fluidic motion.

Settling into deeper engagement

As the superficial wavelets and ripples settle, be aware of the increasing sense of stillness and calmness, the rhythmic motion gradually settling from faster to slower rhythms, perhaps from an initial awareness of cranio-sacral rhythm to an increasing awareness of middle tide motion.

Be aware of any further, more persistent pulls or twists, again allowing the inherent treatment process as your hands are drawn by these more deeply ingrained currents, following the asymmetries to points of balanced tension, points of stillness, feeling the rhythmic motion gradually closing down as it draws into stillness, and staying with your attention at those points of stillness, until resistance softens and release occurs.

Responding to changes in the energy field

As you settle into increasingly spacious engagement with your patient's system, maintain the continuous exploration of levels of physical contact. Feel the energy field within and around your patient's head. See if perhaps it wants to expand or push your hands away, or whether it wants to draw your hands in. Some energy fields may want to push your hands several inches off the body; others may welcome a gentle contact on the surface of the skin. Feel this cushion of energy. Let your hands float on the surface of this fluidic energy field, being pushed out or drawn in or twisted this way and that by the ripples, eddies and currents.

Recognise that the system may want to change from moment to moment, expanding, contracting, twisting, turning. Perhaps it may expand and expand until it reaches a point where it feels comfortable, where it has expanded as far as it needs to go. Wait at that point, and in due course it may flutter, or wriggle, or pulsate, and then melt – and the energy field may soften to allow your hands to settle into a different level, closer to the head, or perhaps onto the surface of the skin, or perhaps opening out into even wider expansion. Be open to a continuous process of fluidic expansion, contraction and other movements, letting your hands float as if immersed in fluidic fluctuating energy.

Perhaps one side will push out, the other side push in – perhaps reflecting a blow to the head from the pushed-in side. The head itself may appear balanced on external observation but the force field will reflect the displacement of energy caused by the blow and still held into the system on that energetic level and affecting function.

Tracing to the source – awareness of the whole person

Perhaps certain patterns of asymmetry or points of stillness may be more persistent and resistant, remaining in a particular asymmetry, apparently reluctant to release. Such patterns may be being maintained by restrictions elsewhere in the body and you can trace them to their source. As you wait within the stillness, let your attention extend along the lines of asymmetry to see where they are coming from. Let your attention project down through the body, observing changes to quality, symmetry and motion as your attention reaches different areas. Perhaps as you identify the source of the imbalance or a key point of restriction, the persistent resistance may soften and release. The source might be somewhere in the cranium, somewhere in the neck, in the spine, in the heart or heart centre, in the solar plexus or diaphragm, in the pelvis, sacro-iliac joint, the knee or the foot, or anywhere in the patient's body or psyche or matrix. When your attention reaches the appropriate focus, the pattern may dissolve, and the system may settle into a more balanced state. As such releases occur, feel them spreading through the whole body, as the system adapts to the changes.

Continue to observe the inherent treatment process as it evolves spontaneously, as it responds to your contact, allowing and enabling the gradual emergence of any resistances, restrictions, or imbalances throughout the cranio-sacral system, throughout the whole person, as reflected through the sphenoid – initially the more superficial patterns, and subsequently ever deeper patterns, until the system settles into a peaceful balanced state, and steady rhythmic motion is re-established. If you are working with a system in which the superficial patterns have already been cleared – as with someone who has received a significant amount of cranio-sacral treatment and is settled in themselves – then you might progress rapidly to encounter deeper levels of the system. If you are working with someone for whom the superficial patterns have not been cleared – like the majority of patients who have not received much cranio-sacral treatment – then you may continue to observe the gradual release of superficial patterns, wavelets and ripples from the system as they arise and dissolve.

Shifting to deeper levels

With each release, the rhythmic motion may become increasingly apparent – clearer, calmer, slower, and more expansive. You may feel shifts to deeper levels of engagement, the rhythmic motion settling gradually from faster motion to slower motion, the quality of the system changing to a deeper, calmer, more spacious quality. If your initial engagement has been with the level of the cranio-sacral rhythm, then at some point, perhaps spontaneously, perhaps following a specific release, you may feel a shift to the middle tide level. As the system continues to adjust and integrate at these deeper levels, you may notice that the manifestations of asymmetry, drawing in to stillness, and release are all being expressed on a subtler level.

Maintain your awareness of the whole person, while at the same time feeling the subtle patterns of reintegration between your hands, as you settle into deeper stillness.

Subtle integration

Be content just to be there, allowing the system to express itself, feeling the process of subtle integration proceeding at ever-deeper levels. Settle into deeper stillness, feeling the process of integration spreading through the whole person. Allow yourself to sink deeper and deeper into a more spacious, profound space, moving through deeper levels of middle tide motion and perhaps to long tide and dynamic stillness where you can simply be with the system in deep dynamic stillness. This may often be all you need to do; this may well be the complete treatment process. Within that deep stillness, you may at some point reach a suitable state of completion, where the system settles into a peaceful, balanced, neutral state, and steady rhythmic motion is re-established. At this point you can allow the treatment process to come to an end.

SPECIFIC RELEASE OF THE SPHENOID

Stimulus

You may not always reach the most profound levels of long tide and dynamic stillness. The system will choose to engage with the appropriate level, within the context of the therapist's level of awareness. The process may come to a point of completion within the middle tide level, or within the cranio-sacral rhythm level depending on the needs of the patient. The system may not wish to settle into deeper levels, or may not want to progress, or may not want to reach a point of conclusion. At such times there are other options available.

At some point, it may become appropriate to offer these further options to the system, offering the stimulus of a subtle invitation to further response, asking the system if it has further imbalances that it would like to release, further patterns hidden under the surface, further resistances that it is not quite able to overcome on its own, for which it needs the focused attention of a practitioner to enhance the inherent healing potential within the system.

Spheno-basilar release

From time to time, you may find that the system draws spontaneously into one extreme of rhythmic motion, drawing persistently into flexion (expansion) or persistently into extension (contraction) and you can allow and follow that, feeling a gradual build-up of pressure or tension within the system, until it reaches a point of stillness and eventual release. In the same way, you may find that that the system draws spontaneously into *compression* at the spheno-basilar synchondrosis – particularly where there is a compressive pattern present within the system – reaches a point of stillness, and releases. This is a *spontaneous spheno-basilar release*.

You can also specifically offer the system the further support and assistance of an *invited spheno-basilar release*. The spheno-basilar release is an invitation to the body to enhance its natural tendency to release patterns of resistance as monitored at the spheno-basilar synchondrosis. It involves two components – an invitation into spheno-basilar compression and a subsequent invitation into spheno-basilar decompression. If it does not arise spontaneously, it can be offered to the system. It could be helpful as a means of:

- helping the body to release specific patterns of compression manifesting at the spheno-basilar synchondrosis
- releasing persistent resistances anywhere throughout the system

- settling an unsettled system, or a restless system
- clearing superficial patterns
- exploring deeper into the system
- helping the system to shift to a deeper level of engagement.

Spheno-basilar compression
Compressive forces

Compressive patterns are often present in the cranium. The spheno-basilar area is particularly prone to compression (see Figure 27.11). This may arise due to the compressive forces of birth, from a fall onto the back of the head, or from a blow to the front of the head. It may be a reflection of compression elsewhere in the system, particularly in the suboccipital area or the lumbo-sacral area, or a reflection of the quality of the system as a whole. It may be the result of persistent emotional tension and contraction, with the whole system drawing in and the membranes tightly held. It may be a reflection of the personality, associated with a state of depression, contraction or withdrawal.

Identifying, recognising and connecting with these compressive forces locked into the spheno-basilar area can help the system to overcome the patterns embedded there, enabling them to unlatch – like the stuck drawer in the chest of drawers.

When compressive patterns are present, the head may be eager to draw into those compressions in order to release them. Sometimes, as mentioned above, this may occur spontaneously and be readily apparent as soon as you take up contact on the cranium. At other times, the patterns may become apparent only when you ask the system whether it wants to enter into compression and offer it that possibility.

An invitation

Maintaining the same contact on the sphenoid and communicating through your thumbs (but not tensing or tightening or *doing* anything with your thumbs), you can ask the system if it feels compressed, if it would like to enter into that compression, if it would like to release that compression. In other words, ask yourself if you feel any sense of your thumbs being drawn posteriorly, as if to draw the sphenoid towards the occiput. (With your patient lying supine, this means envisaging your thumbs being drawn down towards the couch.) As always it is just a thought, not a physical force. Observe the response.

A reply

The system may say, 'No, I'm not interested'. That's fine; of course you're not going to force it or impose on it. It might respond by choosing to go off in some other direction, so you can let it do that. It might say, 'Yes, that's exactly what I want to do', and you may feel your thumbs drawn down towards the couch, perhaps symmetrically, perhaps more on one side than the other, perhaps shifting to one side or moving into a twist or bend as it compresses, perhaps passing through a series of different twists and turns as it compresses. As always, allow and follow the various twists and turns while the system responds to your invitation.

A response

As it draws into compression, you may feel drawn to a particular fulcrum around which that compression is focused, whether within the cranium, the neck or anywhere else in the body. Perhaps familiar patterns that were apparent earlier may become exaggerated or more evident; perhaps new patterns will emerge from beneath the surface. As described previously, you may feel a gradual build-up of tension or pressure in the system, until eventually it reaches a point of stillness, where it doesn't seem to need to go any further. Wait with that stillness. Feel that stillness pervading the whole head, the whole patient, the whole room. In due course, the system may start to wriggle, to vibrate, to pulsate, to rock from side to side. Allow it to do whatever it wants to do, while maintaining the invitation to compression. Take care not to mistake these tiny, wriggling, vibrating movements for a release; stay with the system, with the dynamic stillness, with the sense of compression, until you feel a convincing sense of softening. Eventually the system may release, and it may feel as if the whole head – and the

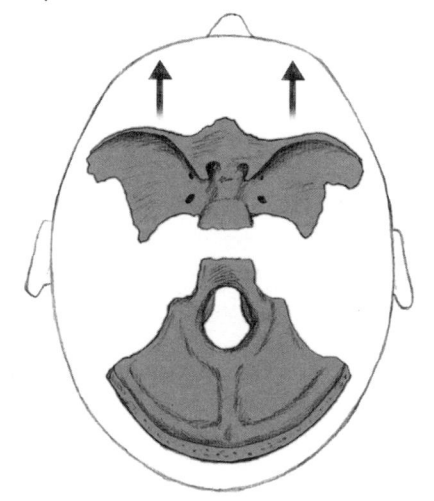

27.11 Direction of compression and decompression at the spheno-basilar synchondrosis

a. Balanced position

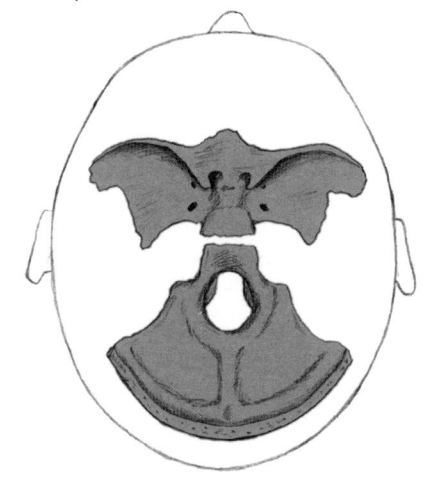

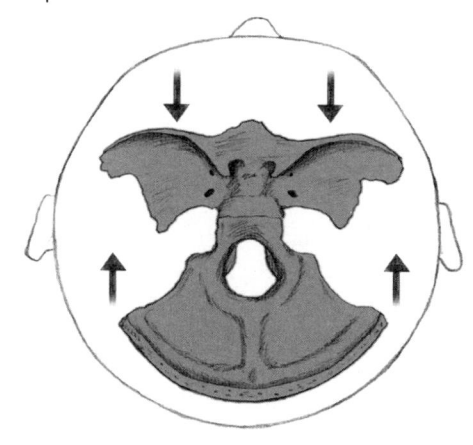

b. Compression

c. Decompression

whole cranio-sacral system – is melting, softening, opening up. Allow it to do so.

Release and reorganisation

Feel the head melting, softening, expanding. Feel it reorganising and rebalancing. Feel that softness and expansiveness spreading throughout the whole system, the whole person. You may feel your hands being pushed off the body as the energy field expands, reaching a point of stillness, releasing and settling back in again.

Allow time for the system to absorb the repercussions of this release, to reorganise itself and adjust to any changes. Allow time for the system to adapt to the release of deeper patterns within. Initially you may experience a sense of disorientation and uncertainty within the system as it resettles itself and reorganises itself. As it becomes settled, you may feel the system settling back into neutral, with the gradual re-emergence of cranio-sacral motion becoming clearer and stronger again.

Neutral

As rhythmic motion re-emerges, feel the softer quality, the more balanced symmetry and greater expansiveness of the whole system. Stay with the system through a few cycles of rhythmic motion.

Be sure to allow the system to settle back fully into neutral – as recognised through the re-establishment of clear, strong, even rhythmic motion.

Completion or continuation

This could be an appropriate place to bring the treatment process to an end. The quality of the system will let you know. If it feels complete, then you can allow completion. But as with the lumbo-sacral area, it is often helpful to follow any compressive invitation with an offer of decompression – in order that the system can make the most of its newly released state to open up into expansiveness, disengaging bony sutures, stretching membranes, allowing the fluids to flow more fluently, allowing the energy field and the whole matrix to expand more freely; and also offering the possibility of different responses through a different stimulus. It can also be helpful in counteracting any vestiges of compression that might remain in the system following the offer of compression. Decompression may occur spontaneously, with the system responding to the release of any compressions by opening up into a broad decompressive expansion. It can also be offered to the system.

Spheno-basilar decompression

A second invitation

Again communicating through your thumbs, once the system has settled completely into a balanced neutral state, with the re-emergence of rhythmic motion, ask the sphenoid if it would like to decompress away from the occiput. Envisage your thumbs floating anteriorly, as if to allow the sphenoid to float up anteriorly away from the occiput. (With your patient lying supine, this means floating up towards the ceiling, off the front of the head.) Remember that it is only your thumbs that are thinking up towards the ceiling, not your whole hands – otherwise you would be inviting the whole head to lift, rather than inviting the sphenoid to lift away from the occiput. See how it responds (see Figure 27.12).

The sphenoid may show no initial response; wait patiently. As you maintain this steady invitation into decompression, it may start to lift gradually off the front of the head. As the sphenoid floats up towards the ceiling, it may float up more readily on one side than the other. Allow it to do so, allowing any responses to be expressed. It may twist superiorly on one side, inferiorly on the other. Allow it to do so, gently maintaining your soft invitation to float up towards the ceiling. As releases occur, you may feel your thumbs, and the sphenoid, lifting more freely with each release, perhaps twisting, turning or pulling, before eventually releasing. Allow the system to express itself in whatever way it chooses. Follow into any pulls, twists and patterns, to points of balanced tension and release.

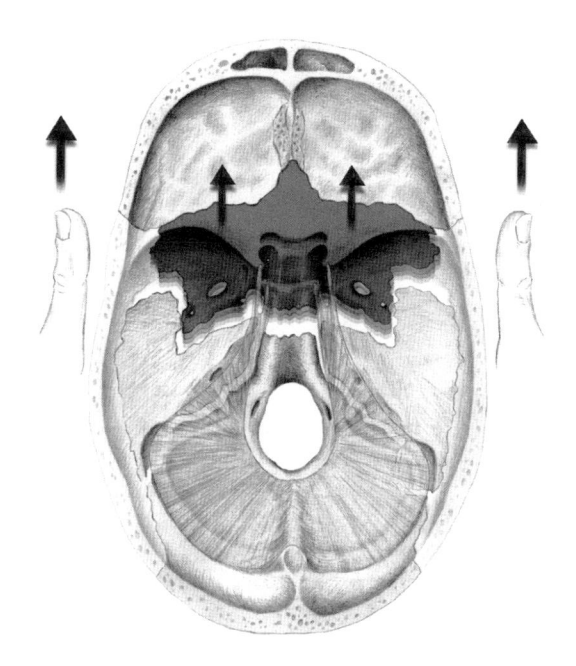

27.12 Spheno-basilar decompression – allow the sphenoid to float up anteriorly away from the occiput

Focal points

As it continues to float up towards the ceiling, your attention may be drawn to particular focal points of resistance, whether local or anywhere in the body – in the bones, the membranes, the energy field or in some more abstract location. As it continues to float up, allow your attention to be drawn to such fulcra, or alternatively you can survey the system to identify any areas of restriction. *Visualise the sphenoid between your thumbs floating up and out from within the head.* Take your attention along the *bony sutures* where the sphenoid greater wings meet the temporals, noticing any changes in quality, symmetry or motion at different areas, waiting at points of resistance, giving your attention to those areas until they soften and release. As the sphenoid continues to float up, take your attention to the *spheno-basilar joint*, or to the *membranes* lining the sphenoid.

Take your attention to the *tentorium*, letting your attention follow those four strands of membrane from their attachments at the clinoid processes, back into the tentorium, identifying any areas of greater resistance or contraction – within the tentorium, within any part of the membrane system, and continuing down through the rest of the *reciprocal tension membrane system* or to anywhere else in the body or through the whole body.

Floating freely

As further releases occur, and your thumbs and the sphenoid continue to lift more readily, you may eventually reach a point where your thumbs and the sphenoid seem to float up into infinity, until they are floating completely freely. Allow them to float as far as they wish, observing the sense of freedom and release within the cranium, within the intracranial membranes, within the tentorium, within the whole system. Continue to allow them to float up until they eventually reach a point where they no longer seem to need to float any further, no longer twisting, no longer resisting, simply floating freely in space. It may feel as if your hands are somewhere up by the ceiling, and if you open your eyes you may be surprised to find that they are still down beside the head. Allow yourself to become fully absorbed into this sense of floating up towards the ceiling.

Gentle release

Take care not to let go of the system too suddenly or abruptly. Although the sense of floating up to the ceiling is only virtual or energetic, it is essential not to let the sphenoid come crashing down onto the cranium again. When the process feels complete, and there is no longer any resistance within the system, gently release any decompressive thought, allowing the sphenoid to float down gently from its elevated state back into the cranium.

Neutral

Once the sphenoid has settled back into place, observe the continuing response of the system. As before, you may find the system initially disorientated by the changes that have occurred. Be content simply to be there, allowing the system to reorganise itself around the changes and releases, reorientating itself to its new state.

As the system settles back into a balanced neutral state, rhythmic motion will gradually re-emerge more clearly and strongly.

Be aware of the looser, softer quality of the system, the more balanced symmetry, the greater expansiveness, and the quality of stillness within the system as a whole. Feel the gradual re-emergence of rhythmic motion and stay with the system through a few cycles of easy, fluent expansion and contraction.

Dynamic stillness

At this stage of the treatment, the system is likely to have settled into a deeper stillness. This is not the end of the treatment, or even the end of this particular process within the treatment. It is an opportunity to move to deeper levels.

With the completion of the spheno-basilar release, you may feel the system shifting to a deeper level. Stay with the system, feeling the process of subtle integration continuing at this deeper level, manifesting locally but reflecting through the whole system. Allow yourself to become more and more deeply absorbed into the process, settling into deeper stillness, deeper spaciousness, shifting deeper into the level of the long tide. Allow yourself to become completely immersed, as if sinking down to the depths of the ocean into a world of silence and stillness, where the material world around you may seem to fade into the background, in which life seems to be proceeding in slow motion. This is likely to be the most profound part of the therapeutic process. Stay with it, content just to be there in deep dynamic stillness.

Chapter 28

The Temporal Area

Introduction

The temporal bones occupy a unique position, caught between the front of the head and the back of the head, and having to adapt to the motion of these two extremes through their distinctive 'wobbly wheel' motion. The temporal area also has many significant and distinctive associations – with the emotional nature of the patient, with specific clinical conditions such as dyslexia, epilepsy and autism, and with recurrent ear infections, glue ear, hearing difficulties and balance – much of which can be understood through its anatomical and physiological relationships.

Location

The two temporal bones form the lower sides of the cranium, relatively intricate bones, housing the organs of hearing and balance (see Figure 28.1).

Each temporal bone consists of:

- a larger, flat *squamous portion*, extending up approximately level with the tops of the ears
- a *mastoid portion*, posteriorly, with a *mastoid process* (which you can feel clearly on yourself as a bony lump projecting down behind each ear) for the attachment of the sterno-cleido-mastoid muscle

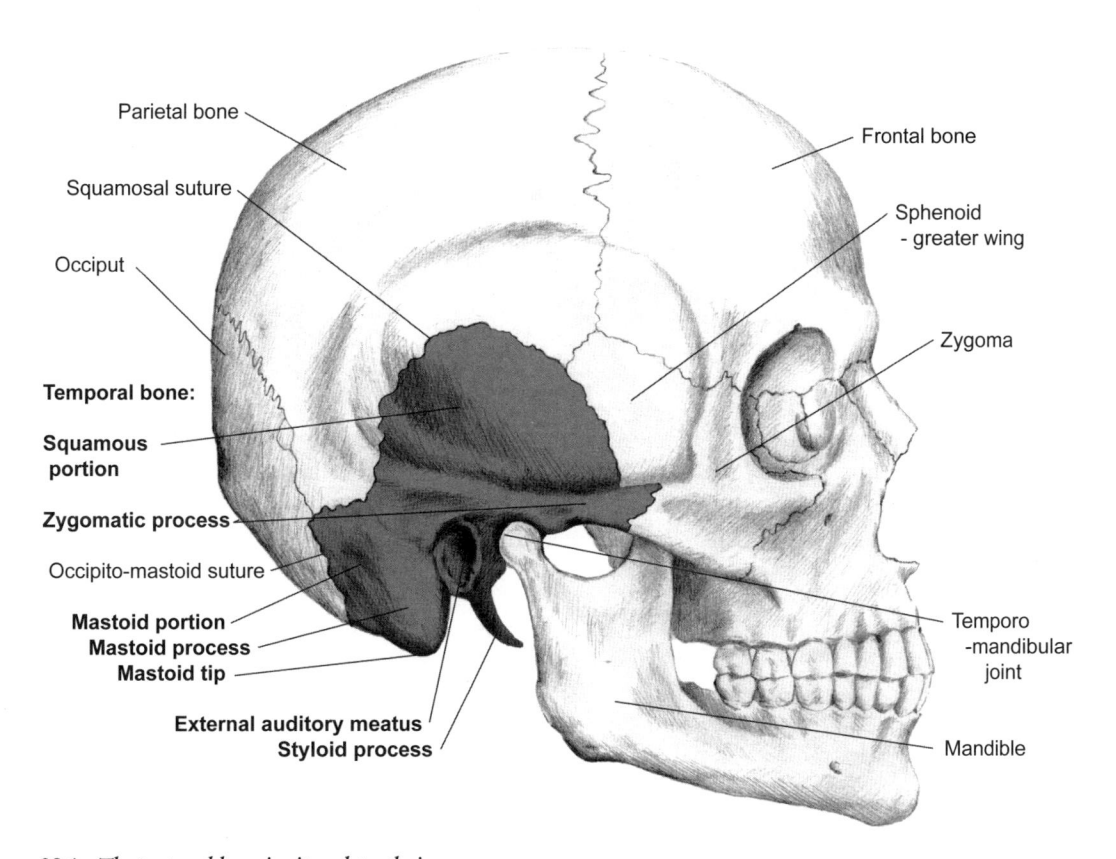

28.1 The temporal bone in situ – lateral view

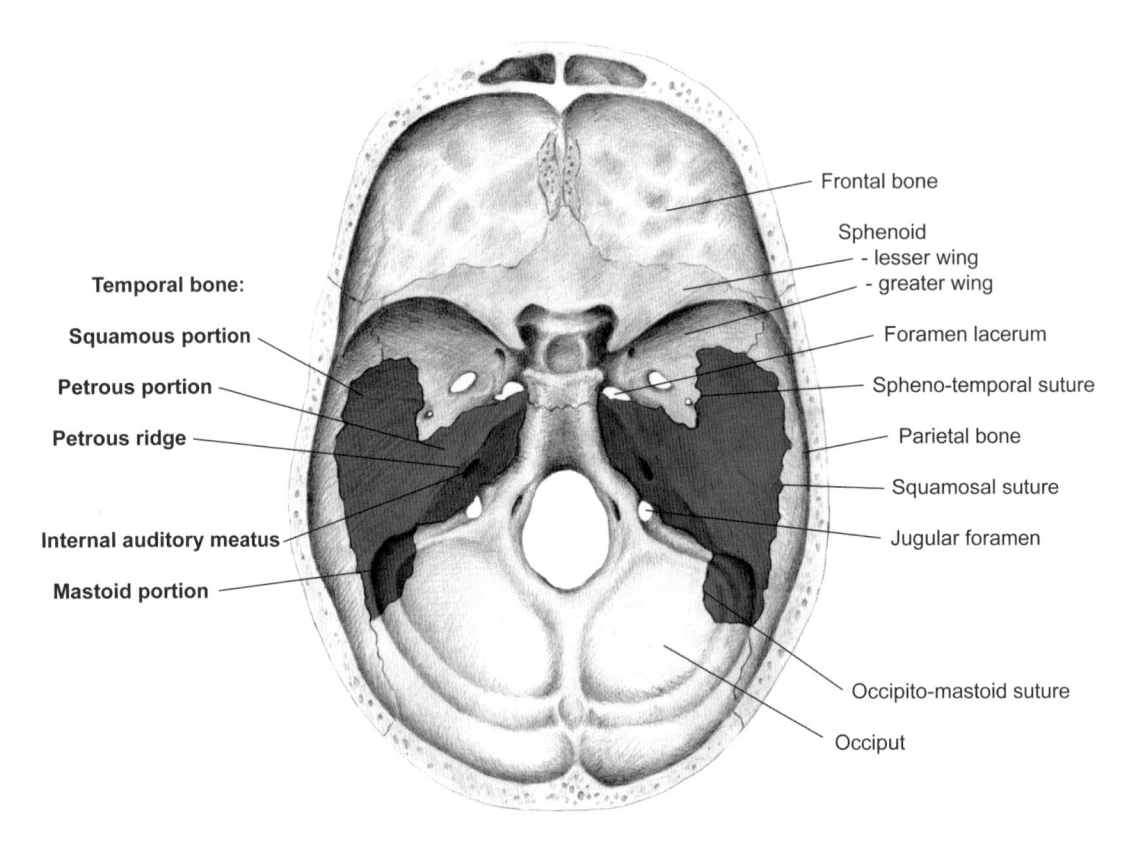

28.2 The temporal bones in situ – superior view of the cranial base

- a *styloid process* – a thin needle-like projection of bone, pointing inferiorly and slightly anteriorly and medially for the attachment of muscles and ligaments (like most bony projections) – in this case the stylo-hyoid muscle and the stylo-mandibular ligament
- an *external auditory meatus* (the earhole) – above the styloid process, in front of the mastoid portion, opening into the external auditory canal
- a *mandibular fossa*, receiving the condyle of the mandible to form the temporo-mandibular joint (TMJ) just in front of the external auditory meatus (this can easily be identified by placing your finger just in front of your ear, and opening and closing your mouth like a fish to feel the movement of the TMJ)
- a *zygomatic process* – a projection of bone passing forward from just above the mandibular fossa, to meet the zygomatic bone (cheek bone) of the face, together forming the zygomatic arch.

Most of these structures are clearly identifiable and palpable on the external surface of the cranium, but there is a substantial and significant portion of each temporal bone which is internal and not palpable. This is: the *petrous portion* (see Figures 28.1 and 28.2). Petrous means rock-like and, as its name suggests, this portion is a solid lump of bone, projecting medially towards the body of the sphenoid and SBS. But this rock is hollow inside, containing the cavities and canals which house the organs of hearing and balance.

Articulations

Each temporal bone (see Figures 28.1 and 28.2) articulates with:

- the *parietal bone* – superiorly (along the squamosal suture – roughly level with the top of the external ear)
- the *occiput* – posteriorly (along the occipito-mastoid suture)
- the *sphenoid* – anteriorly (where the anterior border of the petrous portion meets the posterior edge of the greater wing of the sphenoid at the spheno-temporal suture, the articulation extending out to the external surface at the pterion).

So the temporal bones are wedged between the sphenoid (anteriorly) and the occiput (posteriorly) – a position in which they can become stuck, whether through the compression of birth trauma, the over-zealous use of forceps, head injuries, or membranous contraction drawing the temporal bones medially into the wedge shape (see Figure 28.2).

The temporal bones also articulate with the *zygomatic bones* of the face, and with the *mandible* (at the temporo-mandibular joint) (see Figure 28.1).

Membranous attachments

Each temporal bone is lined with membrane, and also receives attachment of the *tentorium* along the *petrous ridge* – the sharp ridge of bone along the superior edge of the petrous portion. The tentorium is therefore stretching across the back of the cranium from one temporal bone to the other (with the two halves of the tentorium meeting at the midline along the straight sinus) (see Figure 28.3).

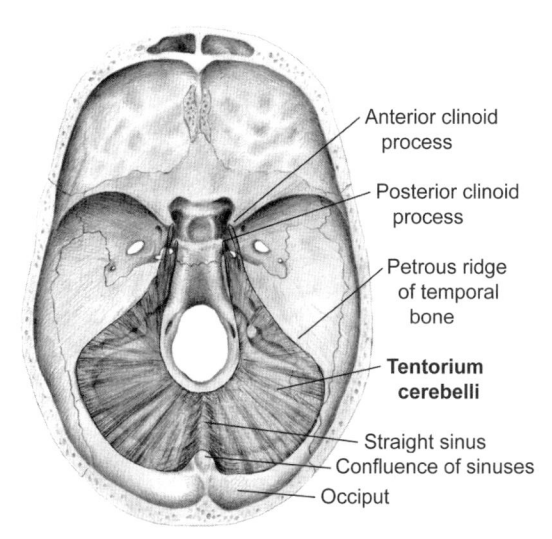

Rhythmic motion

The front of the cranium (frontal and sphenoid) arcs forward and down during the expansion phase of motion. The back of the cranium (occiput) arcs in the opposite direction, tucking under towards the neck.

Where does this leave the temporal bones? Stuck in the middle, wondering which way to go. Should they follow the front of the cranium or the back of the cranium? And how can they accommodate both movements?

External rotation (expansion phase):

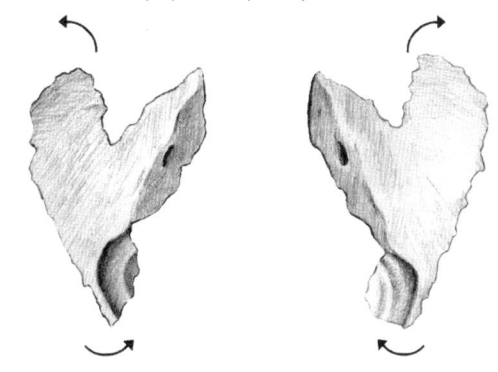

Internal rotation (contraction phase):

28.3 The temporal bones and associated membranes – the tentorium cerebelli

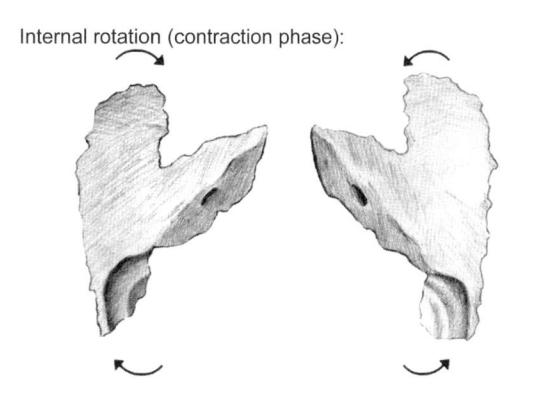

28.4 Cranio-sacral motion of the temporal bones – the temporal bones open out into external rotation during the expansion phase, with the mastoid portions moving medially. They come back into internal rotation during the contraction phase, the mastoid portions moving laterally

Their answer is to exhibit 'wobbly wheel' motion – like wheels rotating on a crooked axle. They rotate forward (together with the front of the cranium) during the expansion phase, but also flare out as they do so (into external rotation), with the mastoid portions moving in medially, thereby accommodating the occipital motion.

In other words, during the expansion phase, the temporal bones externally rotate, the squamous portions rotating forward and out, while the mastoid portions move medially (see Figure 28.4).

The axis for this wobbly wheel motion is the petrous ridge of each temporal bone, thus providing the crooked axle for the wobbly wheels.

Note in particular the *medial* movement of the mastoid tips during the expansion phase. Whereas most bones, including most parts of the temporal bones are widening during the expansion phase, the mastoid tips are distinctive in that they are *narrowing* during the expansion phase.

As the temporals expand out into external rotation, the tentorium flattens as it is stretched laterally, with corresponding consequences throughout the reciprocal tension membrane system.

Contacts

There are several contacts which provide valuable access to the temporal area.

Initial temporal contact

Bring your hands gently in through the energy field towards the sides of the head. Slide your fingers down the sides of the head, with the ring fingers behind the ears, the middle and index fingers in front of the ears – so that the ring fingers are resting onto the mastoid processes, the middle and index fingers resting on the zygomatic processes (see Figures 28.5 and 28.6).

Establish an appropriate level of physical contact. Establish an appropriate level of attention. Allow the process of engagement with the system to evolve and develop. Allow the gradual evolution of the inherent treatment process through the various and variable expressions of the fundamental principles. Observe the increasing emergence of rhythmic motion.

It may be that you *simply rest there*, observing and allowing the various subtle adjustments within the system, or simply feeling the system gradually softening and melting. *Or you may be drawn into a multitude of tiny asymmetries*, brief moments of stillness and release, leading to a clearer more balanced state and an increasingly clearer slower expression of rhythmic motion. As rhythmic motion settles into deeper expression, you may be drawn into more persistent asymmetries, *reaching deeper points of stillness*, leading to more profound releases expressed both at the local fulcrum and throughout the body, and feeling the *return once again to a settled, balanced, deeper neutral.*

As always, this part of the therapeutic interaction may occupy several minutes, gradually progressing to deeper and deeper levels of engagement. Engagement through this initial contact may be all that is necessary and, depending on circumstances, may constitute the complete treatment process.

However, other contacts can also be valuable, whether as alternatives, or as a progressive sequence of different processes relevant to the individual circumstances.

With various contacts, such as the sacrum and the sphenoid, we have explored the possibility of asking the system whether it would like to respond to an offer of compression or decompression. In the case of the temporals, the same possibility arises, but the contacts here have wider implications than mere compression and decompression.

Mastoid tip contact

Lifting the patient's head and gently rolling it to the side (as with the suboccipital release), place your hands under the back of the head, the fingers of one hand crossing over the fingers of the other hand to provide a comfortable support for the occiput (the tips of the fingers extending into the upper neck) (see Figure 28.7).

Rest the *pads* of your thumbs (not the tips) lightly on the tips of the mastoid processes. Settle into the contact, re-establishing appropriate levels of physical contact, attention, and tissue connection. Settle into softness, thinking of your hands as a cushion on which the head can rest, or an ocean on which the head can float. Once again you can *allow the evolution of the inherent treatment*

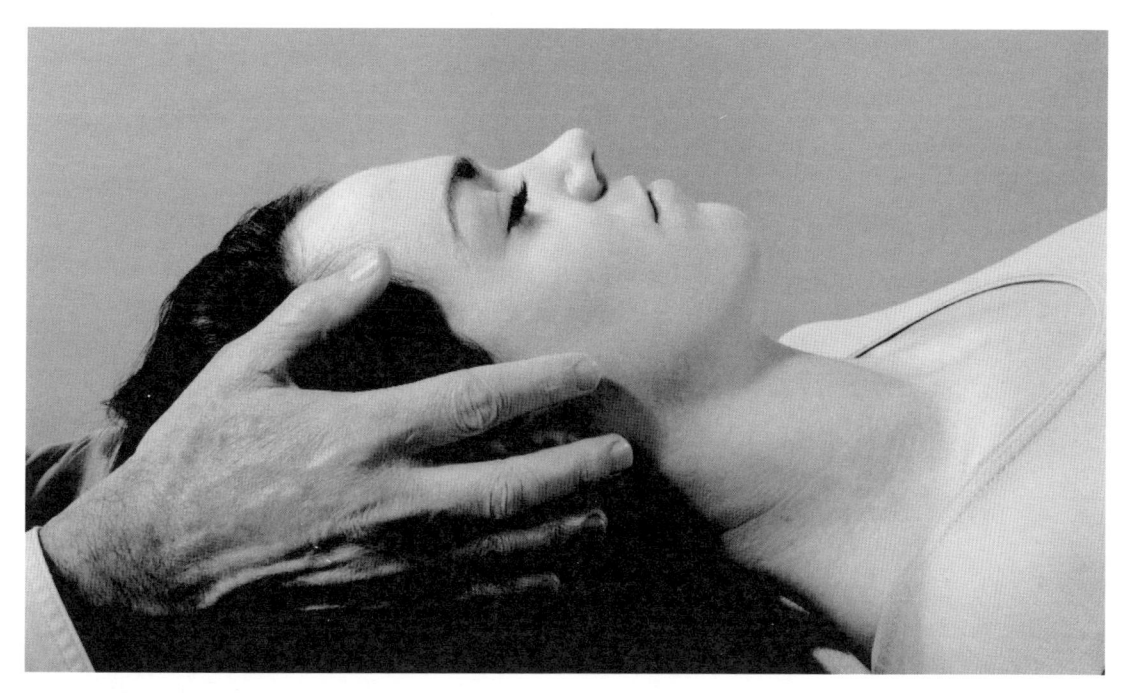

28.5 Initial temporal contact – lateral view

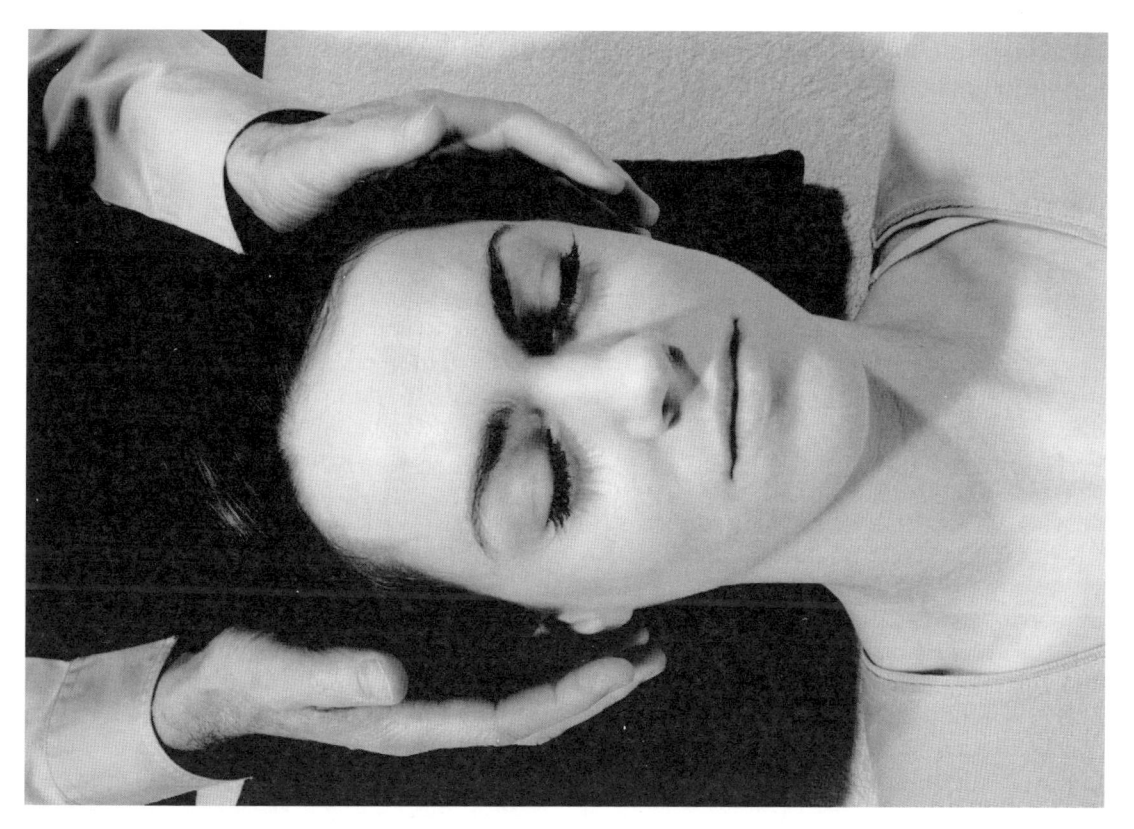

28.6 Initial temporal contact – anterior view

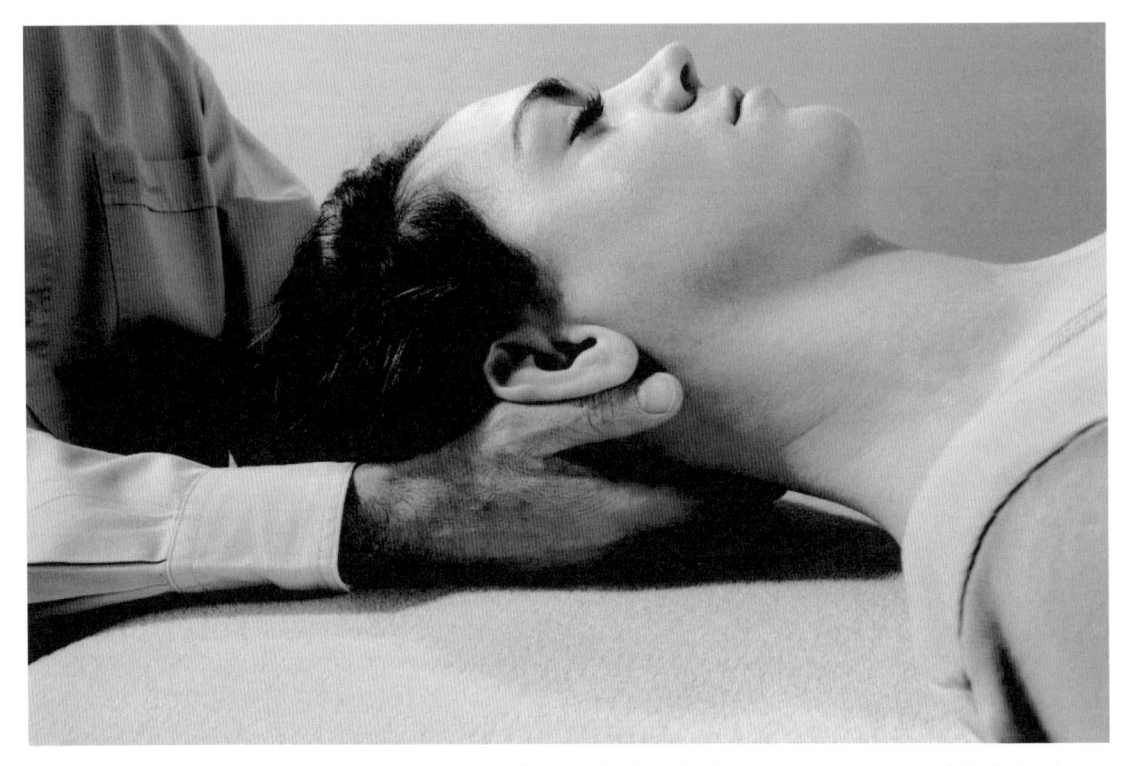

28.7 Mastoid tip contact – think of your hands as a cushion on which the head can rest, or an ocean on which the head can float

process, allowing the system to express itself in whatever way it wants, following wherever it may take you, reaching points of stillness, release and reorganisation.

As the system settles, rhythmic motion may become more clearly apparent. The rhythmic motion may be apparent as cranio-sacral rhythm or as middle tide motion. It may be even and smooth, it may be variable. It may gradually settle into slower more expansive motion. Within the context of the motion, the system may lead you to points of stillness and release, perhaps also drawing into twists, turns and pulls as it does so.

At times, you may find the rhythmic motion specifically drawing more strongly into one phase of motion, and you can allow that. In particular *you may find the mastoid processes drawing medially and your thumbs can allow and follow this motion* further and further into its extreme of motion, maintaining a steady consistent thought medially (but not imposing any physical force) until it reaches a point of balanced tension, a point of stillness, and eventually – whether after a few seconds, or after several minutes – a release, in which you can feel the system soften, the whole surrounding area dissolve and melt, and the system settle out into a calmer, more balanced, more expansive neutral state. Feel the release spreading through the whole body.

With all cranio-sacral contacts, you are engaging with the whole system, and the whole system will respond. So while your contact may be specific to the mastoid tips, your awareness will be enveloping the whole body, as well as the local responses. The releases that result from this process may arise anywhere in the system, but this contact is likely to be particularly influential for certain more specific local and distant effects – releasing the occipito-mastoid sutures, the jugular foramina, the suboccipital area (with beneficial effects on the many significant structures described previously under the suboccipital area), the upper cervical spine, the drainage of the Eustachian tubes from the middle ears – and for the integration of the whole temporal/occipital/cervical region – as well as providing a clear vantage point for a perspective on the dural tube and spine and through the rest of the body.

Consequently, this may have significant effects on a wide variety of conditions related to these structures, including ear infections, tinnitus, torticollis, headaches associated with poor venous drainage through the jugular vein, colic, nausea and the many possible digestive, respiratory and cardiac symptoms that might arise from disturbance to the vagus nerve as it passes through the jugular foramen.

This tendency to draw specifically into the extremes of motion *often occurs spontaneously*. It *can also be offered* to the system. Engaging with the rhythmic motion, you might notice that the system is moving more clearly into medial movement of the mastoid tips rather than lateral movement. Observing this, you can ask the system if it would like to follow that inclination and move further into that medial direction. Maintaining the consistent invitation of medial movement, you can then follow the mastoid tips as far as they wish to go, eventually reaching points of stillness and release.

When taking up this contact on the mastoid tips, it is helpful to *ensure that your thumb contact is appropriate*. First, as already mentioned, it is preferable to *use the pads of the thumbs*, with the thumbs relatively straight – since using the tips of the thumbs with the thumbs bent tends to be potentially more pokey and invasive.

More significantly, it is helpful to ensure that *your contact is on the very tips* of the mastoid processes – not just on the bony lumps behind the ears, but as far down those bony lumps as possible. It may be difficult to determine exactly where the tips of the mastoid processes are, because they are invariably buried to some extent within the sterno-cleido-mastoid muscle which attaches there, but it is helpful to ensure that you place your thumbs well down towards the tips, usually a little below the bottom of the ear lobe.

This is significant, because this process is not intended as a compressive process. If you place your thumbs on the bulk of the mastoid process, the tendency will indeed be to compress the temporals and the occipito-mastoid suture medially towards the occiput. This is not what is desired or intended.

If your contact is appropriately located on the tips of the mastoid processes, then you are encouraging the tips medially. What effect is this having on the temporal bones as a whole?

The mastoid tips move medially during the expansion phase of rhythmic motion. If the mastoid tips are encouraged medially, then this is encouraging the temporals into the expansion phase of motion. As the temporals move into expansion (external rotation) the tentorium will be stretched (see Figures 28.3 and 28.4). This in turn will have effects throughout the reciprocal tension membrane system. So this process can encourage the whole system into expansion, with widespread repercussions throughout the system.

With this in mind, it is also relevant to *consider exactly how you are using your hands under the occiput*. While following the mastoid tips medially (into the expansion phase of motion) there can be a tendency for the heels of the hands (under the occiput) also to be thinking medially (without realising it). This tendency is definitely to be avoided, since this would be compressing the occiput, narrowing the occiput, and counteracting the tendency of the whole system to open up into expansion. So even as the thumbs follow the mastoid tips medially, the heels of the hands need to be softening out laterally into expansion.

As always, you can maintain a constant awareness of the whole system throughout the process, observing responses both locally and throughout the body, and the repercussions of any releases – local or distant – on the system as a whole.

Once the system has moved into its extreme of motion, reached a point of stillness, released, reorganised, and settled back into a neutral balanced state, you can choose whether to complete the treatment there, stay with the same contact to observe and enhance further responses, or move on to a different contact. Your choice will of course be guided by the responses within the patient's system.

As always, staying with the system following a release, and staying with the same contact for a longer period of time, perhaps through several releases, can be one of the most effective ways of moving into deeper engagement. The mastoid tip contact can be a particularly effective contact for enabling this, due to the various associations mentioned above.

Ear hold

The ear hold contact (see Figures 28.8, 28.9 and 28.10) does have more specifically decompressive characteristics, and therefore is a natural sequitur to follow on from the mastoid tip contact. While the mastoid tip contact was not specifically compressive, it will have the effect of releasing compressive forces within the occipito-mastoid suture (which is particularly susceptible to compression, whether due to birth trauma, head injuries or other causes) and elsewhere in the region.

The ear hold contact can therefore be a valuable means of assisting the body to take advantage of its newly found decompressed state to open up into wider expansion and to ease out of its wedged position between the sphenoid and occiput. The ear hold contact may also be used without necessarily preceding it with a mastoid tip contact, but the preparatory release of the mastoid tip contact often enables a far more significant and expansive opening up of the system in response to the ear hold.

The temporal bones, as we have seen, fit like a wedge between the sphenoid and the occiput. Release of the occipito-mastoid suture and the spheno-temporal suture will, as mentioned above, help the temporals to move more freely and thereby express inherent motion more freely and expressively. But specifically encouraging the temporals outwards will also be helpful in this respect. This could be done purely by intention, from anywhere in the body. It could be done simply by harnessing the potential within the system. It can also be done more specifically and effectively by drawing the temporals outwards.

There are no readily available handles on the temporal bones through which to draw them outwards, but we are fortunate enough to have been given ears, which provide the perfect tool for this purpose.

Ears are sensitive, and are best handled carefully – not pinching them between finger and thumb, not pulling them. In order to take up a gentle contact on the ears, rest your hands gently on the couch or cushion at each side of the head. *Curl* your index fingers, so that you can bring the *middle phalanx* of each index finger into contact with the back of the ear, resting the *pad* (not the tip) of each thumb softly inside the front of the ear, as close to the ear canal as possible. In order to enable this more comfortable position, it

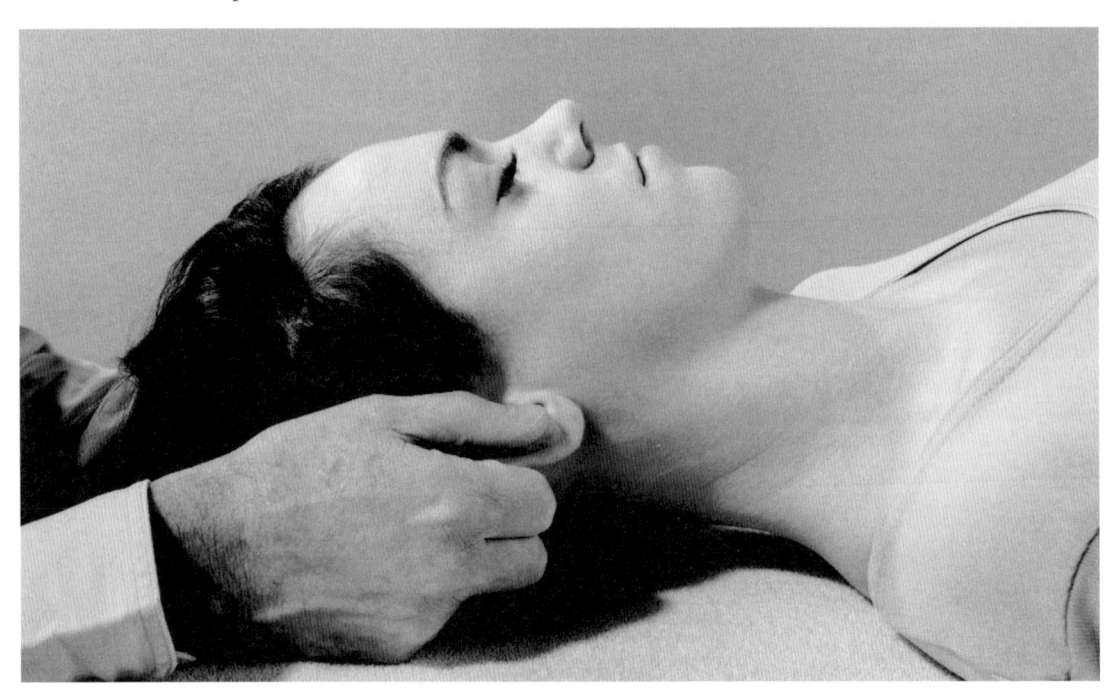

28.8 Ear hold contact – lateral view – curl your index fingers, rest the pad (not the tip) of each thumb softly inside the front of the ear. Keep your contact soft, taking care not to pinch or squeeze

The Temporal Area / 197

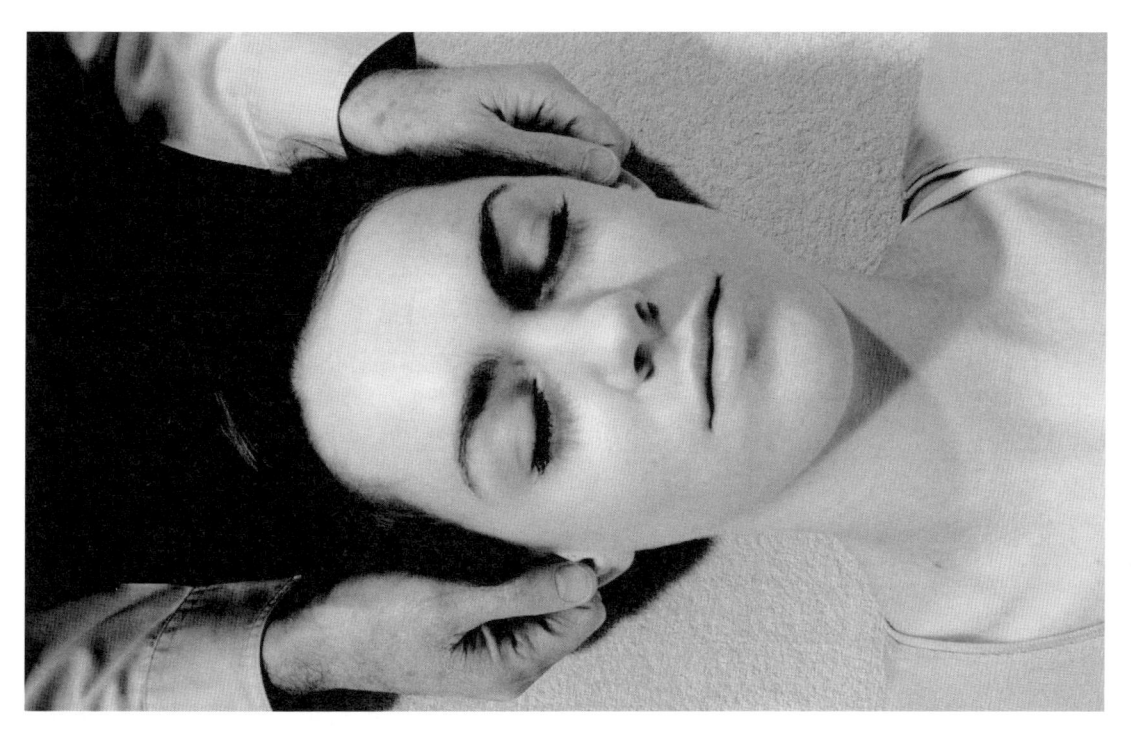

28.9 Ear hold contact – anterior view – the direction of intention is not directly outwards but laterally and slightly posteriorly. With your patient lying on their back, this means that you are inviting the ears to draw out and down – out, at an angle down towards the couch

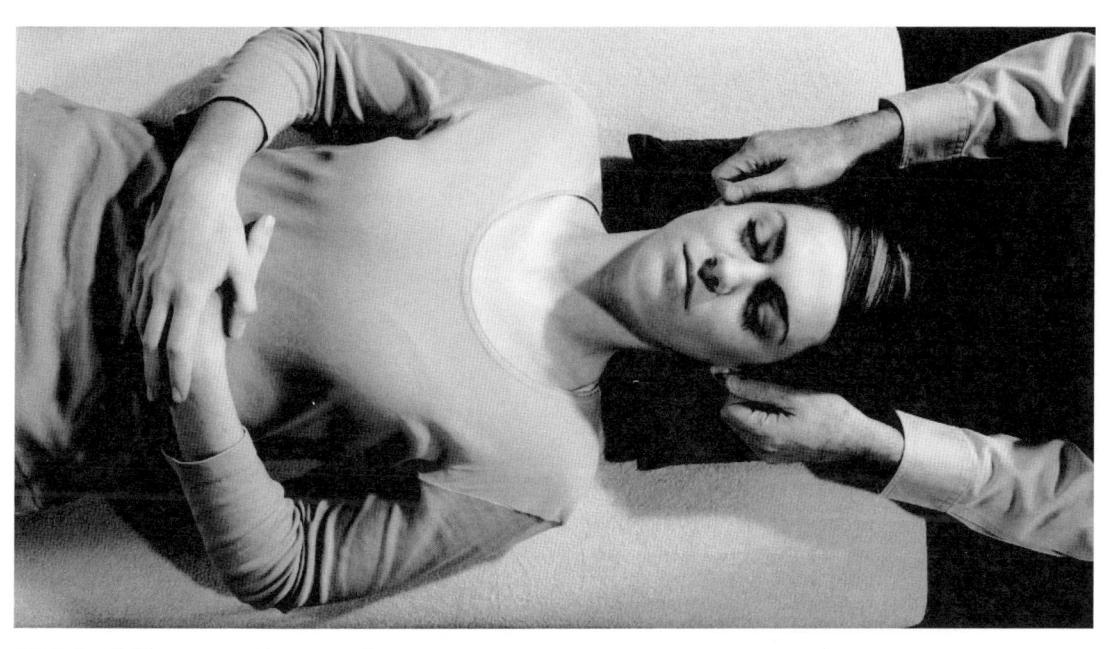

28.10 Ear hold contact – wider perspective

is helpful to keep your wrists straight (not angled outwards) and your hands resting comfortably onto the couch or cushion close beside the head (see Figures 28.8, 28.9 and 28.10).

Keep your contact soft, taking care not to pinch or squeeze. Settle into the contact, taking time to re-engage with the system.

As you feel an increasing sense of engagement, you may feel a variety of responses. You might feel the ears contracting into the head; you might feel the ears expanding out away from the head. You might feel one ear drawing in and the other ear expanding out. You might feel one ear twisting forward and down, the other ear twisting back and up. You might feel any number of variations of different pulls, twists and directions.

As always, allow the evolution of the inherent treatment process, allowing the system to express itself, follow wherever it takes you, perhaps reaching points of stillness, release and reorganisation. If the ears draw you in, follow them in; if they stretch out, go with them. If they twist and turn, let them twist and turn. If they rock from side to side, let them rock. If they roll around, let them roll.

As the system settles, you may find the ears naturally opening out into greater expansiveness and you can let that happen. You can also offer them that possibility, asking the system if it would like to expand. Without any physical force, you can invite the ears to draw outwards. However, the direction of expansion is not directly outwards but *laterally and slightly posteriorly*. With your patient lying on their back, this means that you are inviting the ears to draw out and down – out, at an angle down towards the couch (see Figure 28.11). You may notice that this is the direction in which the ears naturally want to expand anyway, but awareness of this direction will enable you to engage with it more readily, more clearly and more effectively.

The reason for this direction is determined by the structure of the cranium. The direction of movement is along the axis of the petrous ridges

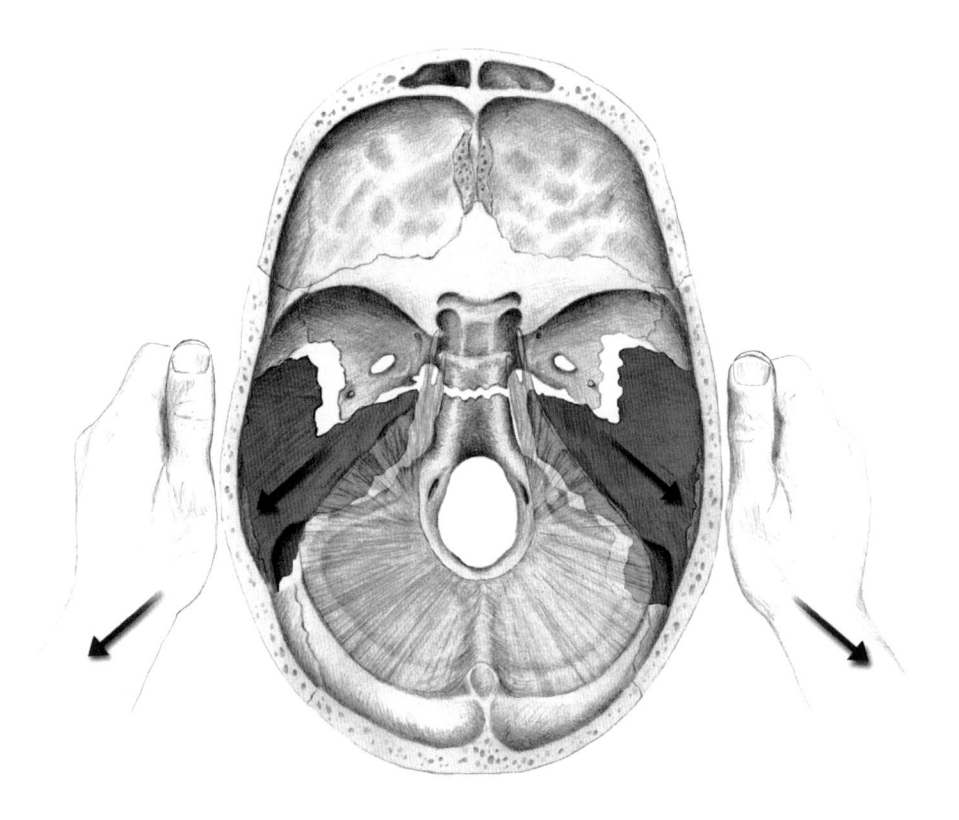

28.11 As you maintain your gentle invitation, you can survey the various associated structures within, observing their response

of the temporal bones, the crooked axle of the wobbly wheels.

As you invite the ears to expand outwards, they may respond eagerly, stretching out readily; they may be resistant or unresponsive, they may contract in against your invitation – in which case, as always, you allow them to contract in, even while maintaining your consistent invitation to expand out. You may find that one ear stretches out while the other contracts in. As always follow whatever the system wants to do.

In due course, having allowed the system to express its various pulls and twists and perhaps encountered various points of stillness and release, you may find that the ears become more inclined to stretch out and down along the axis of the petrous ridges, while still exhibiting twists and turns and various variations of direction and movement.

As you maintain your gentle invitation to traction out, you can also survey the various local structures more directly influenced by this contact (see Figures 28.11 and 28.2). Take your attention to the *muscles and soft tissues* attaching the ears to the temporal bones, feel these soft tissues softening and stretching out. Take your attention to the *temporal bones* themselves, feel the hard quality of the bones, feel how readily they respond and expand. Survey around the edges of the bone, exploring the sutures and sutural restrictions, running your attention along the *spheno-temporal suture*, and along the *occipito-mastoid suture*, observing any points of resistance, any change in quality, symmetry or motion as your attention reaches different areas, waiting at areas of resistance for change to occur, softening, releasing, expanding. As these sutures release, you may feel the temporal bones expanding out more readily, and the *jugular foramina* opening up to greater flow of venous blood through the internal jugular veins, at the same time releasing any compression or restriction on the vagus nerves, accessory nerves and glossopharyngeal nerves.

As the bones begin to feel more free and expansive, take your attention to the *tentorium* as it stretches across the back of the cranium from one *petrous ridge* to the other. Feel the quality within the tentorium; is it loose and free, or tight and contracted? Is it tighter on one side than on the other, or in one area more than another, towards the front or towards the back? Feel the tentorium gradually stretching out on each side, as resistance gives way. As the tentorium loosens, feel the stretching in the *straight sinus* along the midline where the two halves of the tentorium meet. Feel the straight sinus expanding and opening up allowing greater flow of venous blood. The stretching of the tentorium is also likely to open up the *transverse sinuses*, running along the lateral borders of the tentorium, where it attaches to the occiput, with ramifications through the rest of the venous sinus system.

Continue your journey wherever it takes you, up into the *falx cerebri*, down into the *falx cerebelli*, throughout the *reciprocal tension membrane system*, throughout the whole cranio-sacral system. Your attention may be drawn to specific focal points elsewhere in the body – the diaphragm, the pelvis, the TMJ, anywhere – or you might project your attention through the body, identifying specific areas which draw your attention – noticing changes in quality, symmetry or motion as your attention reaches those specific locations, waiting as appropriate for responses from the system, observing how changes can occur anywhere in the body in response to your contact at the ears, and feeling the widespread and far-reaching effects of this gentle ear hold on the whole being.

This process of surveying the internal structures in detail is a highly significant aspect of every cranio-sacral process. The ability to visualise the detailed anatomy within plays a crucial part in influencing the responses of the system. The focus of your attention on focal points of restriction enhances their release.

Your *informed awareness* – the combination of anatomical knowledge and focused attention – is a key component in the effectiveness of the treatment.

Once the ears have stretched as far as they want to go, and the system has expanded as fully as it wishes, to a point where there is no longer any resistance, release any thought of traction. It may feel as though the ears and your hands have stretched several miles away from the sides of the head. Even though you have not exerted any actual pull, acknowledge that feeling of stretching, since on an energetic level that is what has happened. As you release any thought of traction, take care not to let the ears snap back suddenly into place. Release them gradually, gently allowing them to settle back onto the sides of the head. Allow the system to settle back into a balanced neutral state.

You could then return to a general contact on the temporals, similar to the original hold but, rather than sliding your fingers down behind and in front of the ears, you could simply let your hands rest loosely on the sides of the head in the temporal area, around the ears. Re-engage with the system through this contact, evaluate the quality, balance and motion, follow the system through a few cycles of easeful rhythmic motion, and allow the treatment process to continue as appropriate within the context of the overall integrated treatment, whether proceeding to deeper levels of engagement or to completion.

Emotions

It was mentioned previously that there is a specific association between the temporal area and the emotions. Emotional associations can of course be observed and identified anywhere in the cranio-sacral system. The quality of the system as a whole provides a clear indication of the emotional state of the person – both their immediate, current emotional state and their underlying emotional personality. Qualities, asymmetries and movements in any area of the body may relate to and reveal specific areas of emotional tension, or specific emotions held in the body. Certain areas in particular may be specific indicators of emotional holding – the heart, the solar plexus, clenching of the jaw.

Within the context of this overall perspective on emotions held in the system, the temporal area provides a particularly clear view of the emotional state – again both the current emotional state and the underlying emotional personality.

A patient who is emotionally contained, suppressed, or unexpressive will generally have temporals that are contained, contracted, and exhibiting little movement. A patient who is emotionally open and expressive will generally have temporals that are open, free, mobile and expressive. A patient who is emotionally volatile is likely to have temporals that jump around all over the place in response to their emotional volatility.

A patient who is usually open, but who has just had a significant shock which has led them to close down, may have temporals that feel inherently mobile but currently held in contraction and reduced mobility. A patient who is generally contained and suppressed but is currently boiling with anger in response to some recent event may have temporals which feel limited in mobility but which are rumbling like a volcano and struggling to break free and express themselves. And so on.

The temporals provide a particularly vivid insight into the emotional state of the patient. Certain anatomical relationships reveal why this is the case. The temporals are closely associated with the tentorium. The tentorium is a 'transverse diaphragm' – running transversely across the back of the cranium between the two temporal bones. Being a transverse structure, the tentorium relates to, and is affected by, other transverse structures in the body – most notably the thoracic (respiratory) diaphragm, and also the pelvic diaphragm and the other 'transverse structures' described previously within the context of the emotional centres (see Chapter 20) because, like the sympathetic plexi and the chakras, these 'transverse structures' or 'transverse diaphragms' have emotional associations.

Most people alter their breathing according to their emotional state – most commonly holding their breath or breathing more shallowly when stressed, letting go of the breath and breathing more deeply when relaxed, and also breathing irregularly when agitated. The thoracic diaphragm obviously plays a significant part in these responses.

The interrelationship between the various transverse diaphragms means that when the thoracic diaphragm tightens up, so the other associated transverse diaphragms tighten up – including the tentorium – thereby drawing the temporals into medial contraction, into the wedge shape, and holding them in limited mobility.

Hence the contained, suppressed, emotionally unexpressive person, who probably breathes shallowly and holds their diaphragm tight, will have a tight tentorium and contracted temporals. The open, expressive person with a loose diaphragm will have a loose tentorium and expansive temporals, and the volatile person whose breathing changes from moment to moment will have a tentorium that changes from moment to moment and temporals that jump around all over the place.

So when you place your hands on a patient's temporal area, you can read their emotional state – current and underlying, with all the different layers and levels of emotion, and all the various complexities of their emotional life – with profound insight, and greater accuracy than many other psychological or personal assessments. Many times, on hearing a simple description – in cranio-sacral terms of quality, symmetry and motion – of their temporal area, patients will identify with the description very clearly, responding that it describes their whole situation and exactly how they feel at that moment.

Just as the temporal area is an *indicator* of emotions, so it can also be an effective site through which to *influence* the emotional state. When the emotional state is agitated or unsettled, working with the temporals and allowing a gradual settling of the temporals into an easeful rhythmic motion tends to bring the whole person into a settled state, bringing a greater calmness and peacefulness. Where the emotions are suppressed – perhaps someone who has been holding their emotions in and really wants to let go but can't – releasing the temporals can enable that patient to let go, let their feelings out and gain the widespread benefits of letting go throughout their being. With someone who is chronically suppressed, working with the temporals over a long period may gradually enable a corresponding opening up of their emotional nature, as appropriate.

The temporals can be a very appropriate place to bring a treatment to a calm, balanced, settled conclusion and bring a patient to a calm, balanced, settled completion.

Subtle integration

Whether at the end of a treatment, or simply as you conclude your contact with the temporals, you can again settle into increasingly deep engagement with the system. Following the release of various asymmetries, imbalances and restrictions, as the system settles into a calm, settled neutral state, with the re-emergence of rhythmic motion at a slower more expansive rate, so you can continue the treatment process by simply being there, basking in the stillness, flowing with the gentle rhythmic motion, allowing subtle integration, aware of the profound peacefulness spreading through the whole system and through the surrounding environment, settling into deep dynamic stillness and simply being there.

(The associations with dyslexia, epilepsy and autism relate to the associated areas of the temporal lobes of the brain, and will be addressed in greater detail in subsequent volumes, as also will the associations with ear infections, hearing and balance.)

Chapter 29

The Frontal Area

Location

The frontal bone, as its name suggests, is at the front of the cranium, forming the roofs of the orbits, the superior rims of the orbits, and extending up over the forehead to the top of the head (see Figures 29.1 and 29.2).

Articulations

At the top of the head, the frontal bone passes back as far as the *coronal suture*, where it meets the *parietal bones*. Anteriorly, it articulates with the two nasal bones at the *nasion*. On each side it passes down to the *pterion*, where it meets the *sphenoid greater wing*; and just behind the lateral corner of each eye, it forms a bony ridge known as the *zygomatic process of the frontal bone*, articulating with the zygomatic bone of the face. This zygomatic process is a useful landmark when taking up contact on the frontal area (and can easily be identified on yourself).

As well as the visible outer surface, there is a horizontal inner portion forming the roof of the orbits and extending back to meet the *sphenoid lesser wings*. Between the two halves of this horizontal portion, along the midline, is formed the *ethmoid notch*, which receives the ethmoid bone (see Figure 29.3).

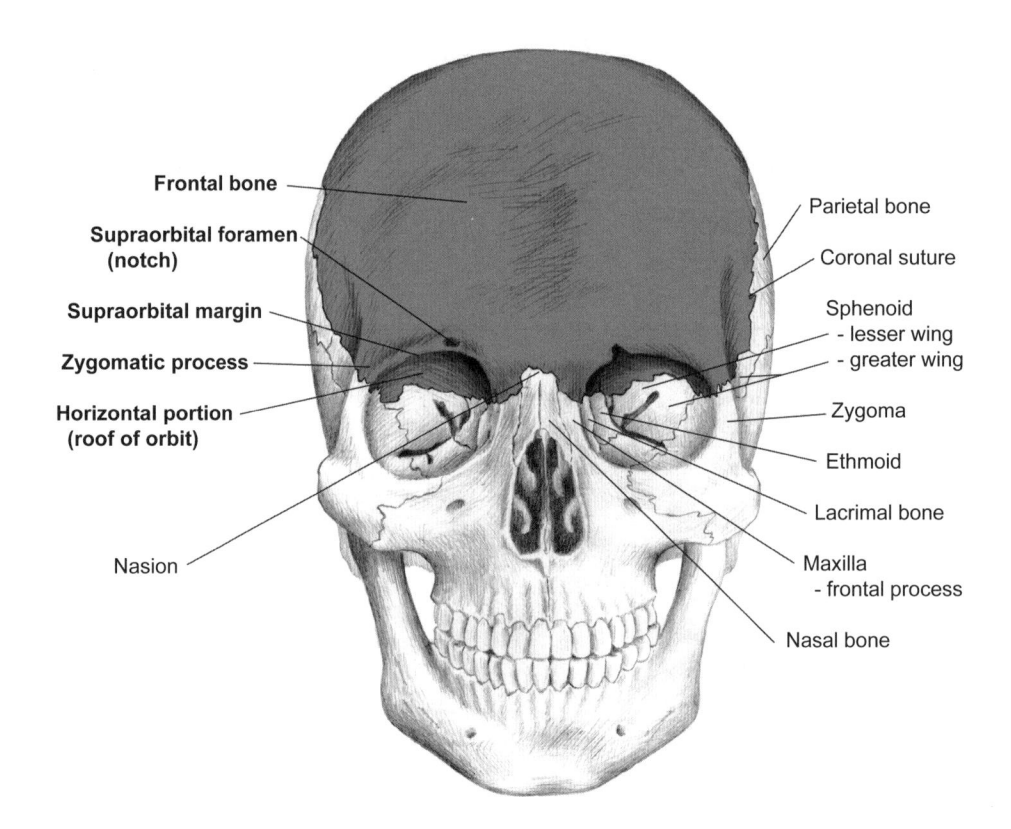

29.1 Frontal bone in situ – anterior view

The Frontal Area / 203

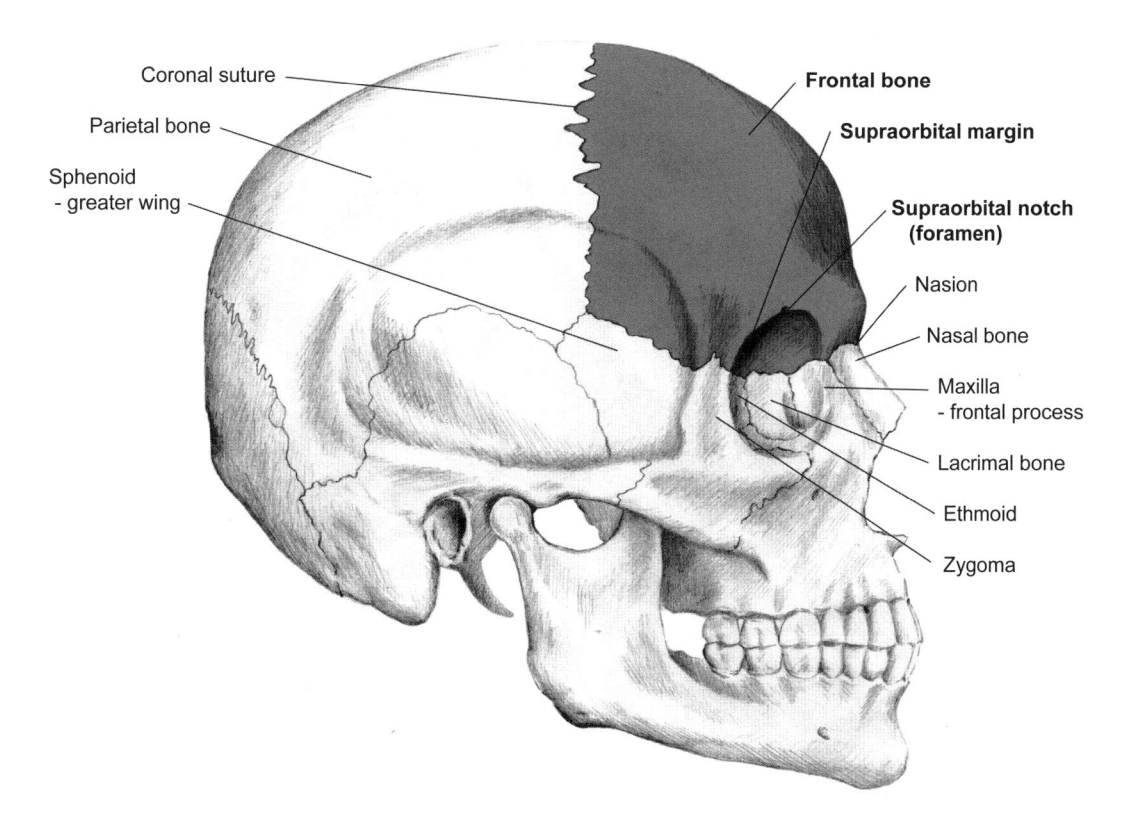

29.2 Frontal bone in situ – lateral view

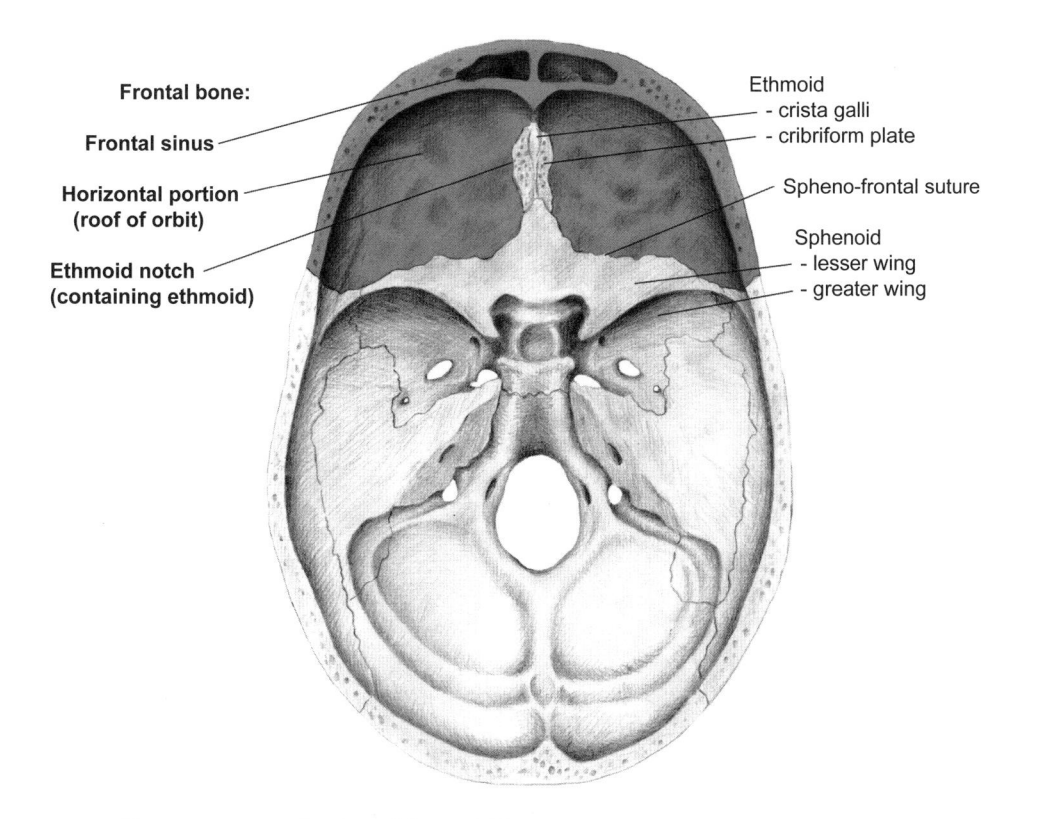

29.3 Frontal bone in situ – superior view of the cranial base

Membranous relations

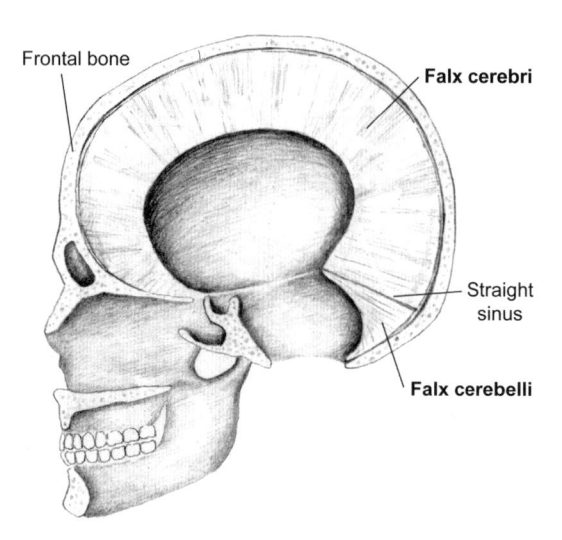

29.4 Membranous associations with the frontal bone – falx cerebri

The frontal bone, like all bones of the cranium, is lined with membrane – so any disturbance to the bone will affect the membrane, and any disturbance to the membrane will affect the bone. The *falx cerebri* passes up along the midline of the internal surface of the frontal bone – where there is a corresponding bony ridge. This line of attachment for the falx cerebri acts as a fulcrum for the rhythmic motion of the frontal area (see Figure 29.4).

Cranio-sacral motion

Embryologically, the frontal bone is formed as two separate bones, divided by the *metopic suture* – a suture which is clearly apparent in the neonate skull, and is only considered to be fully fused around the age of eight years, although it becomes barely detectable long before that. The metopic suture remains patent (open) throughout life in approximately one in twelve people (see Figure 29.5).

During cranio-sacral motion, the frontal area continues to move as if it were composed of two separate bones, hingeing around the metopic suture and the fulcrum of the falx cerebri. (Living bone is of course much more pliable than dry bones – like a living branch of a tree compared to a dead branch – and so is able to express subtle

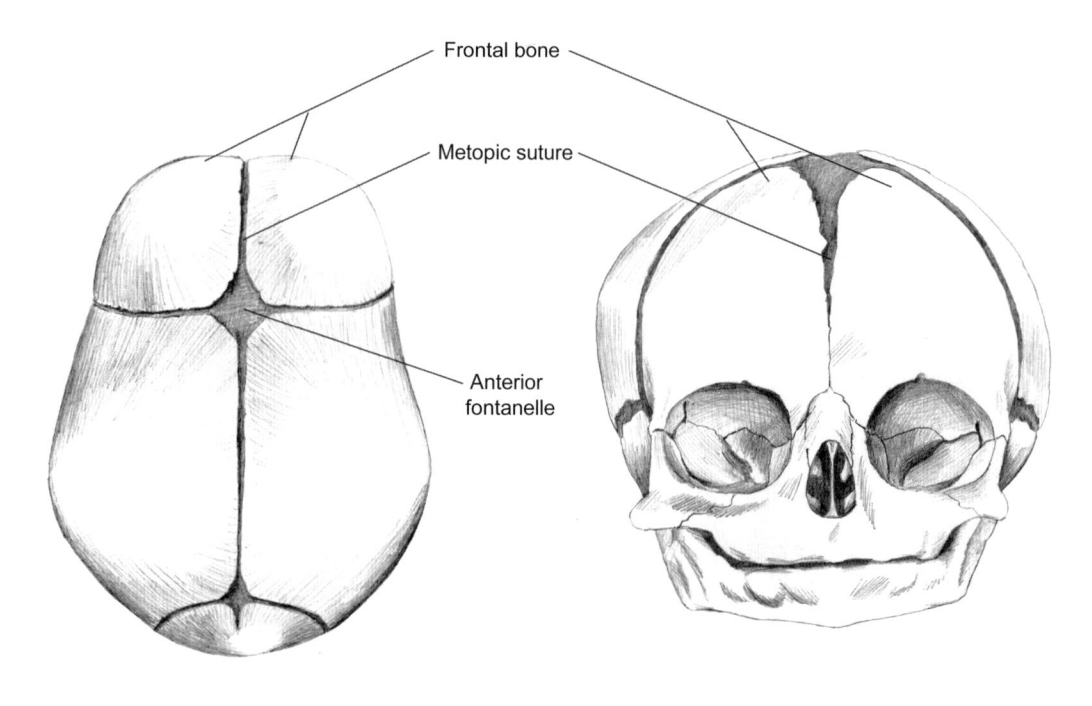

Superior view

Anterior view

29.5 The neonate frontal bone is in two halves, separated by the metopic suture

motion. Of course, although the bone is capable of subtle movement, the movement that we are feeling is not specifically related to bone, but to the expression of vitality.)

There are two aspects to the motion of the frontal area, reflecting the *longitudinal* expansion and contraction of the cranium, and the *lateral* expansion and contraction of the cranium.

Longitudinal motion

During the expansion phase of motion, *the frontal area arcs forward and down* towards the face (following the movement of the sphenoid into flexion) but is simultaneously drawn posteriorly by the falx cerebri. During the contraction phase, the frontal area comes back and up (see Figure 29.6).

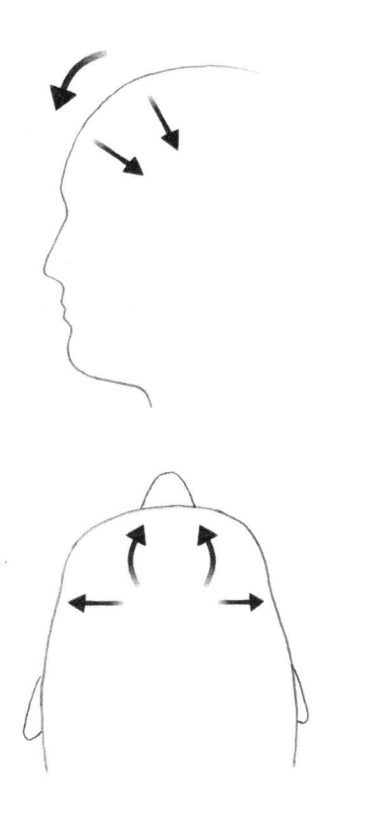

29.6 Cranio-sacral motion of the frontal bone – the frontal area arcs forward and down towards the face during the expansion phase, but is simultaneously drawn posteriorly by the falx cerebri. It also flares – hingeing around the metopic suture and the fulcrum of the falx cerebri

Lateral motion

During the expansion phase of motion, the *frontal area also flares* (widens), hingeing around the metopic suture and the fulcrum of the falx cerebri. During the contraction phase, the frontal area narrows.

Every contact is a window into the whole system

When we tune into the frontal area, we are not merely tuning in to the frontal bone, or simply to the local region, we are, as always, tuning in to the whole cranio-sacral system as reflected through this particular window. There will of course be local characteristics to each area – both inherent qualities and the results of local traumas and tensions. We can acknowledge and address these, and we can also maintain our awareness of the whole system.

Effects of injury

If, for example, a patient has received a blow to the frontal area of the head, this will have various repercussions. Taking up contact on this area, you might feel that *the local area is compressed or contracted*, stuck or solidified, or you might feel that the whole head has been shunted over to one side.

This blow may also have had more far-reaching physiological effects on the body. It may have compressed the cranial sutures. It may have caused the membranes lining the bones to contract. This may have led to damage or restriction of the blood vessels supplying oxygen to the brain, or may have interfered with the flow of cerebrospinal fluid around the brain – all of which may have repercussions on brain function.

There may also be *repercussions beyond the local area*, with effects on the rest of the cranium – disturbing nerve pathways, blood flow, cerebrospinal fluid flow, energy flow; or there may be ramifications in the neck – perhaps causing neck pain or disturbance of the suboccipital region – with consequent compensatory effects on the balance and integration of the whole body, perhaps leading to back pain and other widespread symptoms.

There may also have been *emotional reactions* to the blow – perhaps shock, fear or anger – which may have induced the whole system to tighten up in:
- the solar plexus and in the cardiac and respiratory plexi, causing digestive, respiratory or cardiac symptoms
- the autonomic nervous system, leading to agitation and overstimulation
- the membrane system
- the whole body
- the whole body-mind complex.

All of these repercussions – physical, emotional and energetic – will interact, will be interrelated, and may become mutually perpetuating. They will all create disturbances to the quality, symmetry and motion of the cranio-sacral system and to the free and fluent expression of inherent vitality – reflected in the patient's experience as symptoms and discomforts – with consequent effects on the potential for recovery.

Response to contact

Consequently, when we tune in to the frontal area, there are many different impressions that might come to our attention, arising not only from blows to the head but also from many other different sources.

We might become aware of tensions that are being *transmitted from the membranes* inside the cranium, or from elsewhere in the reciprocal tension membrane system, resulting in contraction of the frontal area, symmetrically or asymmetrically.

We might feel the *consequences of a difficult birth process*, whether due to compression of the cranium during the passage of the baby through the birth canal, or from the more far-reaching consequences of shock and trauma during birth.

We might be feeling imbalances transmitted from *restrictions or injuries elsewhere in the cranium*, imbalances arising from *elsewhere in the system* – the neck, the spine, the diaphragm, the pelvis, the feet. We might feel *systemic characteristics* reflected throughout the whole system as a result of emotional tension, shock, or a systemic disease, such as rheumatoid arthritis.

Through this contact, or any cranio-sacral contact, we are engaging with the consequences of everything that this system has experienced throughout its life; and as always, the appropriate response is to simply be there, with our calm, quiet presence, allowing the natural evolution of the therapeutic process.

Reasons for contacting the frontal area

There may be various reasons why we are drawn to contact the frontal area. There could be *local symptoms* – pain, sinusitis in the frontal sinuses, frontal headaches. (All of these would of course need to be evaluated within the context of the whole person.) There could be a *history of trauma* to the area – a blow to the head, a fall, or a car accident – or symptoms arising from birth. We might be drawn to that area by *pulls or contractions from other parts* of the body, or we might simply want to *check the area* to see what we encounter.

Stimuli

As usual, in many cases the process of tuning in to the area and allowing the system to express itself may be all that is required and all that is appropriate, but as with all areas of the body it is also possible at times, when appropriate, to introduce subtle stimuli to the system in order to enhance the cranio-sacral system's response.

Frontal compression and frontal lift

For example, we could ask if there are *compressive* forces embedded in the frontal area – thereby enhancing the body's ability to engage with compressive forces imposed on the head. Or we could ask the frontal area if it wishes to *lift* off the front of the head.

As the system settles into deeper stillness, more subtle responses will be appropriate to address those subtler levels, until eventually at the deepest level, only the subtlest stimulus of your presence and your attention absorbed in that deep stillness is all that is necessary and all that is helpful at that level.

The Frontal Area / 207

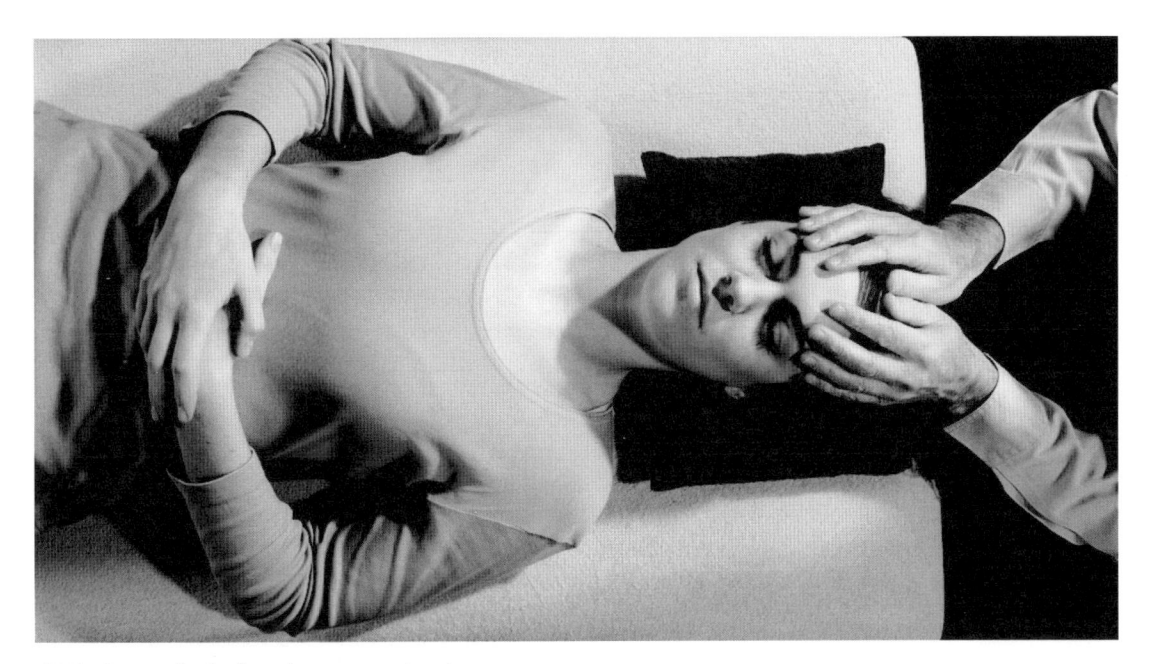

29.7 Contact for the frontal area – anterior view

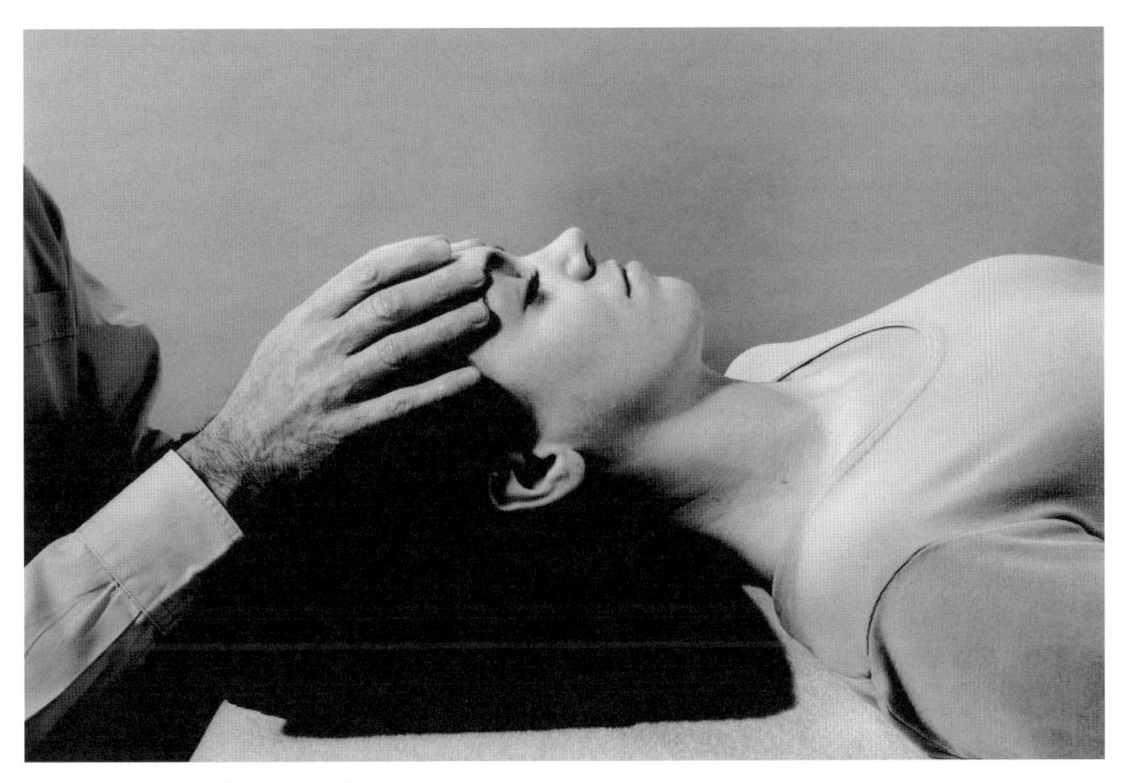

29.8 Contact for the frontal area – lateral view

Initial contact

Sitting at the head of the couch, with the top of the patient's head a few inches from the end of the couch and your elbows or forearms resting on the couch, take up contact. Allow your hands to sink down slowly and gently through the energy field until the fingers and thumbs of both hands come to rest very lightly onto the frontal area with:

- the thumbs parallel, close together at the midline
- the fingers spreading across the frontal area
- the ring fingers just behind the zygomatic processes of the frontal bone
- the fingers pointing down towards the face.

Take care that your fingers don't invade the eyes or eyebrows, as this is likely to be discomforting to the patient.

It is generally helpful to start with your elbows or forearms resting on the couch, to reduce any tendency for your hands to weigh too heavily on the patient's forehead. As engagement develops and the process increasingly takes on a life of its own, you may find that your forearms no longer need the support of the couch and are able to hang loosely from your shoulders, floating freely without weighing heavily.

The process

As you settle into the contact, re-establish your practitioner fulcrums as always, settling into stillness, settling into spaciousness. Establish appropriate levels of physical contact – sensing whether the energy field wants to push your hands away or draw your hands in. Establish appropriate levels of attention. Be receptive to impressions of quality, symmetry and motion.

Allow the gradual evolution of the inherent treatment process. Allow the system to settle into a more balanced neutral state, feeling the emergence of rhythmic motion. Allow the continuing engagement with deeper levels. Observe the repercussions of any changes throughout the body.

This process is likely to constitute the major part of your treatment in this area, eventually leading to a gradual settling of the system into a deeper neutral state, with a more expansive expression of rhythmic motion.

Frontal compression

Within the context of this process, you may encounter a sense of compression, drawing your hands into the frontal area (see Figure 29.9), perhaps as a result of a compressive blow to the front of the head, or to membranous contraction from within – perhaps due to meningitis or emotional tension. Even if such compressions are not apparent, you could explore for underlying hidden forces within, asking the system if there are any forces of compression hidden under the surface and if it would like to draw into compression in order to release them – as always, without any physical force, just an invitation. ('Asking the system' really means asking yourself – can I feel any forces of compression drawing my hands in?) If the system responds to the invitation, allow your fingers to be drawn into compression, feeling the build-up of pressure within the system as it draws to a point of stillness, and waiting for the consequent release, reorganisation and return to a more balanced, expansive neutral state with a clearer expression of rhythmic motion.

Frontal lift

Following any compressive invitation, it is helpful to offer a decompressive invitation; and even without having entered into compression, an offer of decompression may be helpful and appropriate.

With the same contact, you can offer a frontal lift (see Figure 29.9), inviting the frontal area to float up off the front of the head (in other words up towards the ceiling when the patient is lying supine) the subtle thought transmitted through your fingers – as always, without any physical force.

As you maintain that consistent, subtle invitation, the system may respond in various ways. You might feel the system welcoming the opportunity to expand forward and out. You might feel the system contracting. You might feel no response at all. You might feel the whole frontal area readily floating up towards the ceiling; you might feel strong resistance, a sense of stuckness and immobility – which may gradually start to release; you might feel one side floating up and the other side resisting. You might feel an exaggeration of patterns that were already evident from previous palpation. You might feel new patterns emerging. You might feel the system's enhanced ability to overcome resistances that were not releasing before.

Informed awareness

The way in which the system responds will also depend on how you use your attention. Your attention may be spontaneously drawn to specific structures or fulcrums within the matrix. You can also use your attention to survey different structures, patterns, responses, and different levels of being within the system. You can allow your attention to explore different tissue levels – bone, membrane, fluid, energy – and to examine specific structures in detail – sutures, membranous infoldings, foramina, nerves, blood vessels – within the local area or within the body as a whole.

You can let your attention rest at points of resistance, balanced tension and stillness, waiting for them to release. In this way your informed awareness can enhance the body's natural tendency to release and reintegration – gently, subtly, allowing the system to work its way through the multitude of accumulated patterns that have arisen over the years, gradually clearing out the more superficial resistances, encountering deeper resistances, accessing deeper levels and discovering deeper stillness.

As you take your attention to bony levels, you might feel specific bony restrictions within the sutures around the periphery of the frontal bone, whether at the coronal suture, the pterion or the nasion.

You might feel the frontal area being drawn to one side, and you can allow that pattern to be expressed, leading to a point of stillness and release, before returning to a balanced centred neutral.

As solidified resistances release, perhaps reflecting bony restrictions, you might encounter more elastic resistances, perhaps reflecting membranous restrictions, and you can again allow the system to express itself, following the twists, turns and pulls that arise, while surveying the different membranous structures lining the frontal area, or the falx cerebri attaching to the midline of the frontal bone; or perhaps being drawn through the reciprocal tension membrane system to other areas of the cranium, other areas of the body, other areas of the whole system, allowing your attention to be drawn right down through the spinal dura to vertebral restrictions or sacral imbalances, or through other tissues to focal points of restriction in the viscera, in the pelvis, in the legs or anywhere in the body.

Floating freely

As resistances and restrictions soften and release, you may feel an increasing sense of stillness, an increasing sense of symmetry, softness, balance and fluidity; and you may feel that the whole frontal area seems to float freely off the front

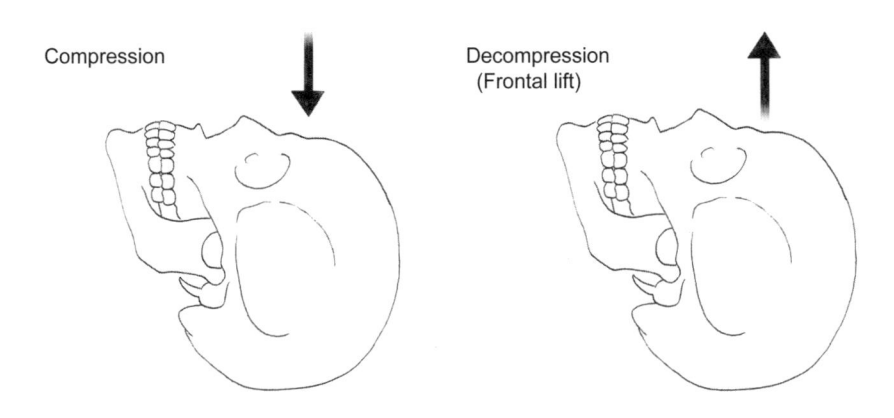

29.9 Direction for frontal compression and frontal lift

of the cranium, no longer twisting, no longer resisting, as if suspended in mid-air.

As the frontal area floats upwards, the sensation in your fingers may feel as if it has physically floated up several feet into the air. As described previously, if you open your eyes, you may be surprised to find that the forehead is still attached to the front of the head, and that your hands are still resting lightly on the forehead. It is helpful to allow yourself to become absorbed into that sense of floating and not to be limited by the gross reality of the visible physical position – because what you are sensing is what is happening energetically and this is what matters in terms of therapeutic effectiveness. The mechanical structural description of bones and membranes is merely an analogy for what is really happening in the matrix.

Once the system has floated freely as far as it wants to go and the process feels complete, you can gently reduce any invitation to expansion and allow the frontal area to settle back very gently onto the front of the head, allowing the system to settle into a neutral balanced state, a state in which many resistances and imbalances have now melted away and disappeared, enabling the system to feel softer, clearer, more balanced, more still; a state in which cranio-sacral motion will be expressed more clearly, more fully, a state in which access to deeper levels of the system will be encountered more readily.

Subtle integration

Having reached that settled neutral state, you can stay with the system, allowing the continuing process of subtle integration on a more profound level, settling into deep dynamic stillness.

When the system expresses a sense of completeness, of resolution, of peace, of stillness, then you can allow the process to come to an end.

Chapter 30

The Parietal Area

Location
The parietal bones form the upper sides of the cranium, the two bones meeting at the top of the head along the sagittal suture. Unlike the frontal bone, the two parietals do not fuse, remaining as two separate bones throughout life (see Figures 30.1 and 30.2).

Articulations
They articulate with the *frontal bone* anteriorly (at the coronal suture), with the *occiput* posteriorly (at the lamdoid suture), and with the two *temporal bones* inferiorly (at the squamosal sutures). They also form small articulations with the tips of the greater wings of the *sphenoid* (at the pterions).

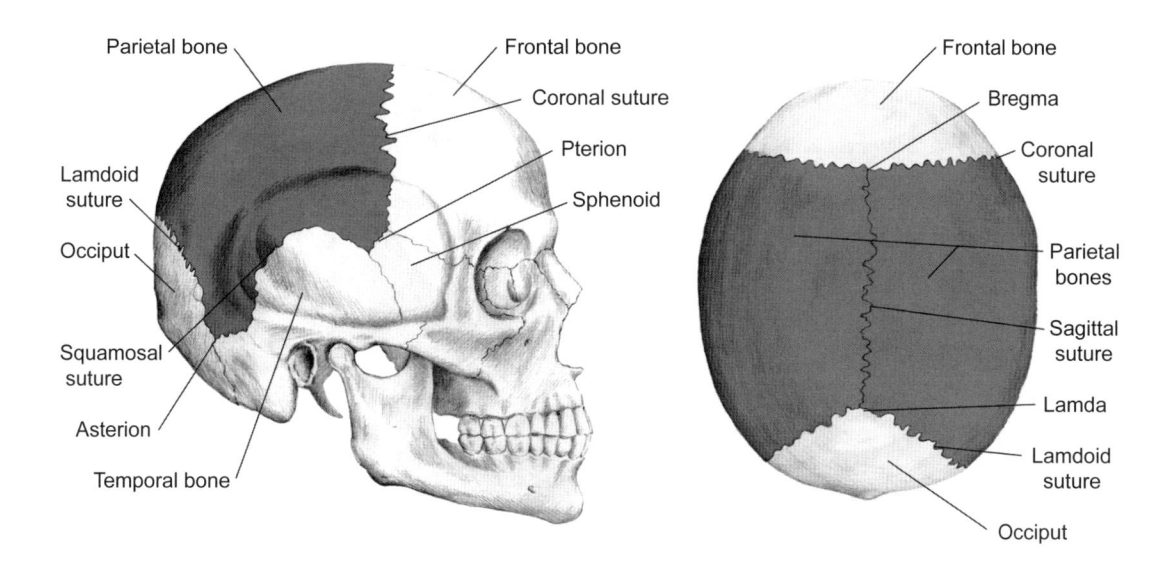

30.1 Parietal bone in situ – lateral view

30.2 Parietal bones in situ – superior view

Membranous relations

Like all bones of the cranium, the parietal bones are lined with membrane.

They also receive attachment of the *falx cerebri* as it passes from front to back inside the cranium, along the midline, beneath the *sagittal suture* (see Figure 30.3). Two bony ridges on the internal surface of the parietals, on either side of the sagittal suture, mark its location, as the membrane separates slightly to accommodate the *superior sagittal sinus*. As with the frontal bone, the falx cerebri again acts as a fulcrum for the rhythmic motion of the parietals.

There is also attachment of a small portion of the *tentorium cerebelli* at the inferior posterior angle of each parietal bone.

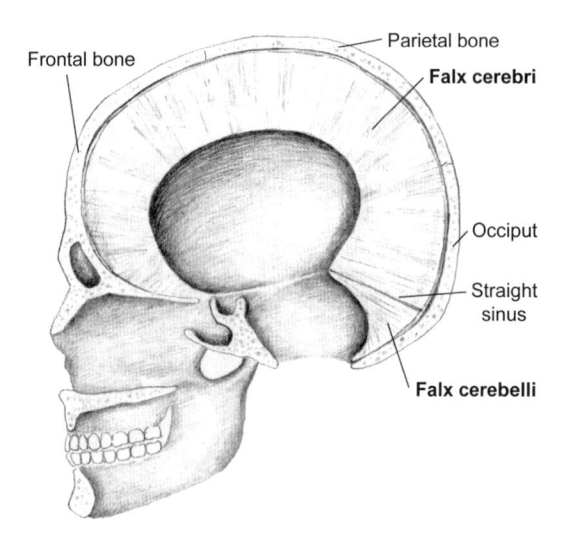

30.3 Membranous associations with the parietals – falx cerebri and falx cerebelli (mid-sagittal section)

Cranio-sacral motion

During cranio-sacral motion, the two parietals flare (during the expansion phase of motion) and narrow (during the contraction phase of motion) hingeing around the sagittal suture and the fulcrum of the falx cerebri along the top of the head. Due to their position at the top of the head, they are only minimally affected by the longitudinal expansion and contraction, being drawn slightly inferiorly at the sagittal suture, thereby flattening the top of the head.

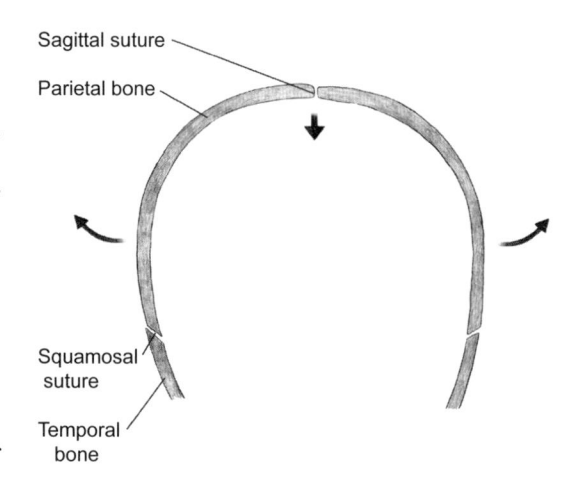

30.4 Cranio-sacral motion of the parietals – the two parietal bones flare and narrow, hingeing around the sagittal suture and the fulcrum of the falx cerebri along the top of the head (coronal section)

All the general points in Chapter 29 on the frontal area apply similarly to the parietal area, and can therefore be taken into account in relation to any contact with the parietals.

Initial contact

Sitting at the head of the couch, with the top of the patient's head a few inches from the end of the couch, allow your hands to sink slowly and gently through the energy field until your fingers and thumbs come to rest lightly on the parietal area, on the upper sides of the head (see Figures 30.5 and 30.6), with:

- the thumbs crossing over at the top of the head so that the pads of the thumbs rest lightly onto the opposite parietal
- the fingers pointing down towards the feet
- the index fingers behind (posterior to) the coronal suture
- the tips of the fingers above (superior to) the level of the squamosal suture (which is roughly level with the tops of the ears).

It is helpful to ensure that the pads of the thumbs are in contact with the opposite parietal. First, this establishes an appropriate guideline position for the appropriate placement of the fingers. Second, it enables clearer monitoring of parietal motion.

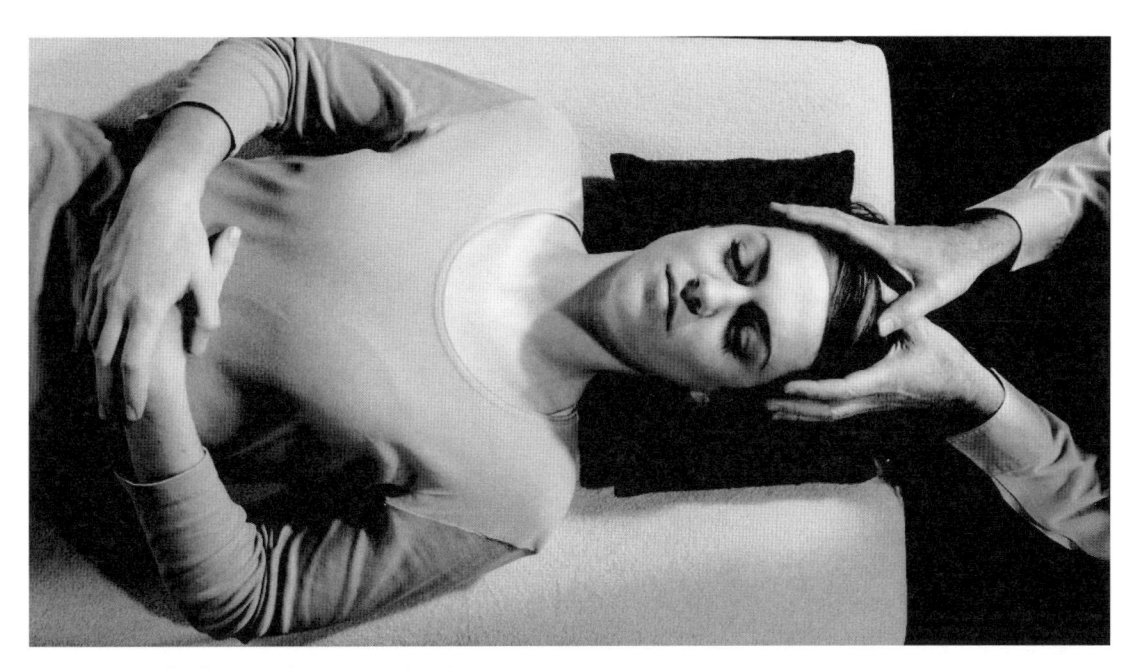

30.5 Contact for the parietal area – anterior view

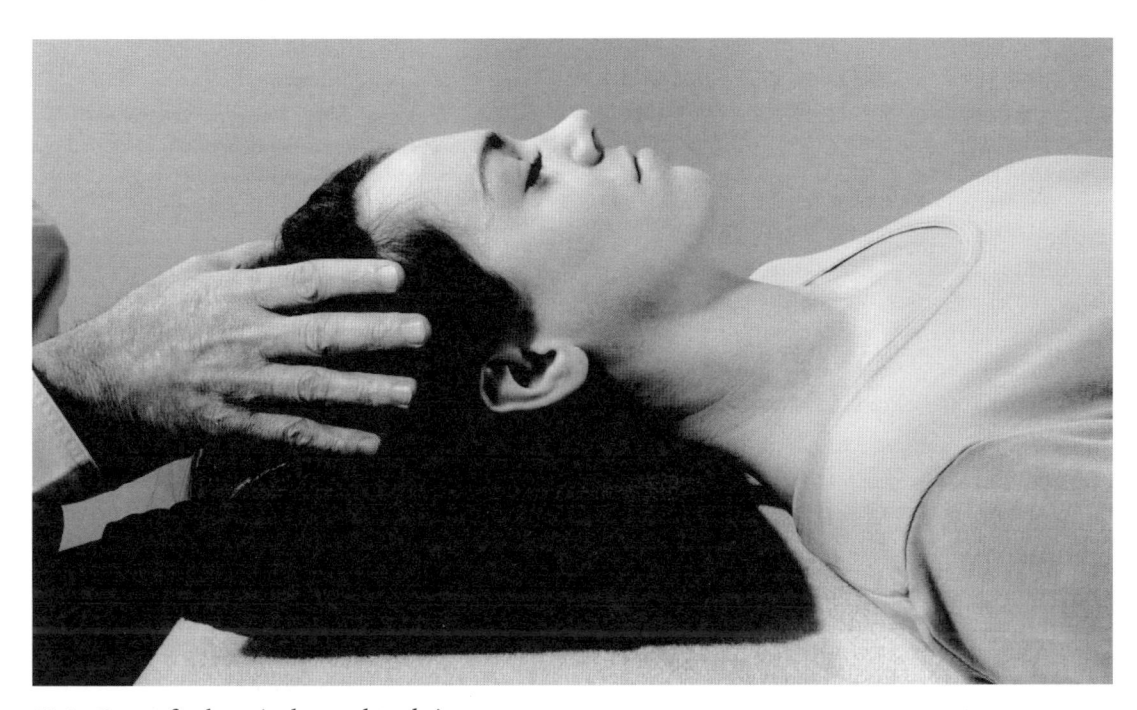

30.6 Contact for the parietal area – lateral view

However, the thumbs should not be pressing on the parietals at all, since this may inhibit the lifting of the parietals off the top of the head.

The position of the fingers pointing down towards the feet (rather than towards the face) helps to ensure that the index fingers are behind the coronal suture – approximately in line with the hairline (depending on your hairline) – and therefore not in contact with the frontal bone.

Keeping the tips of the fingers above the tops of the ears ensures that the contact is above the

214 \ Cranio-Sacral Integration

level of the squamosal sutures and therefore not in contact with the temporal bones.

The process

Establish your own practitioner fulcrums, settling into stillness, settling into spaciousness. Establish appropriate levels of physical contact and appropriate levels of attention.

Allow the gradual evolution of the inherent treatment process. As always, this is likely to constitute the major part of the therapeutic process in this area, gradually moving from initial contact through to deeper levels of engagement over several minutes, allowing the process to evolve and resolve.

Parietal lift

As with the frontal area, having explored the various responses that have arisen spontaneously, we can also offer the parietal area the possibility of lifting off the head – in this case lifting off the *top* of the head, opening up to release the effects of external compressions or of contractile forces from within, inviting the system to respond if it wishes, offering this invitation transmitted through our fingers, and seeing how the system responds.

Due to the nature of the sutures in which the parietals are involved, the parietal lift is most effective when carried out in two separate stages:

1. inviting the parietals to release from the temporals at the squamosal sutures
2. inviting the parietals to lift off the top of the head.

Most of the sutures in the cranium are *interdigitated sutures*, with many tiny bony fingers (digits) interlocking along the length of the suture (see Figure 30.7).

The squamosal sutures, in contrast, are *bevelled sutures*, with the temporal bones overlapping and containing the parietal bones.

Restrictions within the cranium can therefore hold the parietals clamped between the temporals. Consequently, it can be helpful to invite the parietals to squeeze out from between the temporals, so that they can then lift more readily off the top of the head.

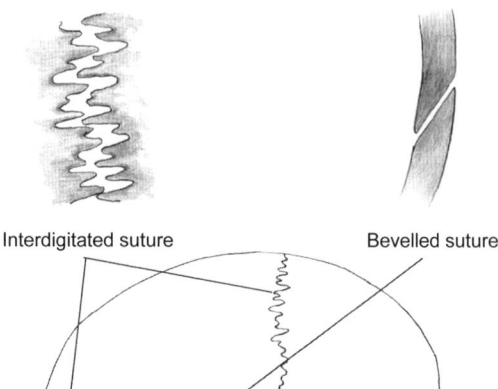

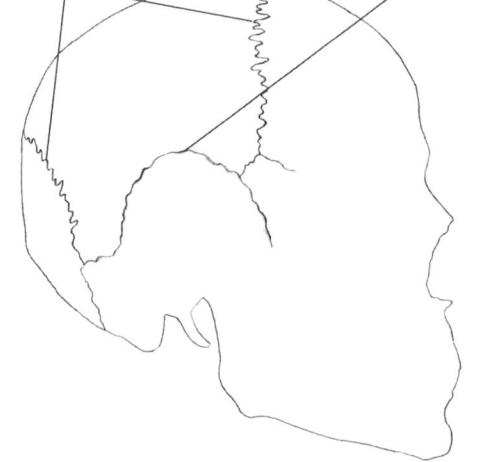

30.7 The squamosal sutures, between the parietal and temporal bones are bevelled sutures, unlike most of the sutures in the cranium which are interdigitated sutures

First stage

Maintaining the same hand position on the parietals, transmitting your thoughts through your fingertips close to the lower border of the parietals, ask yourself if there is any inherent tendency for the parietals to move medially (towards the midline; see Figure 30.8a). Having introduced this gentle question, allow the evolution of fundamental principles in accordance with the individual responses that arise.

The parietals may readily move medially and lift out from between the temporals. They may be resistant and apparently immovable. They may start to wriggle and twist, to rock from side to side, as if to gradually disengage themselves from the temporal bones. They may start to release and lift on one side, while remaining resistant on the other, inducing a sense of bending to one side.

As always, follow wherever the system leads you. If they rock, let them rock. If they wriggle, let them wriggle. If one side lifts, allow that. If the parietals seem to bend to one side, go with that – until eventually a point of stillness may be reached, the second side may release, and both parietals may lift together.

Once both sides have lifted out from between the temporals, creating a softer quality and a greater sense of freedom, release any invitation to medial movement, allow the parietals to settle back into neutral, re-establishing rhythmic motion following the release. Monitor quality, symmetry and motion – feeling the softer, looser quality, the more balanced symmetry, and the more expansive expression of rhythmic motion. Monitor the system through a few cycles of regular rhythmic motion. Once the system feels settled, you can move on to the second stage.

a. First stage - medial

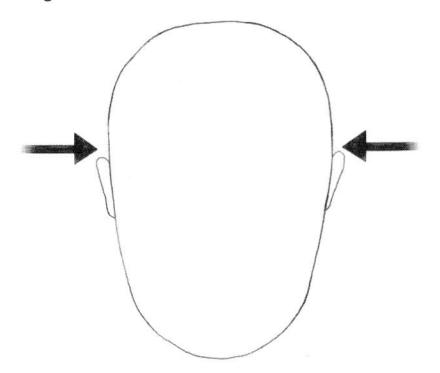

b. Second stage - superior

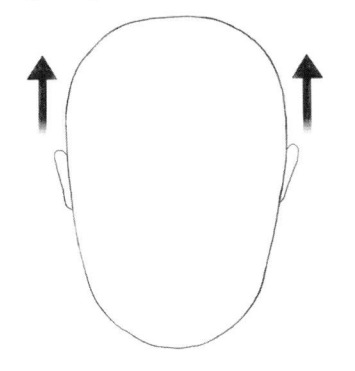

30.8 Directions of intention during a parietal lift

Second stage

With the parietals released from within the temporals, they are now free to lift off the top of the head. Maintaining the same hand position and without any physical force, you can ask yourself if there is any inherent tendency for the parietal area to lift off the top of the head (see Figure 30.8b) (straight back towards you, as you sit at the head with your patient supine). Allow the system to express itself in response to this invitation. Allow the unfolding of fundamental principles in response to the responses within the system, following to points of stillness and release, until the system is no longer twisting, no longer resisting.

As with the frontal area, your attention may be drawn to particular regions, structures, movements, points of resistance, fulcrums; or you can survey the system, taking your attention to different structures – coronal suture, lamdoid suture, squamosal sutures, pterion, asterion, membranous lining, falx cerebri, and down through the reciprocal tension membrane system – through the falx cerebelli and the spinal dura, to the sacrum, pelvis, legs, feet, or any other structures throughout the body, following whatever responses may arise as your attention moves, or is drawn, from place to place, using your informed awareness to enhance the process of release.

As with the frontal area, the sense in your fingers and hands may feel as if the parietals are stretching for miles, even though nothing has visibly moved. Go with this sense, follow it to its extreme – these extremes are the points of greatest therapeutic effectiveness. Also, respect the reality of this extreme sense of stretching – not suddenly abandoning the system at full stretch, leaving it to crash down to earth again (even if only energetically). Once it has stretched as far as it needs to go, and feels soft and loose and free, then gradually reduce any invitation to lift, and allow the parietal area to settle gently back onto the top of the head.

Follow the process through to completion and resolution, allowing the parietal area to settle into a balanced neutral state. Re-evaluate quality, symmetry and motion – feeling the softer, looser quality, the more balanced symmetry, the more expansive rhythmic motion, as the process reaches completion.

As always, following any release, the system is likely to shift to a deeper level of engagement. Stay with the system, appreciating that deeper engagement, allowing the subtle integration of the system at a deeper level. When the process feels complete – settled and peaceful – you can let it come to an end.

Chapter 31

The Falx Cerebri and Falx Release

The intracranial membranes play a highly significant part in the overall balance and integrity of the cranio-sacral system. In day-to-day clinical practice, time after time, attention given to these intracranial membranes has profoundly effective repercussions throughout the system.

This is partly because they act as a fulcrum for the whole reciprocal tension membrane system – particularly around the straight sinus where the various intracranial membranes come together – and therefore for the rest of the system as a whole; when this fulcrum is in balance, the rest of the system can settle into balance around that fulcrum. It is also partly because of their intimate relationship with the flow of venous blood within the cranium, and therefore with fluid flow generally – arterial blood and cerebrospinal fluid as well as venous blood.

The whole cranium is lined with membrane, but the term intracranial membranes is often used to refer more specifically to the infoldings – the falx cerebri, the falx cerebelli and the tentorium cerebelli (see Figure 31.1). All of these have been addressed to some extent through various contacts already described – particularly in addressing the frontal area, the parietal area, the sphenoid and the temporals. An additional process which is particularly powerful and effective is the process known as the falx release.

The term 'falx' is Latin for a sickle or scythe. Both the falx cerebri and falx cerebelli are sickle-shaped double membranes running along the

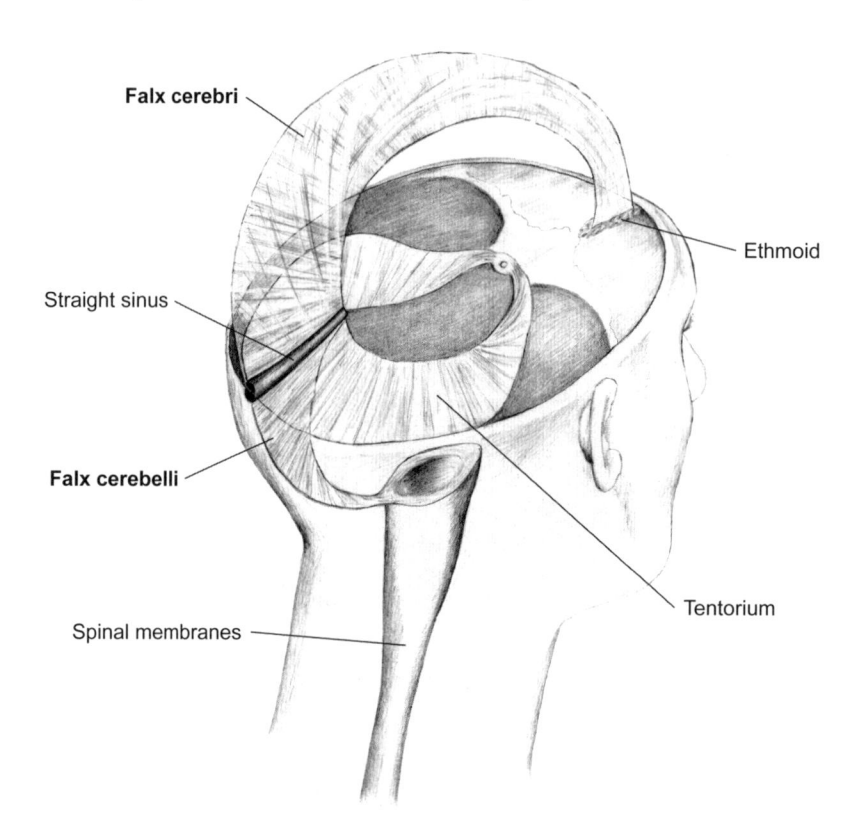

31.1 There is a profound interconnection through the falx cerebri and falx cerebelli to the whole reciprocal tension membrane system down to the sacrum and coccyx

midline of the cranium, partially dividing the two sides of the brain.

Falx cerebri

The falx cerebri stretches from the front of the cranium to the back of the cranium, forming a dividing double membrane between the two cerebral hemispheres – the two halves of the brain maintaining connection via the *corpus callosum*, a bundle of nerve fibres passing transversely below the falx cerebri.

It attaches from the *crista galli of the ethmoid*, along the *midline of the frontal bone*, along the midline *under the sagittal suture*, and down along the *midline of the occiput* – as far as the *internal occipital protuberance* and *confluence of sinuses*.

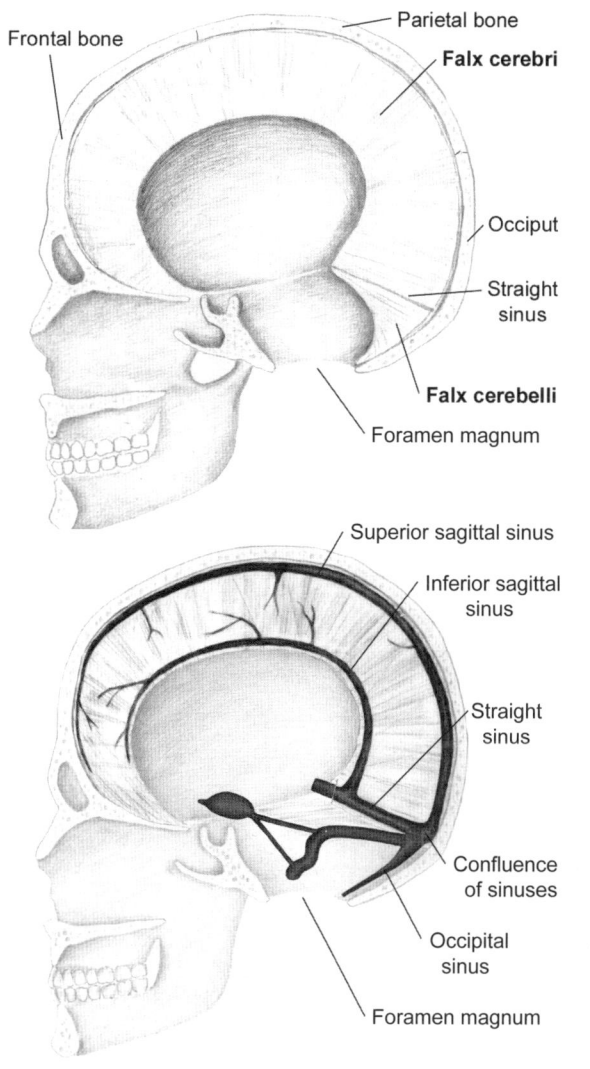

The *superior sagittal sinus* runs along the superior (attached) border of the falx cerebri. The *inferior sagittal sinus* runs along the inferior (free) border of the falx cerebri, deep within the groove between the two cerebral hemispheres (see Figure 31.2).

Many patients describe symptoms that run along the pathway of the falx cerebri. Often they will describe headaches emanating from or following this pattern. In particular, patients who have suffered meningitis often describe a clear pathway of pain and tightness along that region – often slightly one-sided, most commonly to the right hand side, with all the other common associations of the chronic effects of meningitis – headache, neck pain, pain behind the eyes, poor memory, poor concentration, vagueness, tiredness.

Falx cerebelli

The falx cerebelli is a much smaller infolding. It runs along the *midline of the lower occiput*, from the *internal occipital protuberance* and *confluence of sinuses* down to the *foramen magnum* where it blends into the membranes around the foramen magnum and jugular foramina (see Figure 31.1). It forms a double membrane partially dividing the two cerebellar hemispheres. The *occipital sinus* runs along the attached border of the falx cerebelli along the midline of the occiput, draining venous blood up (against gravity) towards the confluence of sinuses (see Figure 31.2).

Again, this is a common site of intense membranous restriction, whether from:

- past inflammation of meningitis, meningisms and other infections affecting the falx cerebelli
- residual effects of birth trauma and other head injuries to this highly susceptible and vulnerable area
- a chronic accumulation of tightness and contraction within the membrane.

This may have consequences spreading through all the surrounding membranes and associated structures, including the jugular foramina (affecting venous drainage through the internal jugular veins, and vagal supply to the viscera, as well as the accessory and glossopharyngeal nerves); the foramen magnum (involving the spinal cord, and the vertebral arteries supplying

31.2 The falx cerebri, falx cerebelli, and associated structures

arterial blood to the brain); the carotid canals (affecting the carotid arteries and sympathetic supply to the cranium). It may also contribute to a vicious circle of mutual interaction between all the structures in the suboccipital region.

Profound connections through the reciprocal tension membrane system

There is a direct pathway of interconnection through the falx cerebri and falx cerebelli down into the membranes around the foramen magnum and the whole suboccipital region, including the membranous attachments to the second and third cervical vertebrae and the membranous attachment to rectus capitis posterior minor. So working with the falx cerebri and falx cerebelli can be a very powerful means of influencing the suboccipital region, and a very effective addition to the suboccipital release, as a means of releasing impingement on the many vital structures in this area.

This interconnection then continues down from the foramen magnum into the spinal dura, with ramifications right down the spine to the sacrum and coccyx (see Figure 31.1).

The falx cerebri (from above) and the falx cerebelli (from below) also blend into the tentorium cerebelli at the straight sinus, with consequent ramifications on these structures and on the reciprocal tension membrane system as a whole and on venous drainage and fluid flow within the cranium.

Working with the falx cerebri and falx cerebelli is therefore potentially very powerful and profound, and has particularly powerful effects on the whole longitudinal membrane system.

Falx contact

This contact involves cradling the falx cerebri and falx cerebelli between the two hands, with a hand at the front of the head and a hand at the back, so that the two falces are extending from one hand to the other (see Figure 31.3).

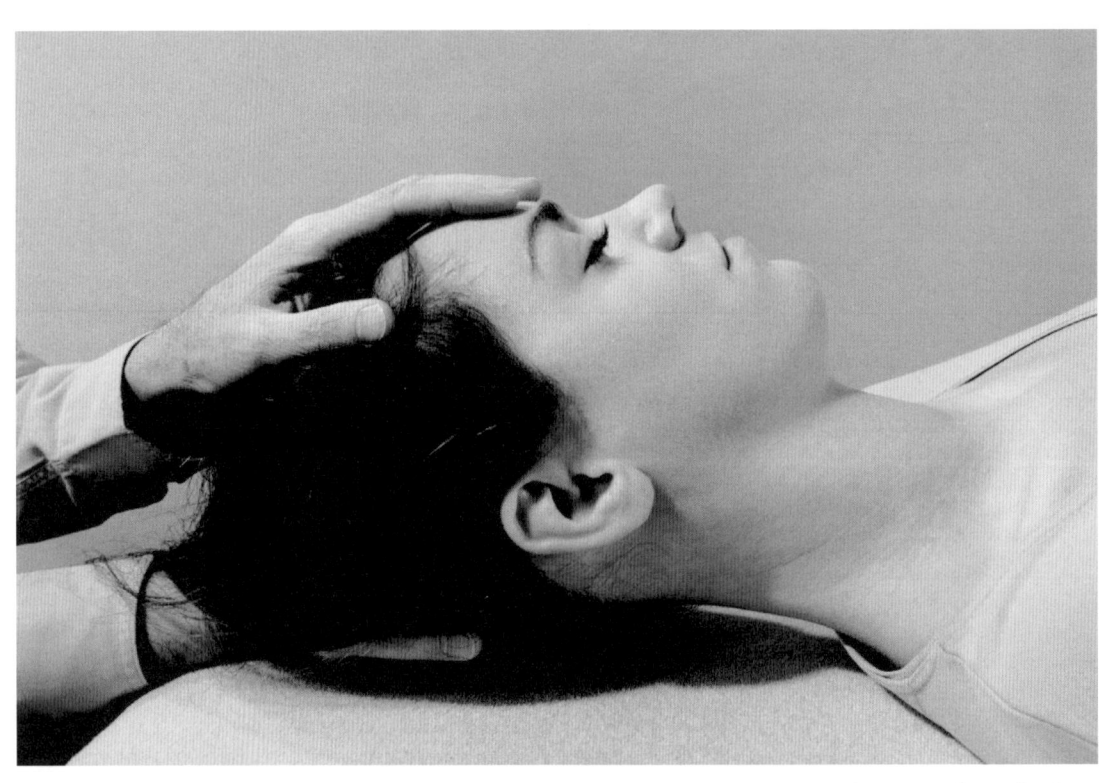

31.3 Falx contact – lateral view – this contact involves cradling the falx cerebri and falx cerebelli between the two hands, with a hand at the front of the head and a hand at the back of the head

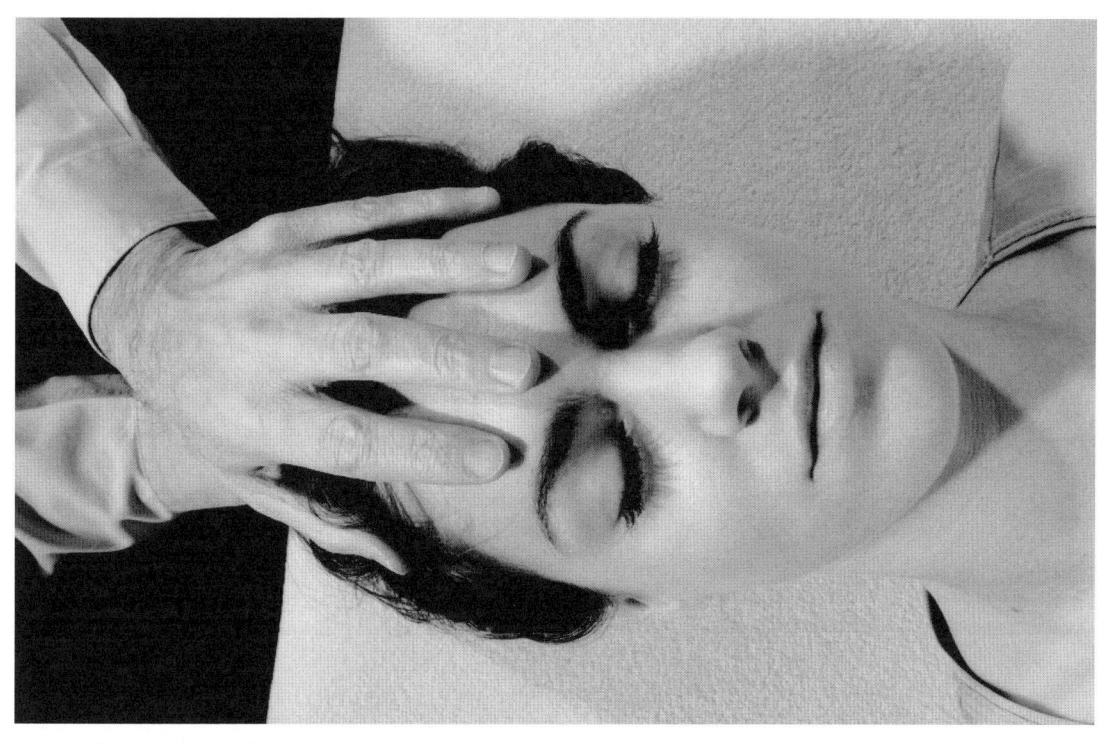

31.4 Falx contact – anterior view

Rolling the head (as with the suboccipital release), remove any cushion, gently sweep any long hair out of the way, and take up contact with one hand under the occiput. This hand needs to be central under the occiput, so that *the curve of the occiput sits comfortably into the curve of the palm of the hand*, with the head well balanced so that it is not rolling over to one side, and so that the practitioner can relax the hand completely without any need to support the head against rolling over. The fingers are pointing towards the sacrum and will probably extend into the neck to contact the soft tissues at the top of the neck; the exact position of the hand will of course vary according to size of hands and size of head. Most of all, the contact needs to be comfortable for both patient and practitioner, with the practitioner able to relax the hand completely.

The contact for the falx release is not a symmetrical contact in terms of the practitioner's position and therefore may need some adjustment to enable maximum comfort for the therapist – and maximum comfort is of course vital in order to enable maximum sensitivity and effectiveness. As you take up this contact, you may find that your arm and elbow feel a bit tucked up into your abdomen, creating a position that is less than comfortable. This can readily be eased by moving your chair slightly to the opposite side (i.e. if you have your right hand under the occiput, move your chair slightly to the left).

Check with your patient that they are comfortable. Having established a comfortable position, bring your other hand in softly through the energy field towards the frontal area, fingers pointing down towards the feet. Let the heel of the hand come to rest around the bregma or crown of the head (depending on size of head and hands) so that the fingers are resting lightly over the frontal area. Take care that the fingers don't invade the eyes or eyebrows.

As you settle into the contact, let your upper hand relax down gradually, letting go of any unnecessary tension. However, take care not to weigh heavily onto the patient's forehead. Some practitioners may prefer to have the elbow of this upper arm resting on the couch to avoid any tendency to weigh heavily. Others may find that they are able to let the weight of their arm hang loosely from the shoulder, so that the hand can rest softly onto the forehead without undue pressure. As you become increasingly engaged with the system, your hand and arm are likely to feel increasingly weightless anyway.

Settling into the contact, apply all the usual prerequisites to treatment – establishing your own fulcrums, establishing appropriate levels of physical contact, attention and tissue connection – acknowledging the system as a quantum energy field, and feeling the gradual sense of increasing engagement with this energy field as you settle into stillness and settle into spaciousness.

As engagement deepens, your upper hand may feel pushed away from the forehead or may feel drawn into the forehead, as the energy field expresses its needs. Respond accordingly, allowing your hand to float freely and be washed this way and that. Both hands may feel subtle pulls, twists and turns, whether in the membranes, the bones, the fluids or the energy field. As always, allow the evolution of the inherent treatment process. Maintain your profound sense of spaciousness, as you allow yourself to be moved by the subtle waves of motion.

With each release, the system will tend to settle back to a balanced, central position. Following a release, you can wait to see what other impressions or patterns may arise, thereby following the system through a series of releases, addressing restrictions in various areas of the system. The points of balanced tension, stillness and release that arise may be local or distant, may be within the falx cerebri or falx cerebelli, within the surrounding membranes lining the cranium, within the membranes around the jugular foramina or foramen magnum, may be within the bones, may be drawing you to fulcrums further down the body, in the neck, the spine, the pelvis, the diaphragm, the solar plexus, the legs, the feet, or in any part of the matrix. Simply allow the system to find its own way through a succession of releases, knowing that the body in its own wisdom knows what to do and where to go in order to bring balance and integrity into the system as a whole.

Up till now we have mostly talked in terms of allowing the system to settle back to neutral after each release. There are other options and this contact provides a good opportunity to explore another alternative, sometimes described as 'taking up the slack'.

Taking up the slack

As the system releases and the tissues seem to soften, melt and dissolve, instead of allowing the system to settle out into neutral, you can follow into the softening, as if your hands are taking up the slack in the newly softened membranes, thereby drawing into the next point of balanced tension, stillness and release. In this way you might take up the slack several times through a series of releases, each time taking you deeper into the system, and perhaps following a series of fulcrums down through the tissues, as your attention and your hands are drawn – perhaps initially to a resistance in the falx cerebri, then taking up the slack to a point perhaps somewhere around the jugular foramen or foramen magnum; as that releases you could again take up the slack to encounter a restriction in the upper cervical region and so on down through the spine, perhaps following a pattern that twists across the body, pivoting around T12, or draws persistently down one side of the body to the sacro-iliac joint. Some of these fulcrums may prove more resistant than others; this may provide diagnostic information regarding their chronicity and indications of which fulcrums are more primary or more deeply ingrained. At some point on the journey, the system may tell you that it doesn't want to take up the slack any more, and wants to release out into neutral. This may particularly occur following the release of the primary source of the pattern, or the release of a particularly resistant restriction.

Once you reach a suitable point of release, reorganisation and settling back to a balanced neutral state, you can allow this phase of the process to come to completion.

This whole process of the system drawing into asymmetries, fulcrums, points of balanced tension, stillness and release will tend to occur spontaneously, and you can follow it as above. You may also find, as rhythmic motion becomes increasingly apparent, that the system is drawn persistently into the extremes of motion, whether into extreme expansion or contraction, and as you follow this tendency, this will enhance the potential for the system to identify, engage with, and release points of resistance, since the power of the system to release restrictions is always enhanced at the extremes of motion.

It is also possible to further enhance the system's natural tendency to identify and release restrictions by *specifically engaging with the system's tendency to follow into the extremes of motion*.

Rhythmic motion

With the hands positioned as described for this contact, with one hand over the frontal area and the other hand under the occiput, you have a clear connection with both the front and back of the head, together with their opposing directions of movement. The frontal area is arcing forward and down during the expansion phase of motion (even though it is being held back by the falx cerebri). Meanwhile, the occiput is tucking under towards the neck so your hands are arcing in opposite directions. The heels of your hands may seem to be arcing away from each other during the expansion phase, and towards each other during the contraction phase.

Following into the extremes of motion

Once the system has settled into a balanced neutral state, with rhythmic motion expressed clearly, whether in cranio-sacral rhythm or middle tide motion, observe to see if the system is naturally drawing more readily into expansion or contraction. Perhaps the system will immediately start drawing into one extreme or the other. If not, you could ask yourself if there is any inherent tendency to follow into one extreme or the other, choosing the direction most favoured by the system.

As you follow the system consistently into its chosen direction, you may feel the usual gradual build-up of tension or pressure within the system. You may feel the system drawing into patterns of asymmetry or towards specific fulcrums. Familiar patterns may become more exaggerated. New patterns may appear. As always, allow the system

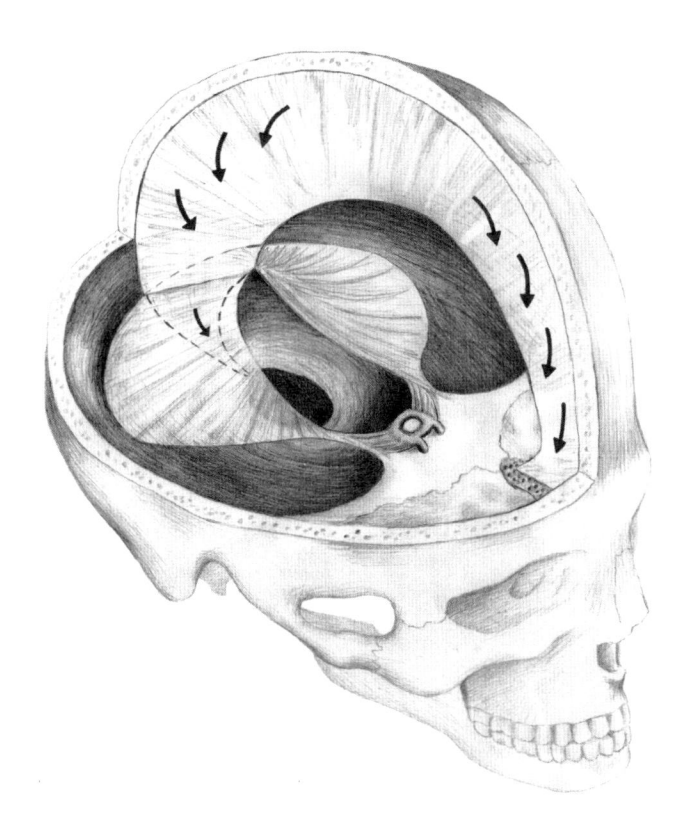

31.5 Cranio-sacral motion of the falx cerebri and falx cerebelli during the expansion phase – your hands are arcing away from each other during the expansion phase, and towards each other during the contraction phase

to express itself, follow wherever it takes you, consistently maintaining this tendency into the preferred extreme of motion.

This approach may not be necessary if the system already has plenty to say. It may happen spontaneously. It may become appropriate after the system has done whatever it wants to do initially.

It may serve as a means of bringing certain patterns more clearly into focus, or enabling the system to address more persistent patterns or restrictions more effectively. It may be particularly helpful in taking up the slack, following the system more fully into an extreme of motion in order to maintain the focus within the tissues. Whatever way it may arise, the healing potency will be enhanced at the extremes of motion.

Settling into subtle integration

Once the system has completed its journey, released whatever patterns of restriction it may want to release, reorganised and settled back to a centred, balanced neutral state, you can stay with it, observing the more spacious quality, the more balanced symmetry, the more settled motion, and the more expansive, freely mobile rhythmic motion. Once again you can settle into simply being there, allowing the subtle integration of the system, settling into deeper stillness, absorbed into the gentle flow of the rhythmic motion, perhaps shifting from middle tide to long tide, allowing the system to settle into deep dynamic stillness.

When the therapeutic process has reached its natural conclusion, with the system feeling settled and expressing even, regular cycles of easeful rhythmic motion, you can allow the process to come to completion. Gently allow your upper hand to float away from the forehead, and carefully release your lower hand from under the occiput, rolling the head over to the side, taking care not to pull the hair, jolt the head, or discomfort the patient in any way. You can then move on to whatever is appropriate next within the context of your overall integrated treatment.

Chapter 32

Completion

Within the context of our four-stage treatment framework, we are now ready for the final stage – completion:

1. Engagement (tuning in)
2. Opening up the system (settling and grounding)
3. Core treatment
4. *Completion.*

Every treatment needs to come to a satisfactory completion, not just come to an end, but come to an appropriately settled and balanced conclusion.

As mentioned earlier, if a patient has been for an operation in hospital and their abdomen has been cut open in order to access their inner organs, it is not generally advisable as soon as the operation is over to send them out into the world without stitching them up, without allowing them time to recover from the anaesthetic and without ensuring that they are ready to return to the fray.

In a cranio-sacral treatment, we are opening up the system, engaging with deep levels of the patient's being, connecting to deep levels of consciousness, potentially enabling profound changes. It is therefore advisable to ensure that the system is sufficiently settled, balanced and ready to go out into the world.

Natural conclusion

Most treatments will come to a natural conclusion. As we have already seen, treatment is likely to consist of a series of episodes through which the system addresses particular patterns, reaches points of release, and then settles into neutral.

Each release and reorganisation is a potential moment of completion. Some will bring about minor changes and resettling locally. Others will bring about more profound changes and a more widespread sense of the whole system resettling. Some will bring a significant shift to a deeper level. Some will lead to a deep dynamic stillness. As a treatment session progresses, the changes and the repercussions of those changes are likely to become increasingly profound, increasingly widespread, increasingly comprehensive.

Any of these moments of resettling could be regarded as a point of completion – completion of that particular phase of treatment, an opportunity to settle into deeper dynamic stillness and subtle integration, or an opportunity to bring the whole treatment session to an end. But certain moments are likely to have a more evident sense of completion – when the whole system feels integrated, with an overall sense of balance, an all-pervasive quality of settledness, no evident extraneous movement, and above all the easeful settled expression of even rhythmic motion. Such moments are particularly likely to occur when an integrated treatment approach has been followed.

The key characteristics that enable you to recognise a suitable moment of completion are:

- the quality – settled, balanced, easeful, peaceful
- rhythmic motion – even, settled, peaceful.

Many opportunities

From this it is evident that the completion of a treatment is determined by the progress of the inherent treatment process itself, not by arbitrary timescales of one-hour or half-hour sessions. There are likely to be many opportunities for a treatment to come to completion, so it is not difficult to find such opportunities within a treatment session, but the priority is that time is not the determining factor, and that the needs of the system are always the overriding factor in determining the completion of a treatment.

Inappropriate moments

Not every moment is suitable; it is not helpful to leave a treatment in mid-process – building up to a point of balanced tension, waiting at a point of stillness, or in any way turbulent or disturbed.

This could leave the patient feeling incomplete, unsettled, or disorientated.

Transient light-headedness or mild disorientation are common immediately after a cranio-sacral session even when the process has come to a perfectly satisfactory completion – this is not a cause for concern, so long as it is transient and mild. Many people, especially elderly people, will feel light-headed after getting up from a lying position at any time, let alone after a cranio-sacral treatment. This does not need to be confused with incompleteness of treatment.

The main guide to the completeness of the treatment is what you feel in the system. If you allow the system to come to its natural conclusion, check the state of the system at the end of the session, and ensure that there is a settled quality and an even rhythmic motion, then the treatment can be regarded as complete.

Incompleteness

So with most treatments you don't need to do anything specific to enable that natural conclusion, other than acknowledging the appropriate moment and checking that the system is balanced and settled.

There will be times when a treatment is not ready to end, however, when the system is still expressing specific requirements, wanting to address unresolved issues, drawing into specific patterns, or expressing turbulence or unsettledness. There is nothing wrong with this; it is simply a matter of being aware of the progress of the treatment process and following it through to completion. Each individual will have different needs which may be expressed and resolved over differing time periods. Simply allow the process to proceed to its natural conclusion in its own time.

The natural process of release inevitably uncovers deeper patterns. These patterns may need time to resolve and settle; they may reveal new asymmetries to be addressed; they may bring up physical or emotional responses in the patient which need time to settle. Again this is nothing to be concerned about, just allow the process the time it needs to follow through to its natural conclusion, and address any emotional needs as necessary, allowing expression, resolution and settling.

There will also be times when you feel so deeply absorbed, so profoundly engaged with the therapeutic process, that you want to stay there longer. It is helpful to work with flexible timescales that allow you to take full advantage of such valuable therapeutic opportunities. Whatever length of time the process may take, you will need to find an appropriate moment for completion, rather than curtailing the session prematurely.

Assisting completion

If for any reason the system does not settle, there are certain processes that can be adopted in order to help it to a point of completion:

1. Simply *wait*, give it time, allow it to find its own natural conclusion.

2. Maintain your own *calm, quiet presence*. This provides a stable fulcrum around which your patient's system can settle, enabling the entrainment of your patient's unsettled system with your more settled system.

3. *Engage with rhythmic motion*, gently allowing and following the rhythmic motion, your attention focused on the rhythmic motion, without being drawn into any extraneous imbalances, encouraging a fluent, settled, even, easeful rhythmic motion. This encourages the system to settle into easeful rhythmic motion, and encourages any extraneous movements to fall into line with the even expression of rhythmic motion.

4. As you engage with the rhythmic motion, you can deliberately maintain a steady stable encouragement into even regular expansion and contraction, specifically disallowing any extraneous movements or diversions, simply insisting on a steady stable even expression of motion. This is sometimes described as *railway tracking* – as if you are providing a straight and narrow railway track along which the system must proceed, not allowing it to go off track into extraneous distractions. In this way you are therefore encouraging the system to settle into this even steady state. This can also be useful at other times during a treatment.

5. You can induce a *still point*.

Chapter 33

Still Point

Spontaneous still points

Still points are occurring spontaneously in all of us much of the time, day and night. They are the cranio-sacral system's means of releasing tensions and restrictions; they are an inherent part of the body's natural mechanism for maintaining health, balance and homeostasis.

They occur particularly at times of ease and relaxation – such as during sleep and during meditation, when we allow our systems to do what they need to do, instead of imposing undue pressures and stresses on ourselves. We tend not to notice them during sleep for obvious reasons, but during meditation one can readily observe still points occurring, noticing the gradual build-up, the point of stillness, and the release, and often the greater degree of ease, balance and harmony in our bodies and minds subsequently.

Spontaneous still points are also an integral part of every treatment process. As we have seen, this will often evolve around a specific fulcrum, leading to release and the re-emergence of rhythmic motion.

The presence of the practitioner enhances this natural tendency. Engagement with the system further enhances the process. The focused awareness of the therapist enhances this spontaneous process even more.

Still point induction

Still points can also be specifically induced by the practitioner, as a means of enhancing the cranio-sacral system's inherent healing potential. This might be appropriate or desirable because the system does not have sufficient resources to utilise its own healing potential – perhaps due to exhaustion, low vitality, chronic illness, severe trauma, shock, or being overworked, tense, or too busy – and therefore needs the presence of the practitioner to enable more effective engagement with that inherent healing potential.

Such a stimulus may also be used for a variety of other purposes:

- to settle a system that is restless or agitated
- to help the system to overcome a particularly persistent resistance
- to help the system clear a multitude of superficial restrictions and imbalances
- to enhance the power of a system that feels feeble
- to address specific clinical conditions – such as inflammatory or immune conditions
- to invite the system to decide for itself what it wants to do with the stimulus
- to help in bringing a treatment process to a balanced and settled conclusion.

Still point inductions can be enabled in various ways:

- By *following the system's spontaneous tendency* to move into one extreme of motion.
- By *identifying a preference* within the system towards one phase of motion and offering it the option of following consistently into that preferred phase.
- Where no preference is apparent, by *selecting one phase of motion* and inviting the system to move consistently into that chosen phase.

If the system responds to your engagement by drawing *spontaneously* into a still point, you can allow it do so.

If the system exhibits a *preference* for moving more readily into one phase than the other, perhaps moving further or more strongly into the contraction phase, and less readily into the expansion phase, you can follow with your attention into the preferred phase.

There will also be times when the system is not drawing into still points, nor exhibiting any preference for one phase of motion or the other, nor identifying restrictions, and not addressing the deeper more persistent restrictions within the system. This could be because it lacks the power to do so, or because it is depleted; it could be because the patient is not in a sufficiently easeful and relaxed state; it could be because the restrictions are particularly ingrained and resistant; it could be because the system is too unsettled and scattered to operate effectively. At these times, even though no preference is shown, you can enhance the body's ability to reach the therapeutic potential of a still point by *selecting one phase of motion* and inviting the system to move consistently into that chosen phase.

The process

A still point can be induced from anywhere in the body, since the requirement is simply to engage with rhythmic motion, and rhythmic motion is present everywhere in the body. The process of still point induction can be summarised as follows:

1. Engage with rhythmic motion.
2. Observe any preference within the system to move more strongly into one phase or the other, or choose one phase or the other.
3. Allow or invite the system to draw consistently into the preferred or chosen phase.
4. Continue into that preferred direction until the system reaches a still point.
5. Wait at that still point until you experience a sense of softening, melting, release.
6. Allow the whole system to reorganise and settle to a balanced neutral state – feeling the gradual re-emergence of rhythmic motion – noticing the enhanced quality, symmetry and motion, and the slower rate and wider amplitude of motion.

In other words it is simply an expression of the inherent treatment process or the fundamental principles.

Variations and observations

When you first engage with the system, particularly if the system is unsettled, you may encounter *various other initial impressions –* qualities, asymmetries, movements, pulls, twists, turns, ripples, vibrations, pulsations. These can be allowed to settle of their own accord by acknowledging them, allowing the system to express itself, and waiting for the rhythmic motion to emerge more clearly. As the rhythmic motion becomes more clearly apparent, focus your attention on this rhythmic motion and stay with it as it becomes clearer and stronger, keeping your attention clearly focused on following the expansion and contraction phases of the rhythm, not giving attention to the extraneous movements.

As the system draws increasingly into its preferred phase, you may feel *a build-up of pressure or tension* within the system. It may feel as if the system is being contained and pressure is building up inside – which is what provides the increased power or potency.

(An analogy for the way this feels is to think of an elongated balloon gently expanding and contracting. As you contain the motion, it is as if you are squeezing the balloon at one end, resulting in a build-up of pressure inside the balloon, and an increased tendency for the balloon to push out more strongly on all sides. This is just an analogy. You do not of course squeeze at all.)

As the process proceeds, the amplitude of the motion becomes narrower and narrower (although the rate of the rhythm generally remains the same at this stage). As it approaches the still point, the amplitude may be so small that it is barely noticeable at all. At this point, precision is necessary to *ensure that you identify any remaining rhythmic motion*. It is possible to think that rhythmic motion has ceased and that you have reached a still point when in fact the system is still expressing rhythmic motion on a barely distinguishable level. If you assume that this is a still point and wait there assuming that you have reached a still point, the system may not address the restriction and no release will occur, and you may be holding at that point indefinitely with nothing happening. So keep a careful watch for every last bit of rhythmic motion, maintaining your intention into the chosen phase, in order to ensure that you reach a true still point.

The *time taken* to reach a still point may vary from a few seconds to several minutes, depending on circumstances.

When you do reach a true still point, It is *not simply a matter of the cessation of rhythmic motion.* There is generally a much more profound sense of stillness, an all-pervasive quality of stillness, a stillness that pervades the whole patient, that spreads through you, that may seem to pervade the whole room with a very deep sense of stillness.

Once a still point has been reached, the system may remain in stillness for some time. In order to establish whether you have genuinely reached a still point, you will need to *evaluate the quality of the stillness*. A true still point will exhibit a dynamic quality, a sense of something about to happen, a profound all-pervasive sense of stillness. If you have not yet reached the still point, there may be a quality of stillness but it may lack that dynamism, that aliveness, that profound feeling – in which case you may need to keep inviting the system into its chosen phase in order to reach a true still point.

As you wait at the still point, *the system may respond in various ways*. Some still points will simply melt away into a release. At other times, the system may wriggle, it may pulsate, it may rock from side to side as if it is trying to break away; it may build up pressure, or it may seem to push your hands away, as if it is trying to escape. *Don't be deceived* into thinking that these are signs of a release and therefore fooled into letting go of your focus prematurely. Be prepared to wait patiently with whatever responses arise, your attention clearly focused on staying with the profound stillness.

Wait until you feel *a very convincing sense of softening* and release. The resistance will melt, the pressure will give way, and the system may go a little further into contraction before releasing out into a long slow expansion phase. Only when you feel this powerful and convincing sense of softening and release, should you let your focus of attention follow the system out into its long expansion phase. Even then, keep your attention still clearly focused on the system, feeling the release through the whole body, as the whole system reorganises around the change and the whole body softens, relaxes and releases.

As the system releases out of a still point, you may notice *a change in the patient's breathing*, becoming a bit deeper and more relaxed. The patient might take a deeper breath just as the release occurs, consciously or unconsciously.

Having contained the system into one extreme of motion, the system is likely to go into *a very long expansion* into the opposite phase (like a pendulum that has been held at one extreme and is then allowed to swing all the way to its opposite extreme).

Continue to follow the system with your attention as it gently settles into easy rhythmic motion – a rhythmic motion which will probably exhibit a greater amplitude than previously, and may feel a little slower and more expansive, with an overall quality of softness and greater expansion throughout the system.

Still points can also provide a doorway or point of transition from cranio-sacral rhythm to middle tide, or from middle tide to long tide.

Once the system has settled into a balanced neutral state and you have followed several cycles of easeful rhythmic motion, you can allow the process to come to completion.

How does a still point induction differ from the still points that occur throughout a treatment session?

They are very similar, but there are a few minor differences. Firstly, the practitioner is making *a deliberate decision* to induce a still point. That does not mean imposing any force, or imposing anything on the body that it doesn't want. It is simply a matter of offering the still point to the system, offering that extra power with which to do whatever it wants, offering it the possibility of enhancing its own natural tendency to enter into still points.

Secondly, when inducing a still point, *less attention is given to asymmetries*, imbalances or focal points of restriction. The focus of attention is on the rhythmic motion, with no specific need to identify any particular fulcrum or to follow into any restriction (although you may choose to focus on a particular fulcrum if appropriate). The still point is generally offered to the system as a whole – knowing that the system in its infinite wisdom will use that power wisely and do whatever it needs to do at that moment in order to bring itself into greater balance and clarity.

How long is a still point?

Still points may occur repeatedly in milliseconds, so quickly that you barely notice them happening, particularly at the start of a treatment when there are many superficial ripples and wavelets to be addressed. They may last *several seconds, or several minutes*.

The time taken for a still point to arise, stay in stillness, and release will generally reflect not only the nature of the restriction being addressed – how deeply ingrained it is, its *chronicity* – but also the level of depth at which you are working. The more deeply you engage with the system, the more persistent will be the restriction and the longer the still points to release them. A still point at the middle tide level will generally arise more slowly, last longer, and be more subtle than a still point at the cranio-sacral rhythm level.

The time taken will also be affected by your *degree of focus*. The more precisely you can focus on the process and the point of stillness, the more effectively it will release. If your focus of attention is vague, unfocused or imprecise (whether through inexperience, lack of concentration, distraction, or lack of precise anatomical location) then the still point may take longer to reach the precise point of balanced tension, or may linger longer due to inadequate focus, or ultimately release with a less effective, less complete release.

Contact points

Still points can be induced anywhere in the body, because wherever you take up contact, you are always incorporating the whole matrix in your still point. Some of the most readily accessible, most commonly used contacts are:

- the occiput
- the temporals
- the sacrum
- the feet.

A sacral still point might be particularly effective for releasing the sacrum, for enhancing the mobility of the sacrum, or for addressing restrictions in the spine.

A still point through the feet might be particularly helpful for balancing the pelvis, addressing joint restrictions in the lower limbs, hips, knees, ankles, or for inflammatory conditions in those joints.

A temporal still point might be particularly helpful for settling emotions and balancing all the transverse diaphragms, and is a particularly valuable way to finish any treatment.

However, all still points will always affect the whole system and have repercussions throughout the whole system. The effect of the still point and the location of that effect is not primarily dependent on the point of contact. It may be determined partly by the focus of the practitioner's attention, and most of all by the body's inherent wisdom.

Expansion and contraction

Still points can be induced into either phase of motion – the contraction phase or the expansion phase. The effects may vary according to which phase you choose. Either phase is likely to be beneficial in most circumstances. The choice of which phase to use is generally determined primarily by the demands of the system. If the system draws more strongly into contraction, it is appropriate to induce a still point into contraction; if the system draws more strongly into expansion, it is appropriate to induce a still point into the expansion phase.

CV4 and EV4

When Sutherland first devised the still point induction, he used the occipital contact – following the occiput into its contraction phase – and he used the term CV4 to describe the process. The term CV4 is an abbreviation for compression of the fourth ventricle, since Sutherland theorised that he was harnessing the power within the system by compressing cerebrospinal fluid within the fourth ventricle, thereby building up pressure within the membrane system, enabling the system to use that increased pressure to break down resistances elsewhere in the system (like squeezing an elongated balloon). The term EV4 is used for a still point into the expansion phase of motion (expansion of the fourth ventricle) and these terms are often used for still point inductions induced anywhere in the system (not just at the occiput) into their respective phases.

As mentioned above, the effect of the still point induction is not primarily dependent on the point of contact, so a still point induced from the feet (or anywhere in the body) with the practitioner's attention on the fourth ventricle might have its effect primarily on the fourth ventricle, or might harness the power within the fourth ventricle, and be termed a CV4. Wherever the practitioner's hands may be, their attention can be focused within the fourth ventricle in order to harness that particular potency. In the same way, they could focus their attention on the third ventricle, a process known as a CV3 (into the contraction phase) or EV3 (into the expansion phase) thereby harnessing a different potential.

Sutherland may have devised the still point induction around the occiput because he regarded the fourth ventricle as a powerful source of potency and vitality, a cistern of cerebrospinal fluid surrounded by crucial neurological structures – such as the respiratory centre and cardiac centre in the medulla.

Some sources suggest various differences in effect between CV4s and EV4s, with still points into the contraction phase building energy at the core, and still points into the expansion phase distributing energy through the system. However, a still point into contraction enables the system to then open out into a more expansive expansion phase, and vice versa, so the effects may be the same either way. In any case, it is preferable to allow the body to decide for itself.

Purposes of still point induction

Still point induction can be used for various purposes at different times during treatment:

- at the start of a treatment, in order to clear superficial patterns so that the subsequent treatment can then focus on deeper issues
- at any point during a treatment when you encounter a particularly persistent resistance which might benefit from the enhanced stimulus of a still point induction
- when the system becomes restless or agitated and might benefit from the calming, settling influence of a still point induction
- when the system becomes quiet or stuck and the treatment process doesn't seem to be progressing, a still point induction may help the body to discover what it wants to do next, or to reveal what it needs
- at the end of a treatment, in order to bring the treatment process to resolution and to invite the body to resolve any remaining imbalances and adapt to any deeper changes that have resulted from the treatment process.

Still points may also be induced for specific clinical purposes:

- when a system feels weak, emaciated, lacking power, with low vitality, or a weak rhythmic motion – for example, in patients who are exhausted, chronically ill, or suffering from some persistent condition such as ME or post-viral syndrome
- in a floppy baby, or a child whose underlying vitality feels feeble
- to reduce blood pressure
- in a chronic inflammatory condition, such as rheumatoid arthritis
- in acute infections or inflammatory conditions
- to reduce a fever
- to boost the immune response.

Various texts may list many other conditions for which a still point may be helpful. Most of these benefits would probably arise from any appropriate cranio-sacral treatment or from cranio-sacral integration in general.

Overall, a still point will, like most cranio-sacral integration, help the system to reach a state in which the whole body softens and relaxes, the nervous system (particularly the autonomic nervous system) is more at ease, the tissues are more relaxed, and consequently the body fluids – arterial, venous, lymph, cerebrospinal fluid – will flow more freely and fluently, thereby enabling the body's various systems – vascular, immune, etc. – to function more effectively.

Summary

- Still points occur spontaneously throughout the treatment process and throughout life (particularly during quiet times such as sleep, meditation and times of rest).
- Still points may occur or can be induced at various times during a treatment for various purposes.
- One common use of a still point induction is for bringing a treatment process to a satisfactory conclusion and resolution.

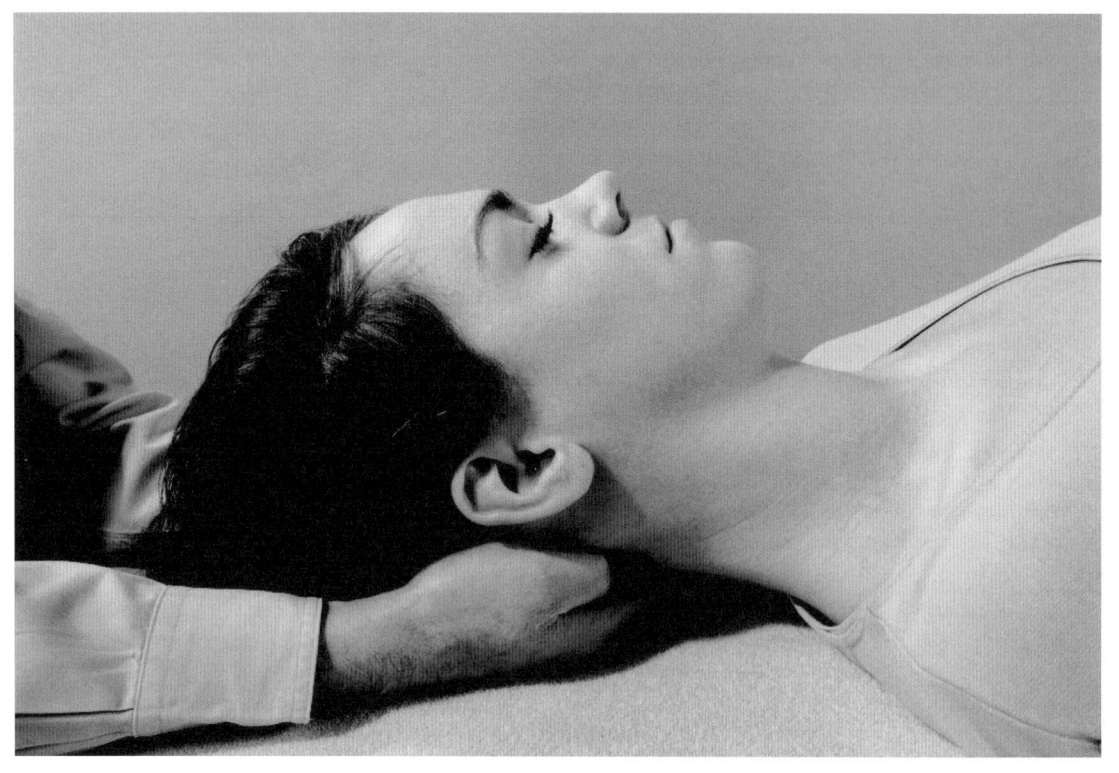

33.1 Contact for a still point induction through the occiput (CV4)

Completing a treatment process

As we have seen, many treatment processes will come to a natural resolution without any need for the specific application of a still point induction. The treatment may reach a conclusion of its own accord. Alternatively, the treatment process may settle into resolution simply by your calm, quiet presence, gently observing even, balanced rhythmic motion. If the system does not settle spontaneously, or if the treatment process feels in any way incomplete, a still point induction provides a very effective means of helping any treatment process to completion.

A still point is an invitation to the system to choose what it wants to do for itself, inviting the system to use the enhanced power of the still point to integrate itself. Still points are the body's natural means of readjusting and reorganising itself. The body in its infinite wisdom knows exactly what to do in order to bring itself into balance – so long as it has the enhanced potential enabled by the presence and awareness of the practitioner.

Still point induction at the occiput

In order to carry out a still point induction at the occiput (see Figures 33.1 and 33.2):

- Place the fingers of one hand under the fingers of the other hand under the occiput.

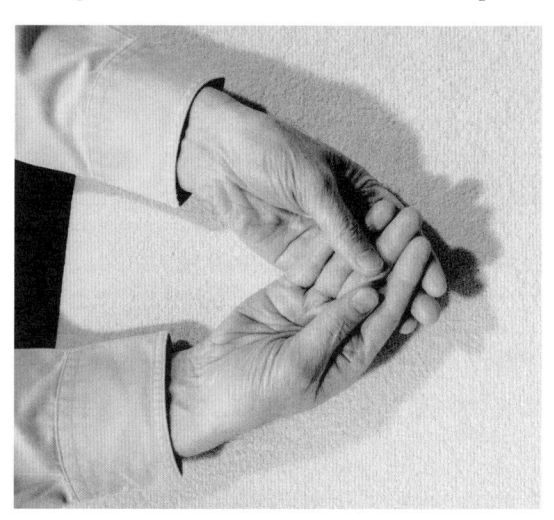

33.2 Hand position for a still point induction through the occiput

- Bring the tips of the thumbs together to form a V-shape into which the occiput can sit.
- Keep your *thenar eminences* (the soft pads at the base of your thumbs) opened out to provide a soft cushion for the occiput (rather than the bony hardness of the first metacarpo-phalangeal joints of your thumbs).
- Allow the system to settle.
- Tune into the emerging cranio-sacral motion, feeling the occiput narrowing during the contraction phase and flaring during the expansion phase.
- Once the motion is clear and settled, keep your attention clearly focused on the rhythmic motion.
- Allow the system to follow consistently into the contraction phases as the occiput narrows, while disregarding any tendency of the occiput to broaden.
- Keep your attention clearly focused on the rhythmic motion as the amplitude steadily diminishes (one advantage of carrying out a still point at the occiput is that the weight of the head sitting into the V-shape of your thumbs will naturally encourage the occiput into contraction, even if you are not aware of the rhythmic motion).
- Keep your attention focused on the contraction phase until the system becomes still.
- Keep maintaining this focus of attention on contraction even when the system appears to be still, in order to ensure that you address every last bit of contraction.
- When you reach a true still point, feel the all-pervasive sense of stillness pervading the patient, pervading you, pervading the whole room (it may take several minutes to reach this point).
- As you remain within that sense of stillness, observe any responses in the system – wriggling, pulsating, build-up of pressure or tension – but keep maintaining your focus of attention into the contraction phase, not being deceived into letting go prematurely.
- When you feel a convincing sense of softening and releasing, keep following the system, as it may go a little further into contraction at this point before releasing out into a long expansion phase.
- Follow the system as it settles and expands out into a long expansion phase, following it all the way, until it eventually settles into easeful fluent rhythmic motion.
- Observe the effects throughout the body.
- Observe the softer quality, the wider amplitude, the slower rate, and the more settled motion of the whole system following the release from the still point.
- Stay with the system through a few cycles of settled, balanced rhythmic motion.
- Allow the process to come to completion.

Chapter 34

Practice
An Integrated Treatment Framework

At this stage:
- We have established *fundamental principles*.
- We have formulated a *flexible framework*.
- We have described various possible *contacts* that might be taken up within a treatment.

We will now look at:
- how to approach practice of these *basic skills* in order to develop the sensitivity and experience to engage more fully
- how all this fits together as an *integrated treatment*.

(We will be looking more fully at how to approach an integrated treatment in Chapter 59 once we have covered some further aspects of the process.)

Practice is essential

Practice is essential for progress. Cranio-sacral integration is not simply a matter of reading a book and applying techniques. It is a matter of developing the sensitivity and the presence to engage deeply with the cranio-sacral system. This only comes through regular and consistent practice.

Practice partners

The ideal practice partners are those in a similar position to yourself, also learning cranio-sacral integration, with whom you can exchange constructive feedback. In the absence of such partners, you can practise on any relatively healthy and willing friends and family, but note the word healthy. It is not advisable to practise on anyone with a significant health issue until you are more experienced. Practise on healthy, stable practice partners.

Cranio-sacral integration is an exceptionally safe therapy, but as with any skill, you need experience before you can apply it in full. Take note of the provisos in Chapter 11, 'To Treat or not to Treat', and as a beginner, avoid practising on babies and children, pregnant women, or anyone who is in poor health or physically, mentally or emotionally unstable.

Those who are experienced in other therapies might be inclined to practise on their current patients. Again this should only be done with clear explanation, information and consent, and understanding of all the ethical and professional considerations.

What to practise
- Engagement.
- Individual processes.
- Complete integrated treatments.
- Other essential skills.

Engagement

Practising cranio-sacral integration is not about techniques, but about principles.

In order to progress, your emphasis needs to be on *engagement*. This needs to be the absolute priority. Nothing else is relevant without engagement, so your practice needs to be primarily orientated around developing the ability to engage effectively.

To this end, the focus of your attention initially needs to be on:
- establishing practitioner fulcrums
- developing your calm, quiet presence
- exploring levels of physical contact
- exploring levels of attention
- exploring different tissue levels
- refining your awareness of quality, symmetry and motion; identifying them, defining them, refining your definitions

- developing the ability to listen attentively to the cranio-sacral system without doing anything, without feeling the need to do anything, and without feeling the need to achieve anything or to make anything happen.

Individual processes

With this in mind, explore each contact at length – tuning in, heart centre, solar plexus, sacrum, subocciput, sphenoid, temporals, and so on – in order to gain familiarity with each contact and to experience how the system feels from different perspectives. Allow time for deeper engagement; you might want to spend 15, 20 or 30 minutes on each contact:

- engaging
- allowing the inherent treatment process to unfold
- allowing the evolution of fundamental principles or whatever variations may be appropriate.

Complete integrated treatments

Practise putting together a complete treatment by:

- exploring how a complete treatment fits together as an integrated unit
- seeing how you can build a complete picture of the whole person
- responding to individual circumstances within the framework of an integrated treatment.

It is clearly not possible or relevant to incorporate every contact into each treatment. That is never likely to be the intention. But it can be useful and therapeutically effective to construct appropriate combinations of contacts to form a cohesive well-integrated treatment.

Practice sessions can usefully combine several purposes:

- maintaining a cohesive overall treatment framework
- practising a variety of different contacts
- allowing sufficient time with each contact to engage deeply.

In order to maintain a cohesive overall framework, each complete treatment session needs to incorporate the four stages of tuning in, opening up, core treatment, and completion.

- Always take time to tune in and engage.
- Always open up the system as necessary, in order to establish appropriate settling and grounding.
- Always ensure appropriate completion.

Within this framework, you can *select different elements of the core treatment*. For example, in one practice session, after tuning in and opening up, the core element might include sacrum and spine and occiput and spine.

In the next session, it might include the sphenoid and temporal areas.

The following session might include the falx release, frontal and parietal contacts, or any other variations according to whatever may be appropriate to the circumstances before continuing to appropriate completion in each case.

At each stage of every treatment and *with every contact*

- re-establish your own fulcrums and allow time for the system to settle back into neutral
- respond according to individual circumstances
- allow yourself to become as fully absorbed into the matrix as possible
- take time to settle into deeper engagement with the deeper tides and with dynamic stillness where possible
- maintain a constant and consistent awareness of the whole picture at all times.

It is this that makes it cranio-sacral integration rather than a series of techniques.

Other essential skills

Within all of this you can also give attention to developing other essential skills:

- *Holding your attention in different places simultaneously* – spacious and local, the wider picture and the detail within the picture – aware of the space around you and of yourself and your patient within that space.
- *Projecting* your attention through the body.
- Identifying *fulcrums*.

- *Diagnosis* – both identification and interpretation of what you find.
- Building the *whole integrated picture*.

A firm grounding

It is helpful to maintain the four-stage framework. It has clear advantages. As a beginner, practise all these basic skills until you no longer need to think about them and the whole process becomes instinctive and intuitive. Beginners should also develop a firm grounding in the overall shape and structure of the integrated framework with all its benefits, so that you will be able to branch out from it with clear understanding and well-established grounding. Within the context of that framework, respond according to individual circumstances.

An integrated treatment framework

The following is a sample *integrated treatment framework* which you might practise, *selecting different elements of the core treatment section during different practice sessions* (for example, 3a and b, 3c, 3d and e). At this stage, a complete treatment session is likely to last approximately one hour (perhaps ten minutes tuning in, 20 minutes opening up, 20 minutes core treatment, ten minutes completion).

1. *Tuning in*
2. *Opening up the system* (settling and grounding)
   - Heart centre
   - Solar plexus centre
   - Pelvic centre.
3. *Core treatment*

a. *The sacrum*
   - Engage and allow the evolution of the inherent treatment process
   - Sacral release (as necessary)
     ○ Sacro-iliac release
     ○ Lumbo-sacral release
   - Projection through the spine from the sacrum
   - Settle into subtle integration.

b. *The occiput*
   - Suboccipital release
   - Engage and allow the evolution of the inherent treatment process
   - Projection through the spine from the occiput
   - Settle into subtle integration.

c. *Falx, frontal, parietals*
   - Engage and allow the evolution of the inherent treatment process with each or any of the following contacts, settling into subtle integration
   - Falx contact
   - Frontal contact
   - Parietal contact.

d. *The sphenoid*
   - Engage and allow the evolution of the inherent treatment process
   - Spheno-basilar release (as necessary)
     ○ Compression
     ○ Decompression
   - Settle into subtle integration.

e. *The temporals*
   - Engage and allow the evolution of the inherent treatment process with each or any of the following contacts, settling into subtle integration
   - Mastoid tip contact
   - Ear hold
   - Temporal balancing.

4. *Completion*
   - Allow the system to settle
   - Settle into deep dynamic stillness and subtle integration
   - Allow the treatment process to come to a natural conclusion
   - Still point induction (if necessary).

With each of the core contacts, engage and allow the evolution of the inherent treatment process as appropriate to the individual circumstances, shifting to deeper levels of engagement as the system allows, settling into deeper dynamic stillness and subtle integration as the system becomes increasingly settled, particularly towards the latter stages of the treatment session.

Always give priority to the needs of your patient's system, rather than to the structure or progress of your practice session.

Always ensure that the system feels settled and complete at the end of a treatment session.

In the rest of the book we will explore how this framework can be adapted substantially to respond to individual needs as you develop increasing experience, perception and understanding, and a wider range of resources.

Part IV
Further Concepts

Chapter 35

The Return of Rhythmic Motion

Entrainment

Rhythmic motion is expressed on various different levels. Each of us will be manifesting rhythmic motion in our own individual way – but this is not an objective absolute value. Like everything, as recognised in this quantum age, it is variable in response to circumstances. Attempts to measure and quantify a particular individual's cranio-sacral rhythm, or to conduct experiments to determine the objective value of cranio-sacral rhythm, are meaningless – because cranio-sacral motion is an interaction, an interaction between observer and observed, between patient and therapist.

When a therapist engages with a patient, the two cranio-sacral systems initially take a little time to adjust to each other – like two people meeting for the first time, going through the formalities of handshakes and small talk. Gradually the two systems get to know each other and start to relate on a more meaningful level; they explore each other's characteristics and find some common ground into which they can settle. Each will have its own expression of rhythmic motion prior to the encounter. The two rhythms (and much else besides) will gradually settle into harmonious interaction, finding a common rate at which they can resonate. Steadily, the calmer, quieter, more expansive expression of the therapist will draw the patient's rhythmic motion to a calmer, quieter expression. This process, as we have seen previously (see Chapter 15), is known as entrainment.

Levels of engagement

What determines the level of engagement and the resultant rate of rhythmic motion?

Various factors – in the therapist, in the patient, in the interaction between them, and in the progress of the treatment process.

The *therapist's inherent characteristics*, which one hopes would be peaceful and quiet, will encourage a tendency towards a calmer, slower rhythm, but this will also be affected by the therapist's level of awareness. If the therapist only ever works with the cranio-sacral rhythm and is unaccustomed to the middle tide or long tide, then he or she may only engage with the cranio-sacral rhythm. If the therapist habitually works with the middle tide motion and avoids the cranio-sacral rhythm, then they are more likely to engage with the middle tide.

But this will also depend on the *patient's inherent characteristics*. If the patient has not received much cranio-sacral therapy and is not naturally settled, their system may be more likely to manifest cranio-sacral rhythm initially and the middle tide motion may not be readily apparent. If the patient has received a significant amount of cranio-sacral therapy or is naturally settled and open, they may readily manifest middle tide motion (or even long tide motion).

This will also be influenced by the *interaction* between them. Just as the two people meeting for the first time may gel quickly or may take time to relate, so different cranio-sacral systems may resonate more readily than others. It is to be hoped that the therapist, having cleared their system and worked on their personal development, will have the ability to relate and respond to a wide range of patients.

A patient who is already well in tune with their middle tide may find a therapist working exclusively with cranio-sacral rhythm inappropriate, and a therapist who works exclusively with the middle tide and deeper tides may have difficulty engaging with a patient whose cranio-sacral rhythm is crying out for attention.

Cranio-sacral integration involves working with whatever arises in the patient and working with that through to deeper levels, not ignoring particular levels, not neglecting anything, without any specific agenda as to what particular rhythm or tide you are going to engage with or how you are going to approach each patient.

The level of engagement will also depend on the *progress of the treatment process*, generally moving deeper as a treatment session proceeds.

Assuming the ability to engage at all levels, it is common for a treatment session to follow a process of gradually deepening engagement, from initial activity, settling into the emergence of rhythmic motion, gradually settling into slower and slower rhythmic motion. This is not simply a matter of cranio-sacral rhythm, middle tide and long tide. There will be many variations and the different rhythms may seem to blend into each other. If cranio-sacral rhythm is being expressed, it may gradually settle to a slower, more expansive expression of cranio-sacral rhythm, particularly following points of stillness and release – but still in cranio-sacral rhythm. At some point, perhaps very soon, perhaps after a while, and particularly following a more significant point of stillness and release, the rhythm may emerge as middle tide motion rather than cranio-sacral rhythm. The distinction between the rate of a slow cranio-sacral rhythm and a faster middle tide motion may be negligible, but the change will generally be accompanied by a significant shift in the whole state of being – the quality of the engagement, the atmosphere, the whole environment.

The rhythmic motion may then again pass through several stages of gradually slower and slower rhythmic motion within the middle tide and may eventually undergo another significant shift into the long tide, with a corresponding shift in level of engagement and atmosphere. Points of stillness and release open the way to slower and deeper expression of rhythmic motion, and particular points of stillness and release may open the doorway to the deeper levels of middle tide and long tide.

As described previously, there will also be times when the rhythmic motion seems to be moving consistently and deeply into one phase of motion (expansion or contraction) for prolonged periods. This can sometimes be mistaken for a shift into a deeper tide, when it is in fact simply drawing towards a long, deep still point.

Working with whatever arises

Cranio-sacral integration involves responding to each patient according to their needs, working with whatever arises in accordance with the state of the patient at that moment. This allows a spontaneous, natural, response to whatever is being expressed. This has the advantage that, not only does it address what is happening at those initial levels, but also it tends to progress more readily and more naturally to deeper levels – so long as you are open to those levels and to that possibility. In this way the treatment process can progress in the patient's time, as appropriate for their system.

When a patient is in a state of shock or extreme trauma, the rhythmic motion may not necessarily be immediately apparent. It is, of course, always present, even if it is not being clearly expressed. In such cases you don't need to be concerned about not being able to connect with rhythmic motion, or concerned that the cranio-sacral process may not be able to proceed, or that you are unable to engage. You can simply engage with the level that is manifesting at that moment – the level of shock. You can allow the system to express its shock in whatever way it needs, and rhythmic motion will appear in due course.

The value of engagement with rhythmic motion

What value is there in feeling rhythmic motion?

- It is an indication that you are *engaged* with the cranio-sacral system. If you can feel rhythmic motion, you are engaged. In order to feel it, you need to be in an appropriate state, so engaging with the rhythmic motion is a way of ensuring that you are in that calm, quiet state that will be therapeutic to your patient, a state that will enable you to connect with the forces of nature, and genuinely engage with the deeper levels of the system – not just putting your hands on the body in an unengaged, superficial manner.

- It demonstrates the *level of engagement* – the level of engagement on which the body is ready to interact, and the level of engagement at which that interaction is taking place – according to whether you are engaged with cranio-sacral rhythm, middle tide or long tide.
- It enables you to *monitor the progress* of the cranio-sacral process:
  - from initial engagement (when you first start to feel rhythmic motion)
  - through points of stillness (when motion ceases)
  - identifying moments of release and reorganisation
  - through to the re-emergence of rhythmic motion as the system settles back into neutral.
- It enables you to *enhance the inherent cranio-sacral process* within the body, by feeling when the system is drawing into a particular phase of motion, drawing into extremes, and reaching still points.
- It enables you to further enhance the therapeutic process by *remaining engaged with the rhythmic motion as the system draws towards fulcrums*.
- It enables you to *assist the body in inducing still points* where appropriate.
- It enables you to recognise the state of *neutral* with the re-emergence of regular, even rhythmic motion.
- It enables you to rest contentedly in neutral, *knowing that you are engaged with the cranio-sacral system and allowing the process of subtle integration to continue.*
- It enables you to feel whether the system is *settled* or unsettled.
- It enables you to *enhance the vitality* by rocking the motion, allowing your attention to follow the system into expansion during the expansion phase and into contraction during the contraction phase, thereby increasing the amplitude of the motion and the vitality and health within the system. This is like swinging on a swing.

Imagine a little girl swinging on a swing. As she moves forward, she can stretch out her legs at the appropriate moment to encourage the forward movement. As the swing moves back, she can fold her legs underneath her to encourage the backward movement – always with the appropriate timing – thereby enhancing the amplitude of swing – as long as she gets the timing right.

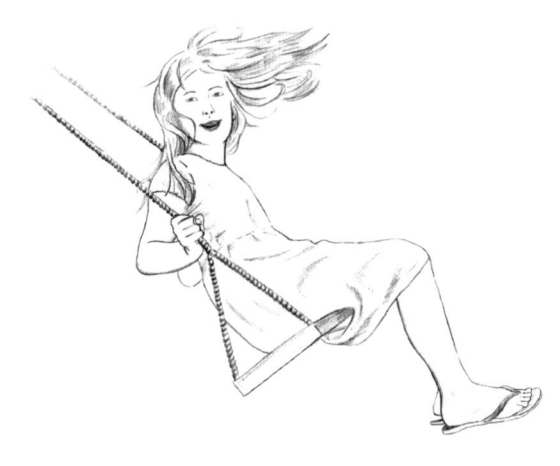

35.1 *By synchronising with the precise moment at which the rhythm changes, you can enhance the power and amplitude of the rhythmic motion*

- This enhancement of the motion can be further developed by *identifying the precise starting point* of the motion.

  Imagine again the girl on the swing. You can help her to expand the amplitude of her swing by giving a gentle push just as she starts the forward movement – the timing is vital, otherwise you will interrupt the flow. The appropriate level of push is also vital, so that you don't knock her off the swing.

  In the same way with the cranio-sacral motion, you can identify the precise moment at which the rhythm changes from contraction to expansion and by synchronising precisely with that moment, you can provide, with your attention, that extra enhancement of the power and amplitude of the rhythmic motion.

- Remaining engaged with the rhythmic motion also helps you to *ensure that you remain in an appropriate state* and with an appropriate level of contact to remain engaged with the cranio-sacral system. If you tighten up, physically or mentally, you may lose touch with the rhythmic motion, so this will send a message to relax and come back to your own practitioner fulcrums. If you start to impose on the system even slightly, or try too hard, or do too much, you may lose touch with the rhythmic motion – again telling you to ease off, to soften, to come back to your own state of ease.

- The rhythmic motion can be crucial in *diagnosis*. As you project your attention through the body or the spine, the rhythmic motion may change or cease, as your attention reaches certain areas. As you take your attention to different time fulcrums, different moments or ages in the patient's life, the rhythmic motion may change. As you follow the system into specific asymmetries, the rhythmic motion may gradually decrease in amplitude as you move closer to the source, eventually ceasing as you reach the exact point of focus. When you ask appropriate questions of the system, it may answer by changes in the rhythmic motion.

- The rhythmic motion is also diagnostic of the *underlying level of health and vitality* within the system – the potency, or fluid drive – powerful, weak, strong, feeble, vital, emaciated, which inevitably reflects the fundamental state of health of the patient and their potential for self-healing.

Engaging with deeper tides

Tuning in

To most people in everyday life, cranio-sacral motion is not apparent. It is subtle and it is not something of which they are aware or to which they are giving any attention. When a beginner first seeks to tune in to rhythmic motion, this may or may not happen easily. Some people feel the rhythmic motion very readily; others not at all. Some feel cranio-sacral rhythm, others tune in immediately to middle tide. Some start to feel more clearly very quickly. Others may not feel rhythmic motion at all for weeks, even months.

This depends on various factors, not particularly on knowledge or technique or previous experience in other therapies, but more to do with the inherent state of the individual – partly their inherent sensitivity, but most of all on their level of ease and relaxation and their ability to settle readily into stillness, softness and spaciousness, both physically and mentally – simply being there.

The 'Tuning In' chapters (Chapters 18 and 19) provide a useful guide for helping to engage with the rhythmic motion along with the other impressions that may arise. From these it can be seen that the principal factors are as follows:

- Relax.
- Breathe easily, letting go completely with every out-breath.
- Feel your whole body relax – taking your attention down through different parts of your body.
- Let go mentally, settling into a more detached, relaxed, meditative state of mind.
- Let go in key areas of your body – heart, solar plexus, head, neck, shoulders, arms, hands.
- Let go mentally into a deeper spaciousness:
  - as if your attention were expanding out into the room around you
  - as if you were looking down on yourself and your patient from above.
- Settle into stillness, softness, and spaciousness.
- Let your arms, hands, fingers and thumbs become so relaxed that they seem to melt into the matrix.
- Maintain a very light touch – barely touching the patient at all, just resting there.
- As well as a light touch, maintain a very soft touch, repeatedly inviting your hands to soften further.
- Try not to be looking for things, not searching intently, not trying too hard:
  - just let any impressions come to you of their own accord (like the kitten).
- Be open to the possibility of feeling rhythmic motion.

- Recognise that it won't necessarily be a very obvious tangible movement:
  - but rather a subtle impression
  - like waves of energy washing through your hands.
- Think of the head, not so much as a solid bony structure, but rather as a soft membranous balloon, or an amorphous fluidic structure with infinite potential to fluctuate gently.
- Engage with the sense of fluidity, rather than with solid structures or tissues.
- Imagine your hands immersed in warm water:
  - and feel that soft fluidity washing over and through your hands.
- Imagine your hands like fronds of seaweed under the ocean:
  - being washed this way and that by the waves, currents, eddies and tides.
- Explore different levels of physical contact.
- Explore different levels of attention.
- Explore different levels of tissues:
  - sensing beyond bones, membranes and fluids
  - recognising that at a quantum level this person is simply a mass of elementary particles, a mass of waves, a mass of energy, a mass of fluidity with infinite potential for change and movement.

As you become more deeply engaged, you are likely to feel rhythmic motion more clearly and feel different levels of rhythmic motion more clearly. You may be encountering cranio-sacral rhythm; you may be encountering middle tide; you may be encountering long tide already if you are in a deep state of relaxation, stillness, softness and spaciousness.

If you are feeling cranio-sacral rhythm, but not experiencing middle tide, there are various ways in which you can enhance your chances of feeling the deeper tides:

- Settle into a deeper, wider, more expansive mental spaciousness.
- Settle into a more meditative space – letting yourself float (but remaining grounded).
- Be open to the possibility of feeling this slower rhythm.
- Maintain a sense of the approximate timing of the middle tide motion (not counting the seconds – that's too cerebral – but having a sense of what it might feel like).
- Be open to the possibility of more subtle waves of motion wafting through your hands.
- You might like to imagine your hands like surfers floating on the surface of the ocean waiting for the next wave to carry them along; let your hands wait for that subtle wave of motion to arrive and softly carry your hands out into expansion, eventually fading away, leaving your hands to settle into contraction.
- However spacious your attention may be, allow it to become more spacious.
- Although your eyes may be closed, imagine that you are looking into the distance.
- Imagine that you are sinking down below the surface into the depths of a deep, deep ocean:
  - to a world where everything is in slow motion
  - to a world of stillness, calmness, silence.
- Allow yourself to sink deeply into this state where the material world may seem to fade into the background, and where time no longer seems relevant.

In this profound state, you are more likely to experience the long tide, and perhaps sink into a world beyond rhythmic motion, a world of pure dynamic stillness – and the deepest healing of all.

Describing this process is relatively lengthy. When first developing cranio-sacral skills, time will be needed to settle yourself into stillness, softness and spaciousness. This can be helped substantially by what you are doing in the rest of your life, clearing your own tensions and traumas through cranio-sacral treatment and personal development, and particularly through meditation.

In time you will increasingly be able to settle more readily into an appropriate state of sensitivity. In due course you will be in a constant and continuous state of sensitivity (but firmly grounded to cope with the insensitivities of the world around you) and able to engage with any system at any time. The more time you spend in the long tide yourself, the more readily you will engage with long tide; the more time you spend in middle tide yourself, the more readily you will engage with middle tide. But you want to be careful that your own state doesn't blind you to other levels, becoming impervious to other levels and only able to relate from a limited perspective. The more you develop your own inner state, your calm, quiet presence, the more readily you will engage with every system, and the greater benefit you will bring to the interactive process of cranio-sacral integration.

Working with the different rhythms

The principles of working with the cranio-sacral process remain essentially the same at whatever level you are working. You will still be engaging with the system, allowing the system to express itself, simply being there. There will, however, be differences in the quality and nature of the process at different levels.

At the cranio-sacral rhythm level you are more likely to feel extraneous movements in various directions; the whole process will tend to occur more quickly; the still points and releases are likely to be more readily apparent, and the changes that ensue from these releases may also be more readily apparent. Although every change affects the whole person, some still points in the cranio-sacral level may feel more local.

At the middle tide level, everything will tend to happen more slowly. The rhythm is slower, there are less extraneous movements, the focus is more on the rhythmic motion itself. Any asymmetries will appear more slowly, everything will seem to be more subtle. Your awareness and level of engagement therefore also need to be more subtle. The build-up to still points will happen more gradually, the system may stay at the still point for longer, the sense of asymmetry may be less obvious but more persistent. The releases may seem to influence the whole body more evidently. The changes may feel more profound and yet at the same time seem more subtle. Still points will seem more all-pervasive, more expansive, more spacious, as if the whole room is becoming still and you and the patient and the whole room are all more deeply absorbed in the still point.

In the long tide, there is a different quality altogether, a sense of being deeply immersed in a world of slow motion, a sense of being simultaneously distant, not quite present on a material level, as if floating in space – and yet at the same time feeling more present, more deeply absorbed and engaged on an energetic level – less present to the material world around you, and yet more present to the sense of profound absorption into engagement with your patient. Extraneous movements are hardly apparent, not much seems to be happening. There may be a sense of the tide rising, rising, rising at great length, and yet the timing of the motion doesn't seem significant. Specific imbalances and asymmetries cease to be relevant. The whole process of allowing the evolution of fundamental principles ceases to be relevant. The healing process is taking place on a different level – enabled by your profound spacious presence and deep engagement rather than by any specific process. You will tend to engage with the long tide when you yourself are in a profoundly spacious state, and your patient is in a deep state of relaxation.

Moving beyond the long tide you can reach a level where rhythmic motion ceases to be relevant – *the level of deep dynamic stillness*. Here, the material world seems to fade into oblivion, time ceases to exist, there is a feeling of deep absorption into a deep sense of spaciousness and connection with the whole universe. Just being there in that profound space is all that matters. There is a profound sense of stillness, yet there is a dynamism to the stillness, something is happening on a subtle level and yet it doesn't need identifying or defining. It just is. It is at this level that the deepest healing occurs.

Chapter 36

Biodynamics, Biomechanics and the Quantum Model

Cranio-sacral therapy involves a light contact, engaging with subtle movements, rhythms and forces within the body, thereby enabling the release of resistances and their associated symptoms and conditions, in order to enhance health.

In a biodynamic approach, we see these forces as coming from external sources permeating the body and establishing a blueprint of perfect health towards which the body will always tend, and the therapist's role is simply to engage with these forces, thereby enhancing their inherent potential to bring about health.

In a biomechanical approach, we see these forces as arising from within the body, and the therapist's role is to release restrictions so that the body's inherent healing potential can be expressed freely in order to bring about health.

Cranio-sacral integration acknowledges both perspectives, seeing them as part of a spectrum, a continuum within which all parts of the spectrum have their significance and can be integrated together.

Spectrum

This spectrum reflects developments in Sutherland's life, the biomechanical concepts reflecting his earlier life and the biodynamic concepts reflecting the latter part of his life. In his earlier days, Sutherland explored the movement of bones, membranes and fluids. In his later days, he was more concerned with the outside forces underlying these movements, which he described as the Breath of Life and also as the external forces of primary respiration.

The differences lie primarily in the perception of the concepts underlying the healing process, although this does of course influence the application of the therapy to some extent.

Neither approach is superior or inferior, deeper or shallower – they are just different interpretations and different parts of a spectrum.

The word

The word 'biodynamic' is not a word that you will find in most dictionaries. The term appears to have first been used in the 1920s by Rudolf Steiner, founder of the Steiner schools and the Anthroposophical movement. He used it primarily in relation to growing fruit and vegetables in a biodynamic manner, similar to what is often described as organic, utilising the inherent forces of nature while minimising the imposition of any artificial additions such as fertilisers and insecticides – a concept which has become increasingly established within the fields of modern-day biodynamic agriculture, gardening and wine production.

The term was again used in the 1960s by the Norwegian psychologist and physiotherapist Gerda Boyesen in her biodynamic psychotherapy, a therapeutic approach which acknowledges not only body and mind but also subtle levels of energetic flow, and particularly the effects of unexpressed emotions and stress held in our digestive organs.

It was also used by the German embryologist Eric Blechschmidt (see Blechschmidt and Gasser 1978) to describe his perception that early embryological development arises through the influence of external forces rather than from genetic influences.

Within the cranial field, the word 'biodynamic' has primarily been developed by James Jealous, an American osteopath, who during the 1980s established a specific Biodynamic Model of Osteopathy in the Cranial Field (BOCF). This model has been adopted by various cranio-sacral therapists under a variety of titles including the word biodynamic.

If we break down the word itself, bio = life, dynamic = forces, biodynamic means life forces. The term biodynamic therefore suggests working with natural life forces. By this definition all cranio-sacral therapy is biodynamic, since all cranio-sacral therapy involves engaging with life forces. If you are not engaging with life forces, it is not cranio-sacral therapy. The difference lies mainly in whether one sees those forces as arising from outside or from within the body, and the extent to which the therapeutic process is guided by those natural forces or by input from the therapist.

All cranio-sacral therapy involves some input from the therapist, since the very presence of the therapist is a potent input, along with any words, thoughts, or engagement on any level that may arise. But there are differing degrees to which input may be introduced. So essentially – all cranio-sacral therapy is biodynamic, but some is more biodynamic than others.

The biodynamic model

It may be useful to distinguish between 'a biodynamic approach' and 'the biodynamic model':

- Biodynamics (working with natural forces) is an inherent part of all cranio-sacral therapy.
- The 'biodynamic model' refers to a particular way of working.

When a cranio-sacral therapist describes themselves as a 'biodynamic cranio-sacral therapist' it generally means that they are working to a 'biodynamic model'. This does not indicate that other cranio-sacral therapists are not working in a biodynamic manner. There are many therapists working in a very biodynamic manner but not describing themselves as biodynamic cranio-sacral therapists, who simply see biodynamics as an inherent part of cranio-sacral therapy. There are perhaps others working to a biodynamic model but not necessarily working in a very biodynamic way. There are also cranio-sacral therapists working in a more biomechanical manner (although not generally describing themselves specifically as biomechanical – simply as cranio-sacral therapists). There are also many cranio-sacral therapists combining biodynamic, biomechanical and other approaches and not feeling any need for a specific title. Most therapists are not concerned with labels and are more concerned with practising effective therapy.

Levels of input

Biomechanical cranio-sacral therapy tends to be described in terms of carrying out techniques, in terms of specific practitioner input, in terms of some degree of physical action – albeit usually minimal – and with a concept of releasing bones, membranes and other tissues.

The biodynamic model tends to be described in terms of the practitioner engaging with the outside forces as the healing force, with minimal practitioner input.

In the biomechanical approach, the level of practitioner input can vary widely, some therapists using significant physical input and following into patterns on a more physical level, others working with subtle intention and minimal input.

In the biodynamic model, the level of practitioner input is minimised – at least on a physical level. There is, of course, always a significant input from the practitioner, through their presence, attention, focus and any augmentation which they may introduce – all of which constitute a potent input. The biodynamic practitioner will not generally follow physically into patterns expressed within the tissues, but through their focused awareness of the system they will be following with their attention – so the level of input is more a matter of degree.

Levels of force

The word biomechanical inevitably suggests something rather more forceful, but the level of force used is usually minimal. The term may also be seen as implying that a biomechanical approach is not utilising inherent (biodynamic) life forces, but in view of the lightness of touch, it is obvious that the results it achieves could not possibly be achieved by mechanical means and must therefore be engaging with inherent forces. As mentioned above, levels of touch and forces used in a biomechanical approach do vary substantially.

Levels of rhythm

The biomechanical model usually revolves around working only with cranio-sacral rhythm – and yet undoubtedly reaches very profound levels of treatment. Engaging with the cranio-sacral rhythm level is constructive, productive and therapeutic.

The biodynamic model tends to focus more on middle tide and long tide levels, with less therapeutic significance attributed to the cranio-sacral rhythm level.

In so far as these different conceptual models exist, they could be summarised as shown in Box 36.1.

Integrating the whole spectrum

Cranio-sacral integration appreciates the whole spectrum of resources and the value of utilising a wide range of resources, in order to engage with different levels of being. This can be helpful in extending the range of effectiveness and enabling a more appropriate response to individual circumstances.

The two approaches – biodynamic or biomechanical – are not mutually exclusive. It is not necessary to choose between practising one or the other. Many cranio-sacral therapists do confine themselves to one or the other, but both approaches are very effective and can be integrated together. There will be times when one approach is more effective or relevant, times when the other is more appropriate. A firm grounding in biomechanical aspects of cranio-sacral therapy is very valuable and relevant to working more effectively with biodynamic forces and vice versa.

Appreciating the value of one level of therapy does not necessitate rejecting other approaches, just as acknowledging quantum science does not necessitate abandoning Newtonian laws. Medication, surgery, psychotherapy, nutrition and many other forms of treatment and bodywork all have their value within the therapeutic field; similarly, the various different aspects of cranio-sacral therapy all have their value and can blend into each other as part of one continuous spectrum of cranio-sacral integration, and treatment can then evolve according to whichever point in the spectrum is most suitable for the patient at that moment.

Box 36.1 Principal features of biomechanical and biodynamic models

Biomechanical model
- Rhythmic motion generated from within (inherent motility of the CNS; rhythmic production of CSF at choroid plexi).
- Healing comes from within.
- Techniques are applied by the practitioner.
- Works primarily with tissues.
- Generally works with cranio-sacral rhythm.
- Applies rationalised techniques and concepts.
- 'Fixes' imbalances and restrictions.
- Tends to treat individual lesion patterns as a means towards integration of the whole.
- Newtonian concepts.
- Based on Sutherland's early years.
- Conventional terminology.

Biodynamic model
- Rhythmic motion generated from external forces (Breath of Life, primary respiration).
- Healing comes from outside.
- The practitioner engages with external forces.
- Works primarily with primary respiration.
- Works primarily with the middle tide and long tide.
- Works with intuition and consciousness – natural forces (Breath of Life, primary respiration).
- Allows the system to resolve imbalances.
- Concerned with integration of the whole – as a means of resolving local individual issues.
- Quantum concepts.
- Based on Sutherland's later years.
- Uses its own individual and sometimes elusive terminology.

Summary

Cranio-sacral integration integrates the whole spectrum of cranio-sacral approaches:

- engaging with the forces of nature to enhance healing and integration within the individual
- acknowledging that different levels of input on the part of the therapist can be appropriate to different circumstances
- recognising that it can be helpful to address all different levels of being
- integrates biodynamics and biomechanics as one inseparable cohesive continuum.

Biodynamics and biomechanics involve different conceptual models and methods. Essentially they are all cranio-sacral therapy and are all profoundly effective when carried out by competent practitioners. The most significant factor is not what label is attached, but the qualities and presence of the individual therapist.

Cranio-sacral therapy and cranial osteopathy

A question that is often asked is 'What is the difference between cranio-sacral therapy and cranial osteopathy?'

They are essentially the same thing, both deriving from Sutherland's original cranial concept. There is considerable overlap between them, and considerable variation within each of them. There are cranial osteopaths working in a biodynamic manner, cranial osteopaths working in a more mechanical manner and cranial osteopaths working with the whole integrated spectrum. Similarly there are cranio-sacral therapists working in a biodynamic manner, in a more mechanical manner and working with the whole spectrum. There are cranial osteopaths with a broad perspective and others with a narrower perspective and there are cranio-sacral therapists with broader and narrower perspectives.

In view of these wide variations and considerable overlap, it may not always be easy to distinguish one from the other. In so far as there is a difference, it is perhaps that cranio-sacral therapists tend to acknowledge and attend to emotional factors more readily and tend to acknowledge energy more overtly. The only definitive distinction is in nomenclature – in that cranial osteopaths must specifically have an osteopathic qualification in order to use the term osteopath, whereas cranio-sacral therapists may come from a wide variety of backgrounds, including doctors, physiotherapists, osteopaths, chiropractors, acupuncturists, homeopaths, massage therapists and many other therapeutic or non-therapeutic backgrounds.

Models

Concepts and ideas, therapeutic or otherwise, tend to involve conceiving a model of some kind. This is understandable as an attempt to explain the concept. But what is a model? The word model indicates that it is 'only a model' not the real thing. In other words the model is just a hypothesis, a theoretical concept, an analogy – often limited by trying to express abstract ideas within the confines of conventional terminology.

The mechanical or biomechanical model is just an analogy. The very idea of calling it biomechanical is unrealistic. In view of the minimal forces involved, and the nature of the tissues, it is clearly not actually a mechanical process. Any influences that are being introduced through the membranes and bones are clearly happening on an energetic level or being transmitted by some other means – but they are not mechanical.

But the mechanical model still provides a useful analogy for understanding the process – because that is the way it feels. We are working with bones and membranes and other tissues – they are after all an integral part of the matrix – but we are influencing them through quantum means, not by mechanical means. (One could perhaps call it quantum mechanics.)

In the same way, the fluid or biodynamic model is also just an analogy. The 'fluid body' is not actually fluid and we are not working specifically with fluids but with energy, with quantum forces. But again the fluid model is useful, because the process feels fluidic and the concept expands our awareness beyond more solid anatomical structures.

What matters is the focus of attention. The models simply provide different frameworks through which to focus the practitioner's attention and consciousness.

Confusion can arise when people become attached to their models. They can tend to believe that the model is real, or that that is the way things actually work. Alternatively, sceptics may dismiss the whole concept because the model isn't entirely credible in reality.

Models have their limitations, but they are also useful. Within cranio-sacral integration, perhaps the most appropriate model is a quantum model.

The quantum model

In the quantum model, we have an individual *matrix* – a coherent mass of *elementary particles and waves* – permeated by the *forces of nature*, generating rhythmic motion and the force fields which determine growth, development and healing.

Chapter 37

Keep Breathing

Have you noticed how your breathing changes in response to – just about everything? Not only in response to the obvious factors like physical exertion, but also in response to thoughts, feelings, emotions, and events going on around you.

It changes when you gasp in surprise, hold your breath in anticipation, breathe more shallowly when anxious or nervous, breathe more deeply and freely when you are relaxed or at ease.

Response to trauma

All these little day-to-day influences affect our breathing. How much greater will the effect be when the causative factor is severe, or prolonged, or persistent? When you are under constant pressure or stress, your breathing may become consistently shallow or quick – creating a habit pattern that is hard to break. A severe trauma may leave the system holding its breath for ever more – held in shock. Breathing patterns may be established by the rigours of a traumatic birth and may stay with that individual for life.

This is not just an incidental point of interest. Breathing not only *reflects* everything that goes on, but also *affects* everything. Shallow breathing means less oxygen intake – less oxygen for the lungs, for the brain, for all the tissues. Shallow breathing also reflects and maintains holding, not only in the lungs, the respiratory muscles and the diaphragm, but throughout the body, resulting in tension, discomfort, restriction of fluid flow, blood flow and nerve supply, and less efficient function.

The diaphragm is one of the 'transverse structures'. When the diaphragm is tight or held, then the other transverse structures tend to tighten up – the pelvic diaphragm, the thoracic inlet, the tentorium cerebelli; and when the tentorium is tight, the whole reciprocal tension membrane system tightens, and so on. As always, when one thing happens, it leads to a whole cascading chain of events throughout the body-mind, particularly when that one thing is something as fundamental as breathing.

Breathing responds to everything and is therefore an accurate guide to the state of the person. Equally, working with the breathing, or consciousness of the breathing can be a profound influence on the state of the person. So we can use breathing in a great many valuable ways as part of the therapeutic process, not just for the patient but also for the therapist.

Diagnosis

Observe the patient's breathing when they first come in, as you talk to them. It can tell you a great deal about their present state, whether due to past trauma, current tension, or apprehension at coming to see you for the first time.

Observe the patient's breathing as they lie on the couch and you tune in. Observe the breathing before you mention anything about breathing, otherwise their breathing will change before you've had a chance to evaluate it. Invite the patient to take a deep breath and let go. Many patients coming for their first appointment with a new therapist will feel slightly apprehensive. Inviting them to take a deep breath (and letting go of it – don't leave them in a suspended state of in-breath) – can help them to relax and let go. Observe how they respond to that suggestion:

- Some patients are unable to take a deep breath.
- Some patients will take one deep breath and then immediately settle back to their usual shallow breathing.

What does this tell you about them?

Depth of relaxation enables depth of therapeutic process

The depth of relaxation in a patient plays a substantial part in the therapeutic process. The more relaxed they are, the more responsive their cranio-sacral system will be; the more they can settle into a deep state of relaxation, the more profound will be the treatment. Helping the patient to let go is therefore crucial, and breathing is one of the most effective ways to enable this.

Different patients will have different needs. Some patients will be breathing easily and freely. Many people breathe relatively shallowly, holding their breath to some extent, never really letting go completely, so most people will benefit from attention to their breathing. Even if they are already breathing freely, attention to their breath can help then to enter into deeper relaxation.

As the treatment session proceeds, continue to observe your patient's breathing and respond according to their needs. Some patients will need an occasional reminder to let go of their breathing. Others will benefit from a continuous process of being guided throughout the session, encouraging a gentle letting go of the breath with each out-breath, establishing new patterns of breathing to replace the usual shallow held breath.

Recognise that there are different approaches to breathing, serving different purposes, and attaining different results. Professional singers have often undergone extensive training and gained great mastery and control of their breathing, with excellent consequences for their singing. This does not necessarily mean that they are good at letting go. Yoga practitioners and teachers have also often given a great deal of attention to their breathing, with substantial benefits. But what we are concerned with here is not control of the breathing, but letting go.

Letting go

Letting go is the essence of this approach to breathing. It is not particularly about breathing deeply. Some patients will respond to any suggestions regarding their breathing by entering into very deliberate deep breathing, which can create more tension than relaxation. The in-breath is associated with holding and control, the out-breath is associated with letting go. Focus on letting go, inviting your patient to let go with each out-breath, again and again. Many patients find this difficult. Letting go may be too unfamiliar to them. They will need to be helped and reminded and encouraged again and again – but if their breathing pattern is deeply ingrained it may not be easy for them to change the habit of a lifetime. It takes time. That's nothing to be concerned about. Don't get tense about not being able to relax! It's perfectly understandable, very common – and just a matter of time and practice.

Attention to breathing should not become an effort or a chore. That would defeat the object of it all. It is simply a matter of letting go, allowing the breath to take its natural course, not trying too hard – but keeping a gentle watchful eye on each out-breath, letting go of the whole body with each out-breath, countering the common deeply ingrained tendency to hold on.

Assisting release

Breathing may change in response to changes in the cranio-sacral system. The breathing may stop or reduce as you reach a still point and then release with a sigh or a deep out-breath as the system releases out of the still point. The patient may think that they have spontaneously chosen to take a deep breath, but the stimulus to breathe is probably instigated by the release within the cranio-sacral system.

Sometimes, when the system is holding into a prolonged still point at a deeper resistance, it may be helpful to ask the patient to take a deeper breath, and as they do so, this may enable a profound release within the cranio-sacral system – but the timing needs to be right, sensing the right moment, waiting for the system to be ready to release, not just using the breath willy-nilly to try and obtain releases.

Sometimes you may feel the patient's system tightening up as the treatment proceeds, for no apparent reason. This can be an integral part of the therapeutic process and you may simply want to let it takes its course. At other times it may be blocking the therapeutic process to some extent. You can invite them to take a deep breath and let go. You can remind them again and again, as a means of maintaining a relaxed open responsive state – as opposed to tightening up, perhaps holding down uncomfortable feelings and suppressing the therapeutic responses, in an unconscious resistance to releases.

At times, reminding the patient to breathe can be a valuable way of helping them to keep in touch with their grounding, of helping them to allow the therapeutic process to evolve rather than tightening up and blocking it – but conversely, there are times when reminding them to breathe can interrupt the process, taking them away from deeper engagement with their process and their feelings. So take care to observe carefully and discriminate when it is appropriate to bring them back to their breathing and when it is helpful to let them stay deeply involved with their feelings and sensations – even when it is disrupting their breathing pattern.

Responding to sensations arising

Sometimes, during the cranio-sacral process, uncomfortable memories, thoughts, feelings, emotions or physical sensations can arise, as past traumas deep within the system come to the surface to be released. At these times, the patient may start to hold their breath or wriggle or become slightly agitated or cry. You can invite them to take a deeper breath and let go, to observe the sensations with equanimity, to let them arise and dissolve away, understanding that they are just past tensions from deep within rising to the surface to evaporate away, welcoming their release and continuing to breathe easily. This helps the therapeutic process in many ways:

1. It enables the process of release to follow through to completion, rather than interrupting it or pushing things back under the surface.
2. It indicates to the patient that you are aware of their responses.
3. It provides the patient with reassurance that what they are experiencing is perfectly OK, safe and nothing to be concerned about.
4. It provides them with a way of dealing positively with any uncomfortable sensations.
5. It provides the patient with a means of dealing with such sensations outside of the treatment setting, whenever they arise in life, helping to change old habit patterns of reaction.

A matter of habit

Habit patterns are difficult to change, whether it be smoking, or patterns of behaviour, or ways of relating to people and to the world around you. Such patterns are often deeply ingrained. They are particularly deeply ingrained when they have been imprinted at an early age, for example by childhood trauma, setting lifelong patterns of behaviour which come to be experienced as the norm – perhaps manifesting as asthma, anxiety, or a withdrawn personality, accompanied by constant holding of the breath or shallow breathing.

Breathing can be one of the most helpful tools in helping to change obstructive habit patterns, whether imprinted by traumatic incidents, upbringing, childhood abuse, or whatever cause which has led to unsatisfactory patterns of behaviour – fear, shyness, lack of confidence, anger, aggression, irritability, feelings of inadequacy, difficulties in dealing with everyday relationships and situations – all potentially leading to feelings of dissatisfaction with life or oneself.

The pattern of breathing will clearly reflect the trauma; it is also something which can be used to change the pattern. It is something which is always with us, day and night, 24 hours a day and therefore something we can use 24 hours a day to create and establish new habit patterns. Of course the trauma will need to be addressed by other means also, through trauma release in various forms; but release of the trauma is not enough if deeply ingrained habit patterns persist, leading the patient to continue repeating their traumatic response out of habit, thereby perpetuating, maintaining and reinstating the physical and psycho-emotional features of the trauma.

Patients can be introduced to new breathing patterns during treatment sessions and encouraged to practise and maintain these patterns 24 hours a day – as they walk down the street, as they sit at a meal, at work or at play, as they drift off to sleep at night (enabling a deeper, less troubled sleep), when they wake in the morning (establishing positive patterns for the day ahead) at times of tension and times of ease. The more they remind themselves to maintain that new habit, the quicker their system will respond. Countless patients have reported that this approach to breathing has transformed their lives.

Pain

Occasionally, pain may arise during a treatment session. It is not a common occurrence, but it does happen and there are different ways of responding to the pain. The first priority is to establish that there is no pathology, or current disease or fracture that needs to be taken into account. Having done so, we can establish that what we are dealing with is therapeutic pain – familiar pain that is rising to the surface in order to release.

The patient's usual response to pain is to tense up, whether as a protective mechanism or simply as a reaction. The first priority is therefore to encourage the patient to relax into the pain, and of course the most effective way to do this is by inviting them to breathe and let go, and to continue to breathe and let go with each out-breath while calmly observing their pain. This enables them to maintain a relaxed grounded response to their pain, allows the process to follow through to completion, and therefore enables the release of the source of the pain. It also prevents the creation of new patterns of tension in response to the pain. As they do so, the pain is likely to pass through its natural evolution, resolve and fade away, and in doing so it is reflecting the release of the deeper underlying pattern which is causing the pain.

An inexperienced therapist's response to a patient's pain might be to back away from it, to ease off, to stop whatever they are doing. This might be an obvious response, but it is not generally helpful. In doing so, you would be avoiding the issue, failing to address the source of the pain, potentially leaving something incomplete and unresolved, and preventing the natural therapeutic process from following its natural course through to completion. A more constructive response is to stay with the process, follow it through to completion until it reaches release, reorganisation and resolution. Of course you will need to clarify for the patient what is happening – which you are doing by inviting them to breathe and let go, as described above, showing them that you are aware of their pain and that it is being addressed, and helping them to develop positive constructive means of responding to pain and avoiding unhelpful responses of tension and reaction.

Where pain is gradually increasing, as might occur sometimes in an acutely painful condition such as when unwinding a frozen shoulder or an acute torticollis, then the most productive approach is to wait at the very edge of the pain, when it first appears and is very slight, encouraging the patient to breathe and let go. As they do so and the pain eases, the system can then draw further into its chosen direction, and if pain arises again, again wait at the edge of the pain waiting for it to ease in response to the patient's easy breathing. This process is not only enabling release, but also changing habit patterns of contraction within the tissues and habit patterns of reaction to pain within the patient, which has wider repercussions and is deeply effective. Many times, patients who have not responded to other approaches have benefited greatly from this approach, primarily due to the use of breathing to help them change the pain-maintaining patterns in their systems. We will see examples of this in Part V on fascial unwinding.

Therapists need to breathe too

Breathing is also vital to the therapist. Some therapists breathe easily and freely as a matter of course, but again many people (including therapists and prospective therapists) are holding their breath, or breathing shallowly to some extent – at least until they have addressed it, and again, even if your day-to-day breathing is relatively free, attention to your breathing can help to take you to a deeper state of ease and therefore a deeper state of engagement.

As a therapist, breathing is valuable first for establishing your own practitioner fulcrums; again it is something that is always with you wherever you are and again it both *reflects* everything that you are feeling, and *affects* everything about you. So paying attention to your breathing not only keeps you in touch with the state that you are in, but also helps you to establish a more relaxed, easeful state, a calm, quiet presence. Bring your attention back to your breathing again and again, time after time.

Keep observing your breathing. You may notice that it changes during treatment sessions. You may find that it changes as you observe your patient's system building to a still point. You may find yourself holding your breath from time to time – an unhelpful tendency that you can eliminate through regular and consistent mindfulness of your breathing. You may find that your breathing changes because the treatment process is bringing up something in your own system – which you need to observe with equanimity, need to process and allow to settle – through your breathing.

Occasionally, working as a therapist can bring up circumstances that are upsetting – severely traumatised patients, babies screaming in pain, tears, disturbing stories of tragedy and abuse. As a therapist you don't want to be impervious to such circumstances, you don't want to maintain a detached impersonal indifference like a scientist monitoring an experiment. You want to be sympathetic, empathetic, caring and understanding, but you also need to be grounded and able to cope. You won't be much use to your patient if you are in floods of tears, nor if you are tensing up throughout your system in an attempt to hold back your own emotions. Through awareness of your breathing (along with extensive personal development) you can maintain an open, relaxed softness which enables you to process your reactions while maintaining a balanced state.

Breathing is also helpful in establishing deeper states of consciousness. This is likely to happen spontaneously to some extent. As you settle into deeper breathing and relaxation, you will naturally tend to settle into a more relaxed, detached, meditative quality of mind and experience connection with more profound levels of consciousness. You can also use this more deliberately, specifically establishing a deeper sense of letting go of your breath and your whole body in order to access a deeper level of awareness, a deeper connection with your intuition, settling into a deeper spaciousness and wider perception, which in turn will help you to engage with the deeper levels of the long tide, dynamic stillness and deeper engagement with your patient's process.

Summary – an invaluable resource

Breathing can be used during treatment sessions from moment to moment to cope with situations that arise. It can be used 24 hours a day to establish a fundamental grounding. It can be helpful in enabling a more positive response to everything that happens to you in everyday life. The more you have established that fundamental grounding 24 hours a day, the more readily you will be able to apply this breathing to the moment-to-moment events during treatment and in life.

Keep breathing.

Part V
Fascial Unwinding

Chapter 38

Fascia

The significance of fascia was frequently emphasised by Andrew Taylor Still, the founder of osteopathy, who provided many well-known comments on the subject in his *Philosophy of Osteopathy* (1899):

- 'We see in the fascia the framework of life, the dwelling place in which life sojourns.'
- 'I know of no part of the body that equals the fascia.'
- 'In every view we take of the fascia, a wonder appears.'
- 'By its action we live and by its failure we die.'
- 'When you deal with the fascia, you deal with the branch offices of the brain, and why not treat it with the same degree of respect.'
- 'The soul of a man seems to dwell in the fascia of the body.'

Fascial unwinding is a very valuable aspect of cranio-sacral integration, expanding the therapeutic horizons to further levels, and extending the range of effective application of cranio-sacral therapy. It is an intrinsic part of the treatment process for many patients, often the most effective approach for specific circumstances, and sometimes the only approach that will effectively address certain conditions. Working with fascial unwinding can bring about therapeutic results that are not necessarily reached without fascial unwinding.

The causes of fascial restriction may stem from many different factors – from everyday sprains, strains, twists and bruises of joints, limbs, trunk or spine to operation scars and adhesions, major car accidents, minor falls, sports injuries, internal inflammation, emotional tension or severe trauma.

The results of fascial restriction are consequently just as wide ranging, depending on the part of the body affected – from headaches, neck pain and acute torticollis to frozen shoulder, writer's cramp and chronically weak sprained ankle, or internal dysfunction – particularly post-operative or post-inflammatory, affecting the digestive organs or causing menstrual or gynaecological disorders. Fascial restriction can also be a significant factor in perpetuating severe long-term debilitation and maintaining chronic patterns of ill health.

Fascial unwinding can also be very valuable in contacting emotional levels and releasing emotional tensions, particularly where the emotional trauma is associated with severe physical trauma.

Fascia

Fascia is a form of connective tissue. It is found throughout the body. It takes various forms, sometimes thicker, sometimes thinner, sometimes tougher, sometimes softer, but predominantly it is a thin membranous sheet which surrounds and envelops almost everything in the body – from the top of your head to the tips of your toes and everything in between. It has been compared to 'clingfilm' – the thin plastic material used to wrap food – and it can be seen when cutting (or eating) meat, as the membranous layers between sections of meat.

Whole body interconnection

Every bone, every muscle, every blood vessel, every nerve, every organ is enveloped in fascia – and yet the fascia is not separate pieces of membrane – it is one continuous unbroken sheet of fascia, extending throughout the body, forming interconnected pockets of fascia enveloping every structure. Fascia therefore provides not only an analogy for the complete interconnected nature of the body, but also an actual anatomical interconnection. The fascia of your ankle is directly connected to the fascia of your neck – so an injury from a sprained ankle many years ago could be transmitted up through the interconnected fascial web to the fascia of your neck, causing restriction of blood supply to the brain.

Fascia forms the periosteum around every bone, the pericardium around the heart, the pleura around the lungs, the fascial sheaths surrounding every digestive organ, the synovial sheaths around every tendon, and is thickened to form the various protective bursae and retinaculi throughout the body – and again these are all connected into, and therefore influencing and affecting, the organs and tissues within and around them – the pericardium of the heart attaching to the fascia of the diaphragm, so that the respiratory movements of the diaphragm are constantly massaging the heart with each breath that you take.

Fascia is also continuous with the membrane system. As mentioned previously, wherever nerves emerge from the central nervous system, the nerve root is initially enveloped in a sleeve of membrane (dura, arachnoid and pia) which is continuous with the epineurium (the fascial sheath enveloping the nerve along the rest of its pathway) which is in turn continuous with the rest of the body fascia. In fact the dura, arachnoid and pia can be regarded as fascia, a very similar tissue, with slight changes in protein structure to provide the different characteristics appropriate to the different tissues; and the whole membrane system enveloping the brain and spinal cord can be seen as 'the fascia of the central nervous system' with complete continuity between membrane and the whole body fascia.

Penetrating to the deepest levels

Not only is fascia *enveloping* every structure in the body, but also it *penetrates* deeply into the tissues. Every muscle is enveloped in fascia, and each bundle of muscle fibres within the muscle is wrapped in fascia. And more than this, each *individual* muscle cell has its own fascial sheath – every miniscule fascial sheath being connected into the surrounding fascia and thus to the whole body fascia (see Figure 38.1).

In the same way, every nerve is enveloped in a fascial sheath (epineurium); every bundle of nerve fibres is enveloped in fascia (perineurium); and every individual nerve cell, *microscopically thin*, has its own individual fascial sheath (endoneurium) (see Figure 38.2).

38.1 Not only is fascia enveloping every structure in the body, but it also penetrates deeply into the tissues

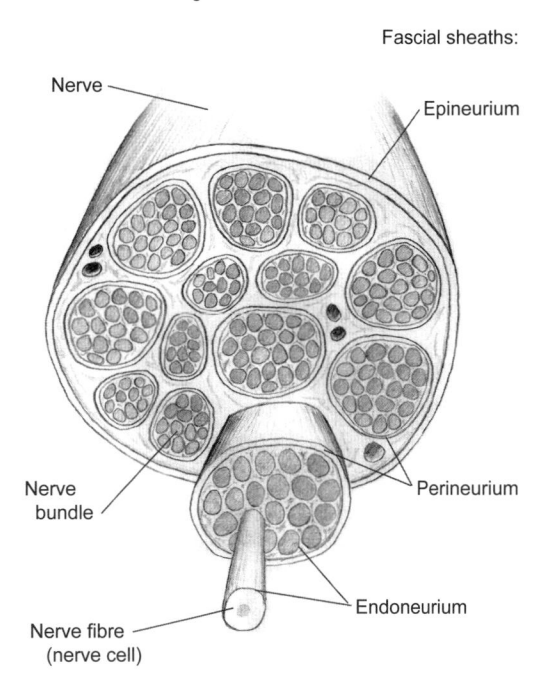

38.2 Every individual nerve cell, microscopically thin, has its own individual fascial sheath

So fascia is all-embracing, connecting the whole body together as one integrated unit, and at the same time penetrating deeply into the microscopic structure of the body tissues.

Functions of fascia

Anatomically, fascia can be classified into two divisions:

- *Superficial fascia* – which forms a thin layer of tissue beneath the skin, attaching the dermis to the underlying tissues.
- *Deep fascia* – with which we are primarily concerned here, forming the many interconnected pockets described above.

Conventionally, its functions are to allow free gliding movement between adjacent tissues (muscles over bones, muscle bundles in relation to each other, tendons over bones, etc.) and to provide a course for interstitial fluid flow.

From a cranio-sacral perspective it can also be seen to be:

- absorbing and maintaining tensions and traumas
- holding these restrictions into the local tissues with potential impairment of function
- transmitting patterns of tension and restriction through the body via the interconnected fascial network.

The degree to which these fascial restrictions will affect other parts of the body will depend on many factors, such as the severity of the restriction, the underlying tension in the fascia generally and the presence of other fascial restrictions or weaknesses imposed on the body by previous injuries or disease.

Rich innervation

Fascia is also very richly innervated, with a massive supply of nerve connections to the central nervous system, particularly through the autonomic nervous system and specifically the sympathetic nerve supply. This has significance in both directions – reflecting the fact that injury, pressure or strain in the fascia throughout the body will feed into the autonomic nervous system, stimulating sympathetic activity; and that sympathetic nerve activity (largely brought about by stress, pressure and trauma) will reflect out into the fascia, both locally and throughout the body, establishing levels of tension in the fascia, with consequent effects on all the tissues enveloped in fascia – blood vessels, nerves, muscles, organs.

This could mean that patterns of trauma – perhaps set up at birth, or by childhood injuries, or persistent stressful circumstances, or car accidents – could instil a deeply embedded, lifelong underlying level of persistent fascial tension that could then impede physiological function of blood vessels, nerves, muscles and organs – with a wide range of possible symptoms, conditions and pathologies potentially arising as a consequence:

- back pain, headaches, migraine, visceral disturbance, poor circulation
- poor coordination, a general level of tension, persistent stress and irritability.

In fact, the list is endless – involving disturbed and limited function of various kinds. This in turn indicates that working with the fascia can have profound effects on the sympathetic nervous system and on the physical and emotional state of the patient.

Principles of fascial unwinding

Same principles

The principles of fascial unwinding are the same as for any other cranio-sacral work – engage, allow, follow, to points of stillness, release and reorganisation. As with all cranio-sacral integration, the essence of fascial unwinding is to enable the release of the inertial fulcrum at the centre of any dysfunction.

There is one small but highly significant difference in fascial unwinding – in fascial unwinding, there is generally a visible degree of movement of the body tissues. We are not simply sensing subtle impressions of movement within the matrix, but actually allowing the movement to be expressed physically and visibly.

It is, of course, perfectly possible to work on the fascia without allowing this visible movement, just as we can work on the bones, membranes, fluids, energy, or any structures in the body without actual physical movement, simply by putting our attention on the fascia and allowing the unfolding of the inherent treatment process – but this would not be fascial unwinding. What distinguishes fascial unwinding is the actual physical movement; and the reason why this is significant is that it addresses a different level of being. Just as working with long tide, middle tide or cranio-sacral rhythm engages with different levels of being, so also fascial unwinding engages with and addresses a different level of being.

Addressing every level

If any one level is neglected – whether long tide, middle tide, cranio-sacral rhythm or fascial unwinding – this can have limitations on the effectiveness of treatment. Each patient is individual and the appropriate level of therapeutic engagement for each patient will vary from person to person. Ideally, every patient would have the benefit of complete integration on every level, but different levels carry different degrees of relevance for different patients, and they may therefore respond more effectively to those specific levels of treatment. For some, the middle tide level will be the most appropriate and effective; for others, engagement with the long tide is most beneficial. For others, the cranio-sacral rhythm level is the appropriate and effective level, and for others fascial unwinding is what they need. And if fascial unwinding is the appropriate level, and fascial unwinding is neglected or not applied, then the patient may not be helped.

Dandelions

If you have dandelions growing in your garden and you wish to eradicate them, it's no use simply mowing them down and cutting off the tops – they will readily grow again from the roots. However, it is equally not adequate to dig up the roots, if you neglect the seedheads, which will rapidly spread new seeds. In order to eradicate the dandelions completely, you need to address the roots, the seedheads and any cuttings from which they might regrow. Similarly in cranio-sacral integration you need to address all levels in order to remove the maintaining factors that may be reintroducing or perpetuating patterns of disturbance.

There are many patients who have received excellent treatment on profound levels, but whose fascia has been neglected and, as a result, their condition has not improved, their pain and discomfort persist (and they may well lose faith in cranio-sacral therapy as a result). Often, a few minutes of fascial unwinding can transform their situation, clear their discomfort, and restore them to health.

All the various levels interact and influence each other. Fascial unwinding has significant influences on cranio-sacral rhythm, middle tide and long tide levels, and each of the other levels can influence the fascial level. Sometimes, addressing one level may be enough to clear issues on other levels – particularly if that level is the source of the matter, and particularly if the injury is recent – but not always. It might be thought that if you treat at the deepest level, the root level, then everything else will be resolved as a result and fall into place accordingly. This is an attractive idea, but unfortunately not necessarily valid – as with dandelions.

There are of course plenty of circumstances where fascial unwinding is not the relevant level, and plenty of patients whose condition will improve without fascial unwinding, so a therapist may have successful results in many patients without the use of fascial unwinding (which might lead them to believe that fascial unwinding is unnecessary). There are also plenty of patients for whom middle tide or long tide levels are not the appropriate level at that particular time. Also, many patients with specifically fascial conditions may feel that their health and vitality have improved significantly as a result of treatment on other levels and even enabled them to cope better with their condition, even though their specific symptoms have not been addressed or resolved. But for those patients for whom fascial unwinding is the appropriate and necessary level, there is no adequate substitute for fascial unwinding, so it is a pity that fascial unwinding is not fully understood, appreciated and utilised by a wider range of cranio-sacral therapists.

When I first graduated as an osteopath many years ago, I happened to set up practice in an area where there were a great many of the most eminent cranial Osteopaths of the day – excellent practitioners. Many of their patients came to see me for treatment. I generally found that their cranio-sacral systems were beautifully fluent and clear; they had obviously received very high quality treatment – so why were they coming to see me? Because they were still suffering from the symptoms for which they had originally sought treatment. Many of them had received excellent treatment on a core level, but the fascial level had not been addressed, and this was maintaining their symptoms and discomfort. Those patients would generally respond very well – because other levels had already been addressed and their underlying vitality was strong. Consequently, simply addressing the fascial level through the specific process of fascial unwinding brought about rapid and successful results.

Many similar situations have continued to arise regularly ever since and continue to arise to this day, with patients who have received excellent cranio-sacral therapy on certain levels, but not received the benefit of fascial unwinding when it was the appropriate approach.

Working with fascial unwinding is an extremely effective branch of cranio-sacral integration and is an invaluable resource for any cranio-sacral therapist.

Movement

Fascial unwinding can be carried out on any part of the body: an arm, a leg, the abdomen, the trunk, a sprained ankle, a tennis elbow, a frozen shoulder, a twisted knee, an old operation scar, a spastic colon, an inflamed pleura or a tense pericardium. As with any cranio-sacral integration, we will be allowing the system to express itself, allowing it to unwind its way to points of stillness and release.

Within the trunk, the degree of movement may be relatively small. When unwinding arms, legs or the neck, the whole limb or neck may be allowed to unravel itself as it performs a slow, gentle dance through the air, tracing the patterns through which it has become twisted and rediscovering the positions in which it was traumatised. It is at these positions of traumatisation that the system is most likely to reach points of stillness and release.

The process is always gentle, just like any other cranio-sacral integration, always simply allowing the body to express itself, not imposing any movements or forces. Even in an acutely painful neck or frozen shoulder, the gentle process of fascial unwinding can be carried out virtually painlessly, to restore full mobility and pain-free movement to the area.

Causes of fascial restriction

Fascial restrictions can arise from a variety of causes, both physical and emotional, as described above.

Since the fascia envelops every nerve, blood vessel, muscle and organ in the body, fascial restriction is likely to cause constriction of blood vessels, impingement on nerves, contracture of muscles and constriction of organs, with consequent reduced blood supply, impeded nerve supply, tight musculature or visceral dysfunction.

Symptoms will of course vary according to the location of the restriction. Fascial restriction in the region of the shoulder girdle, perhaps as a result of a shoulder injury, a fractured clavicle or a local neck injury, could lead to constriction of the brachial plexus and the arterial supply to the arm, resulting in pins and needles, numbness, or weakness in the hands, fingers and arm.

Fascial restrictions in the cervical area as a result of a neck injury, a whiplash injury or chronic tension may affect the arterial supply to the brain through the carotid and vertebral arteries, venous drainage from the brain through the jugular vein and important nerve connections between head and trunk including the vagus nerve supplying most of the thoracic and abdominal viscera, or the sympathetic nerve supply up to the head and eyes. Symptoms could include vagueness, dizziness, poor concentration, loss of memory, weak and photosensitive eyes, headache, migraine, or a variety of visceral dysfunctions.

Restrictions in the lower back as a result of back strain, muscular strains or pelvic twists can similarly lead to sciatica and back pain.

Restrictions within the abdomen or pelvis, perhaps as a result of operations, adhesions or internal inflammation, could lead to disturbed nerve and blood supply to the viscera, with resultant digestive, menstrual or gynaecological disturbances, or pelvic pain.

Fascial restriction may be local – for instance in the wrist, as a result of repetitive strain injury (RSI), carpal tunnel syndrome or a sprained wrist; or may be generalised – as a result of a car accident or emotional tension. Any fascial restriction, however, may potentially have repercussions throughout the body as a result of the interconnected nature of the body fascia.

Fascial restrictions are likely to occur at various times of life in many parts of the body as a result of different injuries, accidents and diseases, leading to an accumulation of fascial restrictions and constrictions, all influencing and affecting each other, gradually weakening the body's resources and potentially causing a variety of apparently disparate symptoms – perhaps arising many years after the original injury.

Operation scars

When an operation, such as appendectomy, cholecystectomy or hysterectomy, is performed (particularly before the days of micro-surgery) the surgery inevitably involved cutting through many layers of fascia. The resultant scarring leads to fibrosis and sclerosis of the fascial tissue (just like scar tissue on the skin) with consequent bunching and reduced mobility of the fascia. This reduced mobility may cause local pain and discomfort but may also radiate out to restrict the free movement of other regions of the interconnected fascial network, with a resultant pull of all the body fascia towards the restricted area.

In this way, fascial restriction around an appendix scar could exert pulls up through the fascia to cause constriction of, for example, the carotid sheath in the neck. The carotid sheath is a tube of fascia passing up each side of the neck, containing the carotid artery, the jugular vein and the vagus nerve. Constriction of this narrow tube – which may arise due to pulls from any fascial restriction anywhere else in the body – potentially affects blood supply to the brain, venous drainage from the brain and produces various effects on the thoracic and abdominal viscera.

Everyday sprains and strains

Common sources of fascial restriction are the many sprains and strains that most of us encounter in everyday life. Many people find after spraining an ankle that, although the ankle may essentially have recovered fairly quickly and might be regarded conventionally as fully recovered, a certain degree of weakness or discomfort remains, with a continuing tendency to collapse. It may be regarded as a relatively minor impairment which just has to be lived with, but in many people it is sufficiently discomforting to prevent them from playing sport or even going for long walks – which can be a frustrating restriction to their life. The reason for the continuing discomfort often lies in the fact that the injury has been imprinted into the fascia, which is maintaining the tendency to twist back into the old pattern of distortion.

I have seen many patients with chronic sprained ankles of this nature, some having put up with it for ten years or more and given up hope of any improvement, not even bothering to mention the fact when they come for treatment for something completely different. In many cases, just a few minutes of fascial unwinding can relieve the condition completely, even when the injury is many years old.

The same principles apply to any joint and any twist or strain or sprain in any part of the body – twisted knees from jumping, dancing or sport, sprained wrists from a fall, a wrenched shoulder from contact sports such as rugby or from everyday incidents.

Many sports injuries leave fascial restrictions which impair performance and may even lead to giving up sport; and professional sports people have had their careers shortened or interrupted by conditions that might well have been relieved by fascial treatment.

The incidents which lead to fascial restrictions can often be relatively insignificant and certainly do not need to be major traumas or dramatic injuries. The incident is often completely forgotten, but the source of restriction can readily be traced and identified through the subtle process of fascial evaluation.

RSI, writer's and musician's cramp

Fascial restrictions can also develop as a result of more prolonged strains and tensions, perhaps due to occupational postures, such as persistent use of computer keyboards or machine operating, leading to repetitive strain injury, writer's cramp, tennis elbow and similar restrictions. They may also arise in violinists, dentists and other occupations where repeated adoption of certain positions or movements may impose patterns of restriction on the fascia, or in anyone who persistently adopts a poor posture.

Charles was a violinist, and quite an eminent soloist, but he was no longer able to perform because his shoulder had gradually become tighter and tighter over the years and not only had lost the flexibility required to play, but also had become increasingly painful, even on lifting his arm. There had been no specific injury; the condition seemed to have arisen simply from the persistent pattern of use. He had received many different treatments, including regular cranio-sacral therapy – but not including fascial unwinding. Fascial unwinding was able to release the restrictions in his shoulder and arm very rapidly and he was soon able to resume his playing career.

Car and bike accidents

Fascial unwinding is particularly relevant following major car accidents, motorbike or bicycle accidents, skiing accidents or any severe fall. Such major traumas can lead to multiple fascial restrictions, which can be very complex and entangled with potentially far-reaching effects, both physically and on personality.

Whiplash injuries in particular are effectively treated precisely because the multiplicity of traumas and forces imposed upon the body is virtually impossible to analyse specifically and individually by any external means of diagnosis. But the inherent wisdom of the body utilised during fascial unwinding enables the tissues to unravel every little twist and turn exactly as required by the body and so restore it to its natural disentangled state.

Severe trauma

Where severe trauma has been imposed throughout the body, a particular process called 'whole body unwinding' can be especially appropriate. In this process, as the name suggests, the whole body is allowed to unwind and unravel all at once. This has a particularly powerful and profound effect, releasing a multiplicity of traumas simultaneously, contacting both physical and emotional levels together, and consequently reaching deeper into the core of the person's being than might otherwise be achieved. This process can also be useful for treating patients in whom emotional tension is being held into the body as a whole, as generalised physical tension. When treating severe trauma, it is of course essential to ensure proper grounding and stability of the patient before embarking on any major release.

There are many other examples of severe trauma, such as rape, mugging and post-traumatic stress disorder, which can be helped through treatment that includes fascial unwinding, again due to the particular ability of fascial unwinding to engage simultaneously with the combination of physical and emotional trauma and the underlying patterns of trauma imposed on the system at a very deeply ingrained level.

Physical and emotional links

Emotional associations with the fascia are of particular relevance in severe physical traumas, such as major car accidents and serious injuries. Very often, the fear associated with such accidents, or the anger of being raped, mugged or beaten, or the apprehension of an operation, will be locked into the body along with the physical trauma. The two components – the physical and the emotional – become inextricably intertwined so that release of one becomes impossible without release of the other.

For this reason, patients may fail to recover, or be very slow to recover from major accidents and operations because, despite excellent physical care, the emotional factors are not being addressed. Similarly, psycho-emotional problems may persist and be unresponsive to psychiatric and psychotherapeutic treatment because the patient is unable to let go until the physical components are addressed.

Often the two components are so intertwined that they will release only when they are addressed simultaneously. It is here that fascial unwinding is especially valuable since it unravels the physical injuries while at the same time contacting the emotional levels associated with those injuries, bringing about a comprehensive process of release – with often dramatic results. Patients may sometimes experience their accident quite vividly at the moment of release – but in the comfort and safety of the therapeutic environment. This process can sometimes be assisted by simultaneous counselling, listening or psychotherapeutic help.

Emotional tensions are very often held in the viscera (organs) and here again fascial unwinding can be very beneficial – for instance, working on a spastic colon to release the combined and interrelated physical and emotional factors held there, or releasing emotional tensions held in the uterus (perhaps due to unconscious fears of pregnancy or as a result of previous terminations) which can be the unrecognised underlying cause of non-conception or repeated miscarriages.

Fascial unwinding can therefore be used specifically for the release of emotional tensions and traumas and also for exploring and discovering the underlying psycho-emotional causes of physical conditions.

Symptoms arising long after the original accident

With time, any fascial restriction tends to sclerose (harden) or fibrose gradually so that the restriction becomes increasingly consolidated and may become increasingly resistant to treatment. This does not mean that the condition cannot be treated, but simply that more time may be needed to enable a complete resolution. As a result of this gradual hardening of the fascia, symptoms may arise many years after the original incident. In such cases, the patient is unlikely even to remember the incident, let alone associate the current new symptoms with some perhaps relatively minor incident many years previously. This process of gradual sclerosis explains why many conditions may appear out of nowhere with no apparent cause, since the cause is long past and the process has been developing insidiously over many years.

Another reason why symptoms may appear long after the original cause is that the body is more pliable and resilient when young and so better able to cope with some degree of fascial restriction, whereas as time goes on the body becomes less resilient, so the effects of restriction become more evident. Also as time goes on, the individual is likely to experience other injuries and fascial tensions, the combination of which will therefore interact and react more.

Chronic emotional patterns

Fascia, as already mentioned, absorbs emotional tensions, particularly through its abundant neurological connections with the sympathetic nervous system. Just as muscles, including the diaphragm, may contract in response to emotional tensions, so the fascia, which envelops them, will reflect that tightening.

Day-to-day tensions, which come and go in response to the various stresses and strains of life, will drop away readily during times of relaxation or during sleep (so long as the sleep is restful). But when emotional tensions are held in the body over a prolonged period of time, these patterns can become ingrained within the fascia, gradually becoming more established and increasingly difficult to release. Even when the source of the emotional disturbance is gone, the fascia may maintain the pattern and reinstate the muscular and emotional holding in a vicious circle of tension. Fascial unwinding can release the fascial and muscular components of the circle, at the same time releasing the emotional level. This may be the most effective (sometimes the only) way to break the cycle of tension.

Fascial unwinding may also bring to light underlying emotional tensions which have not been acknowledged or recognised until then, thereby enabling the patient to deal with emotional tension more effectively. Physical and emotional factors can never be altogether separated and with any injury or illness there is inevitably an emotional component, whether it be an emotional reaction to pain, or frustration at the limiting effects of the illness, or some more dramatic, emotional trauma.

Consequently, the release of any fascial pattern in the body may be accompanied by a corresponding emotional release. It may occur as an almost unnoticed sense of relief or may come as a more profound experience of sadness, fear or anger.

Many people, following a bereavement or broken relationship, do not express their grief fully and may tend to lock up their feelings as physical tension, particularly in the pericardium and the fascia around the heart and the heart chakra, perhaps leading to pain, tightness, discomfort and various referred symptoms (remember Judith from Chapter 12).

Release of this fascial restriction may occur without any corresponding emotional release but will quite often be accompanied by release of the emotional factors held into that area, at a time more appropriate for their release, when the patient is better able to cope with the feelings and in a therapeutic environment appropriate for their release. Such tensions are often not responsive to other physical methods or to psychotherapeutic approaches and may sometimes only be released through fascial unwinding.

The fascia is often the crucial maintaining factor in preventing recovery or causing recurrence of a condition; and its vital interplay between physical and emotional factors enables a uniquely profound process of release.

Engaging with the fascia

As mentioned, it is possible to engage with the fascia without any visible movement. We are, in fact, engaging with the fascia much of the time in any treatment, simply by virtue of engaging with the cranio-sacral system. The fascia is an integral part of the whole body matrix, and just as our attention may be drawn to other tissues within the matrix — bone, membrane, fluid, organs, muscles — so it may also be drawn to areas of fascia which are restricted or unbalanced.

Within the context of an integrated treatment, we can also specifically choose to direct our attention to the fascia. We can also direct our attention to specific areas of fascia — such as the pericardium, the pleura, the fascia involved in an area of scar tissue following an operation, the fascia of a sprained ankle or tennis elbow or frozen shoulder.

As with all cranio-sacral integration, simply identifying an area of restriction, or a pattern of asymmetry, simply letting our attention rest there, and allowing the system to respond through the usual inherent treatment process, will influence the fascia just as it will affect anything else in the system — without any visible movement.

But this would not be fascial unwinding. Fascial unwinding involves a further dimension. When we allow the tissues to express their patterns of restriction and imbalance in actual physical movement, we can connect with a different level of engagement, thereby enabling responses on different therapeutic levels which are not necessarily accessed by other means. The way in which we do this will become apparent as we present the basic skills of fascial unwinding step by step, and subsequently see how these basic skills can be incorporated into the fluent integrated process of cranio-sacral treatment.

Chapter 39

Evaluation of the Fascia

Evaluation of the fascia, like all cranio-sacral integration, involves taking up a light contact, engaging with the system, and identifying the various impressions of quality, symmetry and motion expressed through the body. This can then lead to the unfolding of the inherent treatment process, allowing the system to express itself on a fascial level, drawing to points of stillness and release.

In order to evaluate the whole picture, we can take up contact on various regions of the body (commonly known as the *listening posts*) and identify the various subtle pulls and tensions manifested by the fascia. In this way, an impression may be gained of lines of force drawing towards a specific focal point (the source of the restriction) just as iron filings are drawn towards a magnet.

Taking up contact at the feet

With your patient lying supine (on their back), check that they are lying in a settled, symmetrical and balanced position on the couch. Invite them to take a deep breath and to let go completely as they breathe out, settling into a relaxed state.

Stand at your patient's feet, your weight evenly distributed between your two feet, your knees unlocked, and your body at ease, letting your shoulders drop and your arms hang loosely.

Before taking up contact, establish your own practitioner fulcrums. Up till now, we have worked from a sitting position. As we start to work from a standing position, you may find that you need to give greater attention to your own fulcrums in order to maintain the same degree of ease, relaxation, settledness and spaciousness, when you have the additional demands of standing.

As you continue to establish appropriate physical and mental fulcrums, run your attention down through your own body, from the top of your head down through your neck and shoulders, trunk, pelvis, legs and feet, to feel the soles of your feet firmly grounded on the floor, establishing a suitable balance of spaciousness and grounding.

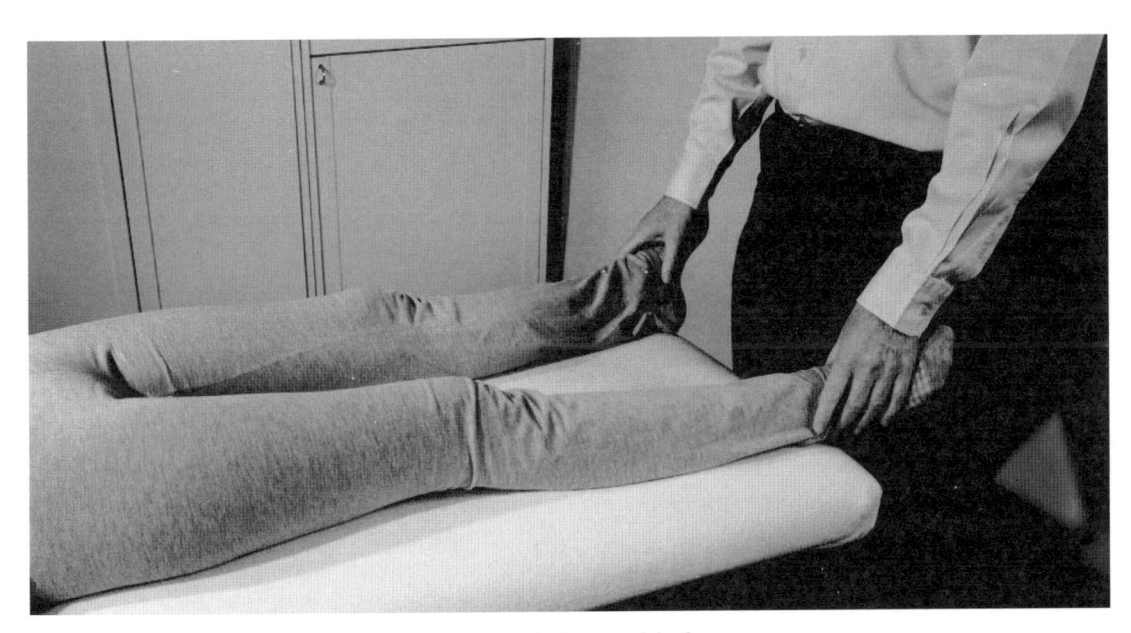

39.1 Allow your hands to come to rest very lightly onto the dorsum of the feet

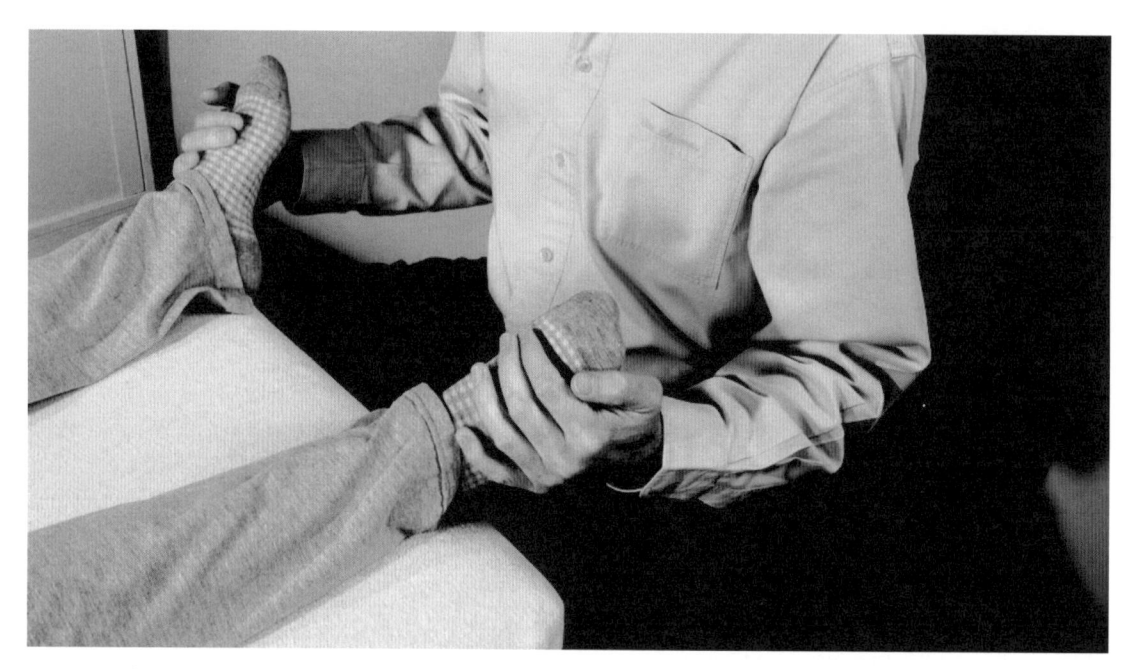

39.2 An alternative contact for the feet

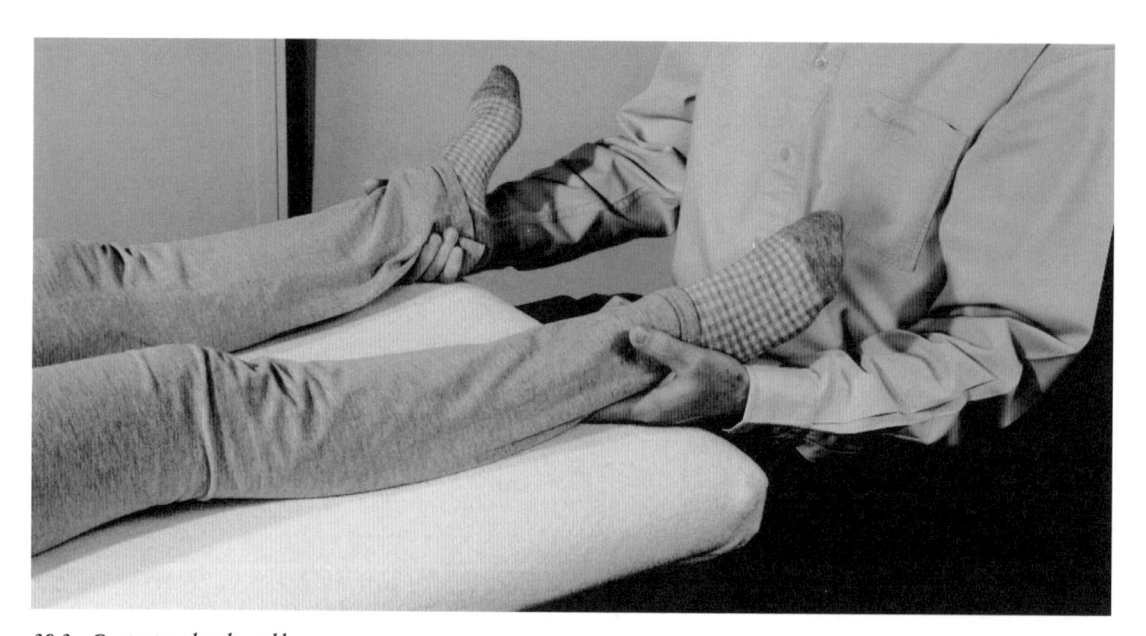

39.3 Contact under the ankles

When you feel suitably settled, take up a gentle contact under your patient's ankles, lift their legs off the couch and gently move them from side to side, together and apart, in order to ease out any superficial tensions. Then allow the legs to rest back onto the couch, slightly apart, and release your contact. (This is not fascial unwinding or evaluation, just a preparatory process to help the patient to relax more completely – but you can use every opportunity to good advantage, so as you move the legs gently, you can also evaluate the patient's response – do their legs move easily and fluently, are they holding them tight, do they resist movement, do they give their legs to you readily, are they relaxed, does one leg move more freely than the other, indicating a restriction or imbalance?)

Bring your attention back to yourself, shoulders dropping, arms hanging loosely by your sides. When you feel ready, allow your hands to move slowly and gently towards the dorsum (upper surface) of your patient's feet. As your hands move to within a few centimetres of the feet, be aware of the energy field around the body and gradually allow your hands to sink down through the energy field, to come to rest very lightly, like two butterflies, onto the dorsum of the feet (see Figure 39.1). Having made contact, allow your hands to relax down, sinking softly into the feet, completely relaxed. Again come back to yourself, checking your own fulcrums. Let your hands be so soft that they seem to melt into the feet, the feet melting into your hands, as if to become one continuous structure.

Evaluate quality, symmetry and motion

As you settle into this contact, feel the gradual process of increasing engagement. As your two systems become increasingly interconnected, be aware of whatever impressions come to you.

Be aware of the quality of the feet, both as a reflection of the overall quality of the whole person and as a reflection of local quality within the feet. Be aware of any differences in quality between the two feet. Does one foot feel tighter than the other? Or warmer, or softer, or any other quality that may come to mind? What does this tell you about the two feet? Does one foot seem more restricted, less alive and if so why? Does the greater tightness in one foot suggest that that foot or leg has been injured, fractured, or is held in restriction in some way.

Be aware of any asymmetry between the two feet. Does one seem to externally rotate or internally rotate more than the other? To invert or evert? Dorsiflex or plantarflex? Does one foot seem to pull up into the leg or towards the hip? Do both legs seem to rotate round to the same side? Observe whatever impressions may come to you, allowing the system to express itself (see Figure 39.4).

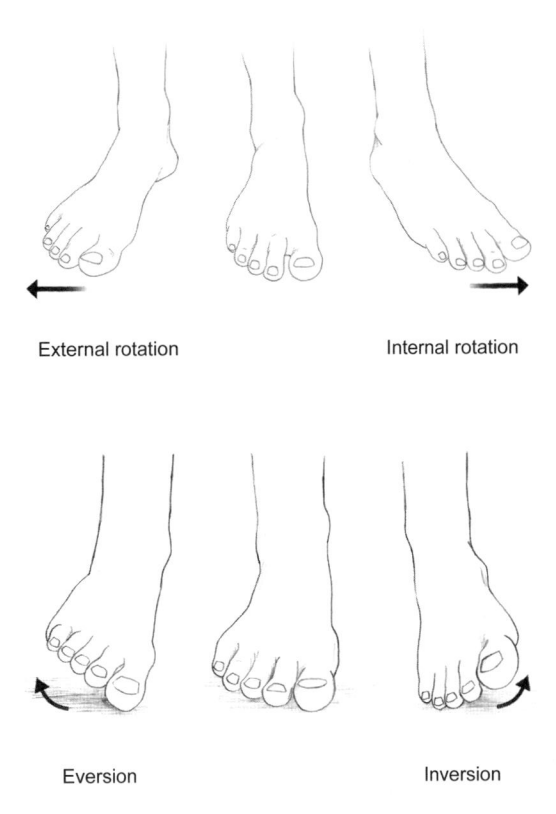

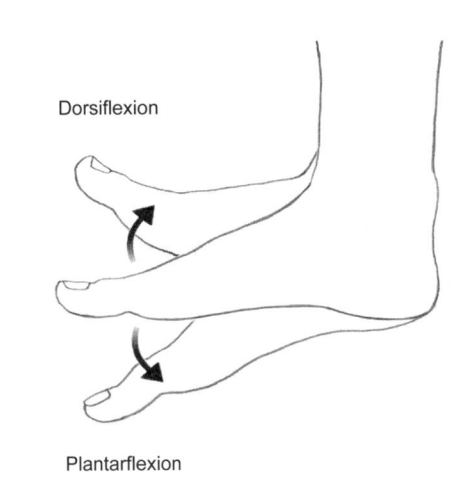

External rotation   Internal rotation

Eversion   Inversion

Dorsiflexion

Plantarflexion

39.4 Movements of the feet

Allow your hands to float freely

Perhaps both feet will feel quite active initially. Be aware of this activity, as if your hands are floating on the surface of a fluid-filled balloon, or immersed in warm fluidity, allowing and following the various subtle movements – ripples, pulsations, shaking, pulling, wriggling – but not of course doing anything, simply being there, letting your hands be washed this way and that by the subtle currents and eddies. Perhaps the feet will move in unison, perhaps they will move independently. Perhaps the whole lower part of the body may seem to twist round in one direction, or shake from side to side. As always, simply allow the system to express itself.

As the initial movements settle, allow the continuing evolution of the inherent treatment process, aware of any more specific persistent patterns, allowing your soft, fluent, fluidic hands to be drawn into any movements, eventually reaching points of stillness and releases, allowing the body to settle into a more balanced and comfortable neutral state.

Cranio-sacral motion

As the system settles into a balanced neutral state, feel the increasing emergence of rhythmic motion, whether in cranio-sacral rhythm or in middle tide motion. During cranio-sacral motion, the feet open out into external rotation during the expansion phase and move into internal rotation during the contraction phase (see Figure 39.5). Be aware of the quality of the motion. Is it broad, slow and expansive, or is it of small amplitude, narrow and restricted? Is the motion more readily expressed in one leg than the other and how does this relate to the other impressions you have gained up till now? Evaluate the potency of the motion. Feel the sense of vitality expressed through the feet and any difference in vitality between the two feet.

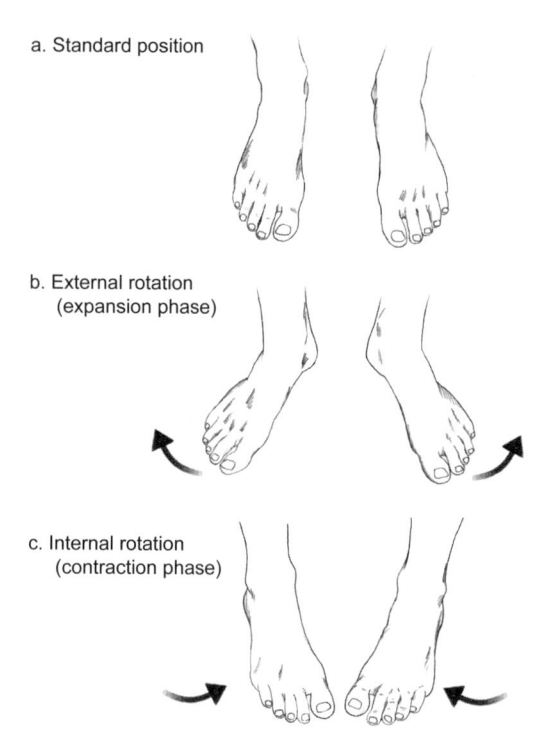

a. Standard position

b. External rotation (expansion phase)

c. Internal rotation (contraction phase)

39.5 Cranio-sacral motion of the feet

Project up through the body

As the system continues to settle, the complex mass of initial movements may clear to reveal more specific persistent patterns. Observe and make a mental note of these patterns as you maintain your contact at the feet. As you identify a particular pull or twist, allow your attention to follow it up through the body to its source, observing whether it intensifies or fades at a particular level or focal point – the knee, the hip, the pelvis – observing any changes in quality, symmetry or motion at the feet.

As your attention is drawn to specific focal points, you may feel the rhythmic motion closing down to points of stillness and release. With each release, as the system settles back to neutral, observe the more expansive expression of rhythmic motion, perhaps shifting from cranio-sacral rhythm to middle tide motion. With each release, notice the softer quality, the more balanced symmetry, the more settled movements.

If no specific pattern or pull is apparent, you could survey through the body. Maintaining your awareness of the rhythmic motion, take your attention up from the feet through the ankles, lower legs, knees, thighs, hips, pelvis, sacro-iliac joints, up through the vertebral column, the viscera and the trunk, up to the neck and head. As you work your way up through the body, be aware of any impressions that come to you as you take your attention to different areas. You may experience these changes as a physical pull up one side of the body, or twisting across the body; you may experience them more as a visual impression, you may experience them intuitively, or you may feel changes in quality, symmetry and motion under your hands at the feet – perhaps experiencing sensations of tightening, loosening, intensifying, pulsating, twisting, or pulling – as your attention moves to different structures.

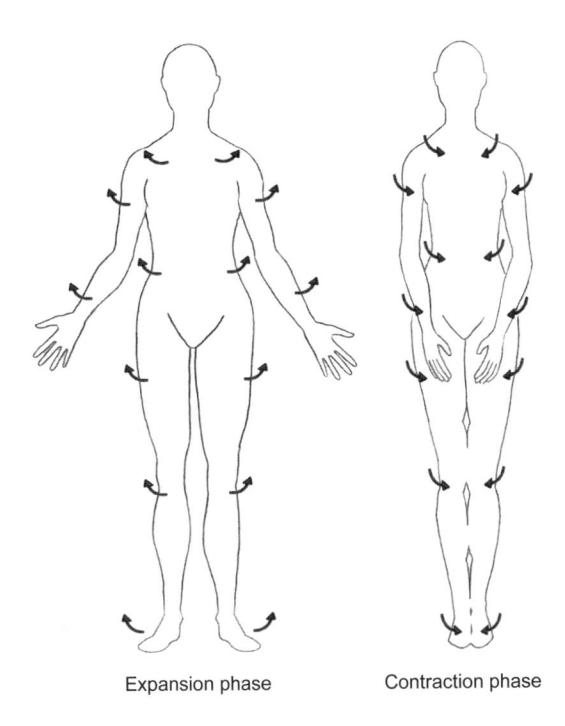

Expansion phase   Contraction phase

39.6 Project your attention up to feel the expansion and contraction of the fascia throughout the body

Interpreting your impressions

If a pull seems to extend up as far as the knee on one side and is then no longer apparent when you take your attention above the knee, it might suggest a restriction in that knee. If the whole lower body seems to twist round to one side as your attention reaches the pelvis, it might indicate a rotation of the pelvis. If, as you take your attention up to the solar plexus, the quality throughout the system (as palpated through the feet) seems to tighten, it suggests there may be tension in the solar plexus. A quality of restriction in one leg which you can follow up as far as the sacro-iliac joint on that side where it intensifies, suggests that the restriction you are feeling in that leg may originate in a restricted sacro-iliac joint. Similarly, a twist or pull or tightness at a particular vertebral level might indicate a restriction at that vertebral level. If, as you take your attention up through the trunk, you feel drawn to the stomach or the heart, then it suggests that there may be some tightness or restriction in those organs.

Identify focal points

In this way, projecting your attention up through the body, identify any focal areas of resistance anywhere in the system, building up a picture of the various twists, turns, pulls and focal points of restriction throughout the whole body, whether from physical injury, emotional tension or whatever cause, and consequently building a comprehensive picture of the whole person. Within that overall picture, as your attention is drawn to specific focal points, again notice the rhythmic motion drawing to still points and release, allowing the system to settle further into a balanced neutral state.

Maintain awareness of yourself

Throughout this process, maintain your own practitioner fulcrums, with a relaxed detached state of mind, not too intently concentrated, and a spacious overview of the whole person, while at the same time focusing on the details within the broader picture. Spend sufficient time at the feet to establish a clear interconnection between your two systems, to allow the initial movements to settle, to allow any pulls, twists and turns to express themselves, to follow into any further persistent patterns until they soften and release, to project your attention up through the body, establishing a view of the whole picture. Then when the system feels ready and has settled into a comfortable neutral state, you can move on through the rest of the listening posts.

The listening posts

The listening posts are a set of standard points of contact which provide convenient places from which to evaluate the fascia from different perspectives. You could use any points of contact, but these listening posts form a framework of positions in key areas which together provide a comprehensive perspective on the whole body.

The standard listening posts are:

- the feet
- the shins – halfway between the ankles and the knees
- the thighs – halfway between the knees and the hips
- the iliac crests
- the lower thorax – over the lower ribs
- the upper thorax – over the upper ribs.

Moving up through the listening posts

Having established a good level of engagement through the feet, and having gained some idea of the patterns of movement and restriction throughout the body, you can move up through the rest of the listening posts more quickly, maintaining your sense of engagement even as you move from place to place. By maintaining your sense of engagement, you will be able to tune in more readily at subsequent listening posts, observing what patterns you feel at the different listening posts, seeing whether they match your previous perceptions, whether they add further detail or confirmation, or whether they perhaps provide conflicting impressions. Each patient will have a mixture of different focal points of restriction, resulting from different injuries, incidents and illnesses throughout life. There may be a very simple picture with one clear focal point; there may be a very complex picture with a multitude of different impressions to be picked up – including conflicting impressions, perhaps arising from different accidents from opposite directions, or from a combination of physical injuries, diseases, and emotional tensions.

As you move from one listening post to another, be sure to move slowly, gently, sensitively – carefully releasing your contact from one listening post, always coming in with the same soft butterfly touch on each new contact, ensuring that your own movements from one place to another do not disturb the fluent continuity of the treatment process, and maintaining your engagement with the patient at all times, through the focus of your attention.

In order to move on from the feet, gently allow your hands to come away from the dorsum of the feet and move up to take contact on the shins – your hands resting softly halfway between ankles and knees, fingers laterally, thumbs pointing medially (see Figure 39.7). You may wish to do this simply by leaning over towards the shins, or you may prefer to come up to stand

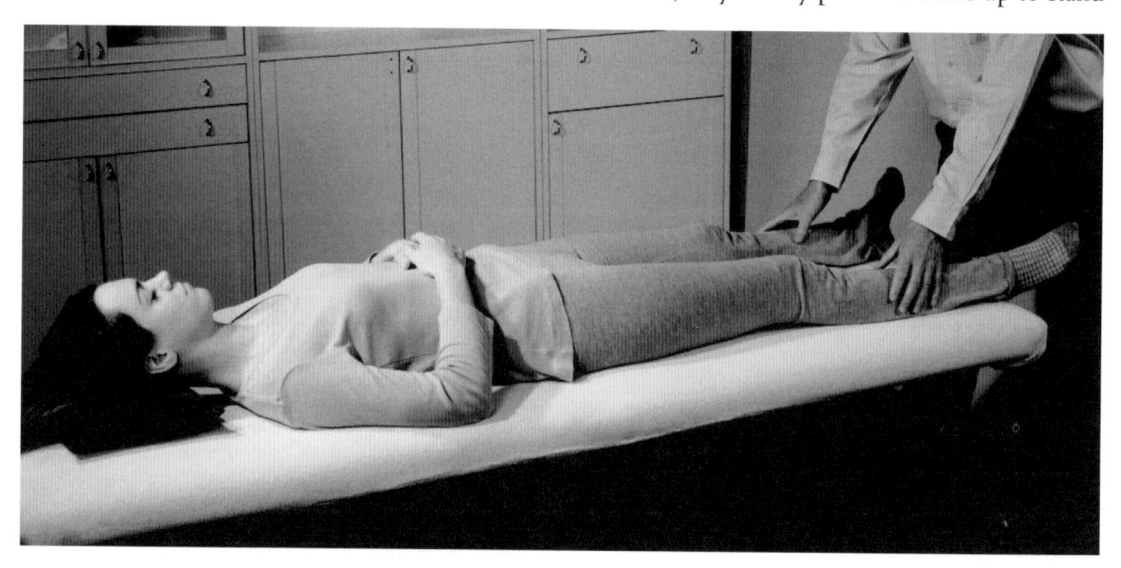

39.7 Contact for the shins – halfway between ankles and knees

at the side of the couch and rest your hands onto the shins from there. In all these contacts on the listening posts it is preferable to use a symmetrical hand contact in order to gain a more symmetrical perspective and symmetrical evaluation of the system.

As you bring your hands to rest lightly onto the shins, maintaining your awareness of yourself, see what impressions you pick up from this perspective. Does the quality differ from your previous contact? Is the overall quality of the system the same, or is there some particular local quality in this area, perhaps suggesting a local injury or restriction? Do the patterns of symmetry and motion match what you felt at the feet or is there some new element to be identified at this point? Is the rhythmic motion being expressed clearly, or is it restricted locally?

For instance, if there were an ankle injury, there might be a pull upwards from the foot but a pull downwards from the shin – the two perspectives combining to indicate a focal point at the ankle.

Having tuned in, and having evaluated the system at the shins, move on up to the thighs – halfway between the knees and the hips (see Figure 39.8). If you have not already moved to the side of the body for the shins, you will certainly need to do so for the thighs, standing beside the couch, level with the thighs, turning your body and feet to face the patient's head, outer foot forward, inner foot back, your body resting lightly against the couch for support and stability thereby enabling you to be more relaxed and to minimise postural strain on your body. You can then place your hands symmetrically on the thighs, thumbs medially, fingers pointing out laterally.

It is not usually necessary to spend a long time at each listening post. Be prepared to trust your first impressions; they are often the most accurate. However, at each point, if you find yourself engaging with some significant asymmetry and being drawn into an imbalance, you can allow that process to evolve, leading to a point of stillness and release. The whole process of working through the listening posts can either be carried out quickly and briefly, simply as a brief diagnostic procedure, or can be used as a more therapeutic process, lingering longer and following into the patterns expressed throughout the system, enabling the system to settle into a more balanced state.

In the same way, move on up through the iliac crests, the lower thorax and the upper thorax (see Figures 39.8, 39.9 and 39.10). At each point evaluate the quality, the symmetry and the motion, always maintaining a sense of the whole

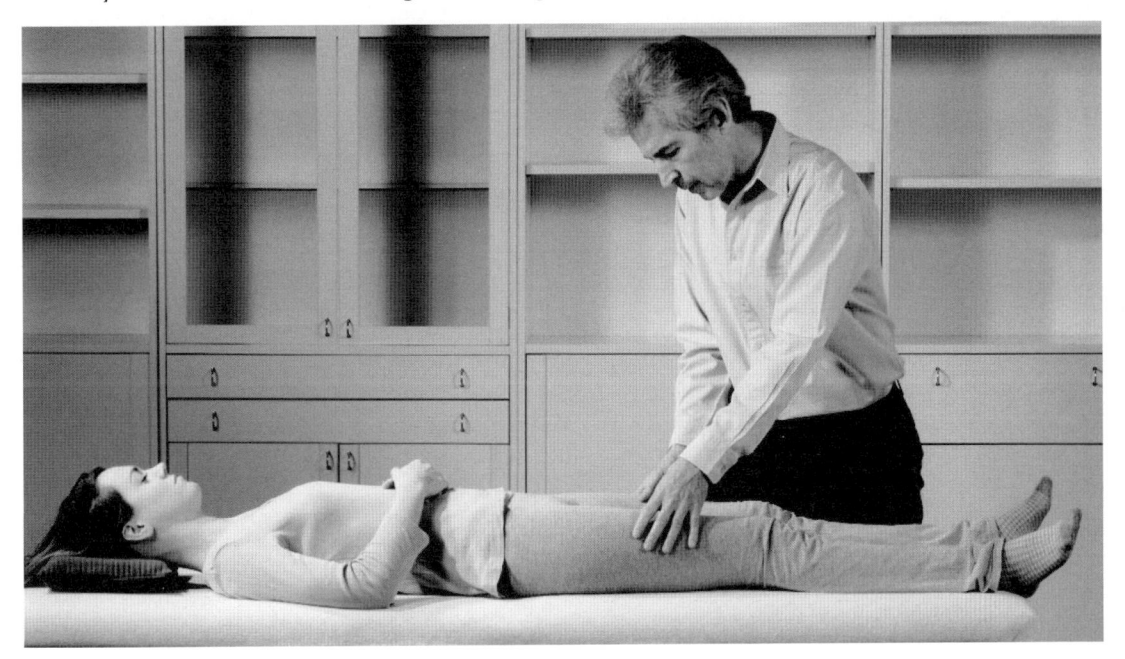

39.8 Contact for the thighs – it is helpful to place your hands symmetrically on the thighs

picture, seeing how the new perspective matches or conflicts with your previous impressions, allowing the responses within the system. See how each new perspective may provide further detail to the gradually emerging picture of the whole person.

The various different perspectives may all lead you to the same predominant focal point of restriction, or they may reveal a number of different focal points of greater or lesser significance. For example, you might feel decreased mobility of the left leg and as you project your attention up through the leg, you might feel that this quality of decreased mobility intensifies as you reach the left knee where you encounter a sense of twist and restriction. As your attention projects further, you might feel the continuing lack of mobility intensifying as you reach the left sacro-iliac joint. Moving your attention beyond that restriction, you might encounter tightness in the thoraco-lumbar junction, agitation in the solar plexus and a pull towards the colon on the left. This might be the picture for a patient with irritable bowel syndrome, involving a combination of an old

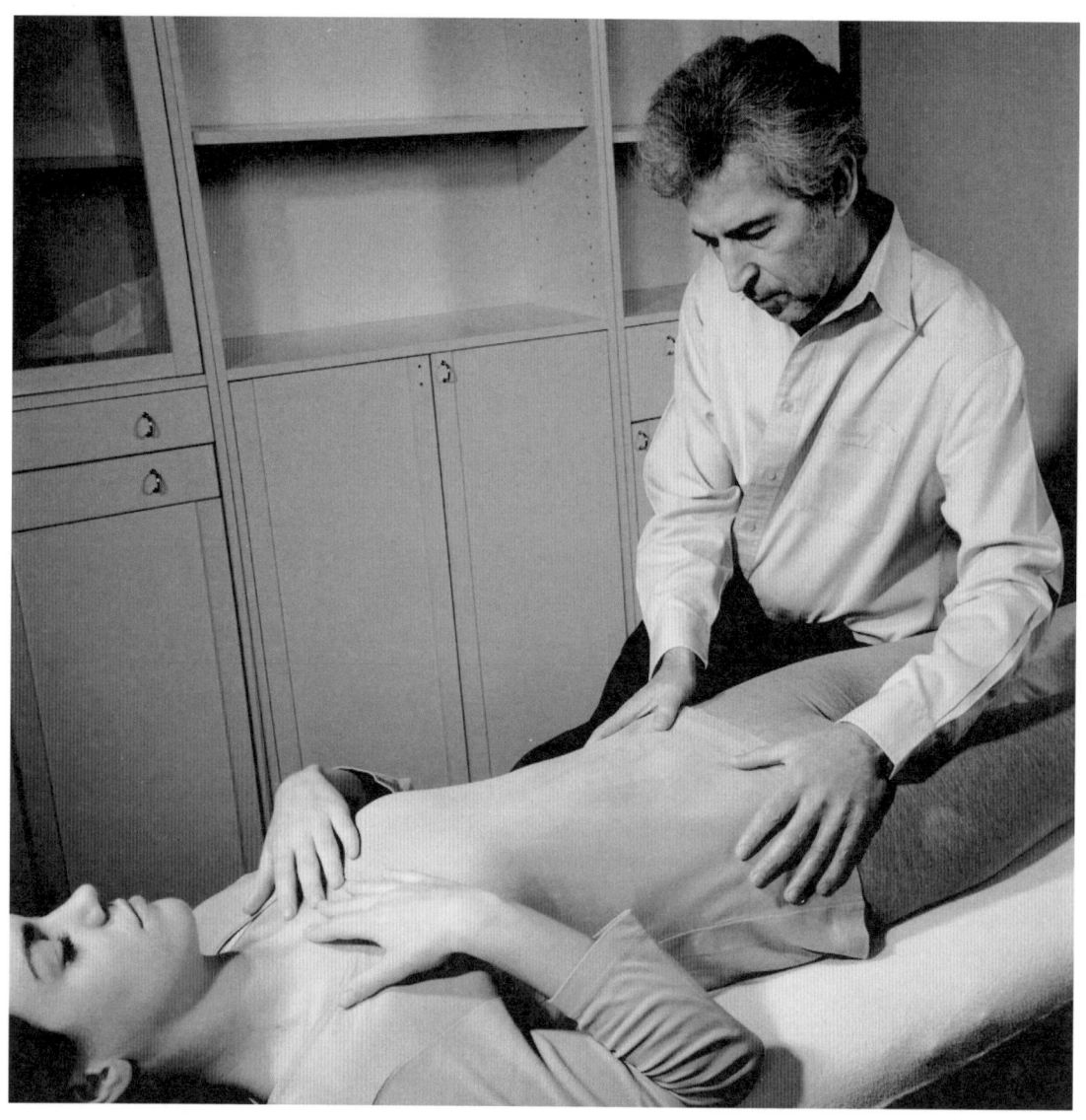

39.9 Contact for the iliac crests – at each of the listening posts, it may be appropriate to linger longer and follow into the patterns expressed throughout the system

knee injury causing compensatory restriction in the left sacro-iliac joint, leading to adaptive strain in the thoraco-lumbar spine compressing the sympathetic nerve supply to the colon, together with emotional stresses leading to agitation in the solar plexus also reflecting into the sympathetic nerve supply to the colon.

As you take up contact on the thighs, let your hands rest at the midpoint of the thighs anteriorly, halfway between knees and hips, fingers extending out laterally, thumbs pointing medially.

At the iliac crests, let your hands rest onto the iliac crests, fingers spreading out laterally, thumbs pointing medially (see Figure 39.9).

At the lower thorax, let your hands rest onto the lower rib cage, fingers extending out laterally, thumbs pointing medially (see Figure 39.10).

In order to take up contact on the upper thorax, stand at the patient's head and let your hands rest over the clavicles and upper thorax, fingers pointing out laterally towards the axillae, thumbs extending down medially towards the sternum (see Figure 39.11).

At every point, maintain awareness of your own comfort, leaning against the couch for support, rather than bending over excessively causing strain and tension in your body, thereby reducing your sensitivity.

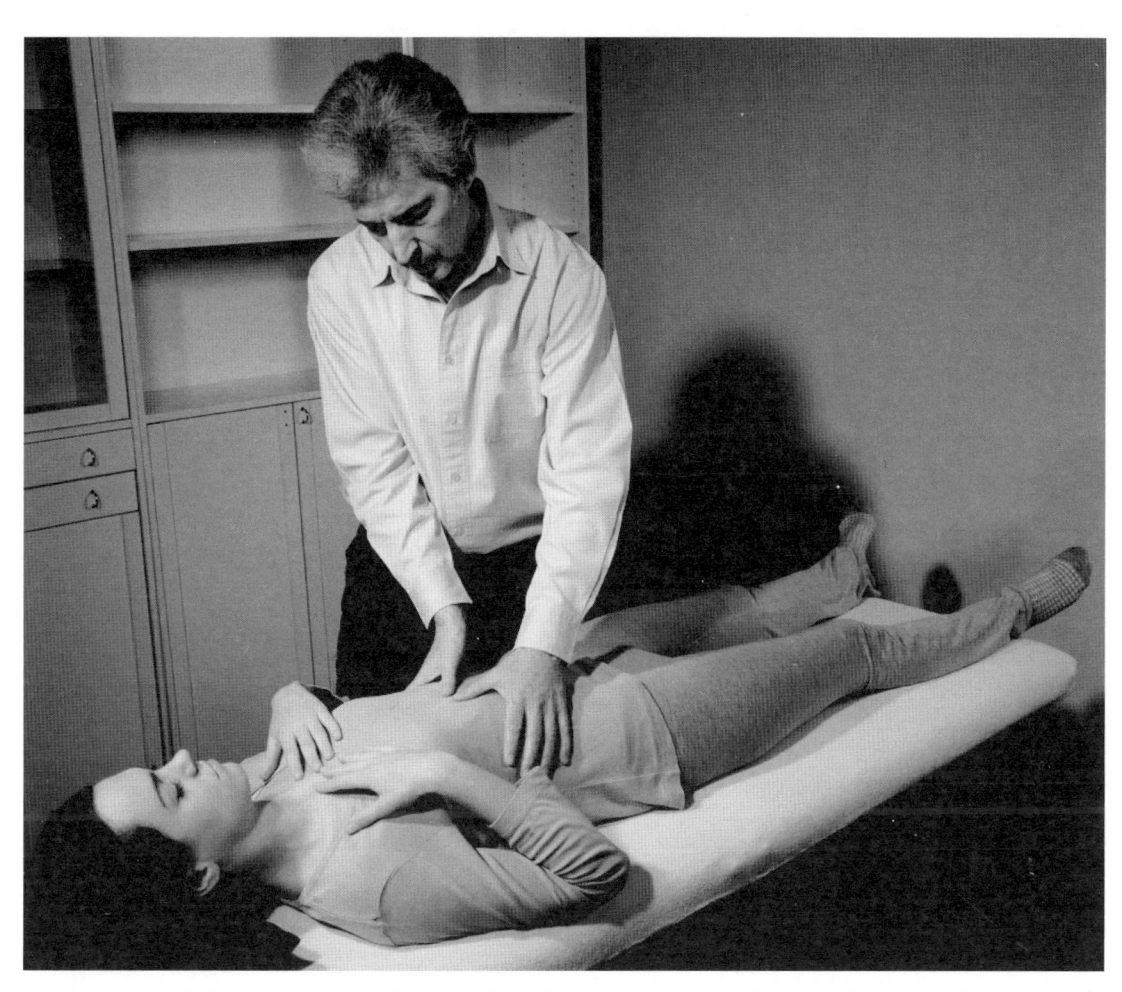

39.10 Contact at the lower thorax – at each point evaluate the quality, symmetry and motion, always maintaining a sense of the whole picture

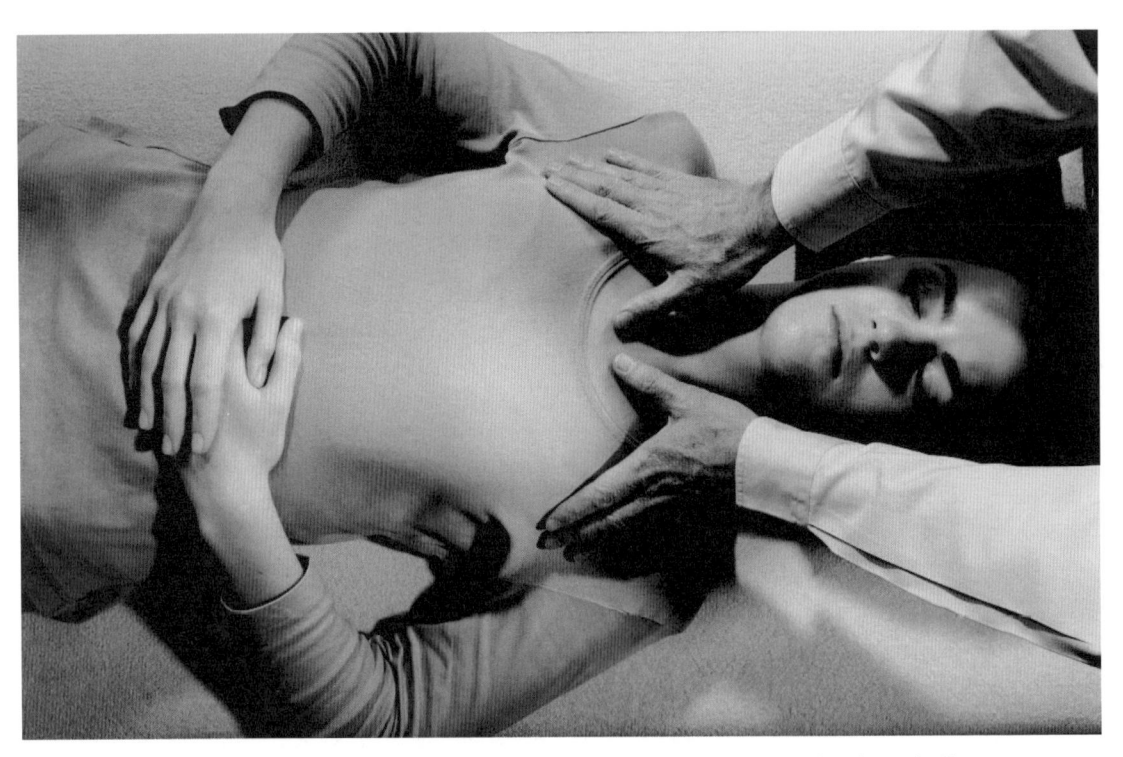

39.11 Contact at the upper thorax – see how each new perspective may provide further detail to the gradually emerging picture of the whole person

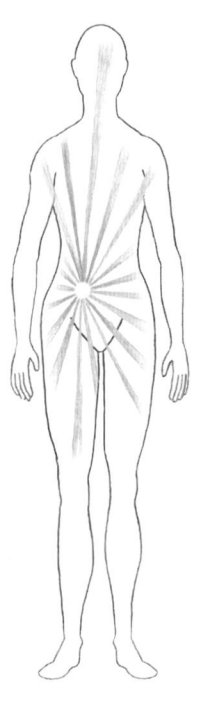

39.12 The various different perspectives may all lead you to the same focal point of restriction – such as an appendix scar

Build up a picture of the whole person

Having evaluated the system from all these different perspectives, you may find an overall picture of your patient's system gradually emerging (see Figure 39.12). By interpreting your findings, you may be able to evaluate the source and the cause of any restriction, and by evaluating the quality and intensity of different focal points you may be able to evaluate the severity, chronicity and relative significance of each focal point.

Having made your evaluation and identified the most significant focal points, you can now move on to take up contact at your chosen focal point or fulcrum of restriction, in order to address it more specifically.

When you first start to evaluate the fascia, it will be helpful to practise evaluating through the listening posts in this methodical way. With practice, you may find that you can see the whole picture clearly just from the contact at the feet, or from anywhere else in the body – although the feet do provide a very valuable vantage point from which to survey and evaluate the whole system and therefore a very good place to start a treatment. Alternatively, you may find that you identify and are drawn to specific fascial fulcrums simply in the course of an integrated treatment process, without using the listening posts at all.

It is possible to address any restriction from anywhere in the body, simply by engaging with the system and letting your attention be drawn to the particular focal point, but significant deeply ingrained restrictions may benefit from a more specific local contact – as we will explore in the next few chapters.

You might encounter a focal point of restriction in an arm – a tennis elbow, an old fracture of the wrist, a frozen shoulder. It might be in a leg – a sprained ankle, a twisted knee, a restricted sacro-iliac joint – in the neck, in the spine, in the trunk, in the viscera. It could be anywhere. We will look at how to address different areas in turn, starting with focal points in the trunk region.

Chapter 40

Fascial Unwinding within the Trunk Region

Identifying a focal point

Having identified a focal point in the trunk region, perhaps by means of the listening posts, or perhaps in the course of an integrated treatment, the exact contact that you take up will depend on the area selected. It might be an organ – the stomach, the liver, the heart, a kidney, an adrenal gland; it might be an area of emotional tension – the heart centre, the solar plexus; it might be an area of scar tissue – from an old appendix operation or hysterectomy; it might be a vertebral segment, or an area of muscular tension such as the rhomboid muscles; it might be a shoulder, or an old rib fracture. The focal point may involve several different structures in combination – the heart, the heart centre, and the vertebral levels associated with the nerve supply to the heart (around T4) – or perhaps the solar plexus, the stomach, and its associated vertebral levels (T6–10).

Taking up contact

Generally speaking, an appropriate contact for fulcrums within the trunk area is with one hand at the back of the body and one hand at the front, so that the focal point of restriction is contained between your two hands. In many cases, the hand at the back of the body may be best placed under the spine at the appropriate vertebral level relating to the nerve supply to the affected structure. For any restriction in or close to the pelvic area, the sacrum is an appropriate contact for the lower hand – since the sacrum is always a powerhouse of energy for the cranio-sacral process.

Having taken up contact on your chosen area, re-establish your practitioner fulcrums, sitting comfortably, re-engaging with your patient's system. As always, don't be in a hurry for anything to happen, simply allow the impressions to come to you in their own time.

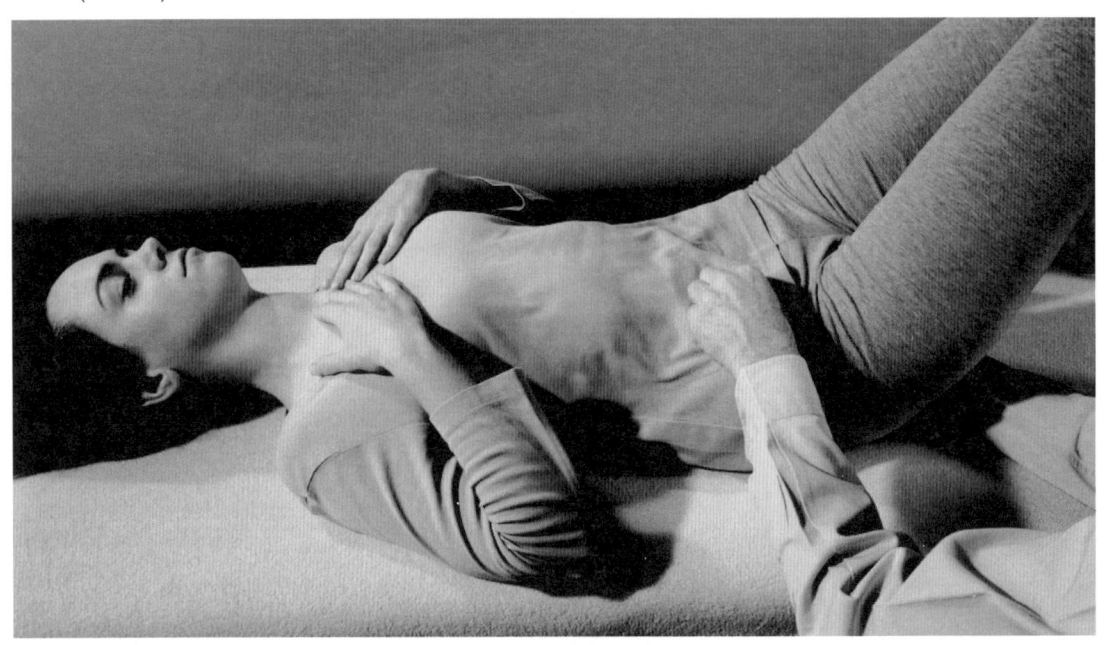

40.1 Contact for working with the right ovary – for any restriction in or close to the pelvic area, the sacrum is an appropriate contact for the lower hand – since the sacrum is always a powerhouse of energy for the cranio-sacral process

Fascial Unwinding within the Trunk Region / 277

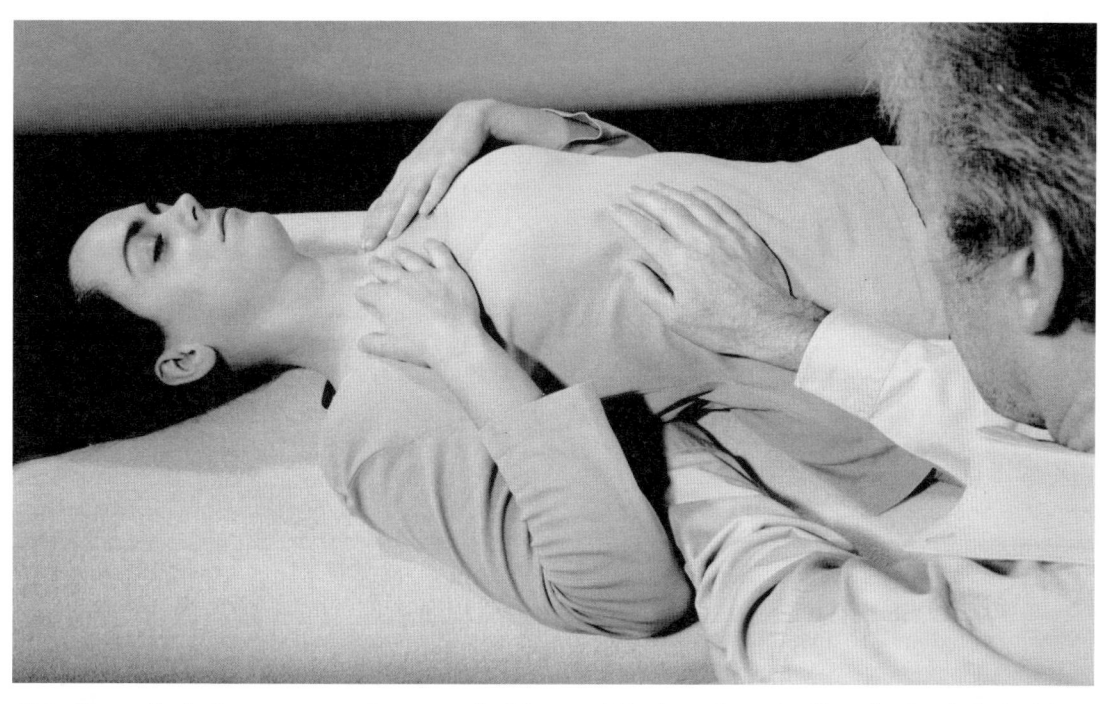

40.2 Contact for the liver – an appropriate contact for fulcrums within the trunk area is with one hand at the back of the body and one hand at the front, so that the focal point of restriction is contained between your two hands

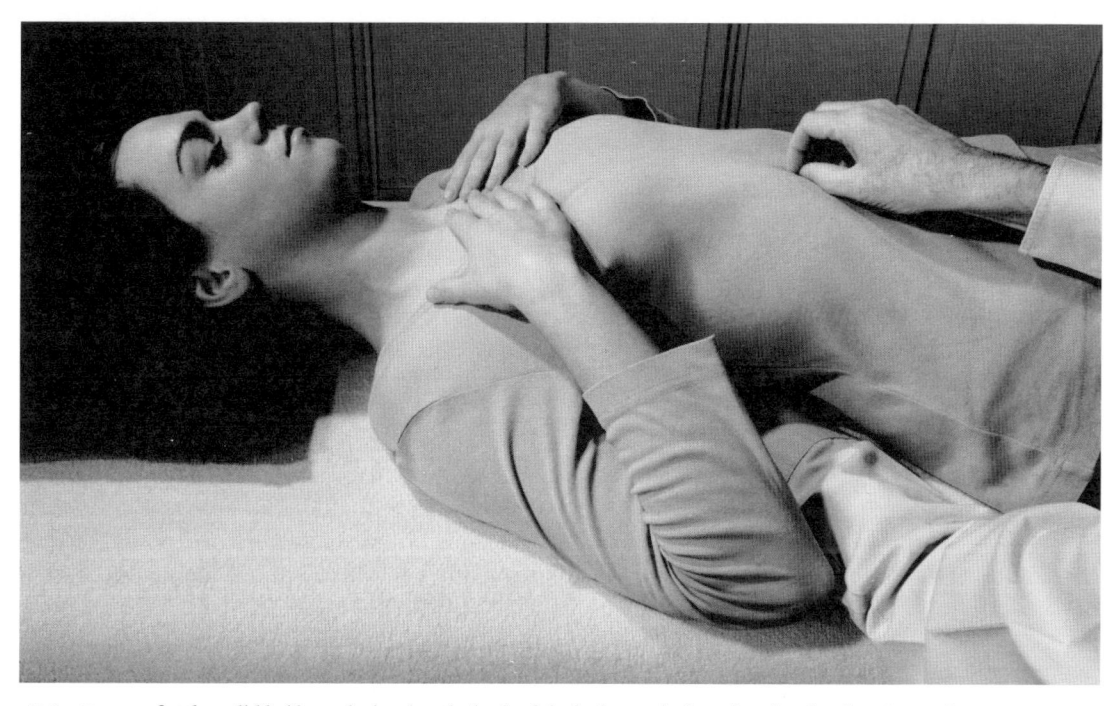

40.3 Contact for the gall bladder – the hand at the back of the body may be best placed under the spine at the appropriate vertebral level relating to the nerve supply to the affected structure

Engaging

Be aware of the quality of the area. Since it is an area specifically chosen as a focal point of restriction, this is likely to be reflected in the quality that you feel.

Be aware of the symmetry of the area. Since you have specifically chosen this area as a focal point, it is likely that the focal point of the pulls, twists and turns will be directly under your hands or between your hands, rather than pulling you elsewhere through the body. Common impressions at this point are to feel the hands drawn directly into the body, to feel both hands twisting round either in the same direction or in opposite directions around a focal point between the two hands.

Be aware of movement. As always, allow the inherent treatment process to be expressed, allowing your hands to float freely on the surface of the body in response to the various movements, or to be drawn into deeper patterns within. As any initial movements settle, be aware of more specific patterns of resistance; and as you allow your hands to follow into these more persistent patterns you may encounter deeper resistances. Stay with the stillness at the edge of these points of resistance until they soften, dissolve and release.

We have mentioned that fascial unwinding generally involves more visible, tangible movement of the body. This will certainly be far more evident as we move on to the arms, legs and neck. When working with the trunk at this stage, we will be working with much smaller movements of the tissues – with the body as a whole remaining relatively still. The tissues under your hands – whether the superficial muscles or the organs deep within – *may* remain still, but they may also wish to express visible movement – twisting, turning, wriggling, squirming, contracting towards a focal point, drawing your hands deep into the body. It is also possible to allow the whole trunk, and in fact the whole body to move into a more active physical unwinding – this is something which we will come back to at a later stage.

Release

As the local area releases, feel the ramifications throughout the body, as the whole body adapts to its new-found state of greater mobility and settles into a more balanced state.

Once a release has occurred, you may feel that the process is complete and be ready to move on, or you may feel that it would be appropriate to follow into further resistances and further releases in that area. Sometimes, the release of a resistance may leave the local area feeling completely free; at other times the release of one resistance may reveal another underlying resistance of a different nature. Other releases may only partially release a restriction, perhaps taking out one layer of a deeply established, deeply embedded, chronic resistance.

It is not always possible to release every resistance completely within a short space of time. When a restriction has been there for a long time, it may have built up layer upon layer of compensatory tensions which will take time to release, and it may be enough simply to release one layer or a few layers of resistance, depending on many factors within the overall picture of the patient's situation. To release too many layers of compensation all at once might be difficult for the body to cope with, so it is best simply to allow the body to release whatever layers it chooses to release.

The appropriate time to bring any treatment process to an end is following release and reorganisation, whether it be a complete or partial release, once the system has settled back to neutral. Following the release, stay with that contact as the whole system settles and reorientates itself around the changed circumstances of its newly released state. Once it feels resolved and settled, gently release your hand contact and move on – to the next area, to reassessment of the whole picture, or to the next part of your integrated treatment process, as appropriate.

Chapter 41

Fascial Unwinding of the Arm

Fascial unwinding of the arm can be appropriate for many different circumstances — tennis elbow, sprained wrist, an old fracture of the arm or of an individual finger, carpal tunnel syndrome, repetitive strain injury, certain cases of neurological symptoms (pins and needles, numbness, pain) in the fingers, various injuries to the arms, or a variety of conditions affecting the shoulder — from frozen shoulder and tendonitis to deeply held occupational and emotional tensions.

But the arm does not exist in isolation. It is of course attached to the trunk at the shoulder girdle and is connected through many muscular, neurological and soft tissue attachments, thereby creating significant reciprocal influences from the arm into the rest of the body, and from the rest of the body into the arm.

Many traumas to the arm — for instance using the arm to save ourselves when falling — are likely to be transmitted not only through the whole of the upper limb but also through the shoulder and shoulder girdle into the neck and trunk, perhaps leading to neck pain, back pain or headache, and potentially affecting the balance, symmetry, mobility and function of the body as a whole, with potential repercussions in any part of the body.

The arm, when it is the source of those repercussions, is often the best place through which to address those forces elsewhere in the body. Fascial unwinding of the arm can also therefore be appropriate for many circumstances affecting or involving other areas of the body — particularly the neck, which carries the nerve supply to and from the arm, and various muscles relating to the arm and shoulder girdle such as the rhomboid muscles, deltoid muscles, the rotator cuff muscles, or latissimus dorsi.

Latissimus dorsi (see Figure 41.1) is a useful example through which to demonstrate the need to maintain an awareness of the integral nature of the whole body. It attaches into the upper arm at the bicipital groove of the humerus and is involved in many everyday arm movements, as well as being involved in many postural and occupational positions and movements — such as playing musical instruments, and a host of other activities. But apart from the arm, where else does this muscle attach?

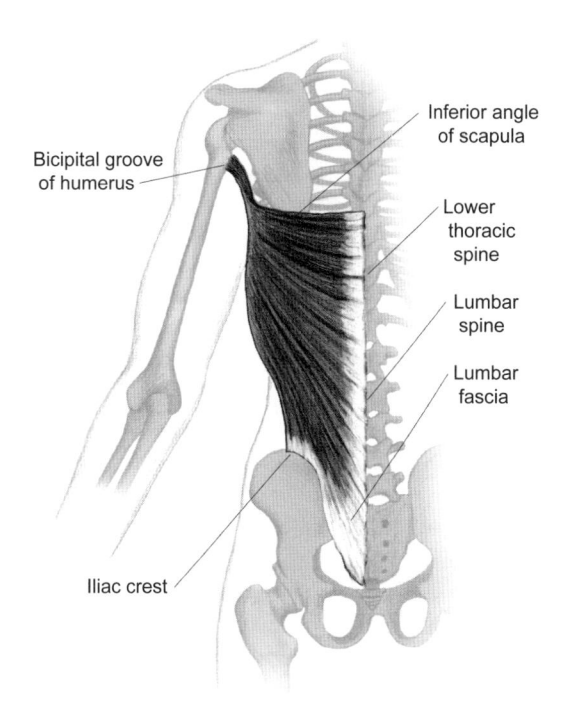

41.1 Latissimus dorsi

The Latin name latissimus dorsi translates as 'the widest muscle of the back'. Not only does it spread across much of the back of the body, attaching into the lower thoracic and lumbar spine and lumbar fascia, but also it reaches as far down as the pelvis, attaching to the iliac crest. It also has a small but significant attachment to the scapula at its inferior angle. All these attachments indicate that tension in the latissimus dorsi muscle can affect the arm, the scapula, the spine, the pelvis and much else besides; and that tension in the arm could cause an imbalance in the pelvis, and that pelvic imbalances can affect the arms. So playing the violin, or falling on your outstretched arm, could create imbalances in the pelvis via the latissimus dorsi muscle, potentially leading to back pain and sciatica among many other possible symptoms. The ramifications are endless and serve to demonstrate again the importance of working with the whole body, the whole person, and trusting the cranio-sacral system, in its infinite wisdom, to guide the therapeutic process, rather than relying on the limited diagnostic skills of the human mind.

Whole person assessment

However specific or local a patient's symptoms may be, we always need to look at the whole picture. We don't simply unwind an arm in isolation.

In every case, whatever the circumstances, we start with an overall *assessment of the whole person* – a case history, tuning in, engaging with the whole system, assessing the underlying vitality, identifying physical injuries and restrictions throughout the body, assessing any emotional component that may be contributing to the condition, evaluating the complete picture, to see what treatment and what levels of treatment may be appropriate in each case.

In every case, whatever the circumstances, *we treat the whole person* – engaging, opening up the system, working with the core, enhancing the underlying vitality as necessary, addressing the overall balance and integration of the system – since every system can operate fluently only if it is fully integrated – and ensuring that the system has the resources to heal itself.

In every case, we make an appropriate *diagnosis of all relevant factors* that might be contributing to the situation – such as the nerve supply to the arm and therefore the state of the neck – associated muscles, emotional factors (such as grief held in the heart) – and address any of these factors as necessary.

The arm receives its nerve supply via the brachial plexus from nerves with their root origins from C5 to T1 (the fifth cervical to the first thoracic vertebrae). Injuries, imbalances and tensions in the neck are therefore a common cause of problems arising in the arm. Injury, trauma and tension in the shoulder, the shoulder girdle, and the brachial plexus region, as well as the heart centre and the whole thorax, are similarly a common cause of symptoms in the arm, and any unwinding process for the arm needs to take all of these factors into account.

Consequently, before unwinding an arm, the treatment process is likely to have addressed many different factors throughout the body as necessary. Within that wider context of an understanding of the whole person, having prepared the way accordingly, and having established for whatever reasons that fascial unwinding of the arm is appropriate, it is then possible to move on to the fascial unwinding of the arm itself, within the context of an integrated treatment of the whole person.

Principles

The principles for fascial unwinding of the arm are the same as the principles for any other cranio-sacral work – allowing the evolution of the inherent treatment process. However, each part of the body has its individual characteristics and the nature of the arm invariably influences the nature of the treatment process.

A more active process

The arm is by nature a more mobile and active part of the body. We move our arms a great deal in many different directions. Consequently, arms may be strained, sprained, traumatised and injured in many different positions and directions. Our arms are also very susceptible to injury and accident.

When we treat the arm through fascial unwinding, the process will reflect this mobility. Not only will we be engaging with the forces held in the tissues, but also we will allow them to be expressed visibly and tangibly, allowing the arm to perform its own intricate dance through the air, unwinding and unravelling the tensions held in the tissues, rediscovering the positions in which it was injured or traumatised, reaching points of stillness at those positions, and waiting at those points of stillness for release. Gradually, the arm will discover, address and resolve the various tensions and traumas contained within the tissues;

gradually it will reach the more deeply ingrained persistent restrictions.

Anne had been suffering from persistent pains in her right arm for more than two years. She had no idea what might have caused it and couldn't remember any injuries or accidents. Various medical tests revealed nothing and several weeks of physiotherapy had not helped. She had lived with it for a long time, but was finding it increasingly limiting and frustrating.

Within the context of overall treatment, I took up contact on her arm, letting it hang loosely in mid-air, free of the couch or any other restriction. The arm seemed to have a mind of its own. It started to twist slowly and to pull back, further and further, far beyond what one might have expected to be comfortable (but with no discomfort) until it was fully stretched behind her back into an extremely twisted position (still with no discomfort). At this point, the arm came to a standstill, the movements in the arm settled into stillness, rhythmic motion reached a still point – and after a few seconds, there was a powerful sense of release and softening. As the arm released, Anne suddenly remembered an incident three years earlier when she had been taking her dog for a walk. The dog had seen a cat going in the opposite direction and had taken off at high speed in the direction of the cat, dragging Anne's arm with it. The forces imposed upon Anne's arm and the patterns of tension set up by the sudden pulling had been held into the tissues ever since, gradually becoming more and more consolidated. Allowing the arm to find its way back to that original position of injury enabled the release of those forces, and as so often happens in fascial unwinding, as the tissues released, a vivid memory of the incident came to mind. Anne's symptoms disappeared immediately.

Allowing the arm to move through the air not only allows it to discover and address all these patterns, but also enables the process to identify the force vectors that were imprinted into the tissues at the time of the injury in that particular position and that have contributed to those patterns – in other words not just dissolving the restriction, but also eliminating the forces that were maintaining, perpetuating or reintroducing those restrictions. This is one way in which fascial unwinding addresses those forces more specifically than other cranio-sacral work.

These forces include external forces imposed by the injury and internal forces due to protective muscular and neurological reactions. These moments of discovery can often be quite dramatic in re-creating the specific combination of circumstances experienced at the time of injury – with the release in the tissues often simultaneously bringing up not only vivid memories of long-forgotten incidents that caused the injury, but also widespread responses of release throughout the body on many levels – emotional, neurological, sympathetic, physical.

Harry was a carpenter. At least he had been a carpenter. He was only in his early forties, but he was no longer able to work because his shoulders and arms had seized up so badly that he could hardly move them and certainly couldn't do his job as a carpenter. He had no explanation for his predicament; it has just gradually developed over the years, steadily becoming worse and worse. Of course he had been to the doctor and had had extensive physiotherapy and osteopathy, but his shoulders and arms simply continued to seize up more and more tightly.

They were certainly very restricted. It was difficult to get any movement out of them, especially the right shoulder. Within the context of overall treatment, I worked particularly with fascial unwinding on his right arm and shoulder. Progress was slow. For the first few sessions, there was only a slight increase in mobility, but Harry felt that there was at least some progress. During the sixth session, we were working as usual on unwinding his arm; as usual there was very little movement, but at least there was a little more each session. We reached a still point, and as so often with Harry the still point lasted a long time. Suddenly he cried out in pain and at the same time he announced:

> *'I've just remembered something very strange. When I was 16, I was an apprentice carpenter, and me and the lads were working on this old house, cutting out rafters from the roof. We had to saw through these thick wooden beams above our heads and it was tough. My shoulder got really painful, but of course I didn't want to look feeble in front of my mates, so I had to keep sawing. I've just felt that very same pain again in my shoulder. It's really weird. I haven't thought about that for years.'*

Harry hadn't wanted to look weak in front of his mates. He had suppressed the pain in order to carry on working. He had suppressed the pain by tightening up the surrounding muscles and he had been doing that ever since, building up layer upon layer of tension to prevent the old injury from rising to the surface, until his shoulder was so tense that he could hardly move it.

As we gradually unwound the layers of tension that had accumulated over the years, we eventually uncovered the original injury. At that point he re-experienced the pain of the injury, and simultaneously experienced a vivid memory of the incident – something he hadn't thought about for almost 30 years – as the tissue memory was released. As that happened, there was a profound release in his shoulder; the tissues softened and his whole shoulder and arm became vastly more mobile. The pain passed fairly quickly and Harry was pleased with the new-found mobility in his shoulder and arm. He needed a few more treatments, but soon he was back at work, able to do his job as a carpenter again after years of feeling that he would never work again.

Pain is not a common or necessary feature of fascial unwinding. In Harry's case, he happened to experience some pain briefly, but the vast majority of fascial unwinding doesn't involve any pain at all. We will explore later how to respond to the emergence of pain.

THE PROCESS

Preparatory articulation

With all unwinding processes, it is helpful to prepare the way with some initial articulation of the appropriate part of the body. Articulation is not a cranio-sacral process; it is widely used in many therapies; it involves moving limbs, joints or other parts of the body in order to loosen them up and enable them to move more freely. In the context of fascial unwinding, articulation helps to relax the patient and to release very quickly a lot of the superficial tensions that may be present, so that the unwinding process itself can focus on more significant, more deeply embedded patterns.

Standing at the side of the patient (who is lying on their back on the couch) gently take up contact – with one hand supporting the upper arm just above the elbow, the other hand supporting the wrist, lifting the arm (and your hands) clear of the couch. Starting with smaller movements, gradually explore and expand the range of comfortable movement of the arm – flexing and extending the wrist, flexing and extending the elbow, loosely moving the whole arm around in various directions to encourage greater looseness and flexibility, to encourage the patient to let go of any tensions.

In some patients, the arm will already be very loose and relaxed and not much is needed in the way of articulation. Others find it very difficult to let go, either through long-standing stiffness and tension, or protective tension around an injury, or simply through an inability to let go. These patients may need a great deal more articulation – and the process of articulation, and particularly helping them to learn to let go can be very therapeutic in itself. But for the most part, articulation is a brief preparatory process lasting around a minute or so.

Loosening and relaxing the tissues is not the only purpose of articulation. It also serves another very useful diagnostic purpose, enabling the therapist to assess the overall quality of the arm, the overall level of tension and restriction in the arm and in the body generally, the ability of the patient to relax and let go, the range of motion of the arm and of the individual joints of the arm, and any specific areas of restriction that may be evident even at this early stage.

Although the articulation may be brief, it is helpful to explore the full range of comfortable movement in order to clear the way as much as possible for the unwinding process itself. Along with the various articulatory movements mentioned previously, a particularly valuable movement is *circumduction* of the shoulder, taking the arm as far up towards the head as is comfortable for the patient, before continuing round, back and down again. In order for articulation to be most effective, it is vital to explore the extremes of comfortable movement. It is at these extremes, when you begin to feel the resistance in the tissues, that the articulation is having its beneficial effect. Otherwise you may just be waving the arm around ineffectually.

Some patients may arrive with a painful condition, or a condition which readily becomes painful on movement – such as a frozen shoulder or an acute tendonitis. It is of course always necessary to check with your patient beforehand to see if there is any acutely painful condition which might preclude such an extensive range of articulation. It is also vital to ask them to inform you if they experience any discomfort – because you don't want your patients to be in pain, and it is on the whole not helpful or necessary for them to go through any pain. It is also therefore wise to check with them regularly throughout the process that they are comfortable – and to observe and monitor the patient's reaction, both during the articulation and during the unwinding, in order to ensure that they are not experiencing any unnecessary pain. The idea is to explore and extend the full range of *comfortable* movement, not to force the tissues to painful extremes.

(Some patients, especially the more stoical elderly patients or more macho men, won't tell you that they are experiencing pain – however many times you ask them to tell you. They will insist that they can cope and that they don't mind going through a bit of pain – but that's not the point. You don't want them to be enduring pain and putting up with it and being brave. Pain is not helpful to the therapeutic process; pain makes the body tighten up, however stoical the owner of the pain may be; you need them to relax and be at ease and to keep you informed of any pain so that you can keep any pain to a minimum and monitor the process more accurately, in order for the therapeutic process to be most effective. So watch your patient carefully, and if you see them clenching their teeth, or screwing up their face in agony, suspect that they might not be telling you the full story.)

Once the articulation is complete, you can gently let the arm come to rest into its original position, with the elbow on the couch and the hand resting on the abdomen. (This is usually more comfortable than placing the whole arm straight on the couch beside the patient.)

Clear distinction between articulation and unwinding

It is helpful to establish a clear distinction between the end of the articulation and the start of the unwinding process – bringing the more active process of articulation to a definite conclusion, and taking time to re-establish your own practitioner fulcrums before entering into a different mode – the more passive, allowing process of unwinding. The two processes might look similar, but they are very different and require a different intention and mindset. It is vital to ensure that any tendency to articulate is not carried through into the unwinding.

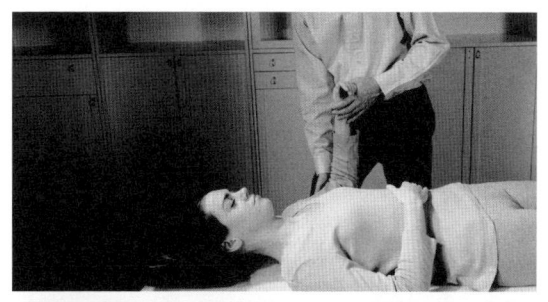

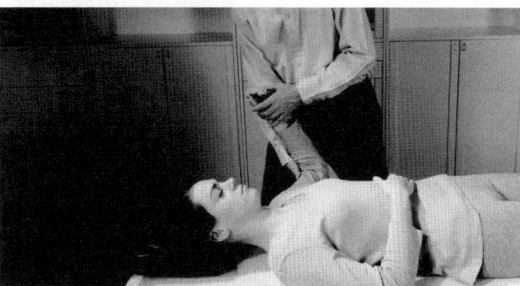

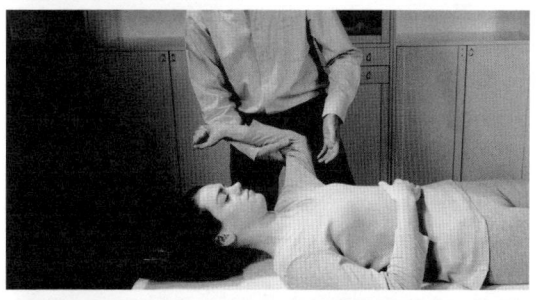

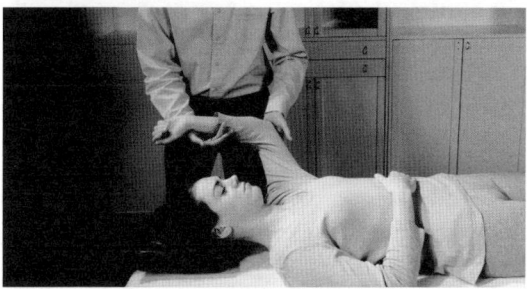

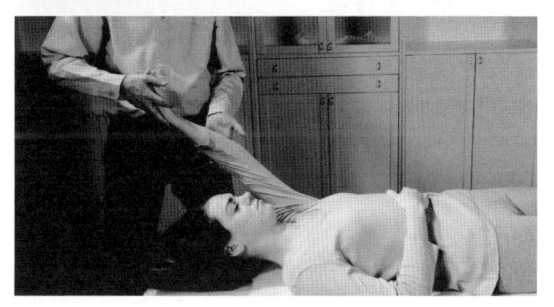

41.2 Fascial unwinding of the arm – allow the arm to perform its own intricate dance through the air, unwinding and unravelling the tensions held in the tissues, re-discovering the positions in which it was injured or traumatised, reaching points of stillness at those positions, and waiting at those points of stillness for release

Unwinding

Taking up contact

Take up contact as before, with one hand supporting the upper arm just above the elbow, the other hand supporting the wrist. Both hands are simply supporting – not holding, gripping, or restricting the arm in any way, simply supporting against gravity. Let the wrist hang limply over your supportive fingers. Let the arm rest softly into your loose, relaxed hand. The arm and your hands need to be completely free of the couch, suspended in mid-air, free to move in whatever direction they may wish.

Establish a balanced, relaxed, starting position for the arm, not over-extended away from the patient's body (incurring resistance), not compressed against the patient's body (leaving them feeling squashed), not lifted up too far or overstretched in any way. Feel the looseness and softness of the arm.

Establishing your own practitioner fulcrums

Having established this loose starting position, re-establish your own practitioner fulcrums – physically and mentally. As usual, most of your attention (90 per cent) needs to be on yourself.

Because fascial unwinding is a more visibly mobile process, and because the practitioner is standing up, it may initially be more difficult to maintain a sense of stillness, softness, ease and relaxation within yourself. It is therefore all the more important to give extra attention to this, throughout the whole unwinding process, checking that your shoulders drop, your arms hang loosely, and that you remain completely at ease, while gently maintaining the contact under the elbow and wrist. (Experience of the Alexander technique can be very helpful in this.)

Having established this starting position and established your own fulcrums, allow yourself to settle into the process of engagement, aware of any impressions that may come to you. Again, because fascial unwinding is a more visibly mobile process, there is a greater tendency for the practitioner to move, to initiate movement, to impose movement, to try and help the process along, and to become more involved in the process. It is essential to counteract this tendency and avoid any tendency to join in, or impose on the body in any way.

Be still

Be patient; don't be in a hurry; simply wait for the impressions to come to you in their own time. Be aware of the quality of the arm, and of the different parts of the arm. Be aware of any pulls, twists, turns or movements of any kind. Be aware of every little subtlety of movement.

The process

As the unwinding process begins, observe the usual evolution of the inherent treatment process – allowing the system to express itself, allowing the tissues to unwind, allowing movement to occur, and gently following the system wherever it may lead you – not doing anything, not helping it along, not joining in – just allowing yourself to be drawn this way and that by the subtle fluidic movements of the system.

Initially there may be no movement at all. Be prepared to wait patiently; the first movements may be very small, subtle, internal movements within the tissues. Be alert to every tiny microscopic movement, since identifying these subtle movements will often be the key that unlocks the way to further more expansive movements.

Take great care not to impose upon the body. Remain soft and fluidic. Again, take great care not to join in with the movements at all. At the same time, however, in your determination to avoid initiating any movement yourself, take care also not to become rigid, thereby blocking the natural inherent movement. It is a fine balance.

As the movements become gradually more expansive, different parts of the arm may be twisting and turning in different directions. Try to follow all the various movements simultaneously, keeping an overview of the whole picture while at the same time following every subtle detail within that picture.

As the process progresses, the arm will perform its slow gentle dance through the air, expressing and releasing the various patterns of tension and restriction held into the tissues.

Moving your own body fluently

At various points, the arm may move in such a way that it becomes necessary for you to adjust your position, in order to accommodate the movements of the arm. First, it may become necessary to change your hand position and you can let your hands glide smoothly from one position to another as necessary, taking care not to disturb or disrupt the fluency of the unwinding process through sudden, abrupt or excessive movement.

As the arm starts to move more expansively, it may become necessary to move your whole body. When this becomes necessary, try to anticipate that need so that you don't find yourself overstretched and unable to move, or at least unable to move fluently. When you do need to move, it is again essential to move fluently and smoothly without disturbing the continuity of the process. The slightest break in continuity may result in losing track of the process and losing engagement. Once you have lost this, it may not be easy to recapture it and it may therefore be necessary to start again. Moving your own body fluently takes care and practice, learning to move one foot first, shift your weight from one leg to the other, then gently move the other foot, always maintaining undisturbed fluency and focus on the unwinding process. (The practice of Tai Chi can be very helpful in developing this skill.)

As you become more deeply engaged with the unwinding process, you may feel an increasing sense of weightlessness in the arm, as if it takes on a life of its own, hardly needing you there at all. Your hand contact can become lighter and lighter, a mere finger contact, softly monitoring the changes in quality and motion as the arm proceeds independently on its own journey of discovery.

Identify focal points of resistance

As the process continues, you will experience different qualities at different times – tightness, looseness, resistance, release, moments of stillness, phases of movement. Keep following the system wherever it leads you until it reaches points of stillness, and stay with that stillness until it softens, melts and dissolves. As always, minor resistances may release within seconds; other more deeply ingrained injuries may take several minutes, or may release partially, layer by layer, coming back repeatedly to the same point, to release further layers until the restriction is completely cleared.

Staying with the stillness

At these points of stillness, you are likely to encounter a significant tendency in the cranio-sacral process, a tendency which is evident in all cranio-sacral work, but perhaps (like many things) more clearly identifiable in the larger scale landscape of fascial unwinding. The cranio-sacral system in its wisdom, knows where to go, how to find resistances, how to lead to those points of stillness and how to release those restrictions. And yet, often when it gets there, it will tend to shy away from those very points that it has chosen to approach, apparently avoiding them instead of addressing them.

This is due to the body's protective mechanisms. It is an indication of a contradiction between two aspects of the body's wisdom. On the one hand it wishes to address the restriction. On the other hand it has protective mechanisms to enable the body to cope and adapt around such restrictions until they are resolved. So one aspect of the system is saying, 'Let's go and address this restriction'; another part is saying, 'Let's avoid that injured area so as not to release those protective layers which are shielding it from feeling pain, further injury, emotion, or painful memories'.

The body needs a little help here to resolve its inner conflict and to make the appropriate therapeutic decision.

The essence of cranio-sacral therapy is to allow and follow, but as we have seen there is also scope for stimulus – and there are times when the body needs a little help to maintain its resolve, to go through with its intentions and to address the restrictions fully, instead of giving in to the unhelpful protective devices that are blocking access to the site of restriction and thereby preventing healing and resolution.

In Harry's case, one aspect of the body's wisdom might have said, 'Let's avoid that area because it might bring up that old pain', thereby condemning Harry to lifelong tension and restriction in his shoulders. By helping the body to hold into the pattern, the resistance was addressed, he re-experienced that brief moment of pain, and the years of tension and restriction were released.

This is a fine line. On the one hand it is essential not to impose on the system, and yet at the same time it is helpful to assist the system in following through with its instinctive intentions. Extensive practice will gradually enable the practitioner to develop a highly refined skill in establishing the exact degree of attention to enable the most effective resolution of these profound therapeutic moments which are occurring constantly throughout the treatment process. As so often, experiencing them during the more macroscopic fascial unwinding process can be very helpful and insightful in recognising the same situations at the more microscopic level within core treatment, and refining your skills through fascial unwinding can again be very helpful in developing a more highly refined skill in core treatment.

Holding at the point of balanced tension

As with any cranio-sacral work, when you encounter a point of stillness, the quality is likely to change. There may be a vibrant, alive, squirming, pulsating, wriggling quality, as if the body were trying to deal with something – all of which is an indication that you are identifying a significant point of restriction. At this point, as always, it is essential to stay with the stillness, holding into the point of balanced tension, not allowing it to escape or shy away, not being fooled into thinking that this is a release. Recognise the value of this dynamic stillness while continuing to identify the tiny subtle movements within the stillness. Be content to stay as long as is necessary, until you feel a convincing sense of softening and release. Following a release, the arm may continue on its journey in search of further points of resistance.

These points of stillness within the broader movements of fascial unwinding are sometimes referred to as the 'eye of the hurricane'. Just as there is stillness at the centre of a hurricane, so there is stillness at the centre of the gentle swirling activity of the fascial unwinding process, and it is these moments of stillness (together with the releases which emanate from them) which are the key therapeutic moments in the fascial unwinding process. Because fascial unwinding involves movement, it is easy to gain the mistaken impression that movement is what it is all about. It is not about movement, it is about stillness. The movements are necessary, but they are only leading to the points of stillness. They are not in themselves profoundly therapeutic. They are just the means towards an end.

Recognise the value of stillness

As in all cranio-sacral work, these points of stillness are the most vital element of the unwinding process – the key moments in the therapeutic process. Failing to stay with these points of stillness sufficiently will render the whole fascial unwinding process meaningless and pointless. It might still feel quite pleasant and relaxing, but without the points of stillness, it is essentially just waving the arm around.

Maintain focus

If the arm is waving around loosely and aimlessly, it is probably not doing anything effective. It is necessary to keep it in focus. This can be helped by maintaining a slight thought of traction throughout the process – just a thought, not a physical pull – in order to maintain a sense of balanced tension within the tissues – not floppy, not overstretched. This is another fine line to maintain. It will help the body to maintain a sense of alert engagement and to identify the points of resistance and the direction which the tissues need to follow.

Reaching a conclusion

Following a significant release, the arm can be allowed to unwind its way back to its original starting position. Many unwinding processes will come to a natural conclusion following the release of a more significant resistance, or following the release of many lesser resistances, with the arm gently unwinding its way back to its original position – elbow on the couch, hand on the abdomen. An appropriate moment at which to let the process come to a conclusion is following a release; it is not of course appropriate to bring the process to an end in mid-process.

Completion

When the arm has found its way back to its original starting position, you can gently let the arm rest back down and release your contacts. Within the context of an overall treatment process, you could then continue with the treatment, or check the balance of the cranio-sacral system as a whole, checking that any changes have been integrated and that the system feels settled before bringing the treatment to an end.

Some further considerations

If the process doesn't start readily

If, at the beginning of the unwinding, when you have taken up contact, the unwinding process doesn't start readily and spontaneously, it may be necessary to explore certain possible reasons for this:

- Check that the patient is relaxed, not tensing up, or holding on. Invite them to take a deep breath and let go. This may also be helpful at various times throughout the unwinding process if the patient is tending to tighten up, as many patients do. In this process we do not want the patient to join in with the movements at all.
- Check that you yourself are completely relaxed and at ease, physically and mentally, and not restricting the process in any way. *This is the most common reason for the apparent lack of progress.* As already mentioned, most (90%) of your attention needs to be on yourself. Remind yourself of this a thousand times over. Breathe, let go, settle into deeper softness and deeper spaciousness, repeatedly softening in your shoulders, your elbows and your hands, consistently, again and again.
- Wait patiently for the process to start; don't try to rush it or impose in any way.
- If there is still no response, you can ask questions of the arm, offer the arm various options – not doing anything, just asking – but asking with your hands. For example, ask if the elbow would like to flex, to extend, to internally rotate or to externally rotate – but always taking care only to invite these options, not imposing them at all – and see if it responds to that invitation. Often the arm will start to respond, and once it gets going, it is likely to proceed of its own accord from there.
- If there is still no response, you could try offering a very gentle thought of traction, as a stimulus in order to bring the process into clearer focus. As with all cranio-sacral stimuli, it is just a thought, transmitted through your hands – the thought of traction is enough of a stimulus.

Using traction to maintain focus

As mentioned, a gentle thought of traction can be used from time to time or throughout the unwinding process, as a way of maintaining the focus and maintaining a balanced tension within the system. The degree of traction must be very finely balanced, taking care not to impose on the system. Excessive traction will create a defensive protective reaction; the tissues will tighten up and the process will stop. On the other hand allowing the arm to become too floppy and loose will result in ineffectual, aimless movements that don't lead anywhere or have any significant therapeutic effect.

In order to gain this fine balance, imagine that you are holding a piece of elastic (or even practise with a piece of elastic). For effective unwinding that piece of elastic needs to be held at just the right point of balanced tension, not overstretched and not allowed to go slack, but maintained continuously at the border line between stretching and slackness.

As the arm continues its journey, it will be necessary to follow very carefully with a high degree of alertness – taking up the slack when it seems to go floppy, taking care not to impose when it becomes more resistant, following every subtlety and identifying every subtle twist and turn within the larger movements. Take care not to impose at all; take care not to get carried away by larger more sudden movements.

Finishing

If, after some time, the unwinding process doesn't want to come to an end, there are various ways of helping it to do so. Firstly, through your intention, give the message that it is time for it to come to an end. Secondly, start to follow only the patterns that lead back towards the original starting position, not following into any new directions. Thirdly, it may be necessary to ask the patient to allow the arm to come back gently to its original position. Whichever way you choose, the arm must be allowed to find its own way back, gently and slowly, rather than simply being put back abruptly or imposed upon in any way.

Pain

We briefly mentioned pain earlier, noting that it may arise during fascial unwinding and noting the need to ask the patient to tell you if they experience any pain.

Fascial unwinding is generally painless, even in acutely painful conditions. There are times however when encountering the edge of pain and hovering gently at the very edge of the pain – where it can be felt mildly but is not excessive – can be the most effective way to address a restriction and enable release (whereas avoiding the site of pain may mean avoiding addressing the issue completely). Teaching the patient to respond appropriately to the pain – relaxing into it rather than contracting against it – can be a highly significant and effective aspect of the therapeutic process.

George had a persistent pain in his left shoulder and arm, a sharp pain in the front of the shoulder which hit him every time he lifted his arm beyond a certain range. It had been with him for years since an injury while sailing. He had received substantial treatment of various kinds, but the pain persisted and he had become resigned to just living with the pain and the restriction that it imposed on his life. Within the context of overall treatment, as I took up his arm, it was very willing to unwind, but as we reached a certain point, George felt the pain and tightened up, preventing the unwinding process from proceeding. Easing off very slightly to the point where the pain was just barely noticeable, I asked George to take a deep breath and let go. As he did so the pain eased, and the arm moved a little further into its chosen direction. Again the pain arose and George tightened up; again I encouraged George to breathe and let go. Again the pain eased and the unwinding proceeded a little further. By now George was getting the idea; each time as the pain arose, we waited at the edge of the pain, George relaxed into the pain, the pain eased, the tissues softened and the unwinding progressed further. In this way the unwinding process was able to proceed gradually but steadily and George's arm reached positions it had not encountered in many years – and without any pain. His pain was soon resolved and George commented that this concept of relaxing into the pain using his breathing had undoubtedly been the factor that had enabled the release of his shoulder, which had been unresponsive to so many other approaches.

A significant part of this particular process is the retraining of the mind and the tissues to respond differently to the experience of pain and to the site of injury – learning to observe the pain objectively, responding to the pain and the injury and any emotional associations with calmness and equanimity.

In doing this, the patient can learn to counteract the inherent protective tendency to react and contract the tissues and suppress the pain – a protective mechanism which can be useful when you have to cope with an emergency out in the wild, but which can prevent access to the source of the injury when the protective tensions become chronically established. So when it is appropriate to work at the edge of the pain, it is helpful to encourage your patient to breathe, relax and let go – and to explain this process to them.

As we have seen with Harry, pain may also arise briefly at the moment of release, perhaps accompanied by memories of the incident that caused the injury. This is usually mild and very transient, and the combination of the release, the memory and the brief reliving of the pain may serve as a clear indication that the injury has been accessed, addressed and released – most evidently because the patient then feels the significant improvement in their condition.

Deirdre had broken her arm two years earlier. The fracture had healed, but she had been left with persistent pain in the forearm and wrist. This was particularly evident whenever she tried to write, at which point the pain would increase rapidly and spread up through her arm into her shoulder, neck and upper back, leaving her feeling tense, uncomfortable and unable to think clearly. She tried to avoid writing, but this was obviously very difficult within the demands of everyday life. She had received various treatments, including cranio-sacral therapy addressing the core, but not including fascial unwinding. Nothing had helped.

As her arm started to unwind, it performed the usual dance, finding its way to the position in which it had been injured. As it reached that point of stillness, Deirdre felt a powerful surge of energy, like a powerful wave surging through the very core of her body and every part of her body; she began to feel very hot; she became very conscious of her diaphragm and started breathing very forcefully; her whole body started to pull into a twisted contorted position, shaking visibly.

The fascial unwinding process had connected with the shock imposed at the time of the original injury and held into her system ever since. As the trauma released, everything settled down. Deirdre felt weak and shaky and warm for a while, but she also felt very loose and felt a huge sense of relief. The quality of her whole body had changed, her face had changed; she felt relaxed and comfortable. The pain in her arm gradually disappeared over the next few days and she was able to write again without any discomfort.

Chapter 42

Fascial Unwinding of the Leg

There are many reasons why it might be appropriate to unwind the leg or some part of the leg. Some of the more obvious situations might include sprained ankles – recent or long past, twisted knees, old fractures, persistent pains and strains anywhere in the leg, restricted hip joints, sports injuries, achilles tendonitis, knee ligament strain.

The legs are also an integral part of the rest of the body, and more significantly, are supporting the rest of the body, in use most of the time in everyday life from the moment we get out of bed in the morning. There is therefore a very significant postural interaction between the legs and the rest of the body (more so than with the arms). Every restriction or lingering imbalance in any part of the leg can have ramifications throughout the body, resulting in postural imbalances and consequent strain in the neck, upper back, lower back, and at various pivotal areas of the spine with potential resultant symptoms of headache and neck pain, or discomfort, tightness and visceral dysfunction anywhere in the body.

Compressive activities such as jogging, jumping and various other sports and also dancing can instil compressive forces through the legs which are transmitted up to the rest of the body with various compensatory effects throughout the body, which may need to be addressed through the legs.

Injuries and pain in the foot, ankle or knee often lead people to shift their weight to the other leg, resulting in symptoms either in the other leg (which is consequently overworking) or in other areas of the body affected by the postural imbalance. This can present a confusing picture, which is often misdiagnosed in therapeutic modalities which follow symptoms rather than causes and which try to address the symptoms in the other leg or elsewhere in the body – not realising that the cause is in the original leg injury (which is no longer displaying symptoms). Appropriate whole body assessment through cranio-sacral integration can readily identify that the underlying cause is emanating from the original leg injury.

Sprained ankles are common; they mostly heal, but often leave lingering effects either in the ankle or elsewhere. Many times I have treated patients with a variety of symptoms in various parts of the body and traced the pattern to a previous sprained ankle perhaps ten or twenty years ago.

Louise was a medical secretary and she suffered from a variety of symptoms. She had lower back pain, upper back pain, neck pain, headaches. When the back pain became uncomfortable it affected her digestion and her neck and shoulders became tight. None of her symptoms were severe, but they were a constant discomfort and, most frustratingly, they had been troubling her for many years. She had received regular osteopathic treatment for years and substantial cranial osteopathy and cranio-sacral therapy. This treatment usually made her feel better temporarily, but the symptoms would always return.

When I tuned in to her system, I was immediately drawn to her right ankle. Restrictions in her ankle were exerting fascial pulls that were drawing her pelvis out of alignment, creating a series of imbalances up through her spine, leading to strain and pain at various points, mostly involving the standard mechanical pivots in the spine and especially affecting the thoraco-lumbar junction (T12/L1 vertebral level) disturbing her digestion and the cervico-thoracic junction (C7/T1 vertebral level) with repercussions on her neck and shoulders.

She hadn't mentioned her ankle, so I asked her about it and she replied that she had sprained her ankle about fifteen years ago but it was so long ago that she didn't think it was worth mentioning; and it didn't trouble her – as long as she didn't run…or play sport…or dance… or go for long walks, which she used to love to do before her ankle injury. It seemed that her whole life had been changed by this ankle injury, but she had simply got used to the limitations, adapted her life and accepted that she would never be able to do any of these things that she loved doing.

The extensive treatment that she had received regularly brought her body back into alignment and felt better for a while, but it wasn't addressing the source of the imbalance, so these fascial pulls from the ankle kept reinstating the imbalance along with the various associated symptoms. No one had treated her ankle. No one had done any fascial unwinding.

Ten minutes of fascial unwinding on her ankle released the restriction. The fascia was no longer pulling her pelvis out of alignment. Her body could settle into a balanced comfortable state again – and stay there. She felt the difference immediately, throughout her whole body. Louise didn't need any further treatment, but she came back from time to time for an occasional check-up, very pleased at being able to dance again and to resume her treasured long walks and all the other activities that her ankle and body were now able to carry out without any discomfort or adverse repercussions.

It is essential in every situation, whatever and wherever the symptoms, first to look at the whole picture, with the understanding that symptoms anywhere in the body may arise from anywhere else in the body, however remote; and second, to integrate the whole person – as the only means to efficient overall function.

This also applies the other way round – in other words it is also essential to establish when symptoms in the legs may be arising due to a cause elsewhere. If a patient has numbness and pins and needles in their foot, it would probably not be an appropriate approach to unwind the foot (where the symptoms are) since the symptoms are probably an indication of sciatic nerve impingement and the cause is more likely to be in the lower back. Similarly, if a patient has painful knees due to rheumatoid arthritis, it would not be appropriate to unwind the joints, since the cause is in the systemic disease of rheumatoid arthritis rather than in local soft tissue strains (one could still treat a patient with rheumatoid arthritis through cranio-sacral therapy but not using fascial unwinding of the knees). Obviously it would also not be appropriate to use fascial unwinding on any part of the body that had recently been fractured (again one can still treat with cranio-sacral therapy but not with fascial unwinding locally).

As with the arm, any treatment of the leg would involve assessing and treating the whole person, and addressing any factors specifically relevant to the legs. This would include the overall balance of the patient, the balance of the pelvis, and awareness of the nerve supply to the legs through the lumbo-sacral plexus, including the femoral and obturator nerves, emanating from the spine at L2, L3 and L4 (the second, third and fourth lumbar vertebrae), passing through the psoas muscle and down to the anterior and medial thigh respectively, and the sciatic nerve with its roots at L4, L5, S1, S2 and S3 (the fourth, and fifth lumbar vertebrae and the first, second and third sacral segments), passing down the posterior thigh to the lower leg and foot.

Principles

The principles for unwinding of the leg are much the same as for unwinding the arm. In order to avoid excessive repetition, it is assumed that the reader has read Chapters 38–41 on fascial unwinding and fascial unwinding of the arm. The main differences occur in the practicalities of handling the leg – which is of course larger and heavier than the arm.

The weight of the leg

In view of its greater size, it is helpful to take up contacts on the leg which minimise the effects of this greater size and weight, thereby enabling the practitioner to focus more specifically on the unwinding process, rather than being weighed down and distracted by substantial gravitational pulls and other aspects of handling a heavy limb.

Focusing on a specific localised region – while maintaining integration

With this in mind, it can be helpful to focus on a specific localised region of the leg – the ankle, the knee, the hip – rather than trying to treat the whole limb at once – always bearing in mind of course the integration of the whole leg, the relationships between different sections of the leg, and the integration with the rest of the system.

An ankle injury may be primarily affecting the ankle but will inevitably have repercussions up through the rest of the limb and into the body as a whole, both through the fascia and through postural compensations. Similarly a knee injury may be primarily localised within the knee but will inevitably have ramifications down towards the ankle and foot and up to the hip, the pelvis, the trunk and the rest of the body. It is always necessary to address all the interrelated influences and interactions between the different parts of the body rather than treating any section in isolation. This is particularly significant where the injury or pattern is long-standing, such that compensations and adaptations may have become deeply embedded through the body, with widespread implications in terms of symptoms and other functional disturbances. If these compensatory factors are not addressed they may act as maintaining factors which perpetuate the condition, leading to recurrence of the local problem in the leg. The whole body needs to be taken into account, but particularly any imbalances of the pelvis or around the L3 vertebra.

There are many different ways of taking up contact on the leg, some of which are more specifically focused on the ankles, some more on the knees, some more on the hip – and some of which will enable a more comprehensive evaluation and treatment of the whole leg.

In order to focus primarily on the ankle, it is not particularly necessary to take up the weight of the whole leg; the leg can remain lying on the couch and contact can be taken up more specifically on the ankle.

When you want to address the hip and its surrounding structures, you can take up contacts which specifically focus on that area.

The most effective contact for integration

When treating the knee specifically, the leg needs freedom to explore the full mobility of the knee in the many directions in which it may have been injured. Greater freedom of movement is therefore necessary for the whole lower limb. Consequently it is this contact for the knee which enables the most effective integration of the whole lower limb.

Injuries and traumas can also occur anywhere else in the lower limb – not just in the ankle, knee and hip – and contacts can be adapted to address whatever factors may be relevant.

The ankle

In order to treat the ankle, first check that your patient is lying comfortably and symmetrically supine on the couch. Check that their feet are within reach of the end of the couch. Invite them to take a deep breath and to relax completely.

Articulation

Start by articulating the ankle in order to release any superficial tensions and restrictions. As always, this articulation can be brief but comprehensive. It can briefly cover all the many different joints within the area, exploring the comfortable extremes of motion in every direction – including dorsiflexion, plantarflexion, inversion, eversion, internal rotation, external rotation, and circumduction (see Figure 42.1). A comprehensive and fairly physical articulation of the whole foot and ankle, mobilising all the tarsals, metatarsals and the toes, can be very therapeutic in itself and is often much appreciated by patients.

Taking up contact

Having loosened up the ankle, sit at the foot of the couch, taking up a comfortable contact which enables a comprehensive connection with the whole foot and ankle.

- Bring one hand from the lateral side of the foot to cradle underneath the ankle.
- Bring the other hand from the medial side of the foot to fit comfortably into the medial arch of the foot, the thumb extending under the sole of the foot, the fingers over the dorsum of the foot (see Figure 42.2).

Practitioner fulcrums

Having settled into this contact, let your hands and arms relax completely, ensuring that your contact is soft, light and gentle. Check your practitioner fulcrums.

Following the process

As you feel an increasing connection between your two systems, wait patiently for any impressions to come to you. Be aware of the quality of this foot and ankle, any differences in quality from one part

Fascial Unwinding of the Leg / 293

External rotation   Internal rotation

Eversion   Inversion

Dorsiflexion

Plantarflexion

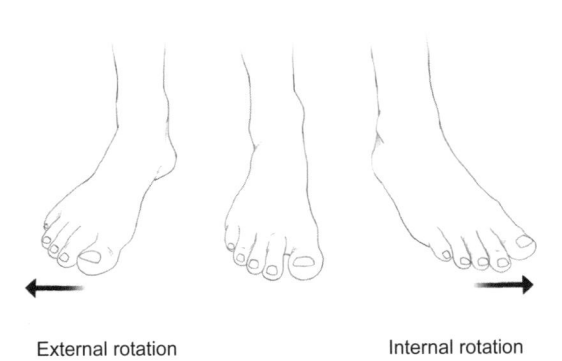

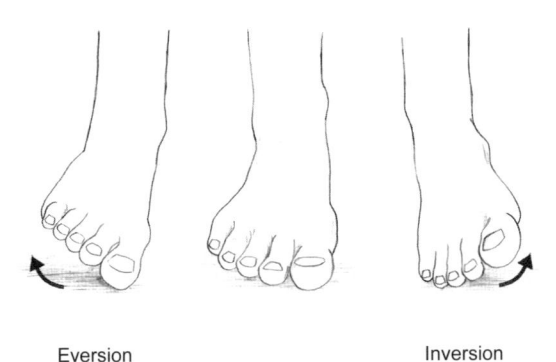

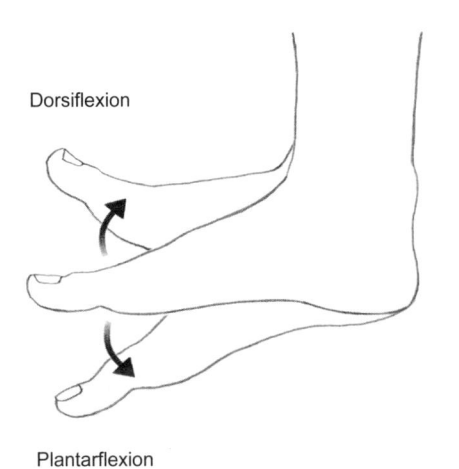

42.1 Articulation of the foot and ankle involves exploring the comfortable extremes of motion in every direction – including dorsiflexion, plantarflexion, inversion, eversion, internal rotation, external rotation, and circumduction

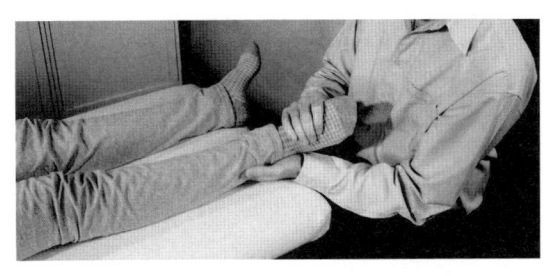

42.2 Initial contact for an unwinding of the ankle – take up a comfortable contact which enables a comprehensive connection with the whole foot and ankle

to another. Be aware of any pulls, twists or turns. Be aware of any tiny subtleties of movement that may unlock the way to larger scale movements.

Within the foot and ankle it is common to find very little in the way of large scale movements but there may be a great deal happening on a subtler level, within the many small joints of the foot and ankle and the many small muscles, ligaments and other tissues, with their various fascial coverings.

Where an ankle has been more severely injured or sprained, you are more likely to encounter a stronger larger scale pull into the direction of injury.

Allow the inherent treatment process to evolve. Allow your hands to float freely on the surface of these movements, allowing patterns of movement to be expressed, encountering points of stillness and release.

There may be a multitude of minor patterns which readily release. As the unwinding process continues, the overall picture may become clearer and more persistent underlying patterns may become apparent.

Projecting through the body

As you follow these patterns and stay with points of stillness, you can use your attention to trace the source of the pattern and the extent of the pattern, either drawn spontaneously to focal points elsewhere, or surveying through the foot and ankle and up the leg, perhaps to the knee, perhaps to the hip, perhaps to the pelvis, perhaps further up the body, observing any changes that occur as you take your attention to different areas and different levels – changes in quality, changes in movement, changes in resistance.

Stubborn resistances

Observe how the pattern may intensify as your attention reaches the source of the resistance, and how it gives way as the restriction releases.

For example, the foot and ankle may be unwinding gently and fluently until they come across a point of resistance within which you feel a tighter quality on, for instance, the lateral side – at which point the unwinding seems to become stuck against this resistance. Take your attention up through the body, while still holding into this resistance, and you may find that the tightness intensifies. Then perhaps at the knee (if that is the original source of the restriction) the sense of restriction may further intensify, start to wriggle and shake, to pulsate and finally to give way, releasing the source of the restriction within the knee, and consequently releasing the restriction all the way down the lateral leg to the foot and ankle. As this release occurs, not only have the foot and ankle released, but also you will have enabled the release of the restriction in the knee – and identified the source of the restriction as being in the knee.

Similarly, with different patterns you may encounter resistances which draw up to the hip, the sacro-iliac area, the pelvis, or somewhere in the trunk, the neck or the cranium. In every case you can project your attention up to trace the source of the resistance, enabling the release of the source of the resistance wherever it may be in the body, with consequent release of the pattern throughout the body. However, if you encounter a strong resistance, particularly from a long established deeply embedded chronic problem, you may decide that it would be more appropriate to leave your contact at the ankle and to go directly to the source of that resistance in order to treat directly at the source.

Completion

Once the foot and ankle have unwound through whatever patterns have manifested and have reached a point of release, and you feel that the process is complete, you can allow the foot and ankle to settle back to a comfortable, relaxed neutral position, check that the quality feels settled and balanced and then gently release your contacts before moving on.

Reassessing

You could then reassess the balance of the whole system through the feet. The contact at the dorsum of both feet (described in Chapter 39 on Evaluation of the fascia) is a very valuable contact for assessing the whole system. It is a contact which is likely to be used frequently.

The unwinding of the foot and ankle is a much more specific process which is likely only to be used where there are specific patterns of restriction arising from that area.

The knee

The contact described here for the knee is the contact which most effectively and comprehensively incorporates the whole of the lower limb. It is therefore a very valuable contact for evaluating and integrating the leg as a whole.

Articulation

It is helpful to precede the unwinding process with articulation, again taking the whole lower limb gently through its extremes of comfortable movement, flexing and extending the knee, flexing and extending the hip, rotating the lower leg in relation to the upper leg at the knee, circumducting the hip, releasing muscular and soft tissue tensions.

Taking up contact in preparation for unwinding

In order to unwind the knee it is necessary to give the leg full freedom to unwind, both below the knee in the lower leg and above the knee in the upper leg. For this contact it is therefore helpful for the whole lower limb to be supported away from the restrictions of the couch and the rest of the body so that it can float freely in space.

Due to the size and weight of the leg, this can create practical problems in supporting the leg, particularly with a heavy leg. These practical difficulties can readily be overcome if certain suggestions regarding the contact are taken into account. However, if these suggestions are not taken into account then the whole process of unwinding the lower limb can be severely hampered by the practical problems of counteracting gravity and the difficulties involved in coping with the weight of the leg.

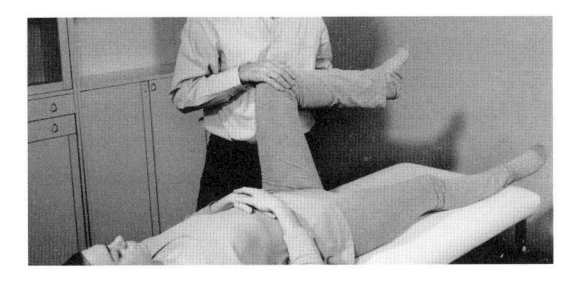

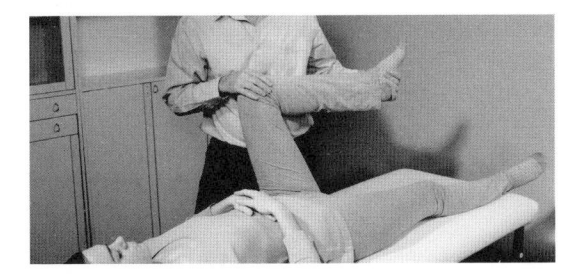

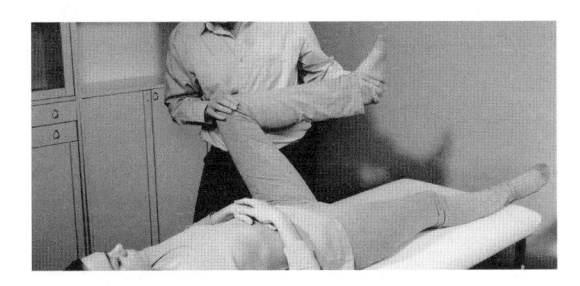

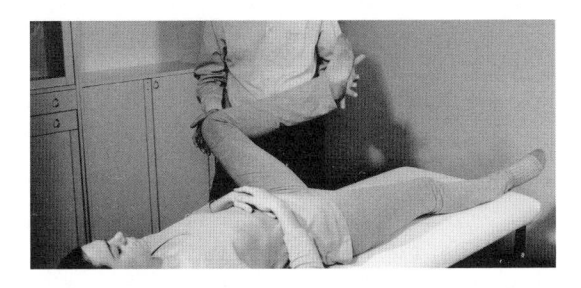

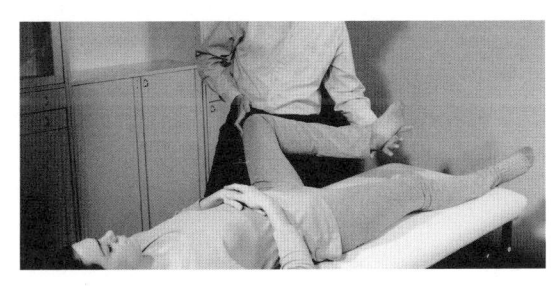

There are four main points to take into account in supporting the leg effectively:

- Bring the thigh up to a vertical position, at a 90-degree angle to the couch. This way the weight of the leg is passing down through the vertical axis of the thigh rather than constantly pulling the leg down to the couch again.

- Bring your own body close in so that the lateral side of the knee is supported by your chest or trunk. This enables the weight of the leg, whose natural tendency is to fall out laterally, to be supported by your body rather than by the strength of your arms. This is also essential in enabling the patient to feel adequately supported so that they can relax their leg completely and let go more fully.

- Place one hand under the sole of the foot (rather than under the heel). This again provides a firmer support, resisting the tendency of the leg to straighten out towards the couch. It also provides a more stable contact than holding under the heel. It also enables a more clear and accurate evaluation of the foot, ankle and lower leg, throughout the whole unwinding process.

- Allow your other hand to come to rest over the anterior surface of the knee with your fingers extending down the medial side of the knee. This hand is not particularly providing support, but with the leg adequately stabilised by the other three points, this hand can remain very relaxed and at ease and in this position can monitor any impressions from the knee. The contact down the medial side is significant, because it is the medial side of the knee that is most susceptible to damage, in the medial ligament and medial meniscus. The fingers of this hand will be able to monitor any stresses, strains and changes in quality in this area.

Minor adjustments to your own body position, both at the start and throughout the process, can also be highly significant in minimising the effort involved and therefore maximising your sensitivity and effectiveness. The inevitable tendency of the leg is to straighten out and down towards the

42.3 Fascial unwinding of the knee – allow the leg to unwind in whatever way it wants, following wherever it needs to go, finding points of stillness and release

couch. In establishing a neutral starting position, you need to counteract this tendency. In order to do so, it is helpful to turn your feet to point towards the patient's head, so that your body weight can easily counter the straightening of the leg, rather than using the strength of your arms, which may then become tired and less effective.

Maintain your practitioner fulcrums
Observing these suggestions should enable unwinding of even the heaviest leg without any significant effort or strain on your own body. If you are feeling any strain, then you are probably not giving enough attention to using and adjusting your own body appropriately. As you settle into the contact, check your own practitioner fulcrums, breathing easily and letting go completely – physically and mentally.

The process
As you settle in, be aware of any impressions that come to you, the quality of the limb as a whole, different qualities in different parts of the limb, any subtle movements that may start the unwinding process and lead you into larger scale movements. Be prepared to wait patiently. Don't be in a hurry for things to get started. It is essential that all unwinding comes from the patient's system and that you don't introduce or impose any movements on the system.

If you have effectively applied the four points mentioned above, most of the weight of the leg should be comfortably supported by those contacts. If you still find the leg difficult to handle, it may be that you are not applying those four points sufficiently effectively. Or that you need to adjust your own body position to enable more effective support. Again, minor adjustments to your own body position can make a significant difference, so be sensitive to your own body at all times, aware of any minor stresses and strains, adjusting accordingly, thereby minimising any effort and strain on your own body.

Even when you do have the leg adequately supported there will always be some tendency for the leg to be constantly trying to straighten out towards the couch. It is necessary to take this into account and to establish a minimum level of resistance which will counteract this tendency – without imposing unnecessary forces on the leg or restricting its freedom to unwind.

As the process unfolds, follow the usual principles of unwinding – allowing the leg to unwind in whatever way it wants, following wherever it needs to go, finding points of stillness, and releasing.

Maintain a constant awareness of yourself.

Maintain an overview of the whole lower limb while at the same time observing the details within different areas. Follow the different parts of the lower limb in different directions as necessary.

Maintain a balance between allowing the unwinding process, while counteracting gravity and the natural tendency of the leg to straighten – taking care not to impose any unnecessary forces on the leg.

Use your attention to survey
As usual, your attention may be drawn to particular pulls, patterns and focal points of resistance. As you encounter these points of resistance, use your attention to observe the extent of the patterns, surveying up or down the leg, feeling the changes in quality as you move your attention from place to place, observing as patterns intensify or fade away, as new pulls and twists appear or intensify, tracing patterns to their source. Use your attention to survey the whole lower limb and beyond, up into the body, to obtain an overall picture of the system while at the same time identifying the various details within that picture.

Move your own body fluently in order to maintain continuity
As the limb continues to unwind, you will need to move your own body to accommodate the movements of the leg. Take care to do this fluently and smoothly, without disturbing the continuity of the unwinding process. Anticipate the need to move, thinking about how you are going to move fluently and smoothly, preparing yourself for movement, moving slowly and gradually while maintaining your focus on the unwinding process. As mentioned, the practice of Tai Chi can be very helpful in enabling this smooth fluent movement of your own body.

As the limb unwinds and you move your body, there will also be an inevitable need to alter your hand contacts. Right from the start, allow your hands to be flexible and adaptable to the needs of the moment, ensuring constant sufficient support for the leg, while moving into whatever positions are most appropriate and comfortable to enable the unwinding process.

The initial part of any unwinding process is simply to allow the system to explore and discover its own patterns of movement. As minor restrictions give way, the pattern of unwinding is likely to become more expansive and more persistent chronic underlying patterns are likely to become more evident.

Be aware of the tendency of the body to lead towards these resistances and then to shy away from them. This may start to create repetitive patterns of movement as the body repeatedly leads towards these same resistances but shies away from them without dealing with them effectively.

Holding into resistances

As the unwinding process approaches these deeper resistances, it is necessary to assist the body in addressing these resistances more effectively. You will need to distinguish the two conflicting tendencies – on the one hand the tendency to draw into that resistance, on the other hand the tendency to shy away from it. Having made that distinction, you need to follow into the resistance, holding into the edge of that resistance, and not allowing the system to escape or to shy away from it continually.

Establishing the right level at which to hold into the edge of any resistance is one of the most crucial factors in effective fascial unwinding. Inadequate holding into the resistance will result in a relatively superficial process which doesn't release the more significant underlying patterns of resistance. Holding in too strongly will induce protective and defensive tensions in the body tissues which will prevent any progress in the unwinding process and any access to those deeper underlying patterns. Finding the right balance requires sensitivity, subtlety and experience and is a skill which you can continue to refine for many years.

Conclusion

The unwinding process may find its way to a natural conclusion – whether following some particularly significant release, or a series of partial releases. Most unwinding processes can continue indefinitely, exploring more deeply as the process proceeds, so it is often up to the practitioner to decide when to bring things to an end, and after which particular release it might be appropriate to finish. As always, it is preferable to bring the process to completion following a release and not in mid-process.

If the leg gradually unwinds down to the couch in a satisfactory resolved way, following a series of releases, this may be a natural point at which to bring the process to an end. However, with the lower limb, the weight of the leg can often bring the process to an end prematurely by pulling down towards the couch simply due to gravity. If this happens too readily, it is necessary to start the process again, establishing a new neutral starting position and starting from the beginning.

If the unwinding process doesn't want to come to an end, you may need to encourage the process to finish, first by initiating the intention of coming to an end, then by following patterns which lead back down towards the couch rather than following new patterns, and ultimately by encouraging the leg gently down towards the couch. As usual you want to avoid imposing upon the leg, always allowing it to find its own way back in so far as possible.

Arabella was 12 years old and her right knee had been painful for a long time – she wasn't sure how long but it seemed like years. It was preventing her from playing sport or running, and even day-to-day activities with her friends were constantly disturbed by her knee pain. Within the context of overall treatment, it was immediately obvious that the imbalance was coming very specifically from the knee itself, but neither she nor her father could remember any injury that might have caused the problem. Since it was evidently appropriate, I included fascial unwinding of the knee in the treatment, and as the knee found its own way to a point of release, Arabella suddenly had a vivid memory of an incident a few years earlier when she had been sitting on the side of a boat with her legs dangling down the side, and the boat had moved up against the quayside, squashing her right

298 \ Cranio-Sacral Integration

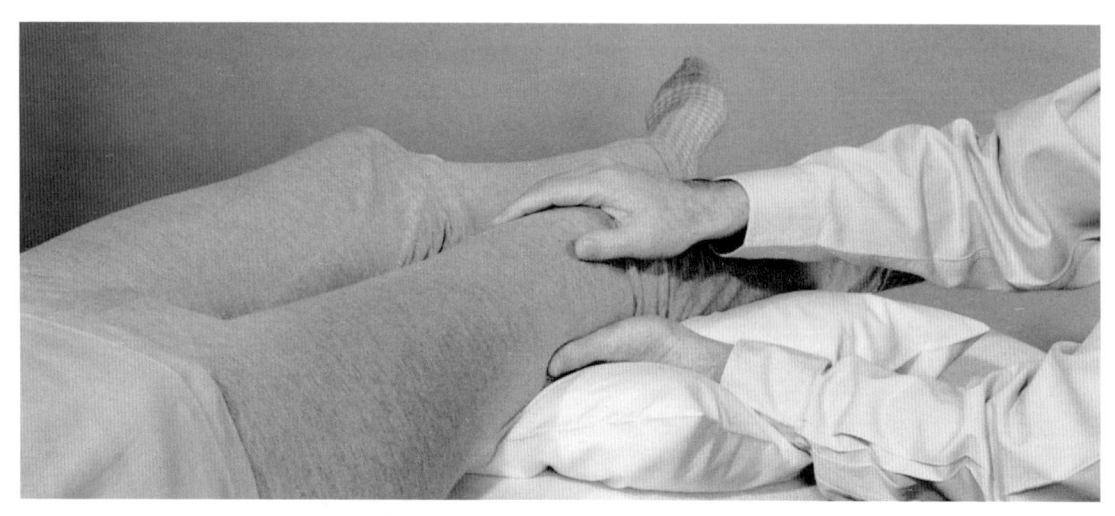

42.4 A contact for more localised integration of patterns within and around the knee

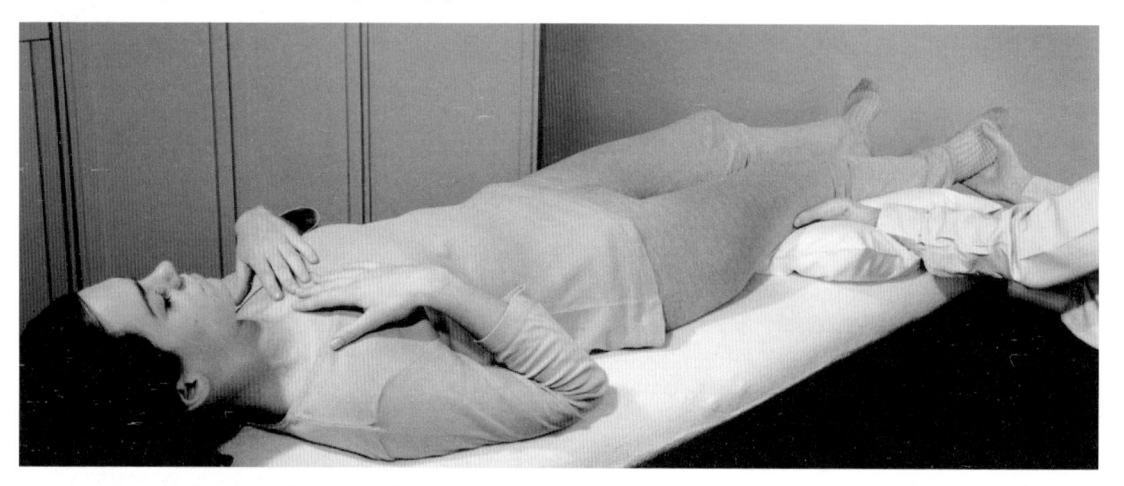

42.5 Integration of the lower leg from the knee to the foot

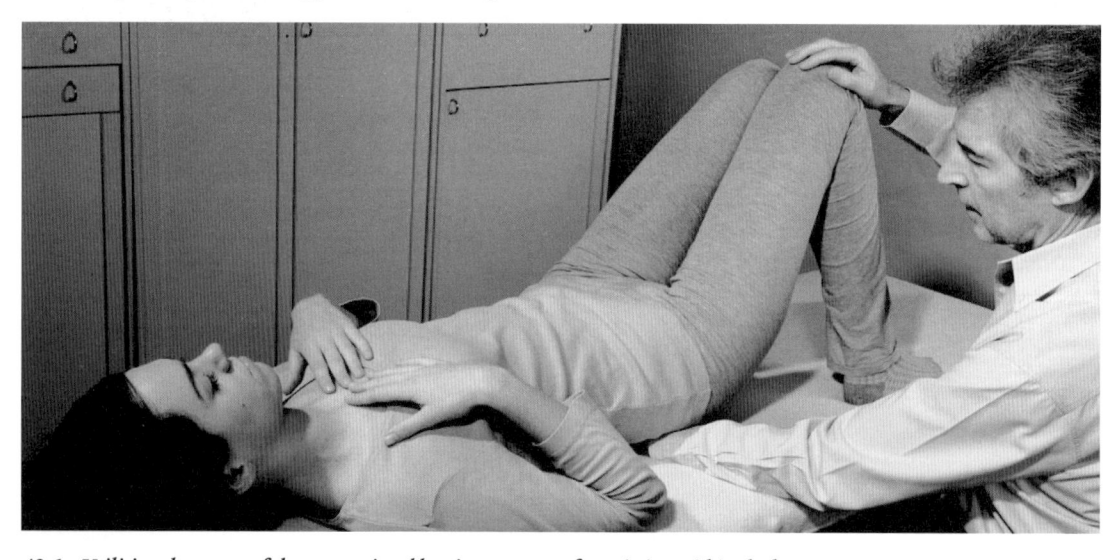

42.6 Utilising the power of the sacrum in addressing patterns of restriction within the knee

knee. It hadn't seemed like a significant injury at the time and it had been several years ago, but that injury had been lodged in her knee ever since, disturbing its fluent function and gradually causing increasing strain on the surrounding tissues. With the release through fascial unwinding, her knee recovered instantly and no further treatment was needed.

The hip and associated structures

Articulation

Articulation follows the same principles as articulation of the knee and elsewhere. The main priorities are to take the hip up into full flexion and out into full extension and, most significant of all, through the widest possible comfortable range of circumduction, taking the hip up and out and round in a wide ranging circular movement, feeling for the gentle stretch of the tissues throughout the perimeter of the circle.

Establishing a focus

It is of course possible to treat the hip without fascial unwinding. Perhaps when you are working at the sacrum, you may become aware of restriction in the hip and you might simply let your attention rest on the hip, or you might move one hand to the hip with the other remaining under the sacrum, or you might move both hands to cradle the hip and allow the inherent forces of the cranio-sacral process to express themselves through a series of points of stillness and release. This may be helpful and effective in some cases.

It is also possible to release patterns of restriction in the hip while unwinding an ankle or knee, with your attention projecting up into a fulcrum at the hip.

There will be times, however, particularly with deeply ingrained long-standing patterns where the mass of muscles and other soft tissues around the hip are deeply set in a pattern of restriction and imbalance, when it will be helpful – and the most effective means of treatment – to take up a contact which can specifically focus the fascial unwinding process on the hip and its surrounding structures.

In order to do this, it is helpful to take the hip well into flexion. This way, the possibilities for

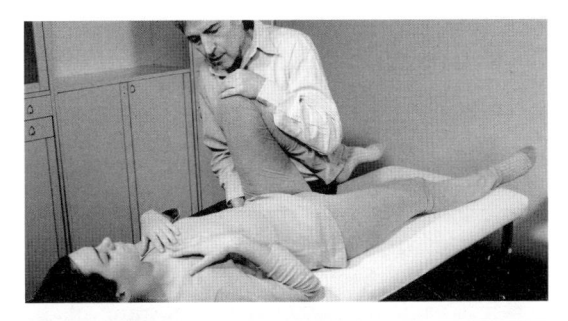

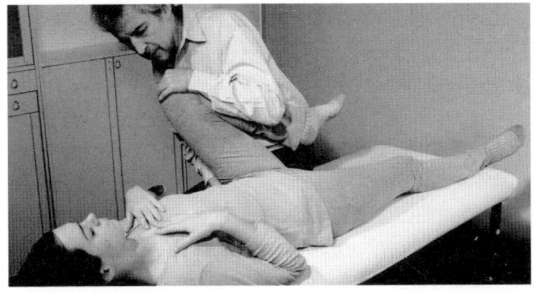

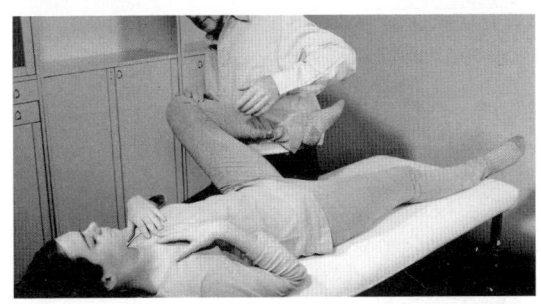

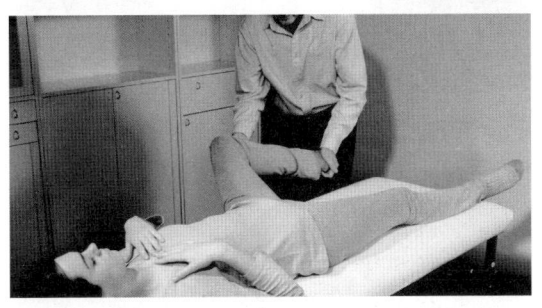

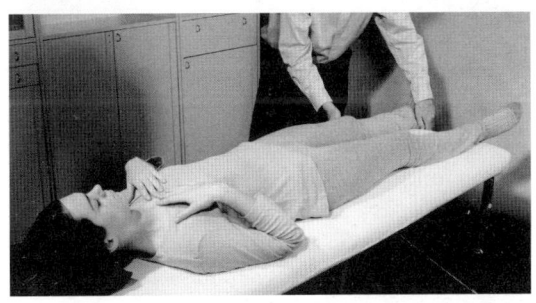

42.7 Effective unwinding of the hip benefits from a degree of containment, holding the hip into flexion in order to focus the therapeutic forces into the appropriate area

shying away from the focus are minimised, and the forces within the tissues are very specifically focused on the hip region.

Taking up contact

If the limb is light, it may be possible simply to hold the thigh into maximum comfortable flexion, with the lower leg and foot falling down towards the buttock. The position of the practitioner here is relevant in stabilising the contact. Standing at the side of the couch a little below hip level and facing up towards the patient's head enables the practitioner to lean into the hip slightly and so support the flexion of the hip up towards the body with minimum effort in the practitioner's hands and arms. The hands and arms can therefore remain more relaxed and free to focus on the unwinding patterns – rather than supporting the leg.

This contact however is inherently less stable than might be desired and, particularly if the leg is heavy, it may be preferable to take the hip into full flexion, let the foot come to rest on the buttock or as close to it as is comfortable, then sit on the side of the couch, facing up towards the patient's head (see Figure 42.7). Lean your chest forward into the leg and thigh so that the weight of the leg is completely supported by your body. Your arms can then remain free to follow the unwinding process. The hand on the medial side can rest onto the knee, so that it can monitor what is happening both in the knee and through the thigh and may also be able to introduce a slight compression if necessary. The other hand, coming in from the lateral side, can pass under the hip and buttock to monitor what is happening and feel the change in quality as the unwinding process proceeds. (If it is uncomfortable for the patient to let their knee flex and their foot drop down towards their buttock, you can support the lower leg over your shoulder. This is a less stable position, but preferable to leaving the patient in discomfort.)

Hips may unwind in various different directions and you can follow the hip wherever it may take you. But once again the inevitable tendency of the whole leg to push out of flexion and try to straighten comes into play. Just as with gravitational pulls, you need to take into account this tendency, recognising that it is not a part of the unwinding, but simply a muscular force. Like gravity, you need to counteract this tendency of the leg to push out, while following the subtle unwinding patterns, recognising the difference between these two forces. As so often, it is a fine line and will take practice in order to differentiate accurately.

If the hip is allowed to come out of flexion inappropriately, the focus will tend to weaken and the whole process may be far less specific. By leaning your own body forward gradually, in order to counteract the tendency of the leg to straighten, you will be able to sense an increasing sense of focus within the tissues until you feel the appropriate quality that tells you that you are in contact with the edge of a resistance, or with that finely tuned point of balanced tension within the tissues. (In this case you are using your body, specifically your chest, rather than your hands, to feel the quality in the patient's tissues.)

As resistances give way, the tissues will slacken and you may need to take up that slack by gradually leaning further into hip flexion in order to maintain the focus within the tissues.

As you lean your body further forward, taking the hip into further flexion as appropriate, so the focus can shift up from the thigh, through the hip, into the pelvis, into the sacro-iliac region, and on into the lower back and trunk. By adjusting the degree to which you lean forward – you can constantly adjust the focus as necessary, finding the precise point of balance that enables optimum engagement with the focal point of resistance. This process also acts as a stimulus to the tissues as well as maintaining a focus.

As with other unwindings, follow the unwinding process while maintaining this stimulus and focus. Allow the system to take you wherever it goes, follow as necessary, adjusting your position and hand contacts to accommodate the needs of the leg. Follow the process through until it feels complete, gently allowing the leg to unwind in whatever directions it needs to go.

This process will not only unwind the hip and issues associated with the hip and its surrounding structures, but can also be extended well up into the back, releasing significant patterns of restriction in the lower back.

Integration and completion

After all unwinding processes, it is advisable to integrate the cranio-sacral system as a whole, and to ensure that it has adapted to any changes. Particularly following the unwinding of the hip it would be relevant to work with the sacrum, enabling the sacrum, the pelvis, and the rest of the system to balance and integrate around any changes that have taken place in the hip, the pelvis, the lower back and elsewhere. It is also always relevant to re-evaluate the cranio-sacral system from the cranium in order to gain a different perspective in ensuring that the whole system has accommodated any changes that have been made.

Cynthia was 82 years old and not very mobile. She was bent over, using walking sticks, and shuffling along somewhat uncomfortably. Her weekly physiotherapy sessions seemed to have done all they could. She had been receiving acupuncture for some time, and she just wondered if cranio-sacral therapy might possibly help at all.

There was a considerable accumulation of tightness throughout her body (82 years' worth), and there was plenty to do in terms of treatment, but her hips were the main source of restriction that were preventing her from walking freely. I treated her once a week and within the context of overall treatment, included some fascial unwinding of the hip. I started very carefully, just a little bit of brief very gentle unwinding, to see how she would respond, and not wanting to disturb years of accumulated compensations and adaptations too suddenly. She responded well. Within a few weeks she was standing upright, had abandoned her sticks and was walking freely and confidently. As we continued the treatments, she commented one day during the hip unwinding, as her left foot floated past her face, 'I think I might take up ballet dancing'.

Some significant points are worth emphasising here, in relation to all treatment, but particularly in relation to osteoarthritic hips. Notice the words 'I started very carefully, just a little bit of unwinding' and even more significantly notice the words 'within the context of overall treatment'.

There are a great many elderly people with osteoarthritic hips, some very severe, some who have had hip replacements. It is not appropriate to think that fascial unwinding is the magic answer to osteoarthritic hips and start unwinding every restricted hip willy-nilly and out of context.

Osteoarthritis develops as a result of wear and tear (as opposed to rheumatoid arthritis, which is a separate inflammatory disease). Most people have some degree of osteoarthritis in their necks, lower back, hips or elsewhere from early adulthood. It doesn't necessarily cause any discomfort. Osteoarthritis shows up in X-rays, so when a patient is in pain and the X-rays show osteoarthritis, the pain is very readily and conveniently attributed to the osteoarthritis. Patients are often told, 'There is nothing that can be done about your osteoarthritis, you'll just have to take pain killers and wait a few years for it to get much worse and then have an operation'.

In fact the pain may not be due to the osteoarthritis at all. After all, osteoarthritis is often painless. Osteoarthritis develops because there is strain on the joints, either as a consequence of injury, or postural imbalance or a combination of both. Osteoarthritis in the hips is often the result of an imbalance in the pelvis and whole lower part of the body – perhaps arising from an original knee injury, a rotation of the pelvis, or a car accident. The osteoarthritis develops within the context of the overall imbalance. The body also develops a great many compensatory and adaptive changes throughout the body to cope with imbalance (perhaps causing symptoms elsewhere). The osteoarthritis does leave the joint surfaces exposed and susceptible to pain, but the cause of the pain is more likely to be due to the imbalance which places undue strain on the joints, rather than due to the osteoarthritis itself.

If you simply dive in enthusiastically and start unwinding that arthritic hip, you will not be addressing the cause, but simply stirring up the compensations and adaptations and adding further strain to a joint that is under strain from the imbalance of the whole body. This is not a good idea.

As we have seen many times, every integrated cranio-sacral treatment involves assessment and treatment of the whole picture. In the case of osteoarthritic hips, the main priority is to bring the whole body into balance in so far as possible, to enable the whole body to become fluent, mobile and adaptable, and only within that context gradually to encourage increased mobility in the hip and its surrounding soft tissues, proceeding slowly, allowing time for the body to adapt gradually from week to week. Overall balance and integration of the pelvis and the body as a whole are the priority.

In this way I have seen countless patients, often in severe pain, supposedly due to osteoarthritis, not only becoming much more mobile but also becoming pain free – by bringing the whole body into balance.

With regard to hip replacements, it is perfectly possible to treat patients who have had hip replacements (or knee replacements or any other surgery) so long as you observe the same principles. After all, it isn't the hip that you are treating, it is the whole person.

Chapter 43

Fascial Unwinding of the Neck

The neck is an area for which fascial unwinding is perhaps most significant, and consequently most commonly used. Unwinding the neck can often bring immediate effects of greater clarity of mind, clarity of vision, clarity of memory. More significantly, it can be profoundly effective in releasing the long-term effects of head and neck injuries and chronic patterns of discomfort in the neck.

Injuries to the neck, frequently as a result of car accidents, can often leave patients with particularly disturbing symptoms, not only causing persistent pain and discomfort in the neck and shoulders and visual disturbance and headaches, but also frustrating disruption of mental faculties and repercussions on general health and ability to cope with day-to-day life.

Patterns of restriction in the neck also arise from many other causes and can disrupt the overall alignment of the body with consequent pain, strain and discomfort potentially anywhere in the body.

Specific applications

Fascial unwinding of the neck has very specific applications in such conditions as torticollis (wry neck), both in the more severe chronic infant torticollis (saving infants from unnecessary surgery) and the acute spasm of adult torticollis. Infantile torticollis generally involves the occipito-mastoid suture, the jugular foramen, the spinal accessory nerve and the sterno-cleido-mastoid muscle along with whole body patterns arising from birth trauma (as we will see in later volumes on birth and babies) and is usually very responsive to cranio-sacral integration within which fascial unwinding can play a significant part.

Fascial unwinding of the neck can also be of great help to elderly patients suffering from dizziness, vagueness and loss of clarity due to vertebro-basilar insufficiency, since the reduced arterial supply to the brain can be largely due to the long-term accumulation of tensions and restrictions in the muscles and fascia of the neck.

It can also be a significant factor in treating patients with migraine – not particularly for immediate relief, but for eliminating the underlying propensity to migraine, particularly where head and neck injuries or the chronic accumulation of tension in the neck are involved.

However, such specific examples should not distract from the overall perspective of the wider picture and the understanding that the neck is such a key area in the overall balance and integrity of the person as a whole.

Wider perspective

As we have seen previously in relation to the suboccipital release, there are many reasons why the neck is significant – the arterial supply to the brain, the venous drainage from the brain, the sympathetic nerve supply to the head, parasympathetic nerve supply to the viscera, the trachea, the oesophagus, and all the many structures connecting and relating the head to the rest of the body and connecting the rest of the body to the head. All of the factors mentioned in relation to the suboccipital release will be relevant to fascial unwinding of the neck, and more besides.

In unwinding the neck we are not merely addressing the suboccipital area, but extending the effects through the whole neck, with widespread consequences through the whole body.

As our influence extends to C3, C4 and C5 (the third, fourth and fifth cervical vertebrae), this may affect the phrenic nerve supplying the diaphragm. Unwinding the neck can therefore release tension in the diaphragm, and engage with complex patterns of interaction between the diaphragm, the neck and emotional tensions reciprocating between them – with inevitable repercussions on other transverse diaphragms and on the body as a whole.

As the effects of fascial unwinding continue down to C5, C6, C7, C8 and T1 (the fifth, sixth, seventh and eighth cervical vertebrae and the first thoracic vertebra) this will affect the nerve supply to the brachial plexus, innervating the arms, hands and fingers, shoulders, chest and back with far-reaching effects down through the body, including the latissimus dorsi muscle extending down to the pelvis.

Fascial unwinding of the neck can also influence the trapezius and sterno-cleido-mastoid muscles with their dual nerve supply both from the upper cervical spine, C2 (sterno-cleido-mastoid), C3 and C4 (trapezius) and primarily from cranial nerve XI, the spinal accessory nerve passing up through the foramen magnum and out through the jugular foramen from its spinal roots at C1, C2, C3 and C4.

As with all cranio-sacral therapy, when you are unwinding the neck, your attention will be aware of the whole person, recognising the relationships between the fascia of the neck and the interconnected fascia throughout the body, tracing patterns of tension and restriction throughout the body, and recognising interactions from one part to another, thereby enabling a more comprehensive integration of the whole person.

The neck extends down to T4

The neck might be thought of as ending at the seventh cervical vertebra C7, since anatomically this is clearly what it does. But in functional terms the neck can be seen as extending at least as far down as the fourth thoracic vertebra T4. In understanding and working effectively with the neck, it is vital to take into account this specific relationship with the fourth thoracic vertebral level and its associations, as well as all the other interconnections through to the rest of the body.

These associations include the connection to the heart centre, the relationship between emotions at the heart centre and tensions in the neck, interaction with the muscles of the upper back such as the rhomboid muscles and any emotional tensions held there, and interaction with the 'T4 syndrome', a complex and fascinating syndrome, which we will explore in Chapter 51.

If you unwind the neck without thinking beyond the cervical spine, your neck unwinding is likely to be less effective, not integrating the full picture, not reaching the source. Not only are the specific associations with T4 very relevant, but as always, awareness of the whole person is fundamental to effective cranio-sacral therapy.

Common site of trauma

As mentioned when addressing the suboccipital region, the neck is also significant because it is such a common focus for tension and injury. Most people hold a significant level of tension in the neck; a great many injuries to all parts of the body tend to gravitate to the neck; and a great many tensions – day-to-day and chronic – tend to accumulate there.

In view of all of this, the neck can be seen to be a particularly vital area for treatment, and significant results are often obtained from fascial unwinding where other treatment (including cranio-sacral therapy without fascial unwinding) has not helped.

Principles

The principles for unwinding the neck are much the same as for any other unwinding process or any other cranio-sacral work. Once again it is the practical considerations specific to the neck which need to be explored in order to make the process most effective.

Articulation

As with all unwinding processes, it is helpful to start with some gentle articulation and soft tissue work on the neck, loosening the tissues and releasing superficial tensions. As always, this doesn't need to take long but it is useful to explore the comfortable extremes of motion, starting with smaller movements so as not to introduce any sudden, abrupt, unexpected positions into the neck, gradually increasing the range into further and further side-bending and rotation – within the limits of whatever is comfortable for the patient, and always starting very gently, seeing how far the neck is happy to move, taking care not to force it anywhere that it doesn't want to go.

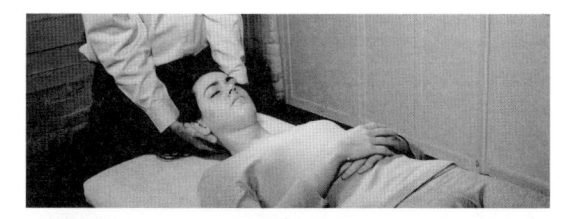

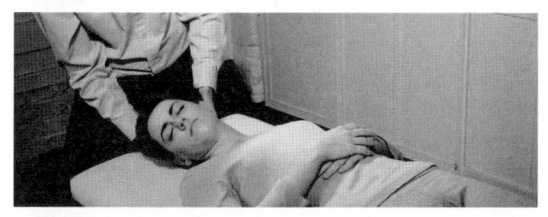

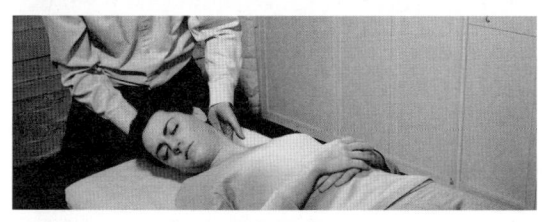

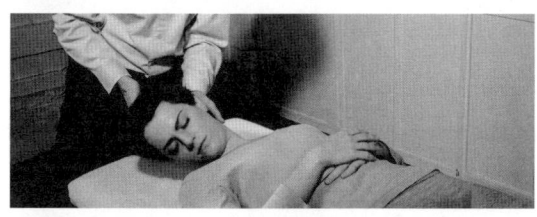

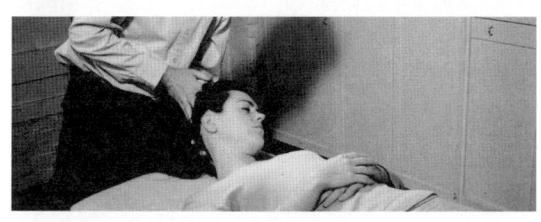

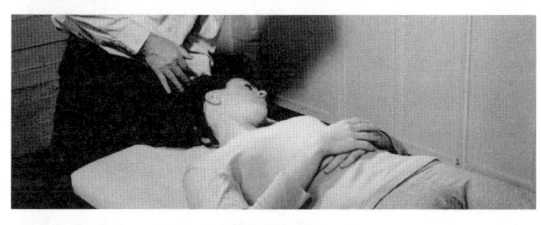

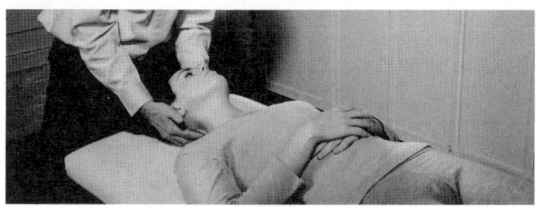

Unwinding

Like any cranio-sacral process, there are many different ways of approaching a neck unwinding and many different ways of taking up contact. Each practitioner will develop their own variations and methods in their own time, but certain guidelines will help to establish useful starting points.

Taking up contact

With the patient lying supine on the couch, with the top of the head close to the end of the couch, stand at the patient's head. When you are ready to take up contact, cradle under the patient's head and neck, with the fingers of one hand underneath the fingers of the other hand, creating a hammock – but not interlocking the fingers, as this reduces your flexibility to move your hands when necessary. It is necessary to support the head and neck fully so that the patient feels comfortable and at ease, without in any way restricting the mobility of the head and neck. The hands therefore need to be at the junction of the head and neck – partly under the occiput, partly under the neck – not so far down that the head is falling back over the hands into excessive backward bending, not so far up that the contact feels wobbly and unstable, but so that the fingers and hands are also well in contact with the neck to monitor and follow whatever patterns may emerge. Feel for the quality of the contact – comfortable, stable, secure, comprehensive, balanced, flexible.

Come back to your own practitioner fulcrums

Re-establish practitioner fulcrums, standing comfortably, balanced between your two feet, your knees unlocked, breathing easily, letting go through your whole body. Establish the right height at which to stand, perhaps by moving your feet further apart or closer together. A 'Tai Chi' type standing position is helpful. Allow your shoulders to drop; allow your arms to hang loosely from your shoulders; allow your hands to cradle the head and neck in a loose, relaxed and comfortable way.

43.1 The neck is an area for which fascial unwinding is particularly significant

Maintaining constant awareness of yourself, gently lift the head and neck – and your hands – off the surface of the couch, to allow complete freedom of movement to the head and neck. Stand upright so as not to put strain on your back, feeling your spine lengthening upwards, your arms hanging to form a loose relaxed hammock, rather than holding the head and neck up high using the strength of your arms and consequently becoming tired very soon.

Follow the usual principles

Having established this position, follow the usual principles of unwinding, waiting for impressions to come to you, waiting for the initial minor movements that will unlock the way to larger scale movements. Follow every subtlety of movement that appears.

Don't be in a hurry to make things move; don't impose upon the body at all.

As the process evolves, follow wherever the head and neck may lead you, allowing your hand positions to adapt to the needs of the moment, allowing your body to move fluently and smoothly without disrupting the continuity of the process.

As always, try to be aware of the whole picture as well as the details within that picture. As you identify patterns of restriction, follow them with your attention to see where they lead you – through the neck and down into the rest of the body.

Initially the head can feel very heavy and you may feel that you need to use some strength to support such a heavy weight. As engagement develops, the head is likely to feel increasingly weightless and the whole process becomes easier. The sooner you can engage, the more quickly the head becomes weightless. If you take too long to engage, or if you put too much effort into it, or if you don't give sufficient attention to your own body use, your arms may become exhausted before you have even got started.

You can adapt to this through greater flexibility in your own body and hand positions. For neck unwinding more than any other unwinding, awareness of the stresses and strains that arise in your own body and adaptability of your own position from moment to moment are more crucial than anywhere else. Remain constantly aware of your own body. Allow your weight to shift from one foot to the other, particularly as the head moves to the side. Allow your hands to glide smoothly into different positions according to the position of the head. As the head rolls into rotation, the weight of the head can be supported entirely with one hand, allowing the other hand to rest, bringing the other hand back in as the head rotates the other way or back to the centre. You can also rest your elbow against your own abdomen for greater support as necessary in order to minimise the effort in your arms. These little details are essential to effective unwinding. If you don't take them into account and explore and learn and develop a multitude of different little ways to adapt and thereby minimise your effort, you are unlikely to be able to sustain an effective neck unwinding.

Extreme positions

You may find that during the unwinding process, the head and neck may move into extreme positions that you might not have thought physiologically possible. It is necessary to follow into these extreme positions as far as is appropriate for the body, because they are likely to be the most significant therapeutic moments in the unwinding process – sometimes reflecting positions into which the neck has been forced by injury or by birth. So long as they are comfortable for the patient then they will be appropriate. So long as you are genuinely following the patterns within the system and not imposing at all, these positions will be comfortable. If at any time, you have concerns that these positions might be uncomfortable for your patient you can always ask your patient if they are comfortable, in order to gain reassurance that such extreme positions are appropriate.

Repetitive patterns of motion

Unwinding of the neck, as with all cranio-sacral therapy, involves following to points of balanced tension at the extremes of motion, and staying with the stillness until releases occur – rather than simply waving aimlessly from side to side, shying away from resistances and avoiding issues.

In any cranio-sacral process, repetitive patterns of motion may not be achieving anything and this principle applies within the neck as well. However, within the neck, due to the structure of the neck, with its symmetrical bilateral pattern of muscles passing down the vertebral column, and through the neck itself, there is a natural inherent tendency for repetitive patterns to manifest. This occurs primarily because, as the neck moves in one direction and releases patterns of tension and restriction on one side of the neck, this will naturally lead to discovering and following matching compensatory patterns of tension and restriction on the opposite sides of the neck, whether at the same vertebral level, or above, or below.

So repetitive patterns are to some extent an inherent part of neck unwinding – whether they are side-bending from one side to the other, rotating from one side to the other, or other patterns of repetitive motion. However, it is still necessary to ensure that these repetitive patterns are therapeutically effective.

This can be gauged by the quality of the process. If it is simply wobbling around loosely in a repetitive pattern, it is probably not doing anything effective. If it is moving to one extreme, reaching points of stillness, releasing and then moving to the other extreme, it is more likely to be effective. If it seems to be moving down the neck through a series of compensatory patterns, this is also an indication that it is probably being effective, as opposed to simply moving from side to side at the same level.

Holding into deeper patterns

Like most unwinding processes, the unwinding of the neck is likely to start with some initial smaller movements, before progressing gradually to larger scale movements. As the more, deeply embedded, persistent patterns become apparent, you may need to hold into these deeper resistances for longer, surveying with your attention, tracing the path of tension down through the body to its source, thereby identifying the origin of the resistance, and therefore assisting the release of the restriction. This could draw your attention to the shoulder, to the heart centre, to T4, to the diaphragm, to the solar plexus, to the sacro-iliac joint on the opposite side of the body, or of course to anywhere else in the body. As your attention reaches the source, you can recognise it by the change in quality – perhaps experiencing a greater intensity of tightness, or a pulsation or a wriggling – leading up to a release. With chronic, deeply embedded patterns, be prepared to stay with the resistance and the stillness for much longer, in order to enable the release.

Recognise the essential value of stillness

Remember that while the unwinding process is often seen as more active, it is the points of stillness at the eye of the hurricane which are the most significant moments therapeutically. Be prepared to stay with those points of stillness for as long as necessary, not feeling the need to move on or encourage movement.

Feel the quality of the stillness; recognise the point of balanced tension by the qualities of vibrancy, vitality, wriggling, squirming, pulsating – the active, alive quality within the tissues, as you stay with the dynamic stillness.

As you stay in that stillness, look for every little subtlety of movement, every tiny twist and turn that may be necessary to help unlock the last little vestiges of that resistance. Stay with it until finally a convincing sense of softening, melting and dissolving occurs.

Following the release, allow the system to continue on its way again, taking care to move fluently from stillness into motion and from motion into stillness. Follow the broader sweeping movements without getting carried away, being prepared for them to come to an end at any moment, identifying all the tiny subtleties within the broader sweeping movements. Be aware of the whole picture as well as the details within that picture.

Integration and completion

Following a series of releases, small and large, minor and major, partial or complete, the process may come to a natural point of completion. At an appropriate point, allow the process to come to an end in a central balanced position, feeling the quality of the neck – loose, balanced, settled and still – feeling the quality of the moment, feeling that it is ready and complete. Once you encounter that stage, allow the head and neck to come to rest gently onto the couch and release your contact. Then check the cranio-sacral system as a whole to ensure that any changes have been integrated and that the whole system feels settled, balanced and complete, and continue with the process of integrated treatment.

Ralph was 67 years old and had been suffering from a headache for over ten years – not headaches, but one continuous headache. He was otherwise healthy and there was no apparent cause for this persistent and debilitating pain.

Naturally, during all these years he had undergone many medical investigations including X-rays, scans and everything else. He had tried many different treatments. Nothing was relieving his headache, nothing was touching it at all. He had been asked many times to go through his whole history and he couldn't identify anything that might have caused or contributed towards his headache.

When I tuned it at his head, there was an evident pattern drawing his head and neck down into his body and twisting to the right. As his neck started to unwind, I allowed this pull to develop; it drew down very strongly; it was very forceful, an exceptionally strong pull drawing deeper and deeper down into the right side of the body. I followed into that pull as far as it wanted to go, which was very deep and very intense over several minutes – checking with Ralph that he was comfortable despite the apparent intensity of the compression. Finally, we reached a point of release at which the whole neck and head freed up, unwound and let go. Exactly at that moment, Ralph suddenly spoke out, 'Of course I was blown up in the war'.

As we reached the fulcrum of his fascial pattern, he had suddenly had a vivid memory. Thrown by a nearby bomb, he had apparently been blown right up into the air, crashing down on his head. This was during the Second World War, when he was 19. The headache had started when he was in his fifties. No wonder he hadn't drawn any correlation – until now. The vivid memory, just at the point of stillness within that compressive pattern clearly demonstrated the relationship; and this was confirmed by the dramatic release in the tissues of his head, neck and shoulder and the immediate improvement in his headache, which was substantially eased by the first treatment and gone within a few further treatments, for the first time in over ten years.

Some additional details on neck unwinding

Unwinding with the head on or off the couch

Neck unwinding is generally carried out with the patient lying fully on the couch, in the usual treatment position. It is also possible to work with the patient moved up the couch so that the head and neck are extending out over the end of the table.

Whist this position does provide scope for a wider range of movement of the neck, particularly into backward bending, my experience is that in the vast majority of cases this is unnecessary; and in most cases it is possible to achieve everything necessary with the head and neck over the table. Consequently, moving the patient up, with the head and neck off the table rarely confers any benefits and it does have disadvantages:

Firstly, the process of moving the patient up and then down the table disrupts the continuity of their treatment process.

Taking the head and neck off the end of the couch also creates greater responsibilities for the practitioner, in that is becomes necessary to support the head and neck from dropping or bending backward too far, and creates further complications to an already sensitive process.

It is therefore preferable only to move the patient up the couch in rare circumstances, where the demands of the unwinding process specifically require it.

Standing or sitting

Neck unwinding can be carried out either with the practitioner standing at the patient's head or with the practitioner sitting at the patient's head. It is useful to be able to do both of these fluently and confidently. Both may be necessary at different times and either might be more appropriate for a particular circumstance and have particular advantages.

Working from a standing position has the advantage of making it easier to lift the patient's head and neck completely free of the couch to allow total freedom of movement for the unwinding process. It enables you to do this with minimum effort in your arms and hands since your arms can hang loosely down from your shoulders and still support the head and neck off the couch. However, this position undoubtedly puts more strain on the practitioner's own body, particularly their back. This in itself can be a useful learning process providing valuable insight into your own body use and how to use your own body more fluently and effectively.

Working from a sitting position is more comfortable for the practitioner, but makes it more difficult to lift the head and neck completely free from the couch. Working on the couch restricts the movement of the head and neck and makes it harder to explore and discover the freedom of movement required for effective neck unwinding.

With experience, a practitioner will be able to work effectively in both positions and to adapt from one to another fluently and confidently without interruption, but initially it is preferable to work in a standing position (learning to overcome the postural strains) and, once you have mastered working in the standing position, to then develop the ability to work in a sitting position.

To articulate or not to articulate

In presenting these various unwinding processes for the arm, leg and neck, we have emphasised the benefits of articulation as a preparation for the unwinding. This is valuable and when choosing to apply an unwinding process, it is generally helpful to start with some articulation.

However, during the course of an integrated treatment, the body may well start to unwind spontaneously, or perhaps during some other process, the relevance of unwinding might start to become apparent. In such cases, the most effective approach is to allow the process of unwinding to evolve spontaneously, and not to be bound by mere technical guidelines regarding the need for articulation.

This is perhaps most common in the neck, where during a suboccipital release, the neck may show some signs of unwinding and you can simply allow this to evolve, following it wherever it may lead you, allowing the subocccipital release to evolve seamlessly into a neck unwinding and then, as the neck unwinding completes, continuing seamlessly back into the integrated treatment process.

It is also useful to recognise, however, that this is not always appropriate. There are times when the system (or the patient) may choose to unwind because it is an easier option, or even as a way of avoiding addressing something on another level. As always, quality is a key factor in identifying this, recognising when the system needs to stay focused on something in the core, and when it is appropriate to allow it to follow into an unwinding. It can often be helpful for the body to unwind first, in order to gain more ready access to an issue on a different level, but if it repeatedly runs off into unwinding somewhat aimlessly and refuses to settle into a clearly identifiable pattern in the core, the therapist may need to focus the system on addressing the core issue, rather than letting it escape into unwinding again.

Chapter 44

Key Factors in Fascial Unwinding

Key factors

Chapters 38–43 have covered a substantial amount of information on the various aspects of fascial unwinding, so it may be useful to review and highlight the key points in the process, particularly for reference as you develop your fascial unwinding skills. Some of these key factors apply more specifically to the use of fascial unwinding for the limbs and neck, but most will apply to other areas as well.

Principles

The *principles* of fascial unwinding are the same as the principles for any other cranio-sacral therapy:

- establish the appropriate state of the practitioner
- establish the appropriate state of the patient
- establish engagement
- allow the evolution of the inherent treatment process leading to points of stillness and release.

Extra attention to self-awareness

Because fascial unwinding is often carried out with the practitioner in a standing position, it becomes necessary to:

- place even *greater emphasis on oneself* and on practitioner fulcrums
- pay greater attention on how you use your own body
- take great care to move with fluency and continuity (helped by the practice of Tai Chi).

This greater attention to oneself can be a very valuable process, rather than merely an extra demand, helping to develop a greater awareness of your own fluency, softness, mobility, flexibility (or lack of it), highlighting the need to work on these aspects of yourself, which can in turn enhance everything you do both on a cranio-sacral level, and in your life generally.

Articulation

Articulation is helpful as a precursor to fascial unwinding, enabling easier access to more significant and deeper patterns. It may be essential in some situations where mobility is very restricted or held. It may not be necessary when fascial unwinding arises spontaneously within a treatment session.

Starting

When starting, it is essential to make a clear *distinction between articulation and unwinding*, so as not to carry any tendency to articulate into the unwinding. They are very different processes and require a very different mindset and intention. It is very helpful to establish a suitable starting point – relaxed, neutral, not compressed, not overstretched.

Take care not to grip or hold tightly.

Identify the tiny subtle initial internal movements – they are the key to engaging with subsequent more expansive movements.

Allow the process to start and evolve of its own accord, not trying to make it happen or encourage it. The movement needs to arise spontaneously from within, not instigated by the therapist.

Utilise as necessary the various options for enabling engagement, primarily taking yourself into deeper relaxation and softness.

Encourage, as necessary, greater relaxation and letting go in the patient, reminding them whenever appropriate, throughout the process if necessary.

As you engage, the limb is likely to take on a 'mind of its own', becoming increasingly weightless.

Take care *not to impose*:
- maintain softness, fluidity and fluency, simply allowing expression rather than imposing any movement
- maintain constant and consistent attention to yourself – particularly relaxing your shoulders, elbows and hands again and again throughout the process
- imagine yourself as an ocean on which the limb or neck is floating
- remember that the more you can keep yourself out of the way, the more effectively the process will evolve.

Maintain focus
Within your calm, quiet, spacious meditative state:
- keep your attention clearly and consistently focused
- remain attentive both to the fine detail and the wider overview
- maintain a fine line of balanced elastic tension throughout – not floppy, not overstretched, dynamic.

Overview
Maintain an overview:
- of the whole limb
- of the whole person
- of the specific detail and the wider picture, simultaneously
- of the subtleties within the more evident movements
- of the connections from the local area to the whole.

Points of stillness
Identify the *points of stillness* (the eye of the hurricane):
- as the essence of the process, the most significant factor
- not just wandering aimlessly
- not revolving round in meaningless circles or repetitive patterns that aren't leading anywhere.

The whole purpose of the fascial unwinding process is to discover still points, but not in a hurry, not forcing it, letting them evolve, letting the body find them for itself (otherwise you will tend to be imposing on the body).

It is easy to think of fascial unwinding in terms of movement, but this is not what it is about. Movement is just the means towards an end, the way towards identifying still points; movement is necessary, but it is not the purpose.

Staying with stillness
- Recognise the points of stillness by the dynamic quality expressed within the stillness.
- Feel the edge of resistance.
- Stay with the stillness, gently holding in, not allowing escape – helping the body to make its choice between addressing or avoiding the issue.
- Feel for the subtle detail within the stillness.
- Allow the gradual build-up of intensity, feeling the dynamism within the stillness.

Ending
Most fascial unwinding processes will reach a natural spontaneous conclusion, following release. Take care not to interrupt in mid-process. Utilise various ways of helping the process to come to an end where necessary.

Fascial unwinding can provide valuable insight into core work and vice versa.

Further reflections on the fascial unwinding process
Memories
Memories may arise during fascial unwinding, as with any other aspect of cranio-sacral therapy – or they may not. It is not something to expect; there is no need to feel disappointed if they don't, or to feel that the process has been inadequate if it doesn't bring up memories. When relevant memories do arise, it can provide satisfying confirmation of the effectiveness of the release and identification of the emotional connection

with the restriction, but it is not something to be specifically aiming for.

Emotions

In the same way, emotions may or may not arise. It is fine if they do, it usually happens gently, it is generally therapeutic, with a sense of relief and lightening, and often with significant changes in the tissues and in the integration of the whole person. All of that is fine, so long as the patient has the understanding that it is simply underlying issues rising to the surface for release – so this may need to be explained and the patient reassured.

It is not necessary to be alarmed by the release of emotion, nor to be over-concerned that this might be traumatic for the patient, as long as the therapist is well-grounded and is providing an appropriate atmosphere of grounding and understanding, and the patient is consequently well-grounded and understands the process.

The release of emotions can be allowed and welcomed, but does not need to be specifically intended, encouraged or expected, nor feeling that the process is inadequate or unsatisfactory without some connection with or expression of emotion. Release of emotion is not the purpose of the exercise, just a possible outcome that may arise in appropriate situations.

There are other therapeutic methods that involve more specific intent to connect with and enable emotional release (including John Upledger's somato-emotional release; see Upledger 1990). Such approaches may involve the patient deliberately moving in to physical positions and patterns with a consciousness of an underlying emotional issue or a specific physical incident or pattern involving emotional patterning. This can be very effective in helping the release of deep emotional tensions and the physical patterns associated with them. This is something which we will explore in a later volume, once the fundamentals of fascial unwinding have been mastered, but it is not what we are concerned with here. The approach to fascial unwinding that we are describing here provides a clear grounding for any emotional process that may evolve from it. A great deal of effective and profound fascial unwinding takes place without any outward expression of emotion, and it can be highly effective for addressing issues that are primarily and ostensibly physical.

All cranio-sacral therapy addresses emotions – whether directly or indirectly. All cranio-sacral therapy may potentially bring emotions to the surface to be expressed and released. Release of emotions is something to be welcomed – so long as it is handled in an appropriate manner, with understanding, within a safe environment, with appropriate grounding and centering of both patient and therapist.

There are different ways of addressing emotions. Some therapists may say that it is not their role to address emotions, which is of course their prerogative. However, physical and emotional are inseparable and to try to treat one without the other is not really recognising the wholeness of the person and can only have limited effectiveness. Some therapists may not be comfortable with the release of emotions, perhaps because they haven't addressed their own emotions and don't feel comfortable with the expression of emotions, and consequently may develop all sorts of rationalisations as to why emotional release is not a good thing. For truly integrated therapy it is essential to acknowledge and address the complete triune unity of the whole person.

How to integrate fascial unwinding into overall treatment

Fascial unwinding has many applications and may be a valuable part of the therapeutic process for many patients – perhaps the crucial key to health in some patients – as has been demonstrated by various examples in Chapters 38–43. But it won't necessarily be relevant for every patient and is not something that you will incorporate into every treatment. There are various reasons why it might be appropriate to include fascial unwinding.

It may arise spontaneously during a treatment – for example, you might be engaged in a suboccipital release, and the neck may spontaneously start to unwind.

Perhaps during a treatment, you might identify a site that feels as if it would benefit from fascial unwinding.

The nature of the injury or symptoms might indicate that fascial unwinding would be appropriate, for example in repetitive strain injury, tennis elbow, sprained ankle, frozen shoulder.

Whichever way it arises, within the context of cranio-sacral integration, you would always incorporate it into a complete integrated treatment – opening up the system, preparing the way, balancing the core and bringing the treatment to a suitable completion – and introducing fascial unwinding into the treatment process at an appropriate moment.

The appropriate moment can vary. The priority is for the patient to be in an open, relaxed and receptive state, not just diving into fascial unwinding out of context, not entering into fascial unwinding when the patient's system is unprepared and unsettled. In other words, like any cranio-sacral therapy, you establish appropriate levels of engagement with the whole system before entering into any specific treatment process.

The most appropriate point at which to incorporate fascial unwinding is generally somewhere in the middle of a treatment, after opening up and before entering into the deeper core treatment and final settling. It is always advisable to integrate the core after any fascial unwinding, feeling how the body as a whole has responded to the unwinding process, integrating any changes into the whole picture, and ensuring that the whole matrix feels integrated and complete.

Fascial unwinding is an invaluable component of cranio-sacral integration and a very valuable aspect of any cranio-sacral therapist's repertoire.

Master keys

Finally, since this chapter is entitled 'Key Factors in fascial unwinding', we will finish by returning to an even briefer summary of the most significant key factors in the fascial unwinding process:

- your own stillness, softness, spaciousness
- the patient completely relaxed, not joining in, or tensing up – helped by articulation and breathing
- allowing, not imposing
- continuity – within the process, within your own movements
- points of stillness – identifying them, recognising them, staying with them
- overview – of the whole person, of the whole matrix, of the detail within the wider picture, of the connection between the local detail and the overall integration of the person.

Part VI
Spheno-Basilar Patterns

Chapter 45

Scales and Arpeggios
Spheno-Basilar Patterns Part 1 – Honing Basic Skills

What's special about the sphenoid?
In Chapter 27, we have seen that the sphenoid occupies a central pivotal position within the cranium. It articulates with every other cranial bone, along with several facial bones. Its pivotal nature is further reflected in the fact that, within its sella turcica, it houses the pituitary gland, the 'master gland' which plays such an important role in regulating function throughout the body. The sphenoid occupies a crucial central role within the cranio-sacral system, and therefore provides an excellent vantage point through which to view the whole picture.

What's special about the spheno-basilar synchondrosis?
The spheno-basilar synchondrosis (SBS) is the joint between the body of the sphenoid (anteriorly) and the basilar portion of the occiput (basi-occiput) (posteriorly). Like the sphenoid, it occupies a central pivotal position. It is the fulcrum around which the whole bony cranio-sacral system moves (see Figure 45.1).

Cartilaginous joint
The spheno-basilar synchondrosis differs anatomically from most other joints in the skull in that it is a cartilaginous joint, whereas most joints in the skull are sutures.

A synchondrosis is a *'primary cartilaginous joint', which starts life as a cartilaginous joint and gradually ossifies. In the case of the SBS, this ossification is considered to be complete around the age of 25 years.*

Sutures are fibrous joints, closely stitched together by a mass of tiny fibres, whereas the SBS, being a cartilaginous joint, starts life with a pliable section of rubbery cartilage between the two bones which form the joint.

Sutures exhibit very little mobility. Cartilaginous joints are able to move a little more freely than sutures (at least in early life). The SBS, being a cartilaginous joint, is therefore more mobile than most joints in the cranium.

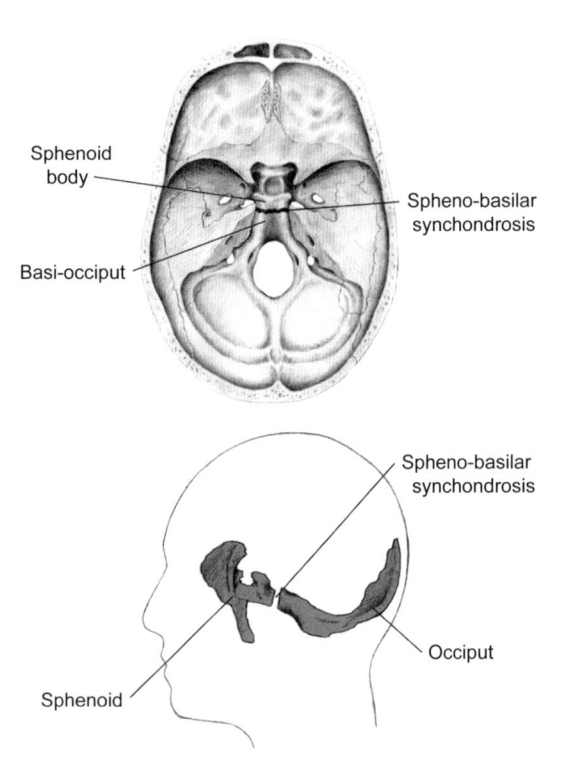

45.1 The spheno-basilar synchondrosis occupies a central pivotal position – it is the fulcrum around which the whole bony cranio-sacral system moves

Why might this be significant?

As a result of its increased mobility, and also because of its central pivotal position, the SBS is more readily affected by patterns of strain, tension and asymmetry from elsewhere in the cranio-sacral system – at least in early life – and this sets up patterns of response throughout life. Twists, turns, pulls and restrictions from all over the body are therefore more readily reflected into this pivotal joint, creating corresponding asymmetrical patterns at the SBS.

The SBS therefore provides a window through which we can more readily read everything that is going on throughout the system – every imbalance, every asymmetry, every stress and every strain. Not only can we read these patterns, but also we can engage with them more readily and thereby enhance the body's ability to resolve and integrate those imbalances.

Based on this theory, Sutherland devised a framework for evaluating the cranio-sacral system. His framework consisted of six patterns, which can be used to explore and assess asymmetries throughout the body, and to enhance the system's natural tendency to come into a greater degree of balance and integration.

Individual patterns

Bulges and twists

If you have been working with the cranio-sacral system, you will probably have noticed that some heads bulge to one side, that others seem to be twisted, and that most heads reveal some kind of imbalance or asymmetry. When we start to explore spheno-basilar patterns, what we are doing is defining those bulges and twists more clearly, identifying and describing those inherent tendencies within the body more specifically, thereby enabling more accurate diagnosis and treatment.

The six patterns described by Sutherland are:
- flexion/extension
- torsion
- side-bending
- lateral shift
- vertical shift
- compression.

This does not, of course, mean that the system can be distorted only in six directions. It simply provides us with a framework within which to view the system. The points of a compass – North, South, East, West – provide us with a similar frame of reference; this doesn't mean that we can only move in those four directions, but it provides us with a frame of reference through which we can describe and define any direction. In the same way, we can describe patterns within the cranio-sacral system within the framework of Sutherland's six patterns. There will of course be many variations.

Complex mass of patterns

As we introduce this concept of SBS patterns, we will start by exploring each pattern individually, in order to gain an understanding of the individual definitions. It will soon become apparent that they don't actually occur individually, or in simple pure form; they always occur in combinations.

In fact the whole system is a complex mass of hundreds of patterns – reflecting all the stresses and strains, injuries, accidents and imbalances in our bodies – everything that has happened to us throughout our life and left its imprint.

So in every one of us, there is a multitude of torsions, side-bendings, lateral shifts, vertical shifts, and compressions, pulling us in a mass of different directions, like a tangled ball of wool, full of knots and twists. Certain patterns are likely to be predominant – either because they reflect particularly severe traumas, or because they happen to be at the surface, or are more accessible at that particular moment.

The body knows what to do

Fortunately, we don't need to concern ourselves too much with sorting out this tangle, or even analysing its complex intricacies in detail. The body, in its own wisdom, knows what to do and – with a little help – will reveal, address and resolve the most immediate patterns, and then each subsequent pattern thereafter. All we need to do is follow the inherent treatment process. Simply by doing this, the system will, in its own time, work its way through a process of disentanglement. As superficial patterns resolve, so further underlying patterns will emerge, to be released and resolved; and so the process will continue indefinitely, moving deeper and deeper, until the system becomes clear, balanced and integrated.

Returning to neutral

Some patterns will resolve easily – superficial, recent, minor patterns. Others will take time – chronic, deeply embedded, severe patterns. As each pattern releases and resolves, the system will tend to come back to neutral, providing an opportunity, either to wait peacefully in that settled neutral state allowing the process of subtle integration to continue, or to wait for the system to reveal some further pattern of imbalance that it wishes to address, or to bring the treatment to an end. In this way, the therapeutic process will proceed in the body's own time, for as long as it wishes – or until the therapist chooses one of those neutral moments to bring the treatment to a suitable conclusion.

Reflecting the whole system

Although we are focusing here on the SBS and describing these patterns in terms of the SBS, we are not simply assessing the bones or the joint. We are, as always, inevitably engaging with the whole system. The patterns that we encounter are a reflection of the whole system. They may be coming from anywhere throughout the system – pelvis, ankle, back, neck, solar plexus, stomach, psyche, personality – anywhere and everywhere.

Basic building blocks

For the moment we will be looking at the individual patterns as defined by Sutherland. Once we have an understanding of these basic building blocks, we will see how we can apply this information in practice, in a more integrated manner.

Concert pianists need a high degree of technical skill in order to be able to perform with fluency, artistry and sensitivity on the concert platform. In developing those skills, pianists might practise scales and arpeggios and other technical exercises. Of course they are not going to go out on to the concert platform and play scales and arpeggios. But the technical skills which they have developed through practice will enable them to become deeply absorbed into the flow of the music, with all the necessary skills at their fingertips to flow with the music without having to concern themselves with the technical aspects. Their fingers will know what to do without thinking.

In the same way, as cranio-sacral therapists, if we develop and practise the basic technical skills and understanding, through study and practice of SBS patterns and anatomy, when we go into treatment, we will have the necessary skills at our fingertips to flow with the therapeutic process with fluency, artistry and sensitivity, without having to think about the technical aspects, deeply absorbed in the therapeutic process – but with the necessary grounding in knowledge and technical skills so that our fingers can instinctively identify, recognise and engage with whatever is going on within the system and flow with the therapeutic process – with informed awareness.

Practical application

As we describe these individual patters, we will use Sutherland's original terminology of flexion and extension:

- flexion, occurring during the expansion phase of motion
- extension, occurring during the contraction phase of motion.

The terms flexion and extension, strictly speaking, refer to the movement of midline bones, rather than to phases of motion. But for clarity in this chapter, it will be easier to refer at times to the flexion phase (expansion phase) and extension phase (contraction phase).

Hand contact

Throughout this process of exploring and evaluating spheno-basilar patterns, we will be using the same contact that we took up for the sphenoid in previous chapters – with the thumbs resting lightly around the tips of the greater wings of the sphenoid, at the pterions or temples, the fingers wrapping round the head towards the occiput, with the little fingers extending to the occiput.

As always, the contact will be extremely light, whether on or off the body. As always, the practitioner's hands – and whole being – will be extremely soft and fluidic. As always, we will establish appropriate levels of physical contact, appropriate levels of attention, and engagement with the system on all the various different tissue levels – bony, membranous, fluid, energy.

THE SIX SPHENO-BASILAR PATTERNS

1. Flexion/extension

Flexion and extension are the usual physiological expressions of rhythmic motion of the cranio-sacral system during the expansion (flexion) and contraction (extension) phases of motion – whether in cranio-sacral rhythm or in middle tide (see Figure 45.2).

During the flexion phase of motion, the sphenoid arcs forward and down (nose-diving) together with the rest of the front of the cranium.

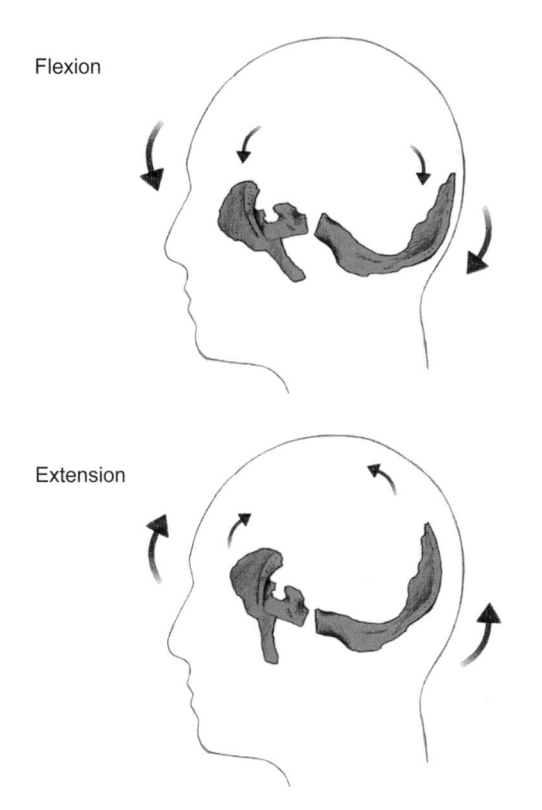

45.2 Flexion and extension at the spheno-basilar synchondrosis

During the extension phase of motion, the sphenoid moves back and up.

At the same time, during the flexion phase of motion, the occiput tucks under towards the atlas (also flaring). During the extension phase of motion, the occiput arcs back and out (also narrowing).

This combination of movements between the sphenoid and the occiput produces flexion and extension at the inferior surface of the spheno-basilar synchondrosis. *(Flexion is the closing or narrowing of an angle. Extension is the opening or straightening out of an angle – as seen for example in flexing or extending your elbow.)*

It is because of the movement at this joint that Sutherland chose to establish the terms flexion and extension to describe the movements of certain midline bones during the expansion and contraction phases of motion of the cranio-sacral system.

Perfect fluency

In a perfect system, this rhythmic movement of flexion and extension will be fluent, fluidic, easeful and balanced.

Imperfect imbalance

Since very few of us are perfect, it is common to find that the system moves more readily into one phase of motion than the other, or may seem to be held into one phase rather the other – either more into flexion, or more into extension.
This could be the result of past trauma – birth trauma, accidents, physical injuries at any time in life – emotional tension, or personality.

Restoring balance and fluency

Using the concept of SBS patterns, we can explore any imbalances with greater precision and accuracy, and thereby enhance the system's natural tendency to restore balance, fluency and integration.

The process

Engage with the system through the standard sphenoid contact.

Feel the natural flow and balance of rhythmic motion.

Observe whether there is any tendency for the system to move more readily into flexion, or more readily into extension.

- Some cranio-sacral systems express a very clear imbalance, drawing strongly into one phase rather than the other, immediately apparent even to casual observation.
- Other systems may not immediately reveal any imbalance on first sight – but closer observation (and *informed* observation) may reveal subtle imbalances that were not apparent on the surface.

So look more closely – but without intensity, remaining soft and spacious.

Continue to observe the natural flow of flexion/extension motion, allowing your hands to be washed gently by the waves of rhythmic motion.

As you observe flexion/extension motion, ask the system whether it prefers to move:

- more readily into flexion, during the flexion phase
- more readily into extension, during the extension phase.

This process does not involve any physical input from the therapist, but simply asking questions. You are not trying to make the system do anything, but simply observing more closely for any subtle imbalances of motion within the natural flow of rhythmic motion.

As always, 'asking the system' can be interpreted as asking yourself whether you can feel any preference or tendency within the system.

- If the system favours flexion, it is described as a flexion pattern.
- If it favours extension, it is described as an extension pattern.

In order to assist the system in addressing and resolving this imbalance, we will, as always, allow the evolution of usual fundamental principles – following the system into its preferred direction – whether into flexion or into extension – until it reaches a point of stillness, release and reorganisation.

This *may happen spontaneously*. The system may naturally want to draw into that pattern, since that is its inherent tendency – its way of resolving any imbalances.

But *often the system needs a little help* – to overcome inertia, to overcome counterbalancing strains, or simply to provide the necessary energy to initiate the response. The very presence of the practitioner's focused and *informed awareness, identifying the pattern, may be sufficient stimulus* to the system to respond and address it – which is why it is helpful to understand these SBS patterns.

Asking questions of the system provides a more specific stimulus, focusing the practitioner's attention more specifically on the relevant pattern, and thereby identifying subtle hidden patterns of imbalance within the system which are not readily identifiable on the surface, again recognising the therapeutic value of informed awareness.

Having identified the preferred phase of motion, we can ask the system again if it would like to move in that direction; and as it takes up that offer, we can again allow it to go there, follow it continuously and consistently as far as it wants to go in that direction, and wait at the resulting point of stillness until it releases.

As the system returns to neutral and rhythmic motion is re-established, you can re-evaluate the rhythmic motion, observing whether there is still any tendency to favour one phase, or whether flexion/extension motion is now more balanced and even. Once the system has settled through several cycles of easeful flexion/extension motion, and the quality, symmetry and motion feel settled, you can move on.

This process can be applied in much the same way to each of the six SBS patterns, so an abbreviated *summary* of the process, applicable to each of the patterns, may be helpful:

Having engaged with the system:

1. Observe any inherent preference in one direction or another – asking the system if it favours one direction or the other.
2. Allow it to go there – following consistently into the favoured direction.
3. Keep following to a point of balanced tension or stillness
4. Wait for release, reorganisation, and settling back to neutral – re-evaluating quality, symmetry and motion.

2. Torsion

Definition

A torsion pattern indicates that there is a twist somewhere in the body. This could be anywhere – a twisted knee, a rotated pelvis, a torsioned vertebral segment in the spine, a twist in the neck, the cranium, the membrane system. It could be the result of a sprained ankle, or a back injury triggered by bending over to lift something heavy in a twisted position; it could have been caused by turning your head too quickly, or by a car accident in which the seat belt pulled the body into a twist; it could be a deeply ingrained pattern arising from birth.

Whatever the cause and whenever it occurred, such twists will have repercussions throughout the body and be reflected in the spheno-basilar area as a torsion pattern.

A torsion or twist manifests at the SBS as the sphenoid twisting superiorly on one side in relation to the occiput – the other side twisting inferiorly.

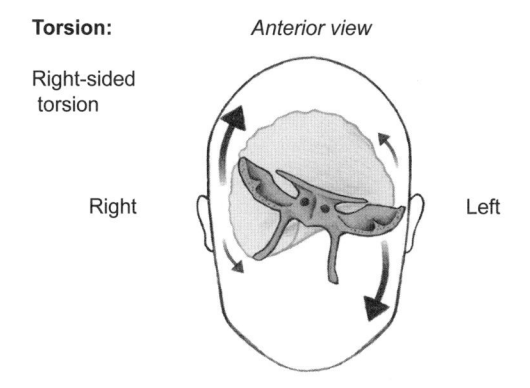

Torsion: Anterior view

Right-sided torsion

Right   Left

45.3 Torsion – in a right-sided torsion, the sphenoid greater wing twists superiorly on the right and inferiorly on the left, relative to the occiput

With the thumbs on the tips of the greater wings of the sphenoid, the therapist will experience this as one thumb twisting up towards the top of the head (superiorly) while the other thumb twists down towards the feet (inferiorly).

(This can feel like twisting a peach in half. You probably eat a peach simply by putting it to your mouth and taking a bite, but if you wanted to cut your peach in half, you could use a knife to cut around the middle of the peach and then twist it in half. Perhaps an avocado is a better example. The feel of an SBS torsion is similar to twisting the peach or avocado in half – at least in terms of direction.)

The torsion is named by the side that is *superior*, in other words; the side on which the sphenoid greater wing is superior – but this does not imply that the source of the twist is on that side. The source could be anywhere in the body, but is resulting in a twist through the body which manifests as a torsion to that side.

Identifying

The process for identifying and addressing a torsion is much the same as described earlier for the flexion/extension pattern.

- Engage with the system, and with rhythmic motion.

- Observe any obvious tendency for the head to twist in one direction or another, i.e. for the sphenoid greater wing to twist superiorly on one side and inferiorly on the other side. This may be immediately apparent, or it may not be evident.

- If no obvious torsion is apparent, explore in greater detail, to see if there might perhaps be some subtle twist hidden under the surface. Ask the system if it would like to torsion to the right (right thumb up, left thumb down) or to torsion to the left (left thumb up, right thumb down).

  As always, there is no physical input, just asking questions.

- It is helpful to ask these questions in time with the rhythmic motion. This is not essential, but it provides a more balanced view if you ask your questions during the same phase of motion each time. In other words:

  - As the system moves into extension, ask if it wants to torsion to the right.
  - As the system moves into flexion, allow it to settle back to the centre.
  - As it moves into extension again, ask if it wants to torsion to the left.
  - As it moves into flexion again, allow it to settle back to the centre.

The advantage of asking in time with the rhythmic motion is that you are establishing 'a level playing field' so that your perception is not distorted by the fact of the system being in flexion for one reading, in extension for another, or somewhere in between flexion and extension for another reading. Another advantage is that it keeps you clearly engaged with the system through its rhythmic motion, thereby guarding against becoming too physically involved, or too mentally intense, or so caught up in the technical aspects of the process that you lose touch with the cranio-sacral system.

You can ask these questions two or three times, until you have a clear response. There may be a clear sense of torsion to one side; there may be a very subtle impression of torsion to one side; or there may be no particular favoured direction. Torsion is not an inherent physiological movement of the system in the way that flexion and extension are, but there is usually a sense of some slight potential degree of torsion in each direction. If this feels equal on both sides, then there may not be any torsion pattern to be addressed at that moment.

Addressing

Where there is a very obvious torsion, the system may be very eager to draw into that pattern spontaneously and you can simply follow it where it wants to go.

In other circumstances, where the torsion pattern is more subtle, or where the system is held by conflicting patterns or other overriding factors, it may benefit from more specific attention on the part of the practitioner:

Having identified a torsion pattern:

- Ask the system again if it wishes to enter into its favoured direction.
- Allow it to go there, following consistently as far as it wishes to go.
- Keep following till it reaches a point of balanced tension or stillness.
- Wait at the point of stillness until you feel a sense of release, reorganisation, and settling back to neutral, with the re-emergence of rhythmic motion.
- Re-evaluate the system to see if the torsion pattern is still evident, whether it has reduced, or whether it is no longer evident – asking questions as before.
- Re-evaluate quality, symmetry and motion:
  ○ perhaps feeling a more settled easeful quality
  ○ a more balanced symmetry
  ○ and a more expansive fluent rhythmic motion.
- Once the system has settled through a few cycles of easeful rhythmic motion, you can move on.

Degree of resolution

Some patterns will resolve completely, others will resolve substantially, others may reduce slightly but remain clearly evident. The degree to which a pattern resolves is primarily related to its chronicity, as mentioned previously. Long-established, deeply ingrained patterns not only will take longer to release, but also may release only partially, so that the pattern remains evident, although reduced. Such patterns may need to be addressed several times, perhaps over several sessions.

One common cause of torsion patterns is as a result of birth patterns in which the baby twists through the birth canal. Such patterns, if they remain untreated into adulthood, are likely to be deeply ingrained in the body tissues, well established within the growth patterns of the whole body, and therefore not likely to disappear instantly. This does not mean that they can't be resolved – just that it is likely to take longer.

3. Side-bending

Definition

A side-bending pattern at the SBS indicates that there is a side-bending restriction somewhere in the body. This could be a scoliosis due to vertebral restriction in the spine, a pelvic imbalance, muscular tension on one side of the body, a contraction of the pericardium around the heart, a head injury or, as always, anything anywhere in the body and reflecting throughout the body.

This side-bending restriction manifests at the SBS as a gapping between the sphenoid body and the basi-occiput on one side, with a corresponding narrowing on the opposite side.

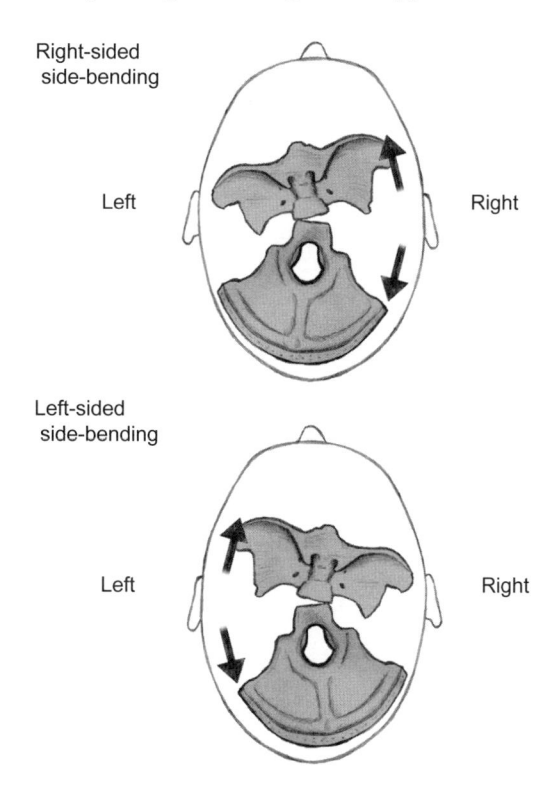

45.4 Side-bending – in a right-sided side-bending pattern, the head bulges on the right

The therapist will experience this as a bulge on one side of the head, with the other side of the head seeming to cave in. This can feel as if you are holding a balloon, which is being squeezed in on one side (as if your thumb and little finger are drawn towards each other) and consequently bulging out on the other side (as if your thumb and little finger are being pushed apart).

The pattern is named by the side that is bulging – which is odd, because it is contrary to common usage for side-bending in other anatomical descriptions, but since that is the convention established by Sutherland, it is clearer to stick with that terminology. So a right-sided side-bending pattern is one in which the head bulges on the right – perhaps most clearly (although more cumbersomely) expressed as a side-bending pattern with bulge to the right – and more commonly and easily expressed as a right side-bending.

Identifying

The process for identifying and addressing side-bending patterns is very similar to the process for torsion patterns:

- Engage with the system, and with rhythmic motion.
- Observe any obvious tendency for the head to bulge to one side or the other. This may be immediately apparent, or it may not be evident.
- If no obvious bulge is apparent, explore in greater detail, to see if there might perhaps be some subtle sense of bulging hidden under the surface. Ask the system if it would like to bulge to the right (while caving in on the left) or to bulge to the left (while caving in on the right).

  As always, there is no physical input, just asking questions.

- As before, it is helpful to ask these questions in time with the rhythmic motion – inviting the bulge as the system moves into extension, returning to the centre as the system moves into flexion.
- You can ask these questions two or three times, until you have a clear response.

Addressing

Where there is a very obvious bulge, the system may be very eager to draw into that pattern spontaneously and you can simply follow it where it wants to go. Where the side-bending pattern is more subtle, you can give more specific attention to the particular detail of the pattern, in order to enhance the body's ability to address the restriction.

Having identified a side-bending pattern:

- Ask the system again if it wishes to bulge into its favoured direction, caving in on the other side.
- Allow it to go there, following consistently as far as it wishes to go.
- Keep following till it reaches a point of balanced tension or stillness.

- Wait at the point of stillness for release, reorganisation, and settling back to neutral – with the re-emergence of rhythmic motion.
- Re-evaluate the system to see if the side-bending pattern is still evident, whether it has reduced, or whether it is no longer evident – asking questions as before.
- Re-evaluate quality, symmetry and motion.
- Once the system has settled through a few cycles of easeful rhythmic motion, you can move on.

Two groups

These six patterns are sometimes considered to divide into two groups. The three which we have described so far are regarded as less severe. They tend to reflect everyday stresses and strains. The causative factors are more often located outside the cranio-sacral system – muscular tensions, minor injuries, reflected into the cranio-sacral system. The symptoms connected with these patterns are usually of a more transient nature, such as headaches or short-term aches and pains.

The latter three patterns more often arise from major trauma directly to the cranio-sacral system, such as a direct blow to the head or birth trauma. These patterns tend to be more deeply ingrained, more chronic and solidified, and therefore more resistant when it comes to treatment. Because the symptoms associated with these patterns are more deeply rooted in the system, they are likely to be more severe. Migraine, autism and personality disorders are examples of the sort of symptoms associated with these latter three patterns.

However, these are fairly broad generalisations. All six patterns can arise from both minor and major trauma and may be transient or deeply resistant, depending on many different factors. These generalisations should therefore be taken only as a broad guideline, perhaps contributing to an understanding of where certain patterns have arisen or why they are so resistant to change, and therefore contributing to an overall understanding of the complete picture.

4. Lateral shift (also known as lateral strain, lateral shear, side-shift)

Definition

A lateral shift pattern at the SBS indicates that there is a lateral shift pattern held somewhere in the body.

Obvious causes might be a blow to the side of the head, or a blow to the side of the pelvis – shunting it to one side, with the whole body adapting to the injured area with appropriate compensatory patterns of lateral shift, at various levels throughout the body.

This lateral shift pattern will manifest at the SBS as the sphenoid shifting directly to one side relative to the occiput.

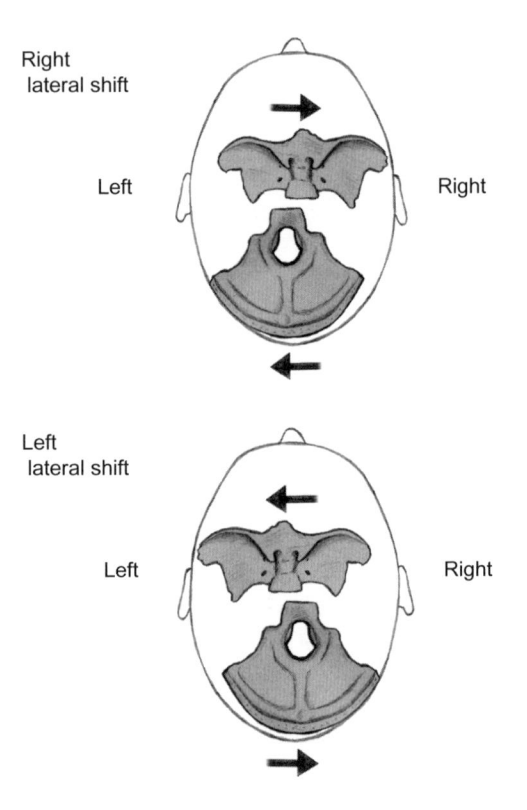

45.5 Lateral shift – in a right-sided lateral shift pattern, the sphenoid shifts to the right, relative to the occiput

The therapist will experience this as if the head were a parallelogram, with both thumbs shifting together either to the left or to the right.

The pattern is named by the direction towards which the thumbs (and sphenoid) are shifting.

Identifying

The process for identifying and addressing lateral shift patterns is very similar to the process for side-bending patterns:

- Engage with the system, and with rhythmic motion.
- Observe any obvious tendency for both thumbs to be drawn to one side, giving the impression of a parallelogram. This may be immediately apparent, or it may not be evident.
- If no obvious side-shift is apparent, explore in greater detail, to see if there might perhaps be some subtle sense of shift hidden under the surface. Ask the system if it would like to shift to the right (both thumbs shifting together) or to shift to the left.

  As always, there is no physical input, just asking questions.

- As before, it is helpful to ask these questions in time with the rhythmic motion – inviting the lateral shift as the system moves into extension, returning to the centre as the system moves into flexion.
- You can ask these questions two or three times, until you have a clear response.

Addressing

Where there is a very obvious lateral shift, the system may be very eager to draw into that pattern spontaneously and you can simply follow it where it wants to go. Where the pattern is more subtle, you can give more specific attention to the particular detail of the pattern, in order to enhance the body's ability to address the restriction.

Having identified a lateral shift:

- Ask the system again if it wishes to shift into its favoured direction.
- Allow it to go there, following consistently as far as it wishes to go.

- Keep following till it reaches a point of balanced tension or stillness.
- Wait at the point of stillness for release, reorganisation, and settling back to neutral – feeling the re-emergence of rhythmic motion.
- Re-evaluate the system to see if the lateral shift pattern is still evident, whether it has reduced, or whether it is no longer evident – asking questions as before.
- Re-evaluate quality, symmetry and motion.
- Once the system has settled through a few cycles of easeful rhythmic motion, you can move on.

5. Vertical shift (also known as vertical strain, vertical shear)

Definition

A vertical shift pattern at the SBS indicates that there is a vertical shift pattern affecting the body.

This will manifest at the SBS as if the sphenoid body is shifted superiorly or inferiorly in relation to the basi-occiput.

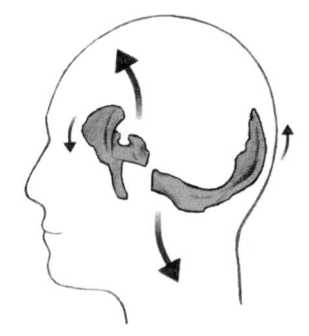

45.6 Vertical shift – in a superior vertical shift pattern, the body of the sphenoid moves superiorly relative to the basi-occiput, while the greater wings (and thumbs) move inferiorly

The therapist may experience this as either the thumbs being drawn straight down towards the feet (superior vertical shift) or the thumbs being drawn straight up towards the top of the head (inferior vertical shift). In both cases the occiput will be shifting in the opposite direction.

You may have noticed that the naming of these vertical shift patterns appears contradictory.

If we look in more detail at what is happening at the SBS, we will see that there is an explanation:

In all of these SBS patterns, the movements are actually more complex than the simplified versions that have so far been described. Rather than moving directly in the directions described, they all involve *rotatory* movements of the sphenoid and occiput, which result in the specific effects at the spheno-basilar synchondrosis. In the case of the vertical shift, these rotatory elements become more significant.

As can be seen in Figure 45.6, when the body of the sphenoid moves *superiorly* (at the SBS), the tips of the greater wings (and therefore the thumbs) move *inferiorly*. When the body of the sphenoid moves *inferiorly* (at the SBS), the tips of the greater wings (and therefore the thumbs) move *superiorly*. So when you feel your thumbs being drawn straight down towards the feet, this is superior vertical shift (at the SBS); and when you feel your thumbs being drawn straight up towards the top of the head, this is inferior vertical shift (at the SBS).

Vertical shift patterns are also sometimes confused with flexion/extension patterns, so it is useful to identify certain significant differences.

Firstly:
- In vertical shift patterns, the thumbs and little fingers are moving in opposite directions. When the thumbs are moving towards the feet, the little fingers are moving towards the top of the head, and vice versa.
- In flexion/extension patterns, the thumbs and little fingers are moving together, arcing down towards each other, or arcing back up away from each other.

Secondly:
- Vertical shift patterns are felt in a straight line between the feet and the top of the head, thumbs drawing straight down towards the feet, while the little fingers are drawing straight up towards the top of the head.
- Flexion/extension patterns are felt as an arcing movement, thumbs and little fingers arcing forward and down towards each other, or arcing back and up away from each other.

Identifying

The process for identifying and addressing vertical shift patterns is similar to the process for previous patterns:

- Engage with the system, and with rhythmic motion.
- Observe any obvious tendency for both thumbs to be drawn in a straight line down towards the feet (superior vertical shift) or in a straight line up towards the top of the head (inferior vertical shift). This may be immediately apparent, or it may not be evident.
- If no obvious vertical shift is apparent, explore in greater detail, to see if there might perhaps be some subtle sense of vertical shift hidden under the surface. Ask the system if it would like to shift superiorly or inferiorly.

    As always, there is no physical input, just asking questions.

- In the case of vertical shift, it is *not* helpful to ask these questions in time with the rhythmic motion, due to the potential confusion with flexion/extension motion.
- You can ask these questions two or three times, until you have a clear response.

Addressing

Where there is a very obvious vertical shift, the system may be very eager to draw into that pattern spontaneously and you can simply follow it where it wants to go. Where the pattern is more subtle, you can give more specific attention to the particular detail of the pattern, in order to enhance the body's ability to address the restriction.

Having identified a vertical shift:

- Ask the system again if it wishes to shift into its favoured direction.
- Allow it to go there, following consistently as far as it wishes to go.
- Keep following till it reaches a point of balanced tension or stillness.
- Wait at the point of stillness for release, reorganisation, and settling back to neutral – feeling the re-emergence of rhythmic motion.

- Re-evaluate the system to see if the vertical shift pattern is still evident, whether it has reduced, or whether it is no longer evident – asking questions as before.
- Re-evaluate quality, symmetry and motion.
- Once the system has settled through a few cycles of easeful rhythmic motion, you can move on.

6. Compression
Definition
A compression pattern at the SBS indicates that there is a compression force held somewhere in the body. As always, this could be coming from anywhere. It could be a specific reflection of a lumbo-sacral compression, or a suboccipital compression; it could be the result of slipping on ice and sitting down heavily – any time in life, recent or many years ago; it could be the result of a blow to the head or a car accident or a sports injury; it could have arisen at birth; it could be a reflection of a generalised quality of compression throughout the body – whether due to physical injury, occupational positioning, postural collapse, or emotional tension; it could be associated with depression.

Whatever the source, the compression can be identified through the window of the SBS, and in addressing it at the SBS, you will be addressing the pattern throughout the body, with all its ramifications and repercussions, physical and emotional.

We have already looked at spheno-basilar compression in Chapter 27, and what we are looking at here is exactly the same, but we are looking at it in more detail and within a wider context.

In a compression pattern, the sphenoid is compressed posteriorly towards the occiput, compressing the joint between the sphenoid body and the occiput (the spheno-basilar synchondrosis).

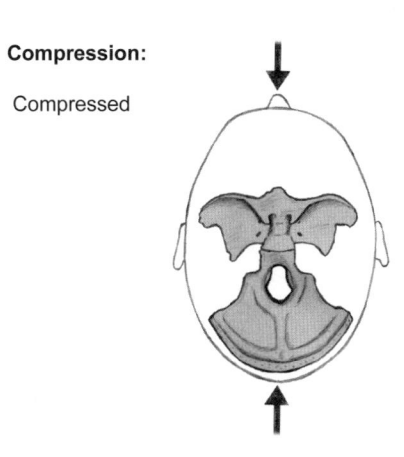

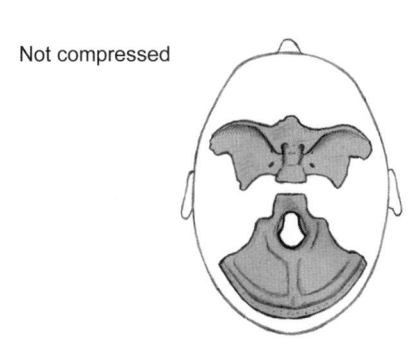

Compression:

Compressed

Not compressed

45.7 Compression – in a compression pattern, the sphenoid is compressed posteriorly towards the occiput, and the occiput is compressed anteriorly towards the sphenoid

The therapist may experience this as both thumbs being drawn posteriorly towards the occiput. In other words, with the patient lying on their back, your thumbs are being drawn down towards the couch.

A compression pattern is named by the presence of compression. Unlike the other SBS patterns, there is no corresponding opposite pattern; there is no 'decompression' pattern, since, if the spheno-basilar joint is not compressed, it is freely mobile, loose and unrestricted (at least in that direction) and therefore does not qualify as a 'pattern' of restriction. Nevertheless, we can explore the possibility of decompression – as an indicator of lack of compression.

Identifying

- Engage with the system, and with rhythmic motion.
- Observe the quality of the system – does it feel stuck, held and compressed, or loose, free and open? Observe any tendency for the thumbs to be drawn down towards the couch (posteriorly), or for the thumbs to feel light, soft, floating upwards towards the ceiling (anteriorly). There may be an immediate strong sense of drawing the thumbs down into the couch into compression, or there may not be any evident indication of compression.
- If no obvious compression is apparent, explore in greater detail, to see if there might perhaps be some subtle sense of compression hidden under the surface. Ask the system if it would like to draw into compression; ask if it would like to float freely up towards the ceiling into decompression.

As always, there is no physical input, just asking questions.

A compressed system will tend to draw into compression and will be reluctant to decompress. A system that is not compressed will tend to decompress readily and will not show any tendency to draw into compression.

These questions *can* be asked in time with the rhythmic motion. However, in the case of compression, it can be helpful to sustain the question over several cycles of motion – inviting compression through two or three complete cycles of rhythmic motion, then inviting decompression through two or three cycles of rhythmic motion.

As with the vertical shift patterns, there is potential confusion between compression/decompression and flexion/extension motion and it is necessary to distinguish them from one another. In compression, the thumbs are drawn directly in a *straight* line down towards the couch (posteriorly), whereas in flexion, the motion is *arcing* forward and down. Similarly, the direction of decompression is in a *straight* line up towards the ceiling (anteriorly), whereas extension motion is *arcing* back and up.

Addressing

Where there is a powerful sense of compression, the system is likely to draw into that pattern readily and spontaneously, and you can follow it wherever it takes you. Where the pattern is more subtle, you can give more specific attention to the particular detail of the pattern, in order to enhance the body's ability to address the compression.

If compression is present (in other words, the system seems to draw into compression and is reluctant to decompress), then once again offer the system compression and this time allow it to go as far as it wants to into the compressive pattern, following it consistently as far as it wants to go. As you do so, you may feel a gradual build-up of tension or pressure within the system:

- Keep following till it reaches a point of balanced tension or stillness.
- Wait at the point of stillness for release, reorganisation, and settling back to neutral – feeling the re-emergence of rhythmic motion.
- Re-evaluate the system to see if the compression pattern is still evident, whether it has reduced, or whether it is no longer evident – asking questions as before.
- Re-evaluate quality, symmetry and motion.
- Once the system has settled through a few cycles of easeful rhythmic motion, you can move on.

Decompression following compression

Although there is no 'decompression' pattern, it is a usually beneficial, following any exploration of compression patterns, to offer decompression to the system. This is helpful for two reasons.

Firstly, it helps to ensure that no hint of compression from the therapist – even the thought of compression is left in the system.

Secondly, and more significantly, it helps the system to make the most of its new-found uncompressed state, to take advantage of its release from any compressive patterns, and to expand more fully into an open, decompressed, freely mobile state.

The process of decompression

Once the system has settled back to neutral following its release from compression:

- Ask again if it would like to decompress.
- If it favours decompression, allow it to go there, following consistently as far as it wants to go – floating up towards the ceiling.

It may feel as if the sphenoid is floating freely several feet up into the air. It is helpful to become fully absorbed into this floating feeling and to follow it right up to the ceiling, as this is what it is doing energetically and it is at these extremes of apparent movement that the most profound therapeutic changes occur.

- Keep following it as far as it wants to go, until it is floating completely freely, no longer twisting, no longer resisting (this may take several minutes).
- Once it has reached a point of stillness, gently allow the sphenoid to settle back down onto the front of the cranium.
- Allow the system to settle back to neutral.
- Re-evaluate quality, symmetry and motion:
  - perhaps feeling a more settled easeful quality
  - a more balanced symmetry
  - and a more expansive fluent rhythmic motion.
- Once the system has settled through a few cycles of easeful rhythmic motion, you can move on.

(See the following page for a summary of sphenobasilar patterns.)

330 \ Cranio-Sacral Integration

Bony perspective	Practitioner's perspective	Lateral view

a. Flexion

b. Extension

c. Torsion - right sided

anterior view
R   L

far side
near side

d. Sidebending - right sided

L   R

head bulging on the right

e. Sideshift - right sided

L   R

not visible from this perspective

f. Vertical shift - superior

g. Compression

not visible from this perspective

45.8 Spheno-basilar patterns – summary

Chapter 46

Opus 27 Number 2
Spheno-Basilar Integration

If you listen to Beethoven's Moonlight sonata, you will hear a profoundly beautiful and sensitive piece of music. And yet much of it is built – both in the opening Adagio and the final Presto – on arpeggios. These basic building blocks of music can be so profoundly effective when incorporated appropriately (and with a little touch of genius) into an integrated piece of music.

In Chapter 45 we have looked at the spheno-basilar patterns as individual patterns, basic building blocks, the scales and arpeggios of the cranio-sacral process. Now we will explore how to incorporate these basic technical skills into a more integrated fluent approach through which we can move beyond mere technique to integrated treatment of the cranio-sacral system, beyond scales and arpeggios to a more flowing expression of music.

We will look at spheno-basilar integration from several perspectives:

1. An integrated approach – working with what's there, rather than looking for specific patterns, or following a routine.
2. An integrated understanding – recognising that patterns occur in combinations, rather than individually.
3. Integration of the concept of SBS patterns into an overall treatment session.
4. Integrated diagnosis and treatment of the whole person through the SBS.

1. An integrated approach

Having examined the individual patterns separately, we can now explore how to work in a more integrated manner with this concept – a manner more in tune with what actually happens in the body.

The approach, as always, comes down to allowing the evolution of the inherent treatment process.

The difference is that, having explored these SBS patterns, we can now tune in with an *informed awareness*. We can allow, follow, reach points of stillness, release and reorganisation. But with this additional knowledge and understanding, your fingers and your attention will subconsciously recognise and identify more subtle detail – and therefore be more precise, more profound and more effective.

In other words, an integrated approach to SBS patterns does not need to involve a methodical examination of each pattern in turn, but is simply allowing the system to express itself, following whatever responses arise – but with greater awareness.

2. An integrated understanding

Initially, we explored the SBS patterns as if they were individual items occurring in isolation. This is helpful in order to learn and identify the basic nature of each pattern.

In real life, SBS patterns don't occur in isolation. They occur in combinations – a complex mass of patterns – reflecting all the injuries, accidents and imbalances that have accumulated throughout life.

Any injury or trauma creates a combination of patterns. There is a multitude of different traumas reflecting our whole history, creating a similarly complex multitude of combined, intertwined, interactive patterns within the SBS, a combination of torsions, side-bendings, lateral shifts, vertical shifts, and compressions, pulling in different directions, like a tangled ball of wool, full of knots and twists.

When you engage with the cranio-sacral system through the sphenoid, you may encounter various different responses:

- There may be a predominant pattern pulling in one direction.
- There may be a number of pulls, twists and movements, all drawing in different directions, the system not quite sure which way to go.
- You might find the system starting to draw in one direction, but with other pulls and twists emerging simultaneously.
- You might feel the whole system solid, stuck, jammed – perhaps because there are so many different pulls drawing in opposite directions, perhaps in direct opposition to each other, that the system is unable to move in any direction, unable even to express fluent rhythmic motion.

Whatever you encounter, the approach to the cranio-sacral system, as always, is:

- engage
- allow the system to express itself.

One predominant pattern

If there is one predominant pattern, you can allow the system to follow into that, to stillness and release – but without any rigid sense of having to stick with that particular pattern or direction. You may find that as the process evolves, things change, the direction of movement changes, different patterns arise and as one thing releases, it leads to another.

A mass of different pulls

If you feel a mass of different pulls and twists drawing in different directions, you can again follow the inherent treatment process – allowing the system to express itself, observing these various pulls and twists and waiting for the system to sort itself out.

In due course, so long as your attention is aware and alert, observing each of these subtle movements and twists, the system may address one pattern after another. As one pattern disentangles, something else becomes apparent; and a process of continuous disentanglement, points of stillness and release, evolves and continues.

As always, all you need to do is be there with the system, in stillness and spaciousness, aware and alert, your attention engaged with the system, thereby providing the stable fulcrum around which the system can respond and disentangle.

INFORMED AWARENESS

The fact that your *informed* attention is specifically identifying and engaging with the patterns within the cranio-sacral system is a major factor in enabling the cranio-sacral process to evolve. It is through *informed awareness* that more effective, more profound, and more detailed responses are enabled.

When concert pianists are playing Beethoven's Moonlight Sonata, they are not thinking about scales and arpeggios, but their fingers are so familiar with these technical skills that they flow with the essence of the music, oblivious to technique. In the same way, as a cranio-sacral therapist engaged in treatment, you don't need to think about torsions, side-bendings and lateral shifts, but your fingers and your attention need to be well practised in how to recognise them, so that they can respond fluently, albeit unconsciously, to all the tiny little details, to all the tangled mass of patterns, all the multitude of torsions, side-bendings, lateral shifts, vertical shifts, flexions, extensions and compressions that arise from moment to moment within the patient's system. A cranio-sacral therapist who doesn't have that firm grounding in technique and basic skills is likely to be more limited in their effectiveness.

Simultaneous patterns

When you find the system starting to draw in one direction, and then other patterns start to emerge simultaneously – simply allow that to happen. Perhaps you find the system drawing into a right-sided twist, then as you allow that to be expressed, the head simultaneously starts to bulge on the same side; and as you allow that to happen so you feel your thumbs drawn into a parallelogram towards the opposite direction. Simply allow the process to evolve.

When several different patterns emerge simultaneously – as happens most of the time – this is described as stacking.

STACKING

Stacking means piling things on top of each other.

Throughout our lives, vast numbers of traumas and tensions are stacked on top of each other, layer by layer, year by year, in our body tissues, in our psyches. The cranio-sacral system reflects this stack of traumas. The SBS reflects this stack of patterns.

As we engage with the system through the SBS, we may encounter this stack of patterns, with several patterns emerging simultaneously stacked on top of each other – perhaps a right-sided torsion, combined with a left-sided side-bending, together with a right lateral shift, for example. Stacking will occur spontaneously, and all we need to do is recognise the various components stacked together and allow their spontaneous release. The body may need to reveal these patterns simultaneously in order to release and move forward – perhaps because they were imposed simultaneously or because they are somehow intertwined and inseparable.

Stacking can also be introduced deliberately. This can be helpful when encountering a particularly entrenched resistance, when the system is not responding readily, when the system appears to become stuck.

In such situations, we can apply our informed awareness to surveying the system, exploring why it is stuck and is not moving forward, identifying precisely which patterns are arising in the stack at this moment, and what precise detail may need to be identified and acknowledged in order to enable the release of this complex and entrenched resistance.

It is in such circumstances that specific application of the knowledge of SBS patterns may be the key to effective release, surveying through each individual pattern, asking questions of the system to see if it wants to reveal some little detail that is hidden under the surface and not responding.

INEXTRICABLY INTERTWINED

As mentioned, when a system is locked and unresponsive, it may be because it has a specific need to express certain combinations simultaneously in order to release restrictions that were imposed simultaneously. A common example might be the multidirectional forces imposed by a car accident.

The patient was sitting in her car in a line of traffic, contentedly listening to the radio. Suddenly, another car crashed into her car from behind at a slight angle, her neck was thrown back then whiplashed forward; the seat belt prevented her from hitting the windscreen but pulled her body round into a twist, at which point her car shunted into the car in front, she was thrown forward and immediately whiplashed back; as she moved back, her head hit the side window. As all this was happening, shock and fear were rising up in an overwhelming wave of confusion.

PRECISE IDENTIFICATION

As all these various factors were imprinted simultaneously into her body, they became inextricably intertwined. When you tune into that patient's system, your informed awareness can enable their disentanglement. But with such complex and entrenched combinations, precise identification of specific detail, again through informed awareness, can be the key that unlocks the combination.

ACKNOWLEDGING EMOTIONAL FACTORS

Recognising and acknowledging the qualities of shock and fear arising in conjunction with the physical twists and pulls can also be vital in enabling the release. The shock and fear held into the tissues may be the factors that are maintaining and perpetuating the patient's debilitated condition – perhaps for years after the accident (probably leading to her being dismissed as a malingerer or her symptoms being dismissed as psychosomatic, instead of having her condition diagnosed and addressed appropriately).

If you don't acknowledge these factors, the system may remain locked. When your informed awareness recognises those emotional qualities, it enables their release. A comprehensive perspective on the whole scene, acknowledging all the aspects that occurred together in that moment – the precise combination of physical patterns together with the emotional component – can bring the whole process to life and enable it to move from a frozen image to a moving picture, from a locked position to moving forward – out of resistance and into free-flowing vitality, from a feeling of being stuck to feeling that your life can move forward again at last.

In the same way, recognition of the emotional components of many different traumas and tensions within the system may be vital to their effective release and resolution.

Stacking occurs spontaneously most of the time. Deliberate stacking is not generally necessary – since the cranio-sacral system will for the most part know what it needs to do for itself. However, deliberate stacking can be helpful at certain times, particularly when specific combinations of patterns are holding the system locked into a particular state – such as following the car accident described above. This is no different from any other cranio-sacral work. It is simply focusing the practitioner's informed awareness more closely on the inherent patterns within the system in order to help the system to overcome persistent resistances or inertia.

A system that is jammed up

When you feel a system that is jammed up, locked solid, that doesn't seem to want to move in any direction, there may be various factors contributing to the situation. It could be due to the 'simultaneousness' of the forces imposed, as in the car accident above. It could be emotional factors. It could be that the system is in shock.

It could also be a multiplicity of different forces, not necessarily imposed simultaneously, but pulling the system in so many different directions that it can't move in any direction. There can also be forces pulling in direct opposition to each other, arising from different injuries at different times (see Figure 46.1).

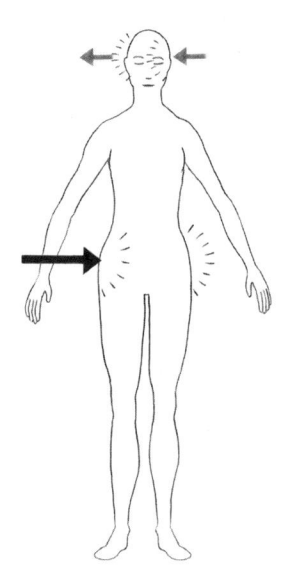

| An impact from the right, shifting the pelvis to the left, may induce a corresponding right-sided side shift at the SBS. The body might adapt and cope reasonably well. | Some time later, a relatively minor blow to the left shoulder, shifting the shoulders to the right, might induce an opposing left-sided shift at the SBS. | The combination of left lateral shift and right lateral shift, although imposed many years apart, may leave the whole system locked up and unable to function effectively. |

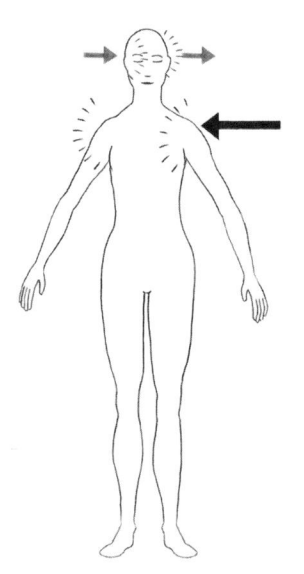

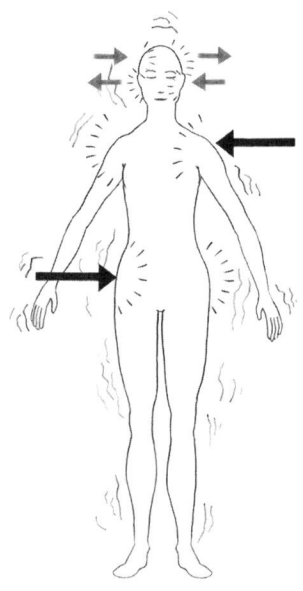

46.1 *A combination of forces acting in direct opposition to each other can leave the whole system jammed up and unable to function effectively*

OPPOSING FORCES

A shunt from the right, shifting the pelvis to the left, might induce a corresponding right-sided lateral shift in the SBS. The body might adapt to that and the patient might cope reasonably well. A few years later, a blow to the left shoulder, shifting the shoulders to the right, might induce an opposing left lateral shift at the SBS. This second injury might be relatively minor, but suddenly the patient's body can't cope at all and starts throwing up aches, pains and other symptoms all over the place – feeling stuck, tight, depressed, unable to think clearly. The combination of left lateral shift and right lateral shift, although imposed many years apart, are acting in direct opposition to each other, leaving the whole system jammed up and unable to function effectively, unable even to express fluent rhythmic motion.

When you encounter a system that is locked solid, the first step is as always to allow the evolution of the inherent treatment process, to wait patiently, to allow the system time to express itself. You will as a matter of course also explore for different sources of the jamming – emotional factors, shock, compression at the lumbo-sacral area or subocciput, birth patterns, other factors anywhere in the system.

In terms of the SBS, having allowed the system time for expression, there are also various other possible approaches:

- The most obvious is to apply the spheno-basilar release process introduced in Chapter 27 in the context of the overall treatment framework – gently asking the system if it would like to enter into spheno-basilar compression, followed by spheno-basilar decompression. This can have a widespread effect of releasing and opening up any system.
- You can also look more closely for subtle details of SBS patterns within the system, surveying the system through each of the six SBS patterns in turn in a more deliberate and meticulous manner, in order to identify any subtle hints of a pattern that might be hidden under the surface – and once you identify some tiny subtle hint of a pattern, this can provide the key to opening up the whole system, step by step.
- You may also encounter patterns that directly oppose each other – as in the example above – where the system seems to want to draw into both left lateral and right lateral shift. In such cases, you can choose to address each of them in turn, deliberately inviting the system to address the left lateral shift, and then, following some degree of release, inviting the system to address the right lateral shift – as you do so, identifying the source in the shoulder during the first release, and the source in the pelvis for the second release. It is likely that the more recent injury will be more accessible and amenable to treatment and will therefore arise and respond first.

3. Integration of the concept of SBS patterns into an overall treatment session

Although for the purpose of explanation, the SBS patterns were described in a separate section, they are not, of course, a separate part of treatment. In real treatment, as with all cranio-sacral processes, the approach to the SBS naturally becomes an integral part of any treatment session.

Every treatment is likely to involve some time spent at the cranium. The sphenoid contact is one of the most fundamental cranial contacts. As you work with this contact, or for that matter with any contact, you will naturally become aware of patterns:

- bulges, twists, parallelograms
- side-bendings, torsions, side-shifts

and you will respond to them appropriately – as a natural integral part of any treatment process.

Through your informed awareness of the fundamental SBS patterns, you will be able to respond to these patterns more effectively – consciously or unconsciously. You won't necessarily be thinking about SBS patterns. You certainly are not likely to be deliberately applying a spheno-basilar routine – unless circumstances specifically demand that. But your informed awareness will enable your hands, your fingers and your attention to identify, recognise and address intuitively the various patterns that arise from moment to moment.

(Intuitively here does not mean working blindly, or that you don't need any knowledge. It means that the profound depth of knowledge gained by extensive study and practice will enable you to engage with subtle and profound details within the system, without necessarily thinking them through logically, or even being consciously aware of them at the time.)

4. Integrated diagnosis and treatment of the whole person through the SBS

In exploring SBS patterns through the sphenoid, we are not looking merely at patterns within the SBS itself. We are reading the whole person as expressed through this particular window. Everything in the body-mind is reflected into the cranio-sacral system as a whole and consequently into the SBS and can therefore be identified and addressed through the SBS. But the degree to which the treatment involves the whole person will depend to a large extent on the way in which you use your attention.

Attention

In all cranio-sacral integration, your attention is constantly aware of the whole person – body and mind. If your awareness is focused merely on the SBS, the treatment will have limited effectiveness. It will still influence the whole person – treating the SBS will undoubtedly have repercussions on the rest of the system. But those repercussions may be limited, or you may encounter blockages or resistances that are not keen to respond and release.

When you extend your awareness to encompass the whole person, your effectiveness will extend and expand accordingly, you will engage with the whole person, you will identify the source of resistant restrictions, and enable more profound and comprehensive release and reorganisation.

Projection

Projection may arise spontaneously or may be introduced deliberately. As you engage with a particular pattern at the SBS, your attention may be drawn to other parts of the body and to fulcrums of resistance anywhere in the body, reflecting the source of the imbalance – perhaps to a particular vertebral level, perhaps down the left side to the stomach, perhaps through a complex pattern of twists and turns.

If your attention is not immediately drawn anywhere, you can also survey through the body, seeing what responses arise as you move your attention from place to place. The more you practise surveying through the body, the more you will develop the skills of projection and find your attention more readily drawn intuitively and spontaneously with less need to survey.

As you engage with the system at the SBS and project your attention through the body, you can identify any responses under your hands, any changes in quality, symmetry or motion as your attention rests at different areas.

- You might feel a contraction, tightness or compression at the SBS as your attention reaches the diaphragm in a patient whose breathing is shallow and whose diaphragm is held tight.
- You might experience agitation at the sphenoid as your attention focuses on the solar plexus of a nervous, worried patient.
- You might notice an increased lateral shift pattern at the SBS, as your attention reaches a pelvis which has been shunted laterally by a blow from the side.
- You might notice the head bulging into a side-bending pattern at the SBS as your attention passes through an area of scoliosis in the spine.

In the same way you could identify everything that is going on in the patient from the SBS, physical and emotional, recent or chronic, their whole life history – in so far as the system is ready to reveal it at that moment.

Spacious perception

When you are engaged in treatment, your attention will naturally be aware of the whole person as well as the specific features within the wider picture. This will happen spontaneously – so long as you are open to the possibility and your perception is sufficiently spacious and broad.

The more completely you can engage with the source of the pattern, the more effective the response to treatment will be. This includes not only identifying the source of the restriction on a physical level, but also picking up any emotional qualities and associations that may arise in conjunction with the pattern, and perhaps even a whole vivid picture of the incident which inflicted this pattern on the body – whether it be a specific accident, an image of the patient as a baby passing through the birth canal, or an image of a particular life situation – such as an abused child cowering in fear, reflecting some repeated childhood experience.

Hugh was 60 years old, suffering from constant pain down the whole of his left side, with particularly severe pain and twitching in his face, accompanied by nausea and agitation in his solar plexus. As I worked at his head, his system went into a strong right-sided torsion together with a right lateral shift. Among other aspects of the treatment, I had an image of a small boy being hit on the left side of the face with a sports implement. As the image arose, the pattern released. At the end of the treatment, I reported this image and Hugh confirmed that he had been hit very hard on the left side of his face with a golf club at the age of seven – an incident which he had completely forgotten until I mentioned it.

The whole picture

As you observe the changing patterns at the SBS, you can engage with the repercussions throughout the body, identifying focal points of restriction, diagnosing vertebral, visceral, emotional, musculo-skeletal or energetic focal points. As you hold into points of balanced tension, and project your attention down through the body, you can identify connections from this point of balanced tension to elsewhere in the body:

- perhaps the source of the restriction
- perhaps a symptomatic area
- perhaps a fulcrum around which this pattern is revolving
- perhaps identifying a number of different fulcra and focal points.

In this way you can make a detailed diagnosis and gain a profound understanding of the patient.

Susan suffered from back pain, especially around the right sacro-iliac area with pain radiating down the back of the right leg. She also suffered from asthma, triggered particularly by episodes of anxiety to which she was prone, and she suffered from right-sided headaches.

Engaging with her system through the sphenoid, the predominant feature was a right-sided torsion pattern. Maintaining a broad perspective, it was evident that this was part of a twist extending down through her whole body, pivoting around the T4 vertebral level – at which point the sphenoid started to feel agitated – and twisting down to the opposite sacro-iliac joint on the left – where the quality became very tight and contracted.

Interpreting this picture, I could diagnose a pelvic rotation focused around the left sacro-iliac joint (the primary focus – identifiable by its deeply ingrained quality of contraction). (Note that Susan's pain was on the opposite side, the more mobile overworked right sacro-iliac – a common – although not invariable – finding.)

This pelvic rotation was causing the twist up though the rest of the body, with a focus of strain, struggle and tension at T4 (a classic pivotal area of the spine). The strain at the T4 pivot was causing overstimulation and facilitation of the sympathetic nerve outflow in this area (identifiable as agitation at the sphenoid), leading to the feelings of anxiety and reflecting out to the lungs, triggering the asthma attacks.

The twist continued up through the neck and into the base of the cranium, where the tension at the suboccipital region on the right was causing Susan's headaches.

How might you address that situation?

Local or remote

All patterns encountered through the SBS can be addressed through the SBS. It is possible to treat this situation and every situation simply by engaging with the system through the sphenoid (or anywhere else in the body). But this may not necessarily be the most effective or efficient way of working.

If the source of the imbalance is a severely restricted sacro-iliac joint, then moving to the sacrum and addressing the restriction locally may prove more effective.

If the source of the restriction is emotional tension, then it may prove more effective to work at the solar plexus, or the heart centre, or to enter into dialogue and other means of addressing the patient's emotional concerns.

In Susan's case, it wasn't necessary to address the emotional components of her anxiety attacks specifically. They were caused by the physical strain on the T4, and her anxiety and her asthma disappeared once the twist in her body was resolved.

Summary

Working with SBS patterns is not a separate process; it is an integral part of any cranio-sacral treatment. Identifying and responding to such patterns will happen as a matter of course, largely unconsciously, during treatment. You will not generally look for specific patterns or follow any routine, but your ability to respond intuitively to such patterns is dependent on your informed awareness, well-grounded in a knowledge and understanding of these patterns; and from time to time, specific application of this knowledge may be pivotal to effective progress.

Whatever the source of any condition, it is essential to make a comprehensive and integrated diagnosis of the whole person, the whole system, the whole body-mind, in order to ensure that you hold, in your awareness, the overall picture and all aspects of the picture, so that you can respond appropriately to each patient according to their needs, always, of course, balancing and integrating the system at the end of the session and bringing each treatment to an appropriate and complete conclusion.

Through this well-established grounding in SBS patterns and a broad spacious perspective, you will be able to flow with the fluent and spontaneous expression of the cranio-sacral system in order to enable a consummate performance, not just of a sonata, but of a whole cranio-sacral symphony.

Part VII

The Nervous System

Chapter 47

The Nervous System
The Basics

Dividing the body into separate systems is artificial. Every system is interacting with every other system, every cell is in communication with every other cell in the body via various means – chemical signals, electrical pathways, biomagnetic fields, vibrational impulses, vascular channels, the perineural system, integrins and the molecular web – so the conventional view of the nervous system as the body's principal means of communication is limited. But the nervous system is still pertinent, it still carries out its functions, is substantially involved in a great deal of disease and dysfunction, and has many significant clinical applications. So it is still relevant to understand the nervous system clearly, so that we can integrate it into a more complete context, not just the integration of the whole psycho-neuro-endocrine-immune system of modern medical science, but a more comprehensive integration within the whole energetic matrix.

For the benefit of the lay reader, we will start with a review of the basics, as a basis for subsequent reference.

A brief introduction to the basics

The nervous system is composed of hundreds of billions of cells, each of which is a complex vibrant living unit in itself. Each microscopic cell is composed of countless subatomic particles in perpetual motion, and each cell is expressing rhythmic motion. We can engage with the dynamic activity at this quantum level. We can also recognise the significance of the nervous system on a more visible tangible level – both levels essential to our healthy well-being.

Nerve tissue

There are two principal types of cell which form the nerve tissue of the nervous system:

- neurons – responsible for the active transmission of messages
- glial cells (also known as neuroglia) – responsible for support, packing and insulation.

Neurons (nerve cells)

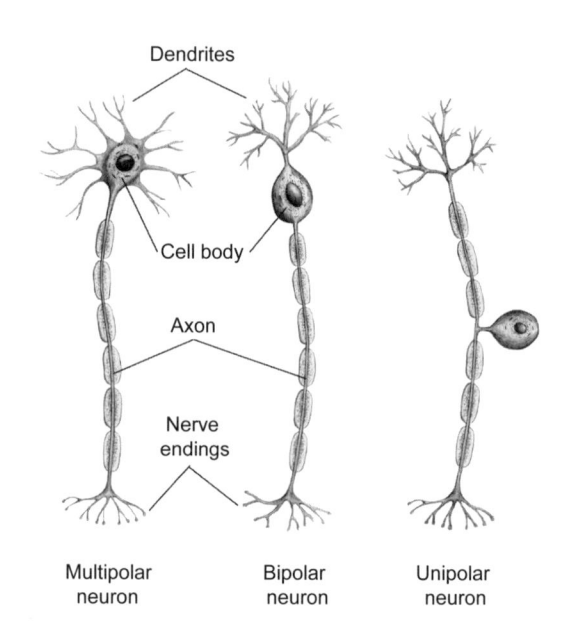

47.1 There are many different types of neuron, varying in their size, shape, function and location

There are many different varieties of neuron, varying in their size, shape, function and location. However, all neurons have a basic form (see Figure 47.2) consisting of:

- cell body
- nerve fibre
- nerve ending.

The Nervous System: The Basics / 341

A typical neuron:

- Cell body
- Nerve fibre (axon)
- Glial cells
- Nerve endings (synaptic terminals)

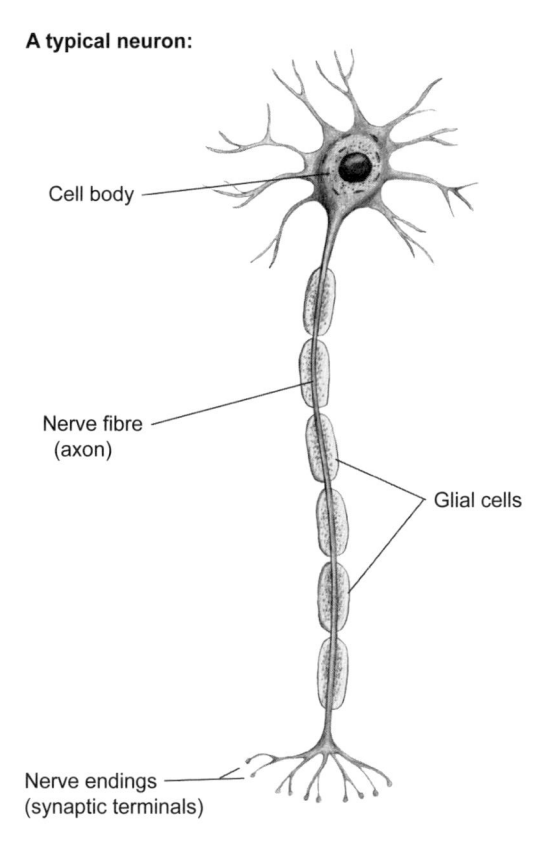

47.2 All neurons have a basic form consisting of a cell body, a nerve fibre, and a nerve ending

Impulses are received by the cell body, travel along the nerve fibre, and are transmitted from the nerve ending to a target organ.

The *cell body* receives incoming information, usually via tiny, branch-like dendrites.

The *nerve fibre* (usually called an axon) is a longer structure emanating from the cell body, along which information travels electrically to its destination. Nerve fibres are microscopically thin and may vary in length from fractions of a millimetre in some cases to more than a metre (as for example in the sciatic nerve).

The *nerve ending* (also known as the synaptic terminal) is located at the end of the nerve fibre. Here nerve impulses are transmitted from the nerve ending to the target organ (effector), which may be a muscle, gland, organ or another neuron.

Synapse

The process by which impulses are transmitted is known as synapse (see Figure 47.3).

The nerve ending at the end of the nerve fibre is known as a synaptic terminal.

The narrow gap that separates the nerve ending from the target organ is known as the synaptic cleft.

When an impulse is transmitted electrically along a nerve fibre to a nerve ending it stimulates the release of chemicals (neurotransmitters) from the synaptic terminal into the synaptic cleft. These chemicals cross the synaptic cleft and stimulate a response (or effect) in the target organ (effector). A nerve impulse is therefore carried both electrically and chemically.

Several hundred billion neurons create billions of interconnections both within the brain and spinal cord and outside in the periphery.

Because neurons are highly specialised for the purposes of transmitting impulses, they lose much of their ability for repair and regeneration. If nerve cells are damaged, there is little potential for repair.

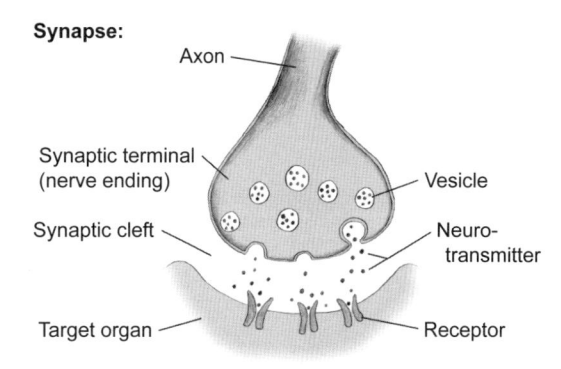

Synapse:

- Axon
- Synaptic terminal (nerve ending)
- Vesicle
- Synaptic cleft
- Neurotransmitter
- Target organ
- Receptor

47.3 The process by which impulses are transmitted is known as synapse

Glial cells (neuroglia)

Neuro means 'nerve', and glia means 'glue'. Glial cells support, nurture and protect the neurons and maintain the ionic and fluid balance of their environment. They outnumber neurons by between five and fifty times and are generally much smaller than neurons. Unlike neurons, glial cells are able to divide and multiply and are therefore able to repair and regenerate. Glial cells produce the white myelin sheaths surrounding nerve fibres, giving the nerve fibres their characteristic white colouration (see Figure 47.2).

White matter and grey matter

White matter refers to the mass of nerve fibres carrying messages from one place to another – the fibres of neurons covered in white myelin sheaths produced by the glial cells.

Grey matter refers to aggregations of cell bodies – the cell bodies of neurons – most evident in the cortex of the brain and in the core of the spinal cord.

a. Coronal section through the brain:

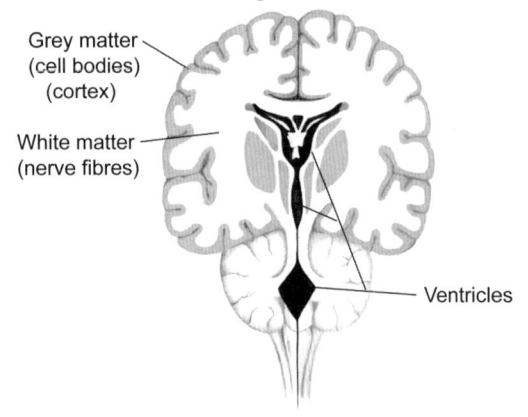

b. Transverse section through the spinal cord:

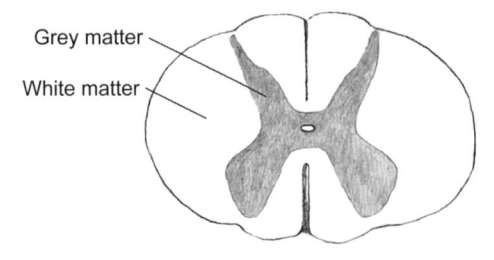

47.4 *Distribution of grey matter and white matter in the brain and spinal cord:*
  a. in the brain, the grey matter is located primarily on the outer surface (cortex)
  b. in the spinal cord, the grey matter is mainly located centrally

A *nerve* is the term for a bundle of many nerve fibres travelling together (see Figure 47.5).

Cross section through a nerve:

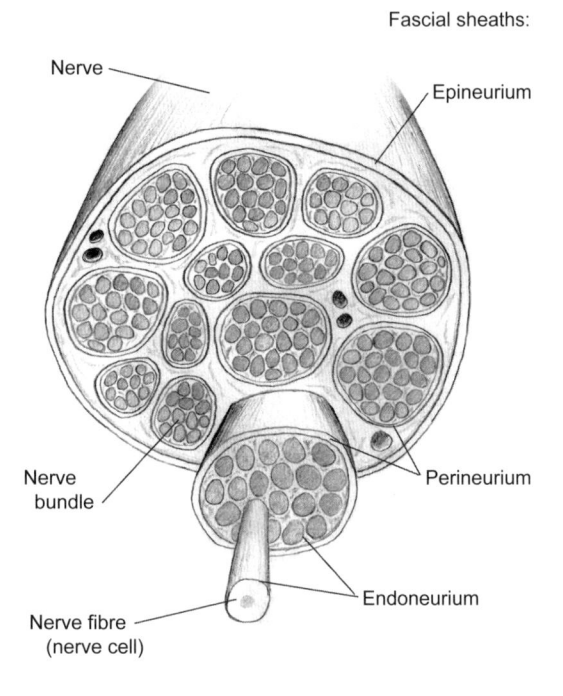

47.5 *A nerve is the term for a bundle of many nerve fibres travelling together*

ANATOMY AND PHYSIOLOGY OF THE NERVOUS SYSTEM

Anatomy of the nervous system

Anatomically (i.e. structurally, in terms of location) the nervous system can be divided into two parts:

- the central nervous system (CNS)
- the peripheral nervous system (PNS).

The *central nervous system* consists of the brain, brainstem, and spinal cord. It is contained within the dural membranes and is bathed in cerebrospinal fluid (CSF). When nerves pass out through the dural membranes they become known as peripheral nerves.

The *peripheral nervous system* consists of peripheral nerves passing out from the central nervous system to other parts of the body (the periphery).

The peripheral nervous system is further subdivided into:

- cranial nerves – which arise within the cranium

- spinal nerves – which arise from the spinal cord.

Despite their different origins, both cranial nerves and spinal nerves are part of the peripheral nervous system, since they are travelling from the central nervous system to areas outside of the central nervous system.

Physiology of the nervous system

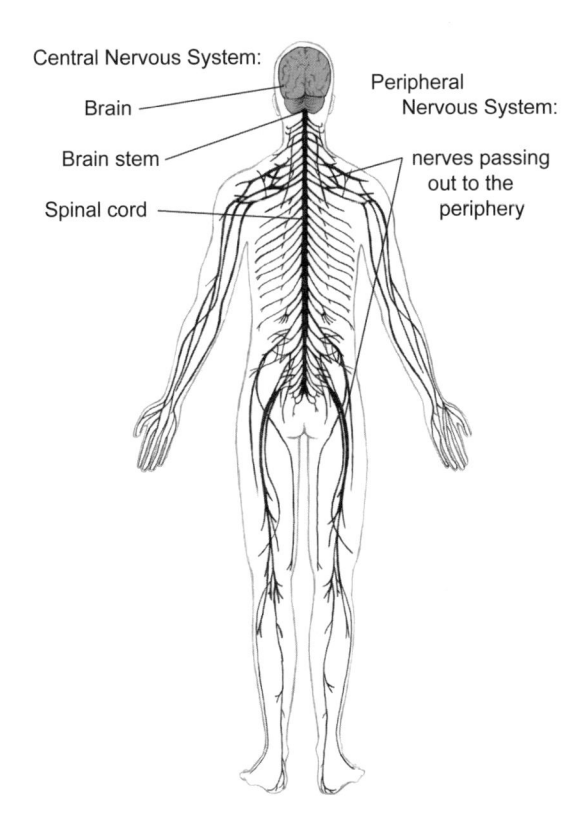

47.6 *The central nervous system (CNS) consists of the brain, brain stem, and spinal cord. The peripheral nervous system (PNS) consists of peripheral nerves passing out from the central nervous system to other parts of the body (the periphery)*

Physiologically (i.e. in terms of function) the nervous system can also be divided into two parts:
- the somatic nervous system (SNS)
- the autonomic nervous system (ANS).

The *somatic nervous system* (also known as the voluntary nervous system) is concerned with voluntary functions which are under our conscious control – such as walking, talking, movement. It is particularly responsible for the innervation of skeletal muscle.

The *autonomic nervous system* (also known as the vegetative or involuntary nervous system) is concerned with those functions which are generally not under conscious control – such as heartbeat, digestion, glandular secretions, pupillary constriction and dilation.

The autonomic nervous system is further subdivided into sympathetic and parasympathetic divisions.

The *sympathetic division* (sometimes referred to as the 'fight-flight-fright' division) is mostly concerned with responses to our external environment and activating the body to deal with external emergencies.

The *parasympathetic division* is mostly concerned with vegetative functions, in other words building up our resources, through digestion, absorption, excretion and more passive activities.

The somatic nervous system and the autonomic nervous system have components located both within the central nervous system and within the peripheral nervous system.

Sensory and motor neurons

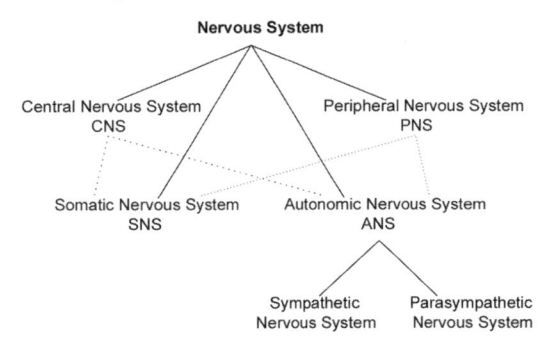

47.7 *Summary of the nervous system*

Neurons (nerve cells) may transmit messages outward from the brain and spinal cord towards the periphery (these are *motor neurons*); or may transmit sensations inwards from the periphery towards or into the brain or spinal cord (these are *sensory neurons*).

Motor neurons, travelling outwards from the core of the system, stimulate an *action* – whether in a muscle, gland, organ or another neuron.

Sensory neurons, traveling inwards from the periphery, carry *sensations* to and into the central nervous system, providing information so that the central nervous system can respond accordingly.

There are both motor and sensory neurons within both the central nervous system and the peripheral nervous system, serving both somatic functions and autonomic functions.

Motor neurons within the somatic nervous system stimulate skeletal muscle to produce conscious voluntary movement.

Sensory neurons within the somatic nervous system transmit impulses from the periphery to the central nervous system, including sensations of pain and temperature, sensations relating to muscle and joint position (proprioception), and information from the special senses (vision, hearing, taste, smell and equilibrium). All these impulses are usually perceived consciously.

Motor neurons within the autonomic nervous system (also known as *visceral efferent neurons*) transmit impulses from the central nervous system to the viscera, in order to regulate visceral activity, stimulating, for example, peristalsis in the digestive system, glandular secretions or cardiac activity. These activities are usually beyond conscious control or perception.

Sensory neurons within the autonomic nervous system (also known as *visceral afferent neurons*) transmit sensations from the viscera to the central nervous system. These afferent signals are not usually recognised consciously, unless the stimulation is particularly intense such as the pain associated with angina pectoris (arising from inadequate blood supply to the heart).

Motor and sensory nerve fibres generally travel together as mixed nerves – nerves containing a mixture of thousands of motor and sensory nerve fibres.

Reflex arc

Sensory neurons entering the spinal cord, as well as transmitting messages to the brain, will also stimulate motor neurons at the local level of the spinal cord via an interneuron. This enables a more rapid response and is known as a reflex arc. For instance, if you touch something hot, you will generally withdraw your hand before your brain is even conscious of the sensation of heat, through messages transmitted via the reflex arc.

This stimulation will affect not only neurons returning to the same organ from which the

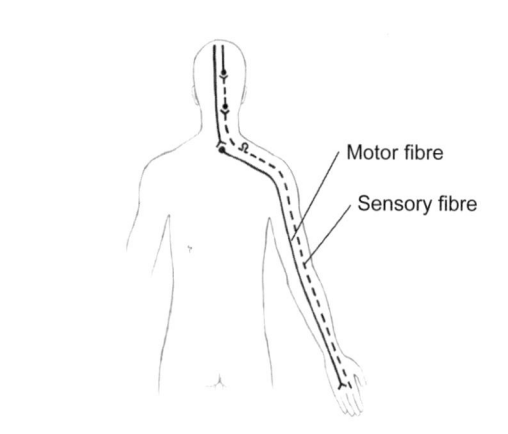

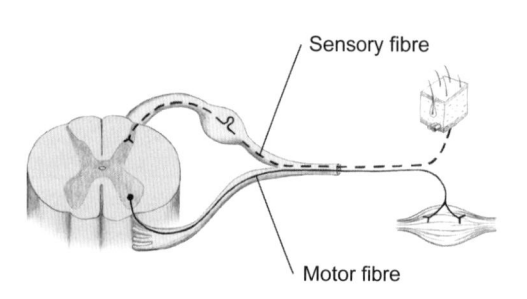

47.8 *Motor and sensory nerve fibres generally travel together as mixed nerves*

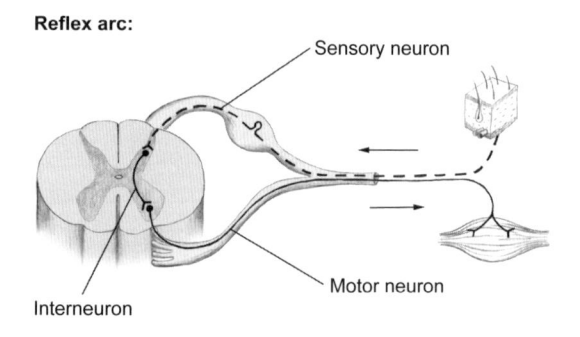

47.9 *Reflex arcs enable a more rapid response, but can also maintain unhelpful vicious circles of activity which can perpetuate patterns of discomfort and disease*

sensation came, but also neurons to other structures supplied from the same vertebral segment, such as surrounding muscles.

Reflex arcs can also be involved in maintaining unhelpful vicious circles of activity which can perpetuate patterns of discomfort and disease.

Box 47.1 The perineural system

The perineural system is a distinct communication system, reaching to every innervated tissue. Perineural cells surround each neuron in the brain, constituting more than half the cells in the brain; and every nerve fibre in the body down to its finest termination is completely encased in perineural cells of one type or another. The perineural system establishes a current of injury that controls injury repair.

The point to point transmission (of the conventional nervous system) allows for very precise control of specific activities, and precise sensory feedbacks. In contrast, the perineural system does not have a specific target, it delivers regulatory messages to every part. It is a global system, integrating and regulating processes throughout the organism.

The perineural system is sensitive to magnetic fields. (*Energy Medicine: The Scientific Basis*. Oschman 2000)

Chapter 48

The Nervous System
Relations with the Cranio-Sacral System

This chapter primarily describes the somatic (voluntary) division of the nervous system. Chapter 49 addresses the autonomic (involuntary) division.

The *border* dividing the central nervous system from the peripheral nervous system is the *dural membrane*.

Central nervous system

The *central nervous system* – consisting of the brain, brainstem and spinal cord – is enclosed within the dural membrane, bathed in cerebrospinal fluid. The health and proper function of the central nervous system is therefore influenced by the balance and integrity of the membrane system and the free flow of cerebrospinal fluid. The cranio-sacral process, encouraging the free and unrestricted mobility of the membranes, the fluent fluctuation of the cerebrospinal fluid, and the integration of the central nervous system, can therefore play a significant part in restoring and maintaining healthy function of the brain and spinal cord, and therefore all the organs, muscles and other structures supplied from the central nervous system.

The spinal cord is shorter than the vertebral column (because the specialised nerve tissue of the spinal cord grows more slowly than the bony vertebral column) (see Figure 48.1).

- The spinal cord (closely enveloped in *pia mater*) ends at the level of the second lumbar vertebra (L2) in an adult (and L4 in a newborn baby).
- The *dura and arachnoid mater* continue down to the level of the second sacral segment (S2), enclosing a space (the lumbar cistern) below the tip of the spinal cord filled with cerebrospinal fluid (see Figure 48.2).

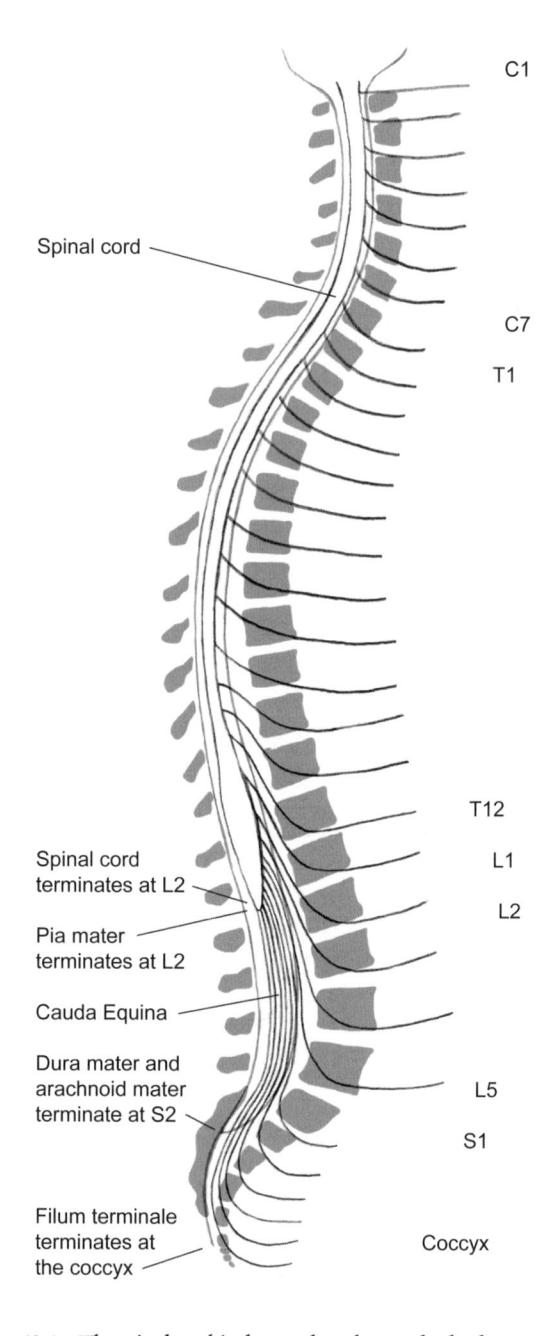

48.1 The spinal cord is shorter than the vertebral column

Box 48.1 Cisternae

Cisternae are areas of accumulation of cerebrospinal fluid within the subarachnoid space, the most notable being the *cisterna magna* (behind the medulla, below the cerebellum) and the lumbar cistern (in the lower spine below the termination of the spinal cord – the site from which CSF is extracted through lumbar puncture).

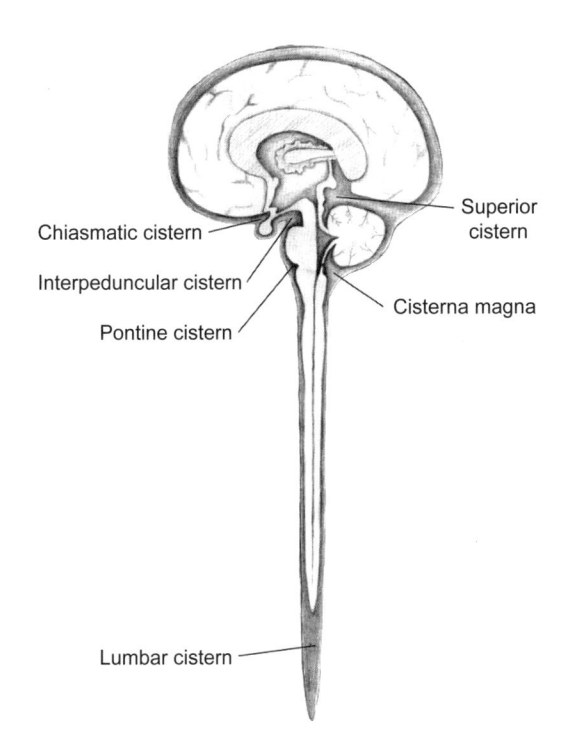

- They exit from the *spinal cord* from levels at or above L2 vertebra (where the spinal cord ends).
- They pass down through the lumbar cistern within the dura as the *cauda equina* (horse's tail), and then penetrate the *dura* down to levels at or above S2 (where the dura terminates).
- They exit from the *bony structure* of the vertebral column from levels at or above the coccyx (this vertebral level being the level by which they are named).

In the practice of cranio-sacral therapy, it may be appropriate to trace with your attention along a nerve pathway, whether from organ to spinal cord or spinal cord to organ, identifying areas of impingement, restriction, agitation or disturbance, whether at the intervertebral foramen, at the penetration of the dura, at the spinal cord level, or anywhere along its pathway. Identification of the precise site of disturbance may in itself play a significant part in the therapeutic response.

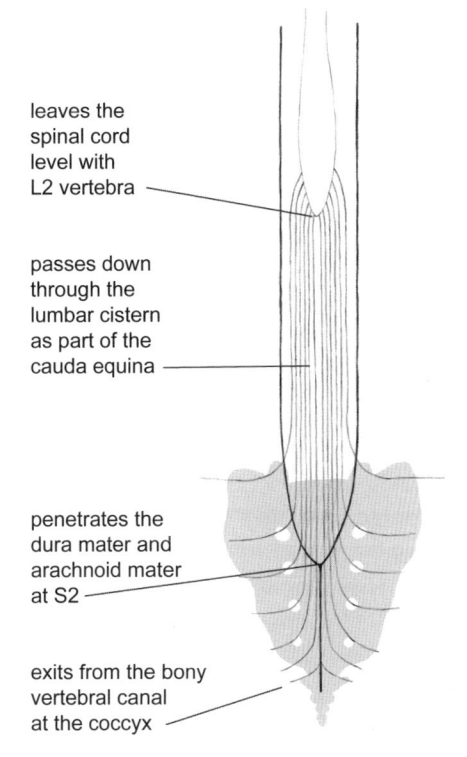

48.2 Cisternae are areas of accumulation of cerebrospinal fluid within the subarachnoid space

- Spinal nerve roots leave the spinal cord at their appropriate *spinal cord level*.
- They then pass down at an increasing angle to their *corresponding vertebral level*.
- Spinal nerves emerge from the bony structure of the vertebral column at their corresponding vertebral level, throughout the spine from the occiput down to the coccyx.
- The lower spinal nerves (lower lumbar, sacral and coccygeal nerves L3–5, S1–5, Co) therefore have some distance to travel between their spinal cord exit and bony exit.

48.3 The coccygeal nerve may be adversely affected by restrictions in various locations along its pathway

For example, the coccygeal nerve could be adversely affected:

- at the coccyx – by a fall or blow to the coccyx
- at its exit through the dura, level with S2 – due to membranous restriction
- at the cauda equina in the lumbar cistern, between L2 and S2 – due to lumbar puncture
- at its exit from the spinal cord, level with L2 vertebra (see Figure 48.3).

Peripheral nervous system

The *peripheral nervous system* consists of:

- nerves *leaving* the central nervous system to be distributed to the periphery
- nerves *entering* the central nervous system from the periphery.

Peripheral nerves penetrate the dural membrane as they enter and leave the central nervous system, and are enveloped in a fascial sheath (epineurium) throughout their pathway to and from the periphery. The balance and integrity of both the dura and the fascia is therefore essential to proper functioning of the peripheral nerves.

From a cranio-sacral perspective, it is clinically relevant to understand the specific relationships and associations between:

- dural levels (and therefore vertebral levels)
- and areas of the body (organs, muscles, limbs, etc.) neurologically supplied from those levels.

For example:

- The sciatic nerve has its root origins at the base of the spine, emerging from the fourth and fifth lumbar segments and the first, second and third sacral segments (L4, L5, S1, S2, S3), so symptoms of sciatica, whether in the posterior thigh, lower leg, foot, or toes, may originate in the lower back (see Figure 48.4).
- The ulnar nerve, supplying the fourth and fifth fingers, has its root origins at the base of the neck, emerging from the seventh and eighth cervical segments and the first thoracic segment (C7, C8, T1), so neurological symptoms (numbness, pins and needles, pain) in those fingers may originate in the neck (see Figure 48.4).

It is also useful to be familiar with neurological pathways, which may be affected by fascial restrictions, since this may in turn lead to dysfunction in distant structures supplied by those pathways.

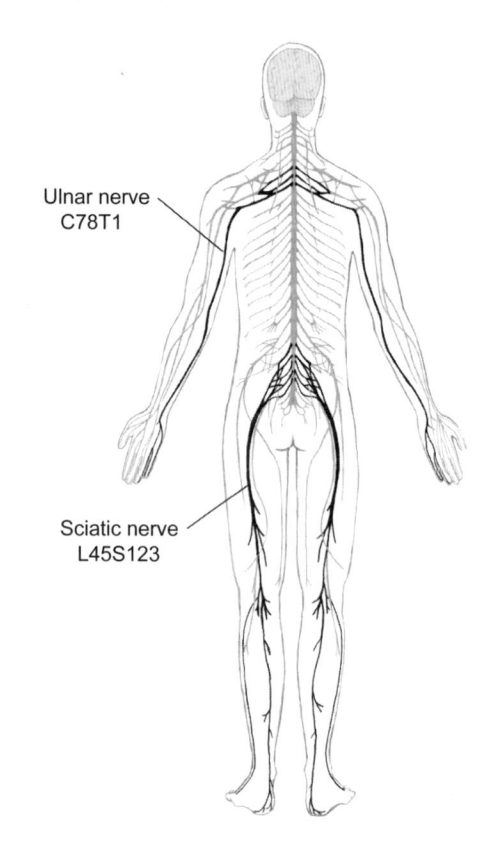

48.4 *It is clinically relevant to understand the specific relationships between dural levels and areas of the body neurologically supplied from those levels*
a. Sciatic nerve
b. Ulnar nerve

Central nervous system associations

The brain

Specific areas of the brain are related to specific functions and specific parts of the body, which may be of value in diagnosis and treatment:

- The frontal lobes are concerned with motor activity and personality.
- The parietal lobes receive sensory information from all over the body.
- The temporal lobes are involved with hearing and speech.
- The occipital lobes are involved in vision.

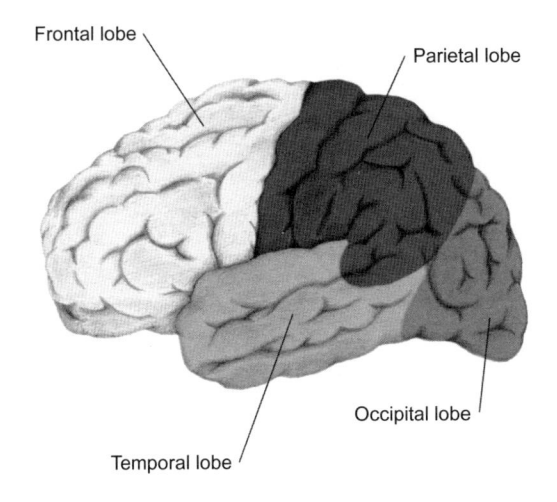

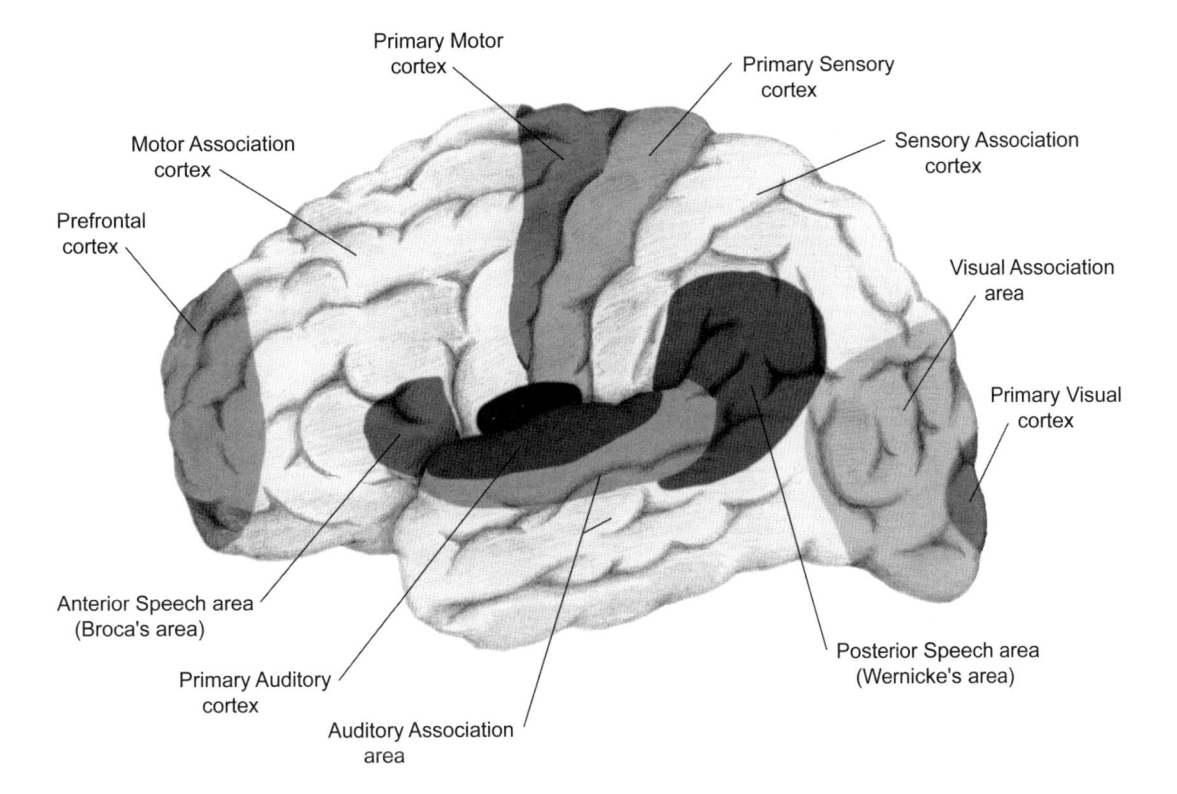

48.5 *a. The lobes of the brain*
       b. Functional areas of the brain

There is clearly a vast amount of greater detail regarding precise relationships between specific areas of the cortex and their associated functions. Specific areas of the brain associated with speech, hearing, writing, reading or motor function could be relevant to the effective treatment of conditions such as dyslexia and dyspraxia (often related to the temporal lobes). Specific dysfunctions may be related to very specific locations within the brain, but the same dysfunction can also often arise from imbalances elsewhere in the system, perhaps far removed from the brain, and often from causes not obviously associated with the condition. As always, healthy function of the system is dependent, not only on local factors, but also on the integration of the system as a whole.

Epilepsy, for example, could be the result of a tumour in the temporal lobe, but could also be due to birth trauma, shock, temporal bone compression, restricted blood supply to the temporal lobe, stress, genetic factors, or a combination of several of these factors. As always, we need to see the complete integrated picture – rather than merely drawing simple associations with specific areas of the brain – assessing the whole system, integrating the whole body-mind, so that the body's inherent healing potential can operate most effectively. Integration is the foundation of all health.

The brainstem

The brainstem (see Figure 48.6) is the bridge between the brain and the spinal cord, extending from the top of the spinal cord into the base of the brain. It consists of three sections:

- the *medulla* – approximately an inch (2.5 cm) long, extending up from the foramen magnum
- the *pons* – the next half inch (1.25 cm) approximately, extending from medulla to midbrain
- the *midbrain* – the top section of the brainstem, continuous with the base of the brain.

The brainstem contains most of the nuclei (aggregations of cell bodies) of the cranial nerves, as well as other important neurological control centres such as the respiratory centre and the cardiac centre, and the neurological pathways passing up and down from the brain to all parts of the body and vice versa.

The fourth ventricle is located posterior to the pons and medulla of the brainstem, with the cerebellum bulging out behind the fourth ventricle into the posterior cranial fossa.

During the expansion phase of cranio-sacral motion, the brain curls in on itself (reflecting its embryological development) shortening and widening, and the spinal cord is drawn superiorly. During the contraction phase, the brain uncurls and the spinal cord sinks down inferiorly.

Peripheral nervous system associations

The peripheral nervous system consists of those parts of the nervous system which carry impulses outside the dural membrane to the periphery. It consists of:

- *cranial nerves* – which arise within the cranium
- *spinal nerves* – which arise from the spinal cord.

Cranial nerves

Cranial nerves (see Figure 48.7) arise from their nuclei (where their cell bodies are located) in the brain and brainstem. Although their pathways are often very short and often stay within the cranium, they are peripheral nerves because they pass outside the dura.

There are *12 cranial nerves, numbered I–XII* in Roman numerals, to distinguish them from spinal nerves. They supply the eyes, nose, ears, mouth, face, throat and neck. The more substantial vagus nerve (the wanderer) Cr X passes down through the body, distributing branches to most of the

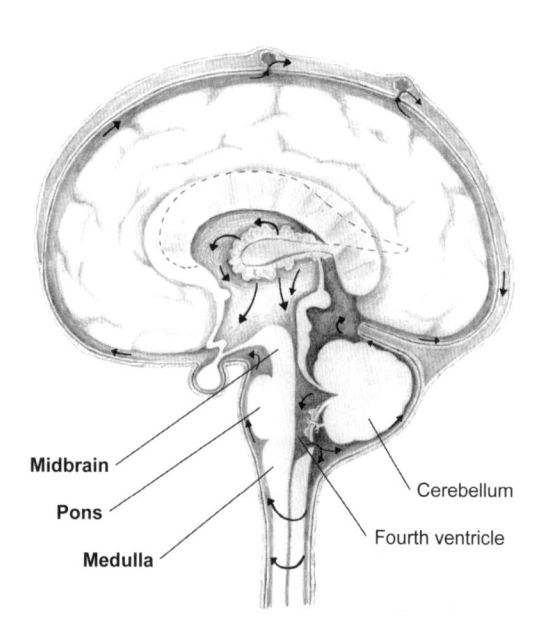

48.6 The brainstem consists of the midbrain, pons, and medulla

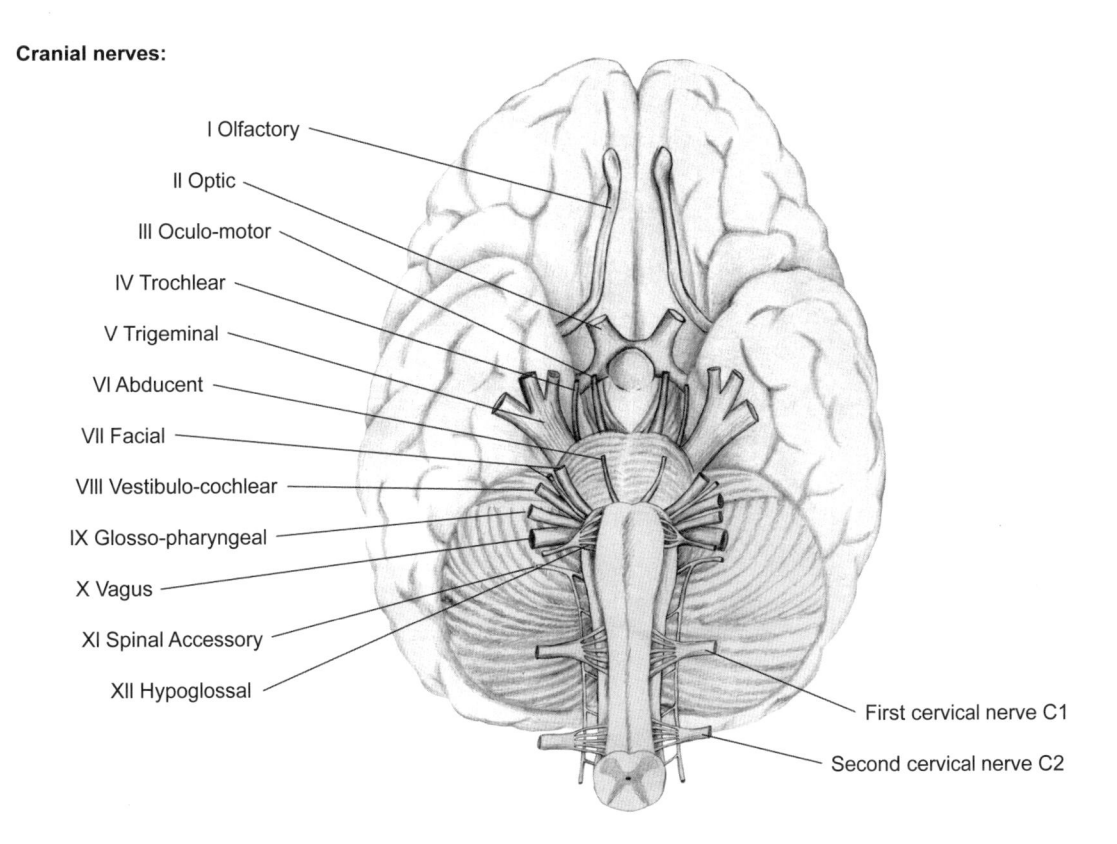

Cranial nerves:

- I Olfactory
- II Optic
- III Oculo-motor
- IV Trochlear
- V Trigeminal
- VI Abducent
- VII Facial
- VIII Vestibulo-cochlear
- IX Glosso-pharyngeal
- X Vagus
- XI Spinal Accessory
- XII Hypoglossal

First cervical nerve C1
Second cervical nerve C2

48.7 The twelve cranial nerves

thoracic and abdominal viscera – including the heart, lungs, stomach, spleen, pancreas, liver, small intestine, and the first half of the large intestine.

Spinal nerves

The spinal nerves (see Figure 48.8) are formed by:
- a *ventral root* (motor) leaving the anterior aspect of the spinal cord, and
- a *dorsal root* (sensory) entering the posterior aspect of the spinal cord.

The two roots join within the vertebral canal to form the spinal nerve. The spinal nerve then penetrates the dura and passes out from the vertebral column between the vertebrae at the intervertebral foramen.

As each spinal nerve penetrates the dura, the first few millimetres of the spinal nerve are enveloped in a sleeve of dura mater, which blends into the *epineurium* (fascial sheath) which envelops the spinal nerve and all its branches throughout the rest of its pathway.

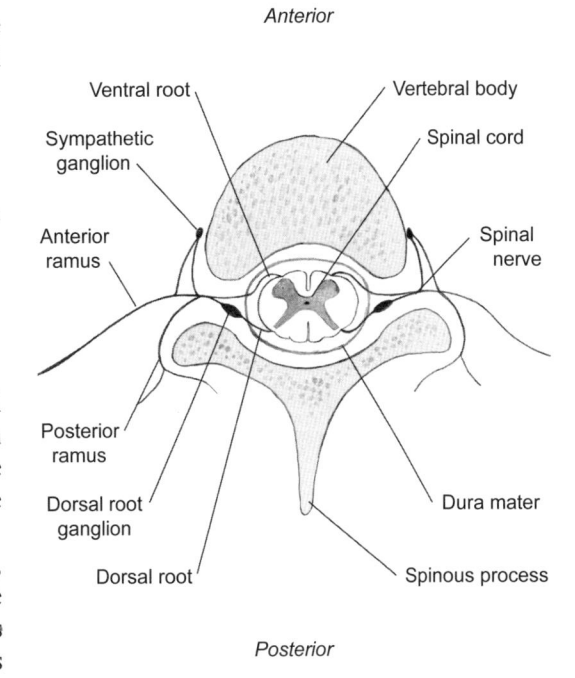

Anterior

- Ventral root
- Sympathetic ganglion
- Anterior ramus
- Posterior ramus
- Dorsal root ganglion
- Dorsal root
- Vertebral body
- Spinal cord
- Spinal nerve
- Dura mater
- Spinous process

Posterior

48.8 Each spinal nerve is formed from a ventral root and a dorsal root

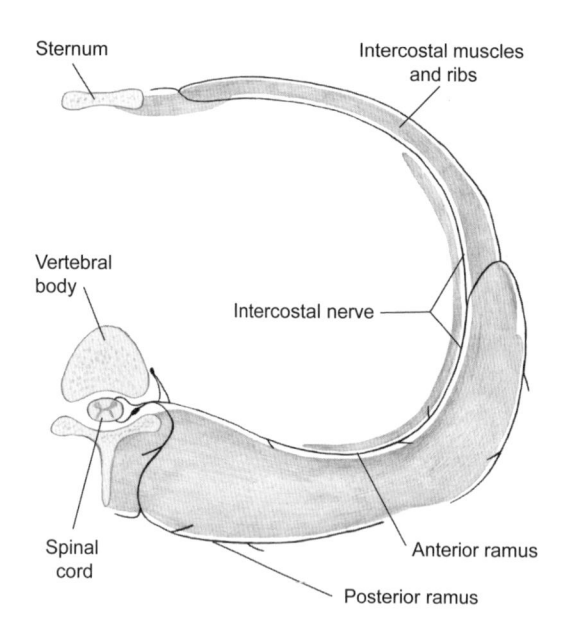

48.9 After emerging from the intervertebral foramina, the spinal nerves divide immediately into a posterior ramus (branch) and an anterior ramus (branch) before travelling to the periphery

There are *31 spinal nerves*, emerging between adjacent vertebrae at the intervertebral foramina: 8 cervical, 12 thoracic, 5 lumbar, 5 sacral, 1 coccygeal (see Figure 48.11).

Spinal nerves are numbered according to the vertebral level at which they emerge. However, the numbering devised by early anatomists is somewhat anomalous:

- Cervical nerves emerge *above* the vertebra of the same number.
- Thoracic, lumbar, sacral and coccygeal nerves emerge *below* the vertebra of the same number.

The nerve which emerges between C7 and T1 is therefore left without a corresponding vertebra and is numbered C8.

After emerging from the intervertebral foramina, the spinal nerves then divide immediately into a posterior ramus (branch) and an anterior ramus (branch) before travelling to the periphery (see Figure 48.9).

The *posterior rami* are short branches travelling directly to a small area at the back of the body around the corresponding vertebral level, supplying muscles and skin within that small area.

The *anterior rami* are longer branches travelling to other parts of the body.

The *anterior rami of spinal nerves from vertebral levels T2–T12*, travel directly from the spine round to the front of the body between the ribs as *intercostal nerves* to supply muscles and skin at the associated intercostal levels ('intercostal' means between the ribs) (see Figure 48.9).

The *anterior rami of all other spinal nerves* form *plexi* (areas of nerve interchange) before being distributed to other areas of the body as combined nerves (nerves containing fibres from several different root origins) (see Figure 48.10).

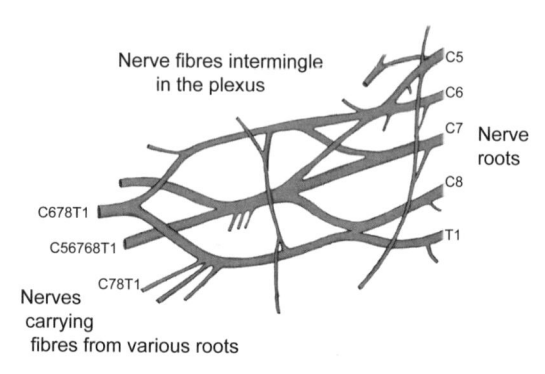

48.10 The anterior rami of all spinal nerves (except those from T2–T12) form plexi (areas of nerve interchange) before being distributed to other areas of the body

These *spinal nerve plexi* (see Figure 48.11) (not to be confused with autonomic nerve plexi) are:

Name of plexus	Root origins
Cervical plexus	C1–C4
Brachial plexus	C5–T1
Lumbar plexus	L1–L4
Sacral plexus	L4–S4
Pudendal plexus	S2–S4

Why do these particular nerves need to contain fibres from various different nerve roots? The nerves from these plexi supply areas of the body which are valuable to survival or effective function (at least for an animal in the wild) – hands, feet, etc. Supply to these areas from more than one nerve root is a protective mechanism. If one nerve root is damaged, this vital area of the body will still be able to function through its supply from other roots.

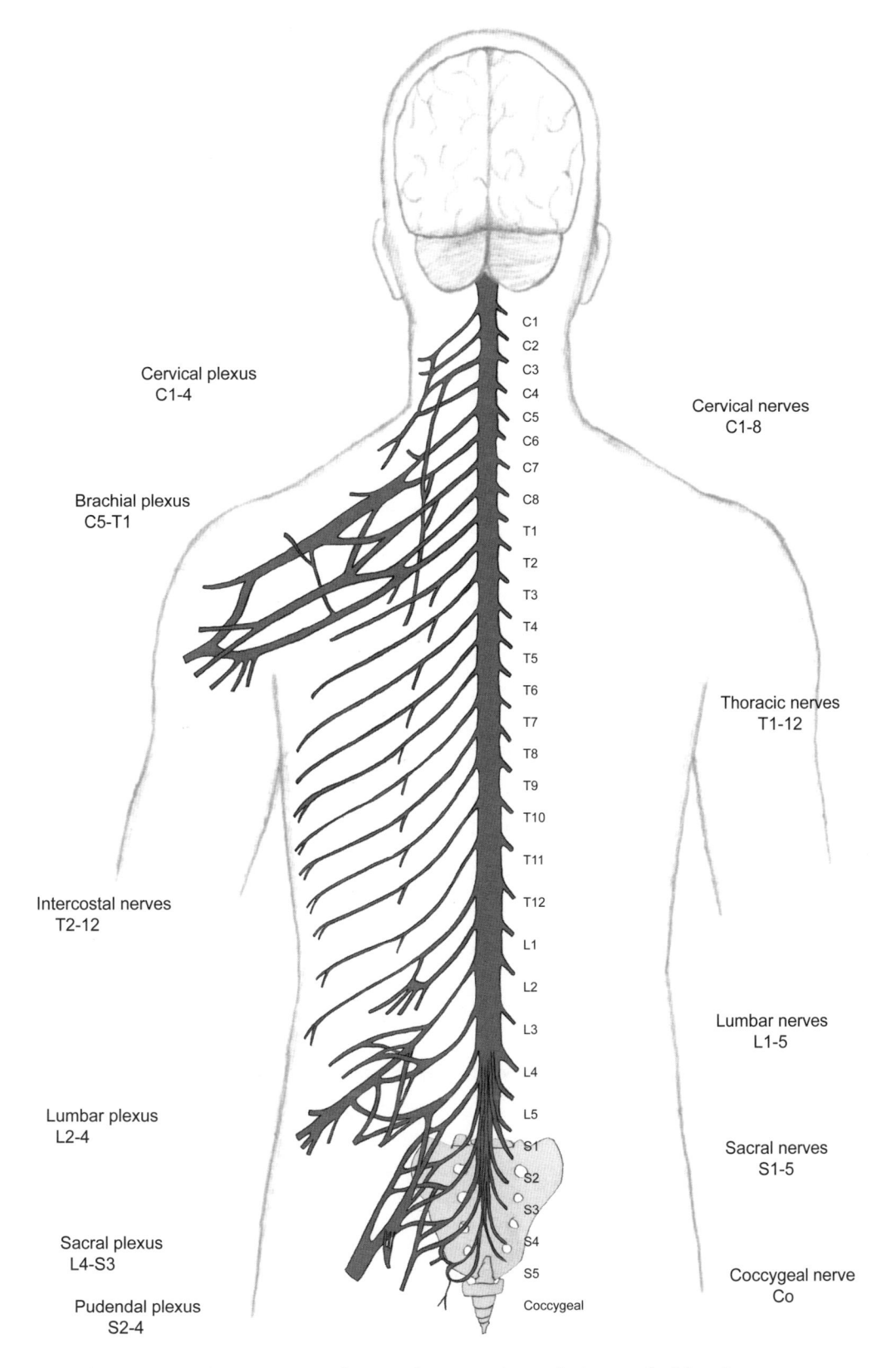

48.11 There are 31 spinal nerves, emerging between adjacent vertebrae at the intervertebral foramina

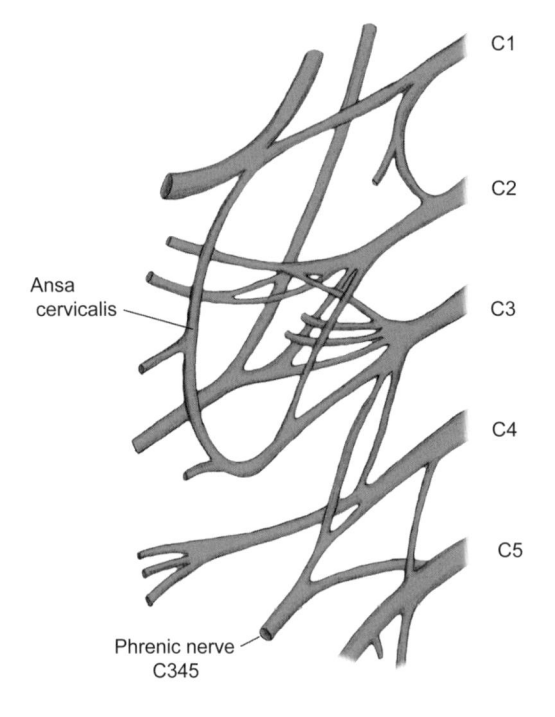

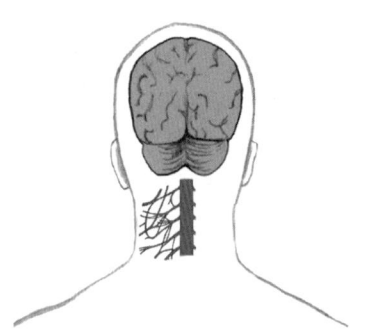

- pectoralis major, pectoralis minor, subclavius
- supraspinatus, infraspinatus, subscapularis, teres minor, deltoid
- levator scapulae, rhomboids, teres major, latissimus dorsi (N.B. it does *not* supply sterno-mastoid or trapezius).

Major nerves:
- axillary: C56 – to the axilla and deltoid
- musculo-cutaneous: C567– to the anterior muscles of the upper arm
- ulnar: C78, T1 – to the flexor muscles on the ulnar side of the anterior forearm and hand (including digits 4 and 5)
- median: C678, T1 – to the flexor muscles on the radial side of the anterior forearm and hand (including digits 1, 2 and 3, and the medial side of 4)
- radial: C5678, T1 – to the extensor muscles of the posterior arm, forearm and hand.

From a cranio-sacral perspective, it is clinically relevant and valuable to:
- understand the relationship between the dural/vertebral levels, and dysfunctions in areas supplied from those levels
- to take into account the fascia and fascial restrictions in areas associated with the nerve pathways, for example, in the case of the brachial plexus: the fascia of the neck, shoulder girdle, arm, forearm and hand, which may be affected by fractures, traumas, tension, inflammation, occupational use, etc.
- to take into account the reciprocity of the whole cranio-sacral system, and compensatory changes which may be reflected structurally or cranio-sacrally or by any other means to distant areas throughout the body.

In other words, knowledge and understanding of neuro-anatomy and the nervous system can be very relevant and valuable, but symptoms and conditions are not always directly related to nerve supply and obvious anatomical relations, and may arise from many different causes, anywhere in the whole body-mind complex.

48.12 The cervical plexus

A summary of somatic plexi
Cervical plexus: C1–C4
The cervical plexus (see Figure 48.12) supplies the muscles of the throat and neck and receives sensation from around the ears, throat, neck and upper chest.

Major nerve:
- phrenic nerve: C345 – to the diaphragm.

Brachial plexus: C5–T1
The brachial plexus (see Figure 48.13) supplies the shoulder, chest, arm, forearm, hand, and upper back, including:

Brachial plexus:

Musculo-cutaneous nerve
C567

Axillary nerve
C56

Median nerve
C678T1

Radial nerve
C5678T1

Ulnar nerve
C78T1

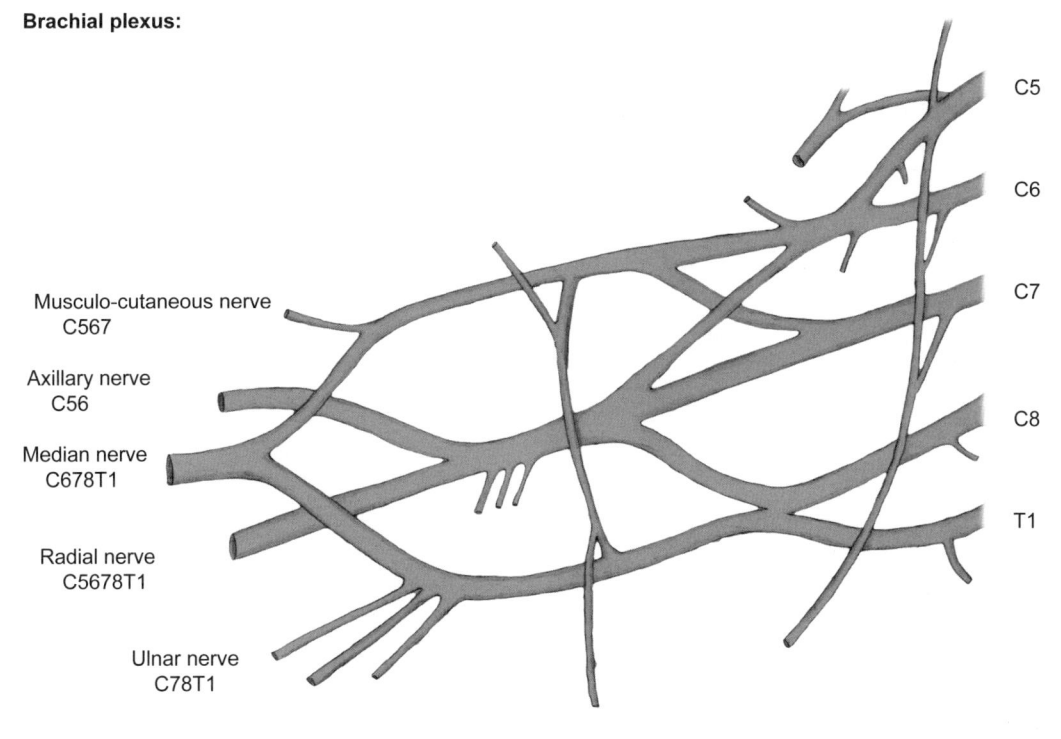

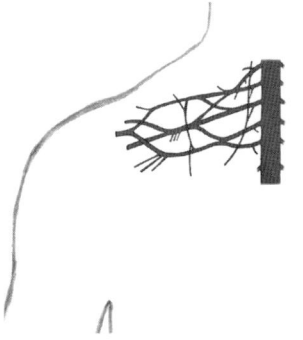

C5
C6
C7
C8
T1

48.13 The brachial plexus

For example, a patient comes to see you with neurological symptoms (pins and needles, numbness, pain, or loss of sensation) specifically in the little finger and ring finger (digits 5 and 4) of their left hand. Your knowledge of the nervous system tells you that the ulnar nerve is involved.

The pathway of the ulnar nerve travels from:

- its roots at C78, T1
- through the neck
- via the brachial plexus (below the clavicle, above the first rib)
- behind the medial epicondyle of the elbow
- its whole pathway passing through the fascia of the neck, shoulder, arm, forearm and hand
- to digits 4 and 5 (see Figure 48.14).

Understanding this pathway enables you more readily to identify possible areas of impingement of the ulnar nerve, whether at:

- the base of the neck – addressing bony, dural and muscular restrictions there
- in the fascia of the neck – potentially benefiting from fascial unwinding of the neck
- in the brachial plexus – possibly affected by a previous fractured clavicle, or tensions and restrictions in the muscles of the shoulder girdle involving the upper ribs and clavicle
- at the medial epicondyle (the 'funny bone') – where the ulnar nerve is particularly susceptible to injury and very responsive to cranio-sacral therapy, particularly including fascial unwinding
- elsewhere along the fascia of the arm and forearm – perhaps due to past injuries, current tensions, repetitive strain injury, or other effects of occupational use.

So it is helpful to understand the neurological pathway in tracing the possible source of the impingement.

But neurological pathways are not the full story. What else could it be?

Neurological sensations in the fourth and fifth digits of the left hand are a possible symptom of a heart condition.

There could be a heart pathology – which might need referral if has not already been checked.

The apparent heart symptoms could also be the result of emotional tension held in the heart and pericardium, such as unexpressed grief.

There could be reciprocal effects from any source – the solar plexus, lumbar vertebrae, pelvic imbalance (via latissimus dorsi), past emotional trauma.

The source could be anywhere – so the neurological information is valuable and helpful, but as always it is essential to look at the whole picture, a well as the valuable local detail.

The following week, another patient comes to see you – and this patient has neurological symptoms affecting the thumb, index and middle fingers, and part of the ring finger (digits 1, 2, 3 and (4)).

Armed with your neurological expertise, you recognise possible involvement of the median nerve.

The pathway of the median nerve is similar to, but not the same as, the ulnar nerve, travelling from:

- its roots at C678, T1
- through the neck
- via the brachial plexus (below the clavicle, above the first rib)
- passing unimpeded through the soft tissues at the front of the elbow
- through the carpal tunnel at the wrist
- its whole pathway passing through the fascia of the neck, shoulder, arm, forearm and hand
- to digits 1, 2 and 3 (see Figure 48.14).

Many aspects of the pathway are similar, but the median nerve is not particularly vulnerable at the elbow. It is however particularly vulnerable and commonly affected at the carpal tunnel, where the median nerve, together with various tendons, passes through a small tunnel on the anterior wrist formed by the flexor retinaculum.

Carpal tunnel syndrome, as diagnosed in this case, is a common condition and it is generally very responsive to cranio-sacral therapy, particularly including fascial unwinding.

Understanding an apparently minor detail, like the fact that the median nerve passes through the carpal tunnel and supplies digits 1, 2, 3 and (4)

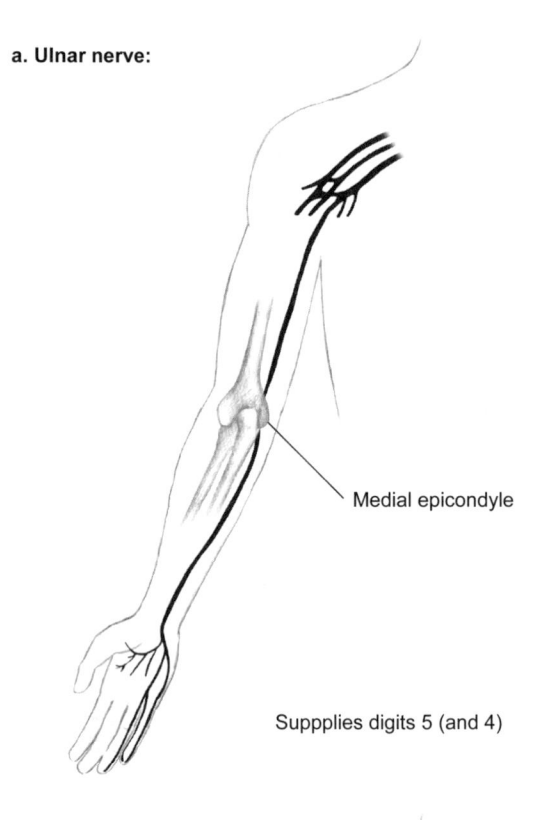

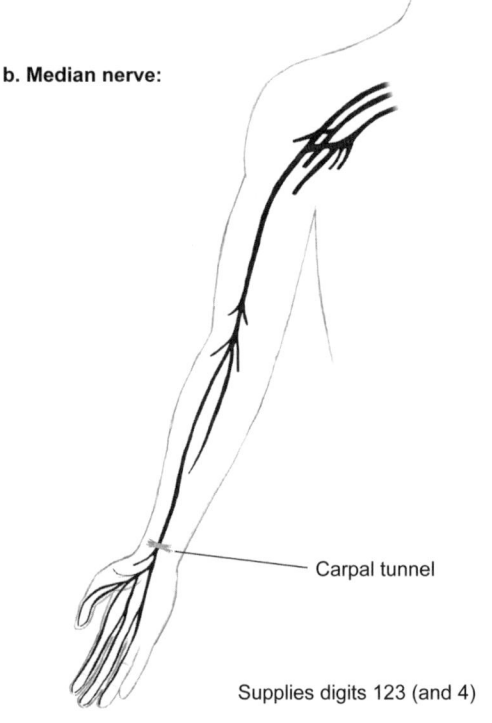

a. **Ulnar nerve:**

Medial epicondyle

Suppplies digits 5 (and 4)

b. **Median nerve:**

Carpal tunnel

Supplies digits 123 (and 4)

48.14 *It is helpful to understand neurological pathways in tracing the possible source of any impingement*
  a. The ulnar nerve
  b. The median nerve

(whereas the ulnar nerve does not pass through the carpal tunnel and supplies digits 4 and 5) can be very significant in enabling accurate diagnosis – in other words, identifying the wrist as the potentially significant area in the median nerve compression and the medial epicondyle of the elbow as the more relevant area in the ulnar nerve symptoms – and consequently more efficient and effective therapeutic results.

It has also been interesting to observe the significant number of patients over the years who have come for cranio-sacral therapy because they have been diagnosed with carpal tunnel syndrome and have been told by their doctor and their orthopaedic surgeon that they need an operation (which they would prefer to avoid if possible) – only to find on simple questioning about their symptoms, that they have symptoms only in their fourth and fifth fingers! Your understanding of the nervous system can save patients from unnecessary operations.

Lumbo-sacral plexus

The lumbo-sacral plexus (see Figure 48.15) is a combination of two plexi:

- *lumbar plexus:* L1–L4
- *sacral plexus:* L4–S4.

It supplies the muscles of the pelvis and lower limbs.

Major nerves:

- femoral: L234 – to the anterior thigh (quadriceps), passing through the psoas muscle
- obturator: L234 – to the medial thigh (adductors), passing through the psoas muscle
- sciatic: L45, S123 – to the posterior thigh (hamstrings) and lower leg, dividing into:
  - common peroneal nerve – to the lateral and anterior leg and foot
  - tibial nerve – to the posterior leg and the sole of the foot.

In identifying the spinal levels associated with these nerves it is helpful to note that:

- these lower spinal nerves leave the spinal cord from levels at or above L2 vertebra

- they then travel down through the lumbar cistern as the *cauda equina*
- before penetrating the dura at levels at or above S2 vertebra
- they then leave the vertebral column at the vertebral level from which they are named.

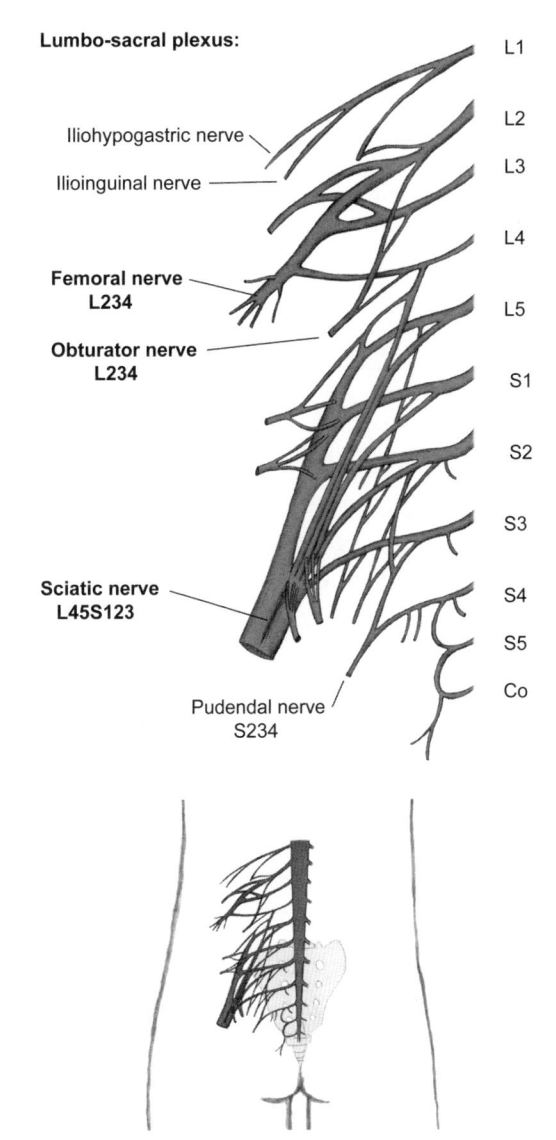

48.15 The lumbo-sacral plexus

Fascial restrictions affecting the nerves of the lumbo-sacral plexus include:

- the fascia of the lower back

- the fascia of the posterior wall of the abdomen (including psoas muscle)
- the pelvic fascia
- the lower limb fascia.

As with the previous examples, understanding the nerve pathways can be crucial in identifying, differentiating and influencing the source of different conditions – whether at the appropriate vertebral levels, at the cauda equina (perhaps due to lumbar puncture) or at dural levels (perhaps affected by an epidural), at the psoas muscle (involving the femoral or obturator nerves), at the fibular head (affecting the common peroneal nerve) or any other relevant areas – neurological or general.

Pudendal plexus: S2–4

The pudendal plexus supplies the genitalia and muscles of the pelvis (in close association with the autonomic nervous system).

In relation to genital function, it is essential to take into account the autonomic nerve supply to these areas.

In identifying neurological restrictions, it is relevant once again to take into account:

- spinal cord levels at or above L2
- dural levels at or above S2
- the exit of the nerves from the vertebral column at S234
- the various implications regarding different sources and causes as described above.

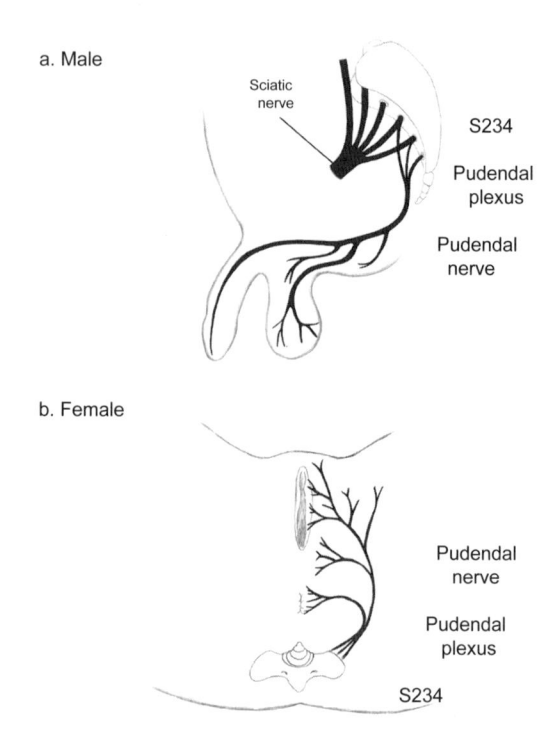

48.16 The sciatic nerve

48.17 The pudendal plexus

Chapter 49

The Autonomic Nervous System

The autonomic nervous system (ANS) is one of the most significant systems in human function. It plays a vital role in maintaining life-supporting organs such as the heart and lungs, as well as all the other viscera. It is one of the principal networks linking the physical body with our emotions and our psyche. It is significantly involved in the majority of health disturbances. It is actively participating in every moment of our lives and is an essential factor in our ability to respond to circumstances from moment to moment in everyday life. It is clinically highly significant. A truly integrated understanding of the autonomic nervous system is invaluable in gaining a proper understanding of health and disease.

We will be looking at the autonomic nervous system in two separate sections:

- firstly, in this section, gaining a basic understanding of the structure and function of the ANS
- subsequently, in Chapter 52, equipped with this basic information, exploring how an integrated understanding of the ANS can play such a vital part in the majority of health conditions, and can be an integral part of everyday clinical practice with almost every patient.

Introduction

The autonomic nervous system is also known as the involuntary nervous system, since it regulates involuntary processes throughout the body.

For example, it regulates:

- the digestive system – through innervation of the gastro intestinal tract (GIT) – innervating the smooth muscle, the glands, and the sphincters, thereby regulating peristalsis and glandular secretion
- breathing – regulating dilation and constriction of the bronchi
- the heart – regulating rate and strength of heartbeat
- blood vessels – regulating constriction (and therefore dilation)
- exocrine glands – regulating sweat secretion and saliva secretion
- the eyes – regulating pupil size and lens accommodation
- the bladder – regulating urinary function
- the genitals – regulating erection, ejaculation, uterine contraction
- pilo erector muscles – raising the hairs on the skin
- the adrenal glands – regulating secretion of adrenalin.

Autonomic nervous system function can be divided broadly into two main categories:

- vegetative processes – digestion, absorption, excretion, etc.
- response to the environment.

The autonomic nervous system has two divisions – roughly corresponding to these two functions:

- *Parasympathetic* – primarily concerned with vegetative processes. This division is anabolic, meaning that it builds up and conserves resources.
- *Sympathetic* – primarily concerned with responses to the environment (including responses to stress). This division is catabolic, meaning that it uses up or expends resources.

The autonomic nervous system is regulated by the hypothalamus. The principal neurotransmitter secreted by parasympathetic nerve endings is acetyl choline. The principal neurotransmitter secreted by sympathetic nerve endings is noradrenalin.

360 \ Cranio-Sacral Integration

Autonomic Nerve Distribution
Schema

Sympathetic division

Parasympathetic division

Cranial
nerves
III
VII
IX
X

T1

L2

Sympathetic
plexi

Sympathetic
chain

S234

49.1 The autonomic nervous system

Anatomy of the autonomic nervous system

General anatomy

ANS neurons pass from their cell bodies in the lateral horn of the spinal cord to the periphery or viscera, in the same way as somatic neurons (see Figure 49.2):

- in other words, motor fibres exit via the ventral root; sensory fibres enter via the dorsal root
- the fibres then travel to their respective destinations.

Autonomic nerve fibres (whether sympathetic or parasympathetic) may travel either:

- with peripheral (somatic) nerves to the periphery – arms, legs, skin, muscles, etc.
- separately to the viscera.

There are sympathetic fibres travelling with almost every somatic nerve to every part of the body. Parasympathetic fibres are less widespread, only travelling with a few specific somatic nerves.

Two neuron pathway

The main difference between the autonomic and somatic pathways is that the autonomic motor pathway is a two neuron pathway (see Figure 49.3):

- The somatic pathway is a one neuron pathway, with a single motor neuron travelling all the way from the spinal cord to its destination in the periphery.
- The autonomic motor pathway is a two neuron pathway from the spinal cord to the periphery or viscera, with one neuron travelling part of the way and a second neuron travelling the remaining distance, the two neurons meeting at a *synapse* in a *ganglion* (the junction where the two neurons meet) somewhere along the path.

Consequently there is a preganglionic neuron (the neuron before the synapse in the ganglion) and a postganglionic neuron (the neuron after the synapse in the ganglion).

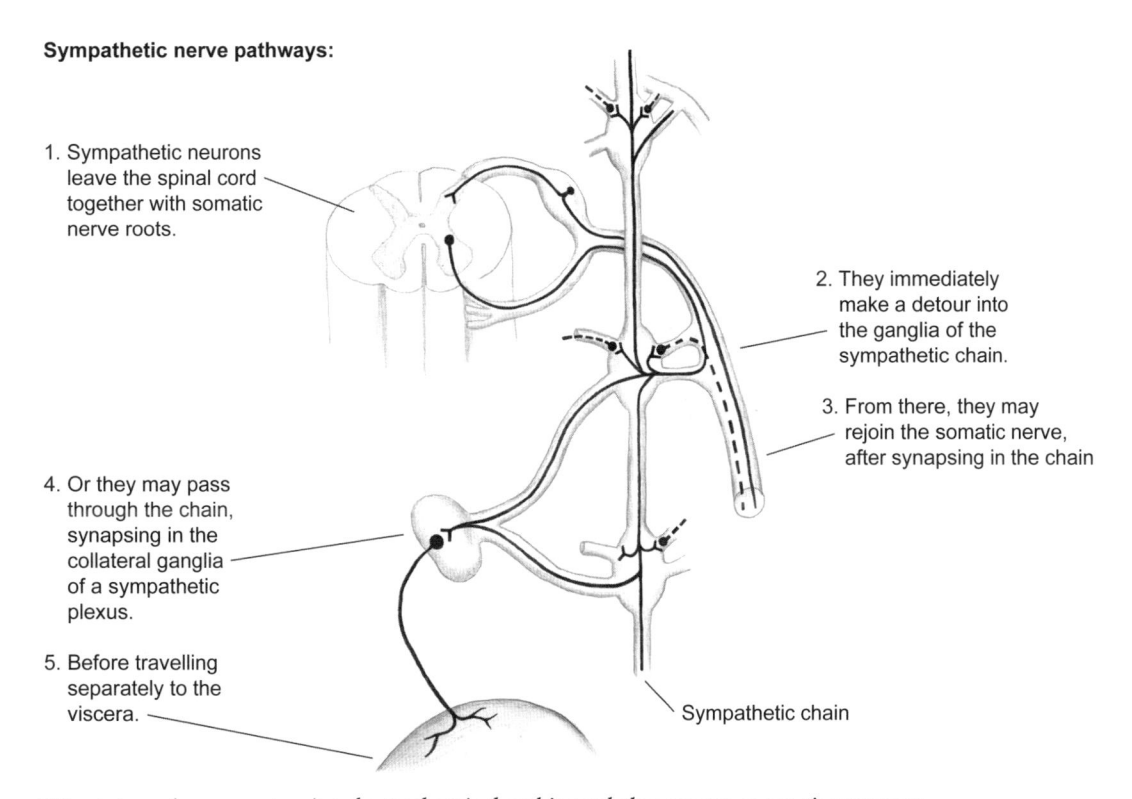

Sympathetic nerve pathways:

1. Sympathetic neurons leave the spinal cord together with somatic nerve roots.
2. They immediately make a detour into the ganglia of the sympathetic chain.
3. From there, they may rejoin the somatic nerve, after synapsing in the chain
4. Or they may pass through the chain, synapsing in the collateral ganglia of a sympathetic plexus.
5. Before travelling separately to the viscera.

Sympathetic chain

49.2 Autonomic nerve roots exit and enter the spinal cord in much the same way as somatic nerve roots

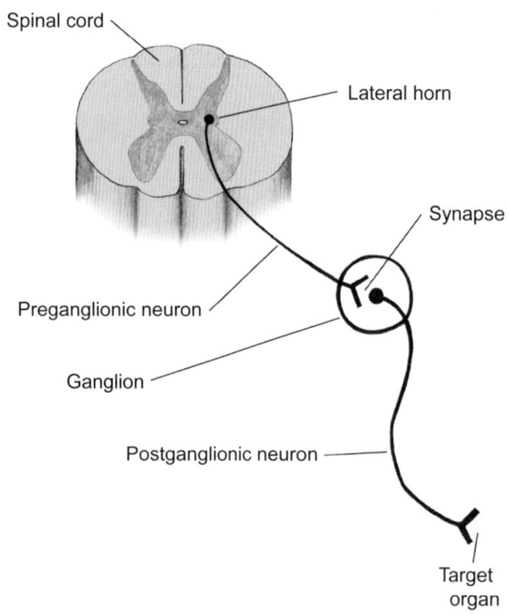

49.3 Autonomic nerve supply follows a two neuron pathway from the spinal cord to the periphery or viscera, the two neurons meeting at a synapse in a ganglion

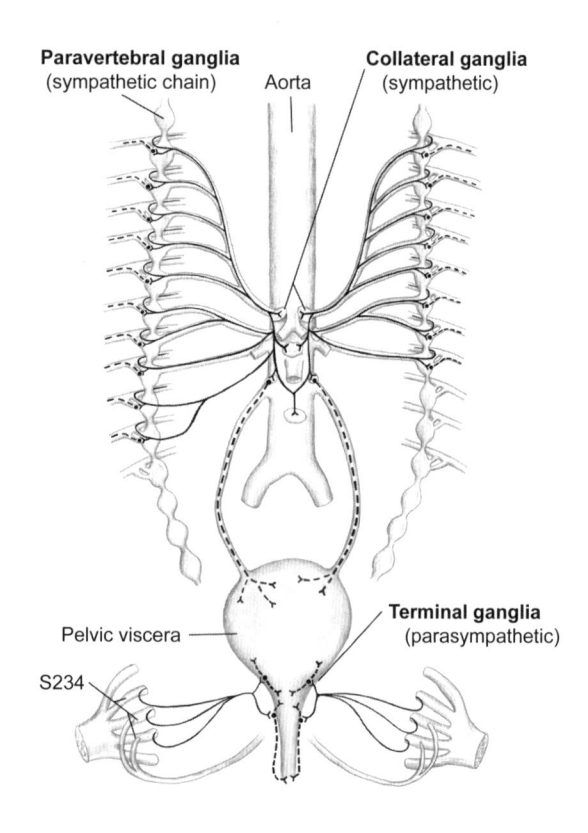

49.4 Ganglia may be located in three places
a. Paravertebral ganglia – beside the vertebral column
b. Collateral ganglia – on the surface of major blood vessels
c. Terminal ganglia – on the organ which the neuron is supplying

Ganglia

A ganglion (in this context) is like a junction box, where neurons meet and transmit messages from one to the other, just as electrical wires might be connected through a junction box. (There is a different type of ganglion, which is a fluid-filled lump growing on a tendon, and which is totally unconnected to these ganglia.)

Ganglia may be located in three places (see Figure 49.4):

1. Paravertebral ganglia – beside the vertebral column.
2. Collateral ganglia – on the surface of major blood vessels.
3. Terminal ganglia – on the organ (target organ) which the neuron is supplying.

Paravertebral and collateral ganglia only contain sympathetic synapses. Terminal ganglia only contain parasympathetic synapses.

- *Paravertebral ganglia* (always sympathetic) form a chain of ganglia on each side of the spine (located on the anterior surface of the transverse processes of the vertebrae). This is known as the *sympathetic chain*.
- *Collateral ganglia* (always sympathetic) form aggregations of ganglia on the surface of major blood vessels. These are known as *plexi* (e.g. the solar plexus/coeliac plexus) (not to be confused with the somatic plexi described previously).
- *Terminal ganglia* (always parasympathetic) form on the surface of target organs (e.g. the bladder).

ANS fibres may pass through several ganglia, but will only synapse once – in one of these ganglia.

Anatomy of the parasympathetic division

All parasympathetic nerve fibres emerge either from the cranium or from the sacrum (see Figure 49.1).

The parasympathetic division is also known anatomically as the cranio-sacral division. This nomenclature bears no relation to the term cranio-sacral therapy, but merely describes the site of origin of the parasympathetic nerves – all of which arise either from the cranium or from the sacrum.

As mentioned previously, autonomic fibres often travel together with somatic fibres along the same pathways. In the case of the parasympathetic division, this involves only a few specific somatic nerves. Parasympathetic nerve fibres travel only with the following *four cranial nerves* and *three sacral nerves*.

- *Cranial nerves: III, VII, IX, X* – with their cell bodies located in the brainstem, their axons travel with these cranial nerves to the eyes, the glands of the face, or with the vagus nerve.
- *Sacral nerves: S234* – with their cell bodies located in the spinal cord, their axons travel with spinal nerves S234 via the cauda equina, emerging from the sacrum to supply the pelvic organs.

Most of these nerves are supplying very specific localised locations, thereby providing fairly limited distribution of parasympathetic supply. However, the vagus nerve (*vagus* means *wanderer*) is the largest nerve in the body and wanders from its origin in the cranium to the majority of the viscera – including the heart, lungs, stomach, spleen, pancreas, small intestine, half of the large intestine, liver, kidneys – thereby providing a very widespread distribution of parasympathetic supply.

Anatomy of the sympathetic division

All sympathetic nerve fibres emerge either from the thoracic or lumbar spine between T1 and L2 (see Figure 49.1).

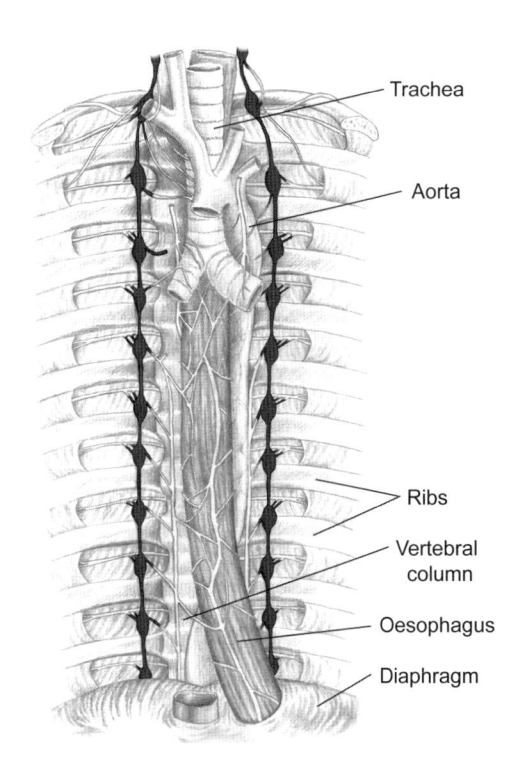

49.5 The sympathetic chain – paravertebral ganglia form a chain of ganglia on each side of the spine

The sympathetic division is also known as the thoraco-lumbar division, because all sympathetic nerves originate from the thoracic and lumbar segments of the spine.

Origins

Sympathetic neurons have their cell bodies located in the lateral horns of the spinal cord from T1–L2.

Pathway

See Figure 49.2:

- Axons *emerge* from the spinal cord together with the somatic motor fibres.
- They then *diverge* from the somatic fibres and take a *short detour into the paravertebral ganglia* of the sympathetic chain.
- Some of them will then *re-join* the somatic fibres on their way to the periphery.
- Others will *travel on independently* of the somatic fibres.

Paravertebral ganglia

Paravertebral ganglia form a chain of ganglia on each side of the spine (the sympathetic chain) (see Figure 49.5). Having entered the paravertebral ganglia, the sympathetic fibres may travel to various locations (see Figure 49.2):

- up the chain to the head
- up and out to the arms (with somatic nerves)
- straight out to the periphery (re-joining the somatic nerves)
- straight through the chain to the viscera (via collateral ganglia)
- down the chain and out to the legs (with somatic nerves).

Although sympathetic neurons emerge from the spinal cord only between T1–L2 (where they have their cell bodies) they can then pass up or down the sympathetic chain, and so join up with any peripheral nerve from any level, and so pass to any part of the body.

Almost every peripheral nerve to every part of the body also has sympathetic fibres travelling with it.

Although sympathetic neurons emerge from the spinal cord only between T1–L2, the sympathetic chain extends:

- up above T1 into the neck where there are three further ganglia on each side (see Figure 49.6):
  - the *superior cervical sympathetic ganglion*
  - the *middle cervical sympathetic ganglion*
  - the *inferior cervical sympathetic ganglion*
- down below L2, where there are several lumbar and sacral ganglia
- the two chains meeting at the coccyx to form the *ganglion impar*.

So the sympathetic chain extends above T1 and below L2, but only makes connections to the spinal cord between T1 and L2.

Extent of the Sympathetic Chain:

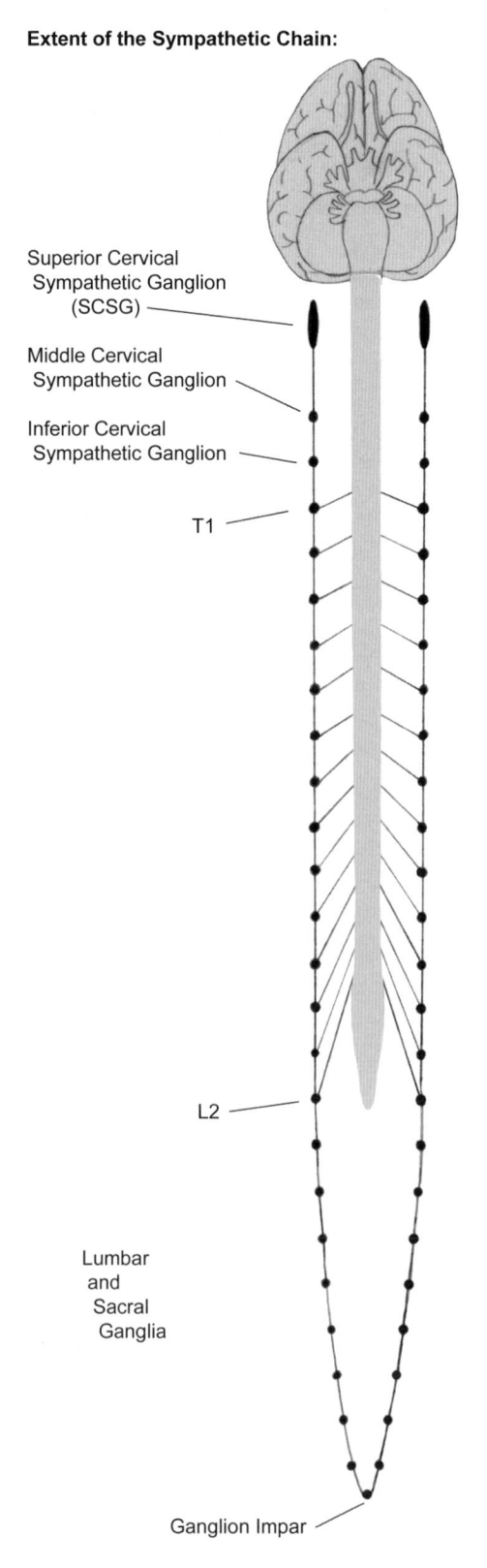

49.6 *The sympathetic chain extends above T1 and below L2, but only makes connections to the spinal cord between T1 and L2*

Collateral ganglia

Collateral ganglia are located in aggregations on the surface of major blood vessels (such as the aorta and its main branches), forming *plexi*.

These plexi are located in various places, such as:

Name of plexus	Associated chakra
Cardiac plexus	Heart chakra
Coeliac plexus	Solar plexus
Superior hypogastric plexus	Base chakra
Pelvic plexus	Root chakra

These plexi are important as:

- nerve centres/energy centres
- areas for regulation of ANS function
- areas where you may feel stress, agitation, emotional responses
- areas equivalent to the chakras.

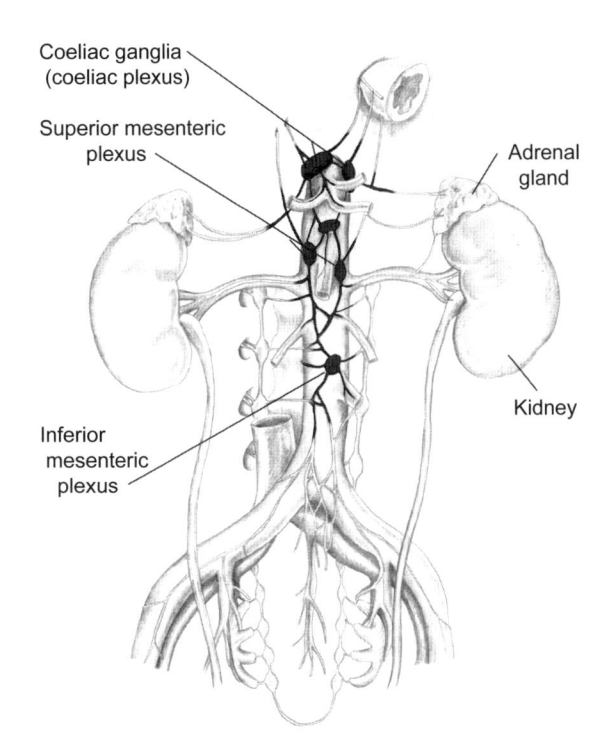

49.7 Collateral ganglia are located in aggregations on the surface of major blood vessels such as the aorta forming autonomic plexi

A single synapse

Preganglionic neurons pass from the central nervous system and synapse either in the paravertebral ganglia (beside the vertebral column) or in collateral ganglia (on blood vessels) from where the postganglionic neuron travels to the periphery or the viscera. The pathway may *pass through several* ganglia, including both paravertebral and collateral ganglia, but will *only synapse once*.

Autonomic nervous system function

Parasympathetic function

Parasympathetic fibres travelling with *cranial nerve III* supply the *eye* and regulate:

- pupil constriction (via the iris muscles)
- lens accommodation (via the ciliary muscles).

Parasympathetic fibres travelling with *cranial nerve VII* supply the *glands of head and face* and regulate:

- the lacrimal glands
- the nasal glands
- submandibular glands, sublingual glands.

Parasympathetic fibres travelling with *cranial nerve IX* supply the *parotid glands* and regulate:

- the secretion of saliva.

Parasympathetic fibres travelling with *cranial nerve X* (the vagus nerve) and comprising the bulk of the fibres of this nerve, supply the majority of the *viscera of the thorax and abdomen* and regulate:

- coronary blood vessels (constriction)
- heart muscle (decrease rate)
- bronchi (constriction)
- digestive system (peristalsis, glandular secretion, sphincter relaxation) as far as the first half of the colon.

Parasympathetic fibres travelling with *sacral nerves S234* (also known as the pelvic splanchnic nerves) supply and regulate:

- descending colon (peristalsis)
- rectum
- bladder (emptying, contraction, sphincter relaxation)
- genitalia (erection, vasodilation).

Summary of parasympathetic function:
- Anabolic function – building up resources.
- Regulates digestion, absorption, and excretion.
- Vegetative function.
- Balances sympathetic function.

Sympathetic function

The sympathetic nervous system is primarily concerned with responses to the environment, notably:
- temperature regulation (through vasoconstriction)
- stress response – preparing for action: the fight/flight/fright syndrome.

Sympathetic fibres travelling to the head regulate:
- pupil dilation
- raising the upper eyelid
- vasoconstriction
- sweat gland secretion.

Sympathetic fibres travelling with every spinal nerve to the periphery regulate:
- vasoconstriction
- sweat gland secretion.

Sympathetic fibres travelling to muscles regulate:
- vasodilation.

Sympathetic fibres travelling to the viscera regulate:
- heart muscle (increases rate and strength)
- coronary vessels (dilate)
- bronchi (dilate)
- digestive system (contract sphincters)
- adrenal gland (adrenalin secretion).

Summary of sympathetic function:
- Catabolic function – preparing for fight/flight/action.
- Closes down digestive system.
- Dilates bronchi.
- Increases heart rate.
- Produces adrenalin.

Dynamic balance

Parasympathetic (anabolic) and sympathetic (catabolic) tend to work by balancing each other with opposing functions, thereby creating a dynamic balance (homeostasis), constantly changing according to the needs of the moment. For example, when the parasympathetic nervous system is stimulating digestive function, the sympathetic nervous system reduces its tendency to contract the sphincters in the gastro-intestinal tract.

Ideally, in a perfect world, the two divisions work together, constantly changing according to the needs of the moment.

Dysfunctional imbalance

In our pressurised modern society, however, the two divisions are often set against each other, creating conflict and dysfunction – for example, eating a rushed meal under pressure of work, or living under persistent pressure and stress, leading to exhaustion of the ANS and confusion and malfunction of both divisions.

This dysfunction may manifest:
- in the organs – as indigestion, ulcers, asthma, irritable bowel
- in the nerves – causing overstimulation, potentially affecting all the body systems
- in and around the vertebral levels associated with the entry and exit of the nerves – leading to facilitated segments (to be described shortly)
- in the muscles of the back surrounding the associated vertebral levels – leading to back pain and tension
- in the central nervous system – leading to disturbed function
- in the psycho-emotional state – leading to agitation, anxiety, irritability, exhaustion.

Physical causes of ANS disturbance

Autonomic nervous system dysfunction may be caused by stress. It may also have physical causes such as visceral pathologies, vertebral restrictions, injuries, infections.

The results (and therefore the symptoms) of the dysfunction may be localised or generalised, and may be reflected or referred to other structures or parts of the body.

For example, localised dysfunction such as a bladder infection might lead to disturbance in the local organ itself, neurological feedback into the associated sympathetic plexus, disturbance along the nerve pathway from that disturbed organ to the spine and disturbance in the localised spinal segment associated neurologically with that organ (causing excessive stimulation of the localised segment), thereby establishing a 'facilitated segment' affecting surrounding tissues.

A more generalised dysfunction such as a severe car accident might create disturbance throughout the sympathetic nervous system, with activation of sympathetic reactions in various sites of physical injury, together with excessive production of adrenalin, leading to agitation, overstimulation, stress, vasoconstriction, poor temperature control, emotional disturbance.

A digestive disturbance brought on by an infectious organism may lead to symptoms of widespread autonomic dysfunction, mediated through the autonomic nerve supply to the digestive system, with agitation in the solar plexus, emotional reactions, and other autonomic responses.

Parasites (often undiagnosed) may lead to persistent symptoms of unsettled digestive and emotional reactions, which may be misdiagnosed as stress-induced.

A back injury or restriction around the T4 vertebral level may activate sympathetic supply to the cardiac and pulmonary plexi, stimulating the heart and lungs, bringing on feelings of anxiety, panic attacks and palpitations or respiratory disorders including asthma.

A back injury around T9–12 might lead to persistent overstimulation of the adrenal glands, with consequent chronic over-secretion of adrenalin and a permanent state of overstimulation, hyperactivity, stress, agitation, and all the other potential responses to adrenalin – a potential lifelong state of fight-flight-fright.

Autonomic nerves and nerve fibres are enveloped (like all nerves) in a fascial sheath (epineurium), and autonomic nerves (like all peripheral nerves) penetrate the dura as they enter or leave the central nervous system. Autonomic nerve activity is therefore reflected through the dura and fascia, influencing the qualities and characteristics (quality, symmetry, motion) of the cranio-sacral system, and is similarly influenced, settled, and reintegrated by integration of the cranio-sacral system as a whole.

The fascia is very richly innervated with sympathetic fibres and is therefore significantly affected by autonomic disturbance, with excessive sympathetic stimulation potentially leading to chronic tightness of the fascia, with associated tension in muscles and other tissues and constriction of blood vessels and nerves. Fascial unwinding can therefore have a profound influence on the state of the autonomic nervous system.

Autonomic relationships with vertebral levels

A clear understanding of the relationship between dural levels (and therefore vertebral levels) and the organs or structures supplied from those levels is obviously helpful in the diagnosis and treatment of visceral dysfunctions and dysfunction generally.

However, the anatomy of the sympathetic nervous system and its plexi is such that there is a great deal of interaction and overlap of nerve supply. Most organs will therefore receive innervation from many different nerve roots, and most nerve roots will supply many different organs. Consequently, the relationship between organs and vertebral levels is less precise and more widespread than in the somatic nervous system. This broad and diffuse distribution is further exaggerated as the sympathetic nerves pass through plexi (cardiac plexus, coeliac plexus, etc.) where a great deal of further interaction, interchange, and redistribution occurs.

The precise distribution of the autonomic nervous system is therefore very complex, but a succinct (if imprecise) summary of vertebral levels in relation to autonomic supply is useful for clinical application, and is summarised below.

A brief summary of the autonomic nervous system

The autonomic nervous system is divided into two divisions:

- *Sympathetic.*
- *Parasympathetic.*

Sympathetic division

The *sympathetic* division is primarily concerned with preparing the body for action – for fight or flight – increasing blood supply to the muscles for increased muscular activity, increasing heart rate and strength, increasing production of adrenalin, responding to danger, emergency, or stresses, responding to the environment, expending resources.

Parasympathetic division

The *parasympathetic* division is primarily concerned with building up resources, through the vegetative functions of digestion, absorption, excretion, and preparing the body for less active more restful function.

In gaining a clinically invaluable understanding of the relationship between sympathetic levels and their associated viscera, it is helpful to remember the following points:

Sympathetic distribution

The *sympathetic* division, while supplying all parts of the body, communicates with the central nervous system (and therefore penetrates the dura) only between vertebral levels T1 and L2.

- The *uppermost sympathetic nerves* (those to the head and eyes) emerge from the central nervous system at vertebral levels T1 and T2.
- The *lowest sympathetic nerves* (those to the pelvic organs and feet) emerge from vertebral levels L1 and L2.
- The *remaining sympathetic nerves* emerge between these levels, roughly in accordance with the level of the structures supplied.

Sympathetic ganglia

The sympathetic ganglia (points of synapse or nerve interchange) are clinically significant sites since they are focal points of sympathetic nerve activity, and are therefore relevant both for diagnosis and for treatment.

These ganglia are located in a chain (the sympathetic chain) running alongside the vertebral column on each side throughout its length from C1 to the coccyx, and also in the plexi such as the cardiac plexus, coeliac plexus (solar plexus), pelvic plexus, etc.

Superior cervical sympathetic ganglia

The *superior cervical sympathetic ganglion* (SCSG), located at the top of the sympathetic chain, bilaterally, at vertebral levels C1–4, just below the cranium, is of particular significance, both in view of its location in the suboccipital region, and in view of its function, being the pathway and area of synapse for sympathetic supply to the head and eyes.

Plexi

All the *plexi* along with the ganglia (particularly the SCSG) reflect sympathetic nerve activity, and are therefore important indicators of stress and sympathetic stimulation, both locally and generally.

Parasympathetic distribution

The parasympathetic division emerges from the central nervous system (and therefore through the dura) only at S234 and via cranial nerves III, VII, IX and X. *There is no communication with the central nervous system at any other vertebral level,* although the vagus nerve (cranial nerve X) passes down beside the vertebral column bilaterally, giving off branches to the viscera of the thorax and abdomen, down to the level of the first half of the colon. The lower half of the colon and the pelvic organs receive parasympathetic supply from the sacrum S2, 3 and 4.

Box 49.1 A brief summary of autonomic nerve root origins

Due to the diffuse nature of sympathetic nerve distribution, this brief summary can only present a broad approximation, rather than exact precision in relation to sympathetic nerve origins. This summary can, however, serve as a valuable point of reference in terms of clinical application.

Sympathetic levels: T1–L2

An even briefer, and therefore less precise but more memorable summary, is as follows:

Level	Structure	Brief summary
T1–2	Head	T1–2 Head
T1–5	Heart	
T2–6	Respiratory tract	T2–6 Thoracic viscera
T4–6	Oesophagus	
T6–10	Stomach, Liver, Gall bladder, Pancreas, Spleen	T6–10 Abdominal viscera
T8–11	Small intestine	
T10–L2	Large intestine (colon)	
T10–L2	Adrenals, Kidneys, Ureters, Bladder, Genitalia	T10–L2 Pelvic viscera
T2–8	Blood vessels of upper limb	
T11–L2	Blood vessels of lower limb	

Parasympathetic levels

Cr III	Eyes
Cr VII	Glands of face
Cr IX	Parotid gland
Cr X	Organs of thorax and abdomen (including first half of colon)
S2–4	Organs of pelvis and second half of colon (pelvic splanchnic nerves)

We will return to look at the overall integration of the autonomic nervous system in greater detail, once we have explored some other factors which contribute to the picture.

Chapter 50

Double Contacts with the Sacrum

Preparatory release

The word sacrum derives from the same root as the word sacred, reflecting the fact that the profound significance of the sacrum has been recognised since long ago.

As we have seen previously, the sacrum is a powerhouse of cranio-sacral energy. Its mobility is essential to free, healthy function of the cranio-sacral system as a whole and consequently to the underlying health and vitality of the individual.

In order to ensure the free mobility, symmetry and motion of the sacrum, various contacts can be used to assist the release of patterns of restriction and tension that are inhibiting its mobility and free expression, particularly around the sacro-iliac and lumbo-sacral joints and the pelvic muscles. These have been described previously (in Chapter 26).

Working with the sacrum – a powerful means of integration

Working with the cranio-sacral system from a freely mobile sacrum can be a powerful means of enabling a greater degree of balance, symmetry and integration through the system as a whole, enabled as always through the unfolding of the inherent treatment process.

As we have seen previously, this may include projection through the spine, with attention to the vertebral column, the vertebral canal, the spinal membranes, the spinal cord, the spinal nerves emanating from the spinal cord, the whole core of the system, the midline, as well as to rhythmic motion, vitality, fluid drive, focal points of restriction, still points and other responses within the system.

Ramifications to all parts of the body

This in turn can enable improved function in the various organs, glands, muscles and other peripheral structures supplied neurologically by the spinal nerves emerging from the spine, when impingement or irritation of nerve roots entering and leaving the spine is released.

It can also enable enhanced vitality and balance throughout the system, reflecting out energetically from the integration of the vital core of the system at the midline.

Persistent resistance

In projecting up through the spine, you might have identified certain areas, focal points, restrictions – some of which will have responded readily to your attention.

However, certain restrictions and resistances may remain more persistent and resistant, particularly the more deeply entrenched, consolidated, solidified, chronic resistances that have been established over a greater length of time. The release of these more persistent resistances may be enhanced through the use of *double contacts* between the sacrum and the spine.

Double contacts

The term double contacts simply means taking up contact with two hands on two different areas of the body. This establishes a specific focus at one or both of those points of contact, and creates a channel for the enhanced flow of vitality between those two points. At times, this flow of vitality may simply be allowed to flow between the two hands, as both hands engage with the cranio-sacral process. At other times, one point of contact may be regarded as a source for harnessing the flow of inherent vitality within the body, and the other point as a target area to which the therapeutic forces can be directed. This can of course be done simply by directing your attention to a particular area, but the presence of the second hand at a target area provides a focus which can enhance the reception of that energy – like a satellite dish receiving electro-magnetic radio waves.

Harnessing the potency

Double contacts can be used anywhere in the body. They are particularly effective when one of the contacts is a powerhouse of cranio-sacral energy such as the sacrum, harnessing the potency within the sacrum, which can then be directed towards the focal point established by the second contact. They are particularly valuable as a means of integrating the vitally significant function of the spine.

The vital spine

The spine plays an essential part in enabling, supporting and integrating function throughout the body. It is the vital core from which health emanates to all parts, irrigating the rest of the system both neurologically and energetically. The bony vertebral column, lined with dura, arachnoid and pia mater contains and protects the vital spinal cord. It allows the passage of the spinal nerves emanating from the spinal cord and penetrating the membranes to pass out through the intervertebral foramina to supply the organs, muscles, glands and other peripheral structures throughout the body. The flow of vitality runs through this vital core from sacrum to cranium and cranium to sacrum, thereby enabling the flow of vitality to all parts of the system. The integrity of the spine is crucial in maintaining the essential flow of vitality.

The spine is also vulnerable. Like many significant areas of the body, it is particularly susceptible to injury and restriction (as indicated by the common occurrence of back pain throughout most populations). Proper integrated function of the spine is essential to proper function of the system as a whole. The use of double contacts involving one hand under the sacrum and a second hand taking up various contacts along the vertebral column is a profoundly effective way of assisting this integration.

Taking up contact

Contact can be taken up with one hand under the sacrum (as described previously in Chapter 26) vertically orientated, with the fingers pointing up towards the cranium. (In fact it is just the fingers that are under the sacrum, in order to avoid a squashed hand.)

The other hand is placed under the back; ask the patient to arch their back a little, so that you can slide a hand under their spine, transversely orientated (across the back), with the vertebral column sitting into the palm of your hand.

Key areas

This second contact may be taken up anywhere along the vertebral column according to the individual needs of the patient, but certain key areas are particularly significant in the overall functioning of the system and these are the areas most likely to demand attention.

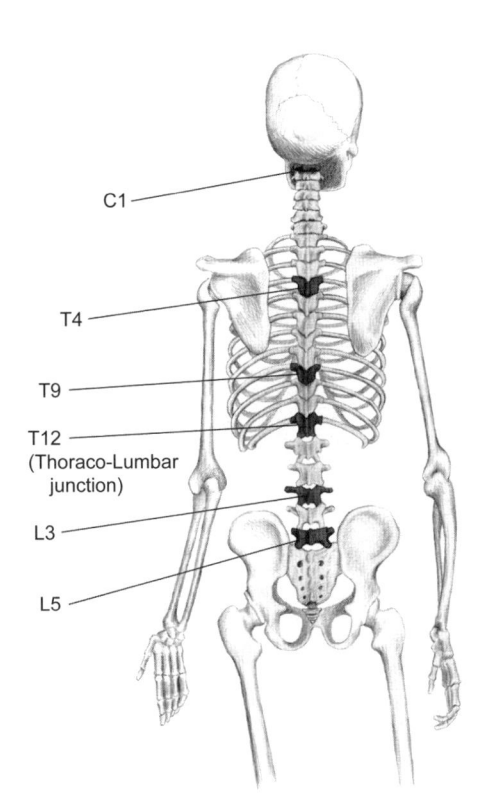

50.1 Some significant pivotal areas in the spine

These areas can be identified by their vertebral levels – although their relevance is by no means restricted to their bony or mechanical relationships (see Figure 50.1):

- L5
- L3
- T12 (the thoraco-lumbar junction)
- T9
- T4
- the cranium.

The significance of these specific areas may relate to the mechanics of the spine, postural stresses and strains, muscular attachments and tensions, areas of neurological outflow and input – particularly sympathetic outflow, associations with specific viscera (as we have seen in exploring the autonomic nervous system) or associations with emotional centres, energy centres or chakras. The specific significance of each of these areas can be summarised as follows.

The fifth lumbar vertebra: L5

Mechanical associations

The lumbo-sacral region (L5/S1 vertebral levels) is a particularly vulnerable part of the vertebral column:

- It is the junction between the mobile vertebral column above and the more solid foundation of the pelvis below.
- It carries the weight of the whole vertebral column above.
- The angle between the L5 and S1 vertebrae is particularly acute, with a vulnerable wedge-shaped intervertebral disc that is more susceptible to damage due to the stresses exerted upon it.
- It is accommodating a major part of the stresses and strains of standing on two legs (rather than standing on four legs as it was originally designed to do – a process to which the human body is still adapting. There have been land animals for 400 million years, but we have been walking on two legs for less than 1% of that time).
- It accommodates a great deal of the twisting, turning, bending and mobility of the body in normal everyday activity.

Neurological associations

It is also one of the principal sites of outflow for the sciatic nerve (whose roots emanate from L45, S123). This region is therefore likely to be involved in cases of sciatica and in many cases

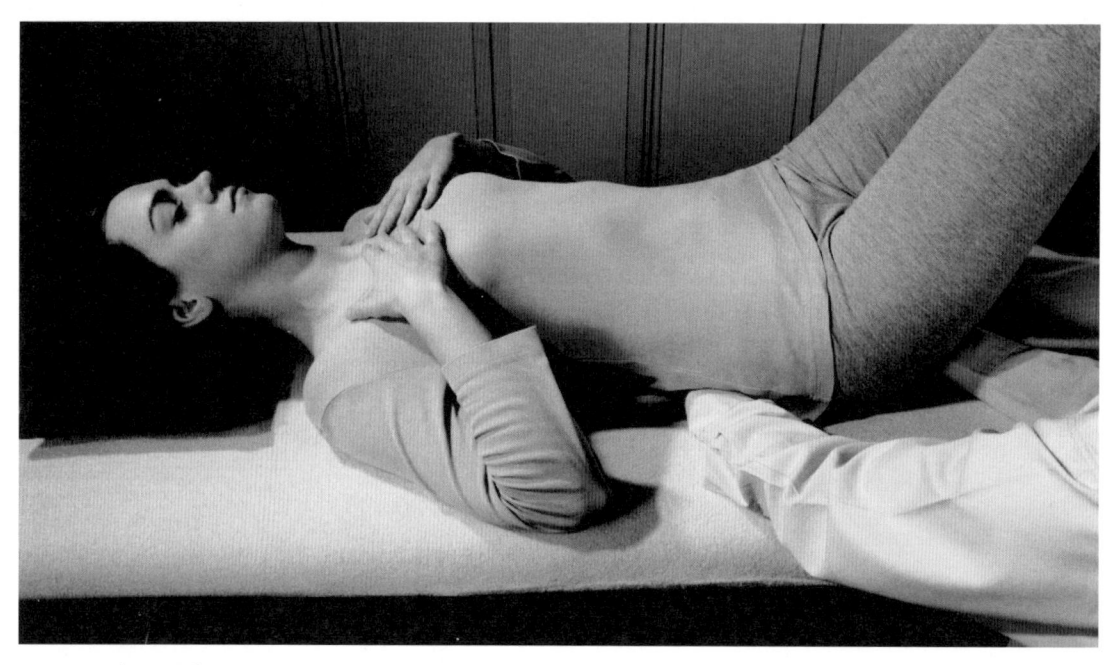

50.2 Lumbo-sacral contact

of low back pain, and is also significant in the overall relationship between the vertebral column and the pelvis. It is also an area that is easily disturbed by compressive injuries, such as a heavy fall on the buttocks.

The third lumbar vertebra: L3

The L3 vertebra is in the small of the back approximately level with the umbilicus anteriorly and with the iliac crests. It is significant in the mechanics of the body in that it forms 'the apex of the lower triangle'. This triangle (see Figure 50.3) is part of a system described by the pioneering osteopath Martin Littlejohn (1865–1947) in which various pivotal and mechanical associations and interrelationships have been defined. This lower triangle associates the L3 vertebra with the sacro-iliac and hip joints as a unit whose unified mobility is vital to the integrated function of the lower parts of the body.

Any disturbance to the mechanical workings of the lower parts of the body – the sacro-iliac joints, the hips, the knees, the ankles – is likely to reflect into the L3 vertebral level; and similarly any disturbance at the L3 vertebral level is likely to reflect out as a disturbance in these lower structures. Consequently:

- Knee injuries may lead to disturbance at the L3 vertebral level.
- Knee injuries may persist because of a disturbance at the L3 vertebral level if it is not addressed.
- Symptoms in the knee may arise without any injury or trauma as a result of strains emanating from the L3 level, together with an imbalance in the whole lower body.

Understanding these points can be crucial in identifying the source of a condition, making an accurate diagnosis, putting together a more complete picture – and consequently in providing effective treatment and potentially avoiding unnecessary surgery.

It is therefore always relevant to integrate the overall functioning of the whole lower part of the body, including the lower triangle with its apex at L3, particularly in any condition with persistent symptoms involving the knees, ankles, hips, or sacro-iliac joints, or involving pelvic imbalances.

The thoraco-lumbar junction: T12/L1

Mechanical associations

The thoraco-lumbar junction is significant first from the mechanical point of view as:

- the transitional area between the thoracic spine above and the lumbar spine below
- the junction between the thoracic kyphosis above and the lumbar lordosis below.

Consequently it is an area of postural stresses and strains. It is another area which particularly takes the strain of standing on two legs. It is another area which particularly absorbs compressive forces, whether from specific sporting activities such as horse-riding, jogging or playing in a rugby scrum, or from compressive injuries from falls or sitting down heavily.

It is also the area of attachment for the *crura* of the diaphragm. The word crura means legs

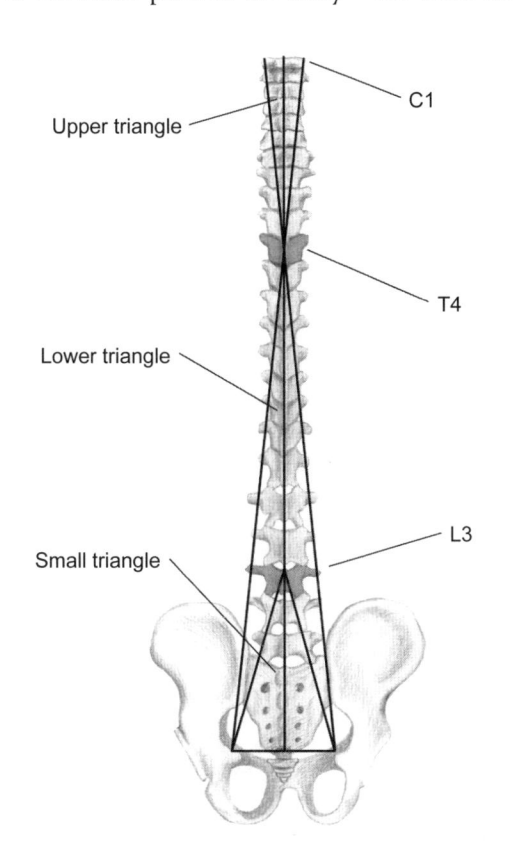

50.3 Littlejohn's triangles (simplified)

and the crura of the diaphragm are the tendinous legs through which the diaphragm attaches to the vertebral column around the thoraco-lumbar junction. Tension in the diaphragm (very common in association with the shallow breathing and emotional holding prevalent in so many people) can therefore tend to compress this region; and similarly compressions, restrictions and asymmetries within the thoraco-lumbar region may exert pulls upon the diaphragm.

Neurological associations
Most significantly, the thoraco-lumbar junction is the area of major sympathetic nerve outflow to many of the surrounding viscera, including the kidneys, the adrenals, the bladder, the small intestine and the large intestine (colon) and also to the uterus, ovaries, prostate, genitalia and other pelvic organs.

It is therefore an area of crucial importance in a wide variety of conditions affecting these various organs, including:

- menstrual disorders
- irritable bowel syndrome or spastic colon
- kidney disease
- bladder conditions such as cystitis.

In cystitis, the infectious focus may lead to irritation of the nerve roots in the thoraco-lumbar region, which may create a chronic, vicious cycle of neurological activity. This in turn may play an important part in reinstating the symptoms of recurrent cystitis even when the infection has passed and no infectious organisms are present. Awareness of the relevant areas of the spine and the neurological pathways can play a crucial part in effective treatment of recurrent or persistent cystitis and many other similar circumstances. An integrated understanding of all these anatomical and neurological relations and their integrated, interconnected interaction is vital to an overall understanding of health.

The ninth thoracic vertebra: T9
Mechanical associations
From a mechanical point of view, T9 is the apex of the thoracic curve and is therefore subject to strain due to anterior-posterior postural imbalances.

Neurological associations
More significantly, it is the vertebral level most associated with the solar plexus and the coeliac ganglia of the sympathetic nervous system. It has also been found (by Littlejohn) to have an important empirical relationship with the adrenal glands.

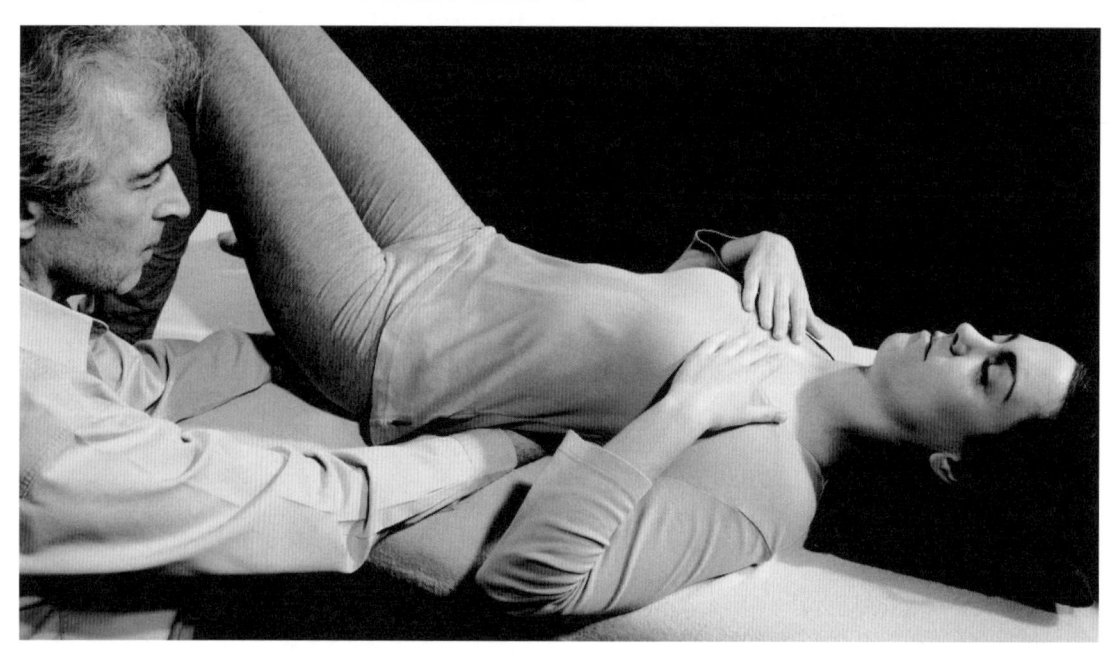

50.4   Double contact between the sacrum and the thoraco-lumbar junction

The T9 vertebral level is therefore particularly significant in conditions of prolonged stress and pressure involving excessive stimulation of the sympathetic nervous system, excessive secretion of adrenalin and excessive activity within the solar plexus. Patients who are under a high degree of stress will very commonly be found to have a significant focus of tension and restriction around this T9 level.

The fourth thoracic vertebra: T4

Mechanical associations

From a mechanical perspective the T4 vertebra is the root of the neck. While anatomically, one might think of the neck as finishing at the base of the cervical spine with C7, functionally the neck extends down to the T4 vertebral level (forming Littlejohn's Upper Triangle; see Figure 50.3). Any condition involving the neck needs to be integrated down through the thoracic spine at least as far as T4 (as well as through the system as a whole). Failure to take this into account in attempting to treat neck conditions is likely to limit the effectiveness of treatment. Once again, this is a two-way relationship in which conditions of the neck can feed into the T4 vertebral level, and conditions of the upper thoracic spine to T4 can affect the neck.

T4 is also the junction between Littlejohn's Upper Triangle and Large Triangle, a crucial junction in the overall balance of the body – a meeting point at which stresses and strains, injuries and imbalances from above and below all come together. Any injury or imbalance from below is likely to feed into the T4 area; any injury or imbalance from above is also likely to gravitate to the T4 area, the various forces from above and below intertwining at this crucial junction creating potentially highly disturbing conflict, with widespread whole person ramifications.

Neurological associations

The T4 level is also the focal area of sympathetic nerve outflow both to the heart and to the lungs. It is therefore likely to be involved in conditions affecting the heart and to a whole range of lung conditions including asthma. Asthma is a complex condition involving many factors, but in any asthmatic condition there is likely to be an involvement of the upper thoracic spine around T4.

T4 is also the level associated with the heart chakra and cardiac plexus and is therefore intimately involved with their associated anxieties and stresses (again contributing to the asthmatic picture). A great many patients with significant levels of anxiety will be found to have a focal point of restriction and agitation around this level.

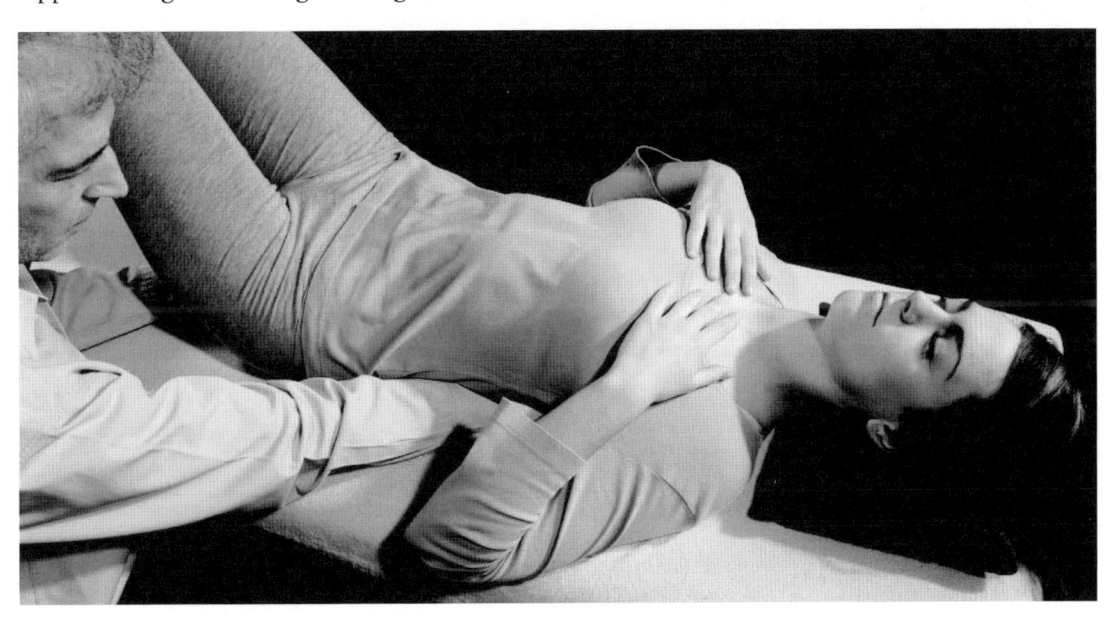

50.5 Double contact between the sacrum and T4

The combination of factors coming together at T4 is particularly significant – sufficient to merit identification of a specific 'T4 syndrome'. This is a syndrome recognised on a partial physical level in physiotherapy and other physical therapies, but which has much more profound implications not generally acknowledged which deserve a section of their own later (see Chapter 51), in order to fully appreciate the integrated effects of all the physical and emotional interactions involved.

The cranium

A double contact between the sacrum and the cranium is a very powerful means of integrating the whole system. In taking up this contact, you are cradling the whole system, wrapping the whole person in your gentle, caring embrace.

In order to take up this contact comfortably, it is necessary to adjust your hand position and your sitting position (midway between sacrum and cranium) in order to avoid being uncomfortably overstretched (particularly with long patients).

Adjust your hand under the sacrum so that it is turned transversely and resting lightly against the coccyx and buttocks (rather than under the sacrum), so that your contact is extremely light and does not have any weight pressing on your hand or fingers.

Move your chair so that you are sitting halfway between sacrum and cranium, so that you are not leaning to one side or stretching with either arm, leading to disruptive discomforts in your own body which will reduce your sensitivity and focus.

For the second contact, bring the palm of the other hand gently through the energy field, until it comes to rest lightly across the frontal area of the head, the centre of your palm over the centre of the forehead. You can allow your forearm or elbow to rest on the couch for support, in order to avoid holding on to any unnecessary tension in your arm and shoulder.

Alternatively, you can take up your second contact over the crown of the head, with the centre of your palm over the centre of the crown, again resting your forearm or elbow on the couch for support. Another option is to place your second hand under the occiput.

This contact is enveloping both ends of the cranio-sacral system, the cranium and the sacrum, and consequently integrating the whole

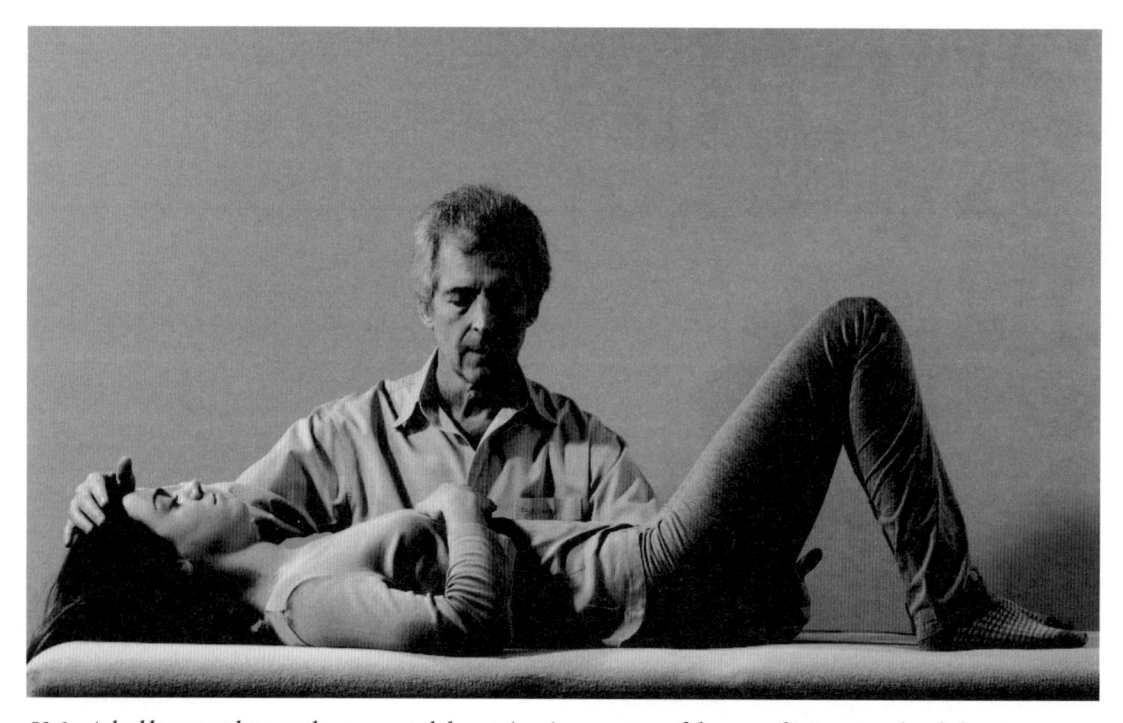

50.6 A double contact between the sacrum and the cranium is a very powerful means of integrating the whole system

cranio-sacral system from the crown chakra to the root chakra. It provides an excellent perspective from which to view the system as a whole.

You can project your attention through the whole body from top to bottom and from bottom to top. You can explore the detailed anatomical structure within, projecting through the bony system, the membrane system, the fluid system and the energetic system, the vertebral segments, the intervertebral foramina, the nerve roots, and any focal points of restriction or irritation in any of these. You can allow the system to express any twists, turns and pulls, viewing the whole picture throughout the body. You can identify twisting patterns through the whole body (a common birth pattern) allowing them to draw to points of stillness and unravel. You can identify fulcrums or focal points of restriction anywhere throughout the body between your two contacts. You can allow the whole system to unwind between your two contacts and you can follow the rhythmic motion as it is expressed through the whole system, surging up towards the cranium and ebbing away towards the sacrum.

It is an excellent contact for integrating a baby's system following the rigours of birth. It can equally be used to integrate an adult's cranio-sacral system. It is an excellent way to finish off any treatment as a final integrative process.

WORKING WITH DOUBLE CONTACTS

Any contact involving both hands could be called a double contact. Double contacts can be taken up anywhere in the body. They may be taken up at any time during treatment. Double contacts through the spine are of particular significance, because they are integrating the vital core of the system.

These double contacts between the sacrum and various regions of the spine may often be taken up as an integral part of any treatment process. As you work at the sacrum, you might identify a focal point somewhere in the spine and introduce a second contact as appropriate *specific double contacts* may be taken up in response to specific patterns of restriction and the major part of a treatment session might involve remaining at one specific point of double contact. Alternatively, you may choose to work your way up through all the double contacts described above as a means of integrating the whole core from bottom to top. *Working systematically through the system from bottom to top* will enable a profound integration of the whole spine, clearing resistances throughout the system while at the same time addressing specific restrictions step by step.

The contact for most of these double contacts on the vertebral column is much the same, with the fingers of one hand under the sacrum, the other hand transversely under the appropriate vertebral level (see Figures 50.2 and 50.4).

However, for *the T4 contact*, it is helpful to adapt the position to accommodate the scapulae. For this contact, place your second hand vertically orientated, the fingers extending up between the scapulae (see Figure 50.5). This is more comfortable for the patient, rather than having your hand digging in to their shoulder blades, and more comfortable for the practitioner, rather than having the scapulae squashing your hand and fingers. It therefore enables more comfortable and deeper engagement with the system. It does, however, involve twisting your arm or wrist significantly in order to establish the appropriate position, a position which may initially feel a little awkward.

The process

Take up contact under the sacrum, releasing the sacrum as necessary to enable a freely mobile sacrum (as described in Chapter 26). Once the system is settled and you feel engaged, *take up a second contact* under the spine.

Allow the system to *settle into neutral*, evaluating quality, symmetry and motion:

- at the sacrum
- at the second contact
- in the system as a whole.

Allow the gradual evolution of the *inherent treatment process*:

- allowing the system to express itself
- following any spontaneous responses (with both hands)
- leading to points of stillness and release

- observing reorganisation throughout the system
- settling back to neutral.

As rhythmic motion becomes clearer, engage more fully with the *rhythmic motion*:
- as it sweeps through the system
- as it sweeps through the core
- feeling the flow of rhythmic motion between your two hands
- feeling the rhythmic waves of motion flowing up repeatedly towards the second contact, tending to dissolve any resistance.

As you engage more deeply and superficial resistances dissolve, you may find the system drawing spontaneously into the extremes of motion, feeling the sacrum drawing consistently and persistently into flexion, as if being drawn up towards the second contact, *harnessing the power* of the system. You may feel a build-up of tension or pressure in the system, focused around the restriction at the second contact, perhaps simultaneously drawing into some imbalance or asymmetry. Follow this process as it builds to a point of stillness, eventually releasing, reorganising and settling back to neutral.

This process is likely to arise spontaneously, but if it doesn't, you can enhance the body's potential by offering it the same possibility, inviting the system to draw into the extremes of motion. Assess whether the sacrum is drawing more readily into flexion or extension. Invite the system to *follow consistently into its preferred phase of motion* to a point of stillness. As you do so, *be aware of the responses*:

- at the sacrum
- at the second contact
- between your two hands
- throughout the system.

Maintain a *constant awareness of the whole system*, as well as the detailed responses within that overall picture. As the system releases, feel the ramifications of the release spreading through the whole system.

This process may happen repeatedly of its own accord; you may invite it repeatedly; it may occur repeatedly at the same focal point in order to address a particularly ingrained chronic resistance, or you might repeat the process at various different points of double contact throughout the spine.

At each point of contact and with each release:
- allow the process to come to *resolution*
- settle back into *neutral* before moving on.

As you take up each *new contact* allow time for re-engagement and for the system to settle again into neutral before proceeding.

Fluent fluidic flow

As the system becomes more integrated and settled, following a succession of releases, gradually the whole spine, the whole core, the whole system may take on a more fluent, fluidic, expansive expression of rhythmic motion and vitality.

If the initial activity is at the cranio-sacral rhythm level, then certain releases might lead to a significant shift into the middle tide level. As the system becomes increasingly settled, the whole process may become more subtle, the build-up to still points developing more slowly and remaining in stillness for longer before dissolving into deeper levels of release. In due course, perhaps following a particularly significant release, the rhythmic motion may settle further and you may feel the emergence of a long, profound shift into the long tide, if circumstances are appropriate. As the system becomes more settled, allow the whole process to settle into deeper stillness, allowing the process of subtle integration, feeling the microscopic adjustments of the system, at the sacrum, at the second contact and everywhere between and around, feeling the whole system settling into deeper engagement, expanding your perception to observe the repercussions throughout the matrix and settling into deep dynamic stillness.

As you settle into the sacrum-cranium contact, *feel the fluent, fluidic flow through the whole system*. Allow the continuing process of subtle integration, settling into increasingly profound levels of long tide motion and deep dynamic stillness, content just to be there in deep absorption with the whole matrix.

Chapter 51

Facilitated Segments and T4 Syndrome

Facilitated segments

The word *segment* in this context refers to a vertebral or spinal cord segment – the area where two vertebrae meet, with nerve fibres passing in and out through the intervertebral foramina between the two vertebrae, through the dura, arachnoid and pia, providing input from the periphery to the central nervous system, and output to the various structures, local and distant, which are supplied neurologically from that segment.

The word *facilitation* means that something happens more easily. In this context, facilitation indicates that this segment, along with its nerve fibres and associated structures, are in a reactive state where they are more easily activated, sparking off neurological messages along the various pathways emanating from that segment (see Figure 51.1).

In other words, a facilitated segment is an area of the spine or spinal cord in which the threshold of response has been lowered, so that a standard level of activity, excitement or stimulation, which the body would usually cope with perfectly well, activates it causing undue reaction and symptoms. In the area of a facilitated segment, the surrounding muscles may be tight and the local skin slightly tender.

A segment may be facilitated because of an old back injury or vertebral restriction, or as a result of a persistent input from any of the structures feeding into that segment – a digestive disorder, a muscular injury or tension, or emotional tension. Anything that feeds into that local area can induce and perpetuate a facilitated segment.

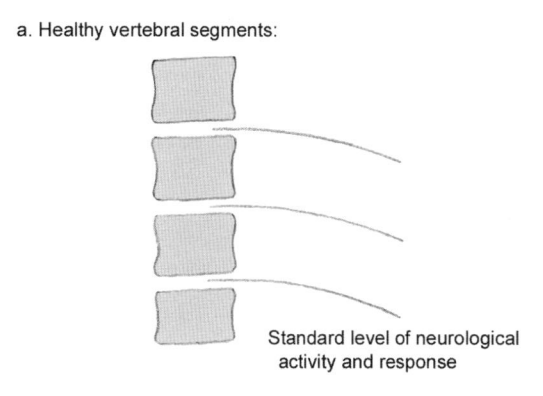

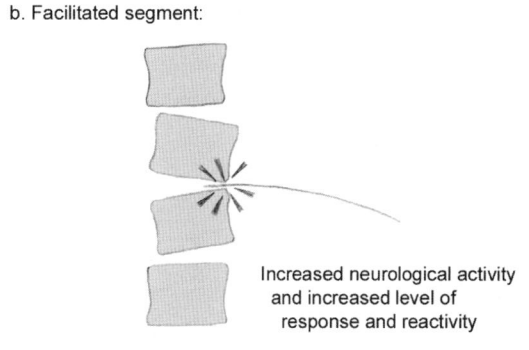

a. Healthy vertebral segments:

Standard level of neurological activity and response

b. Facilitated segment:

Increased neurological activity and increased level of response and reactivity

c. Reflex arc:

Stimulation (e.g. pain)

Reaction (e.g. spasm)

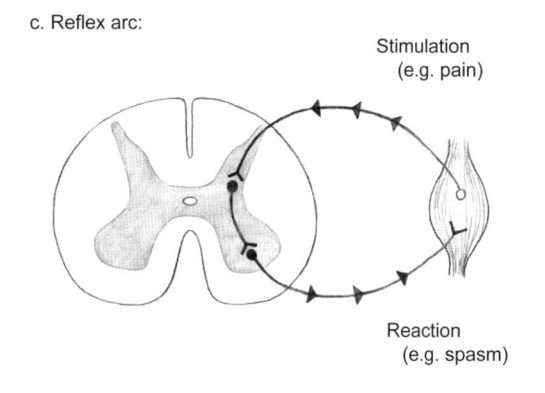

51.1 A facilitated segment – a segment may be facilitated as a result of any persistent input feeding into that segment

Easily sparked off

When a segment is facilitated, it becomes a weak spot which can easily be sparked off by a variety of different factors – not only local factors feeding directly into the segment, but any factor that disturbs the balance of the system, such as lifting something heavy, turning awkwardly, eating (in segments related to the digestive system), dust or pollen (in segments related to the lungs), stress, excitement, or a minor injury or illness of any kind.

So a minor movement or knock can set off a major reaction, as a facilitated segment is reactivated, with the return of old symptoms, apparently from nowhere. Patients will generally experience a facilitated segment as an area where they repeatedly or persistently experience symptoms, often triggered by no identifiable cause.

Ideally, one would wish to eliminate the facilitated segment and restore the area to healthy function, so that it is not persistently or repeatedly activated. But facilitated segments are often there due to a deeply ingrained pattern which is not readily resolved.

Appropriate and inappropriate responses

In addressing a facilitated segment there are therefore several factors to consider:

- To what extent is the facilitated segment itself resolvable?
- To what extent are current symptoms arising from the facilitated segment?
- To what extent is the current activation of the facilitated segment being activated by factors from elsewhere?

In many therapies, therapists are readily drawn to treating a local symptomatic area. In a deeply embedded facilitated segment which is being activated by factors from elsewhere, this is clearly not a good idea. It will simply add further input into an already facilitated area and activate further facilitation, potentially aggravating symptoms, while failing to address the causative factors. Even if it relieves symptoms in immediate terms, it may be aggravating the underlying weakness so that symptoms return more readily.

The first priority is to identify any new or current input from elsewhere and address that – this should reduce the strain on the facilitated area and ease symptoms. In the longer term, you can then see to what extent you can resolve the facilitated segment itself, with a comprehensive understanding of the many factors that might be contributing to and perpetuating it – structural, postural, visceral, emotional.

Essentially this means comprehensive integration of the whole system, identifying and addressing factors throughout the whole person on every level and allowing the cranio-sacral process to reintegrate the whole system through its inner wisdom.

A tropical holiday

For example, you travel abroad, enjoy a wonderful holiday in a tropical country, but unfortunately you contract a nasty 'tummy bug'.

Sensory input from your stomach feeds into the associated vertebral segment (around T6) instigating various reactions: activation of the local reflex arc; activation of other nerve fibres in this segment (both somatic and autonomic); tightness in the back muscles around the local area of the spine; stimulation of the local dural membrane; activity in the solar plexus; feelings of agitation.

All of these may, in turn, have effects on other areas of the body, other weak spots, other facilitated areas which have up till now been settled:

- *The tight muscles exerting pulls on the spine may induce compensatory pulls elsewhere in the spine, drawing the body into postural tensions or scolioses and creating further facilitated segments.*
- *The dural stimulation may exert pulls through the membrane system to any part of the reciprocal tension membrane system, potentially activating any other weak spot anywhere in the body.*
- *The solar plexus agitation may induce emotional disturbance and restlessness.*

The stomach infection may be dealt with, whether through antibiotics or by naturopathic means, and medically there may be nothing further to be done – and yet the activation often remains. Your stomach never feels quite the same again, the restlessness in the solar plexus remains in the background and the tightness in the muscles of the back persists. These discomforts may settle to some extent and you learn to live with them, but any time you find yourself under any minor pressure, or any physical exertion, the whole cycle may start up again – solar plexus, stomach, back, etc. – and you may find that your stomach has become more sensitive and that you have to be careful what you eat. The area has become facilitated and may remain so indefinitely, and may be activated by any other subsequent injury or illness.

If the infection is dealt with fairly promptly and the original source is eliminated and wasn't too severe, then the whole cycle may dissipate and settle back into a healthy state. The longer any stimulus remains in the system, the more likely it is that the pattern will be imprinted into the system, into all the structures within the vicious circle, so that the process becomes self-perpetuating, even when there is no longer any infectious organism present.

Parasites (again most commonly picked up on a tropical holiday) can be a particularly intransigent cause of facilitated segments, since they are often not readily diagnosed or treated and the symptoms are therefore often wrongly attributed to other causes such as stress.

Other sources

This particular example started with a tummy bug. But the original source could be anything, anywhere. It could be a *back injury* – the vertebral bones impinging on the nerves, causing local muscle spasm, and stimulating associated organs and associated plexi. The *muscle spasm* maintains the *vertebral restriction*, which maintains the *nerve impingement*, which maintains the muscle spasm etc., in a perpetual vicious circle. If the vertebral restriction is released quickly, whether through manipulation or other means, then the system may settle. If it persists, or if the back injury is severe, or if the segment is left hypermobile due to excessive manipulation, the cycle may become imprinted and it may remain persistently facilitated.

The source could be *psycho-emotional* – stress creating activation in the solar plexus or cardiac plexus, feeding into the localised vertebral segment at T9 or T4 respectively, causing muscular tension and consequent back pain, and reflecting out into the associated organs, causing digestive disturbances or asthma attacks. A brief episode of stress might cause temporary agitation, some butterflies in the stomach, transient bowel and urinary reactions and might then settle once the stress passes. Persistent, prolonged stress sets up a cycle of reaction, the cycle becoming established so that even when the stress has gone, the system has become so used to behaving in that way that the cycle persists, which in turn creates further stress and worry and further perpetuates the cycle.

Ramifications

Facilitated segments can occur anywhere in the spine. Inevitably, they occur most frequently at the classic mechanical pivots such as T4, T9 and T12, and in the upper cervical spine, with all their many mechanical, vertebral and neurological associations; and the pivots of course take the most strain in response to any structural or postural imbalance, brought on by any movement, or lifting, or secondary injury.

In the upper cervical spine, a facilitated segment may be caused by head injury, neck injury, or a strenuous birth, and whenever it is activated by whatever minor cause anywhere in the system, it may lead to headache and neck pain, or stimulation of the superior cervical sympathetic ganglion and sympathetic pathway up into the head, causing visual disturbances and feelings of tightness, pressure, congestion, and vagueness in the head – sparking off migraine attacks or headaches.

A facilitated segment at T9, perhaps from an old back injury, could activate persistent – even lifelong – over-secretion of adrenalin, causing hyperactivity, stress and pressure, and overstimulation of the whole autonomic nervous system. At the same time it could lead to persistent visceral disturbances in any or all of the abdominal organs with consequent digestive disturbance and food reactions, back pain, and agitation in the solar plexus. There could also be repercussions throughout the system, transmitted mechanically up through the spine (activating other facilitated segments in weak areas with associated consequences), or induced chemically throughout the system through the secretion and distribution of adrenalin – again all potentially sparked off, perhaps repeatedly, by any minor physical or stressful event activating the facilitated segment.

With multiple facilitated segments (such as from a car accident, or from a series of different injuries), combined with chronic stress or significant shock, it is also possible for the whole system to be facilitated. This will spark off reactions all over the place and leave the patient in a state of constant reactivity, struggling to cope with day-to-day life, needing to take inordinate care in looking after themselves – a common finding in patients with multiple symptoms and persistent ill health which hasn't responded readily to other treatment.

T4 syndrome

A facilitated segment at T4 is one of the most common and most significant areas of facilitation. As we have seen, T4 is a significant *mechanical pivot* – not just another of the pivots, but a key pivotal area; not just the apex of a triangle or of a curve, but the junction between the upper triangle and the lower triangle; the place in the body towards which all the mechanical stresses and strains tend to gravitate, whether from the lower part of the body or the upper part of the body, whether from the pelvis, legs and feet, or from the head and neck. T4 takes the brunt of every imbalance throughout the body.

We have also seen that T4 is a principal source of *sympathetic supply to the lungs and heart*. It is therefore implicated in asthma and many lung conditions, and also in many heart conditions, from palpitations and emotional reactions, to severe cardiac pathology.

We have also seen that T4 is a focus for the *emotional centre* which we call the heart centre – the area of the cardiac and pulmonary sympathetic plexi, and therefore an area that reflects and holds various emotional responses including anxiety, grief and other stresses.

It is no wonder that *T4 is readily facilitated*, whether by mechanical imbalances, local injury, visceral input from the heart and lungs, or psycho-emotional stresses or – most often – by all of these interacting and coming together to create a tangled jumble of stimuli and reactions:

- sparking off asthma attacks, panic attacks or palpitations
- stimulating feelings of anxiety and stress
- causing upper back pain, neck pain, or headaches
- or transmitting reactions to other areas of the body and sparking off facilitated segments elsewhere.

T4 is also the focus of many *postural strains*. Many people hold tension, both physical and emotional, in their shoulders and upper back, whether through emotional tension, postural collapse at desks and chairs, or occupational strains. Many occupations, such as sitting at a desk typing all day, will tend to create a focus of strain around T4.

Working with T4 and the heart centre can enable widespread release – through T4 with all its associations relating to the heart, the lungs and the emotions; through the upper thoracic spine with its associated neurological supply; through the cervico-thoracic junction; which is often compressed and collapsed due to injury and postural strain with ramifications into the brachial plexus and the arms and hands, with profound implications up through the neck and into the head influencing blood supply to the brain and sympathetic supply to the head, with a wide range of possible symptoms and consequences.

The term T4 syndrome is in common use, particularly within the field of physiotherapy, but it is usually confined primarily to a physical understanding of the mechanical and musculo-skeletal stresses and strains in this area.

The perception of T4 syndrome described here is of something much more far-reaching – a syndrome which incorporates all of the above, a syndrome which is very common and which has widespread consequences for patients caught up in a cycle of facilitation due to mutually perpetuating stimuli.

Asthma is a common example of a condition arising from T4 syndrome, with the combined input of allergens, anxiety, lung weakness and vertebral restriction (either due to an injury, compression at birth, or persistent tension).

Deeply ingrained

T4 syndrome can arise from any or all of these sources. Depending on the origin of the cycle, how deeply ingrained it is, how complex it is, and many other factors, it may be possible to release the source more readily or less readily, changing the pattern, breaking the cycle, and restoring health.

Where there is a deeply ingrained chronic physical injury, the underlying weakness may not be easy to resolve, and managing the system in order to maintain as much balance as possible may be the priority, through integration of the whole system.

When a chronically facilitated segment is activated, stirring up often familiar symptoms, the priority is to identify the source of the new activation and to integrate the whole. T4 as we have seen will take the strain from all over the body. When symptoms are prevalent at T4, it is not generally helpful to keep treating the local area at T4, thereby simply increasing the facilitation, weakness, vulnerability, and reactivity of the area; it is better to integrate the rest of the system, thereby removing the strains which are accumulating at T4 from all over the body.

Facilitated segments can be dormant and trouble-free while the system as a whole is in balance, but may arise again and become symptomatic at the slightest disturbance anywhere in the system. The segment itself may need to be settled, but the priority is to identify and address the source of the activation. There may be several facilitated segments, all potentially aggravating each other or activated simultaneously by minor disturbances.

Resolution – through integration

Many people will have facilitated segments somewhere in their spine, as a result of old injuries. Identifying the new input, often minor and unrecognised, is most relevant in immediate terms, and may alleviate any symptoms or acute discomfort. But most of all, reintegration of the whole person is the solution to maintaining balance and integrity, both in terms of relieving the immediate symptoms set off by the disturbance to the facilitated segment, and in the long-term maintenance of integrity and, where possible, resolution of the facilitated segment itself.

Chapter 52

Autonomic Nervous System Integration

The autonomic nervous system (ANS) is coordinating every moment of our lives. Each moment of excitement, joy, love, fear or irritation is expressed in our bodies through the ANS. Every subtle change in temperature, every thought, every feeling, every stimulus of any kind involves the ANS. It is one of the principal means through which we process our responses to the outside world – including responses to stress. It is the dynamic link between our emotions and our body and it is working to keep us in a state of physiological balance and homeostasis at all times. If we are out of balance, the ANS is out of balance. If we bring the ANS back into balance, we help to bring our health and well-being into balance. Consequently, the ANS plays a very significant part in the vast majority of health conditions. Understanding the ANS is vital to a deeper, more integrated understanding of human health and function.

Dynamic balance

In an ideal, harmonious world, the two divisions of the autonomic nervous system – the sympathetic and the parasympathetic – work together cooperatively to create a dynamic balance – constantly changing according to the needs of the moment. For example, the parasympathetic division stimulates digestion whereas the sympathetic division closes down digestion in order to focus on more active pursuits.

In modern society, conditions are not always ideal. Many people feel under pressure and cerebral decisions as well as emotional needs often override and suppress natural physiology, so the two divisions may end up in conflict rather than cooperation. For instance, many people who are busy at work, operating to deadlines and never having enough time, may end up eating a rushed meal while working under pressure. This leaves the parasympathetic division welcoming the sandwich and preparing to settle into a peaceful relaxed period of digestion, while the sympathetic division is closing down the sphincters in the digestive tract ready for action and inhibiting digestion in order to focus on getting the work done. Conflict ensues!

The body can cope with this now and again, but if it becomes a persistent habit (as it is with so many people) and if the digestive system is constantly under pressure and therefore constantly under sympathetic stimulation, the digestive system starts to complain, and in due course these complaints turn to disease and pathology. And that's just the digestive system. What about the rest of the body – the heart, the lungs, the immune system – all of which may be similarly under constant strain, persistently under pressure?

Continuing pressure and stress lead to a continuing excess of sympathetic activity affecting the whole body, physically, chemically, mentally and emotionally. A continuing excessive secretion of adrenalin leads to a vicious circle of overstimulation and over-activity – stimulation releases adrenalin, adrenalin leads to further stimulation – in which the person is increasingly caught on a merry-go-round of adrenalin-fuelled stimulation. The continuing conflict between the sympathetic and parasympathetic divisions, as they both do their best to maintain peace and harmony, leads to both divisions working harder and harder and ultimately becoming exhausted.

Fight/flight

The sympathetic nervous system is often described as providing the 'fight/flight' response. In nature, when an animal is confronted with a stressful situation such as an attack, its sympathetic system is activated in order to enable the animal either to fight back or to run for its life – its heart beats faster and pumps more strongly, its breathing increases, adrenalin pumps through its arteries, its whole body is primed for action.

A bear or a tiger might choose to fight. An antelope might choose to run away. In either case, it is the sympathetic nervous system which enables the body to respond appropriately.

In humans, where society is more structured, rationalised and controlled, this fight/flight response is not always expressed so freely. For instance, if you are confronted by your boss at work, your sympathetic nervous system will almost certainly be stimulated, but it is not generally advisable to express your feelings by fighting back and hitting him or her, since this might lose you your job and lead to worse pressures and conflicts. Nor is it generally appropriate to run away, since this might also lose you your job, so the natural responses of the sympathetic nervous system – the fight/flight responses – are suppressed, leading to a build-up of pressure, tension and adrenalin in the system, which in turn may lead to physiological disturbances and dysfunctions.

Autonomic discharge

This accumulation of sympathetic responses needs expression. The antelope will use up adrenalin in running away and even once it has escaped and the chase is over, it may continue the process of autonomic discharge by shaking uncontrollably. Humans generally find themselves not only unable to dissipate the adrenalin by running away, but are also, on the whole, reluctant to shake uncontrollably – particularly in public.

However, humans can find other means of autonomic discharge and of expressing the accumulation of sympathetic activity or stimulation. They might go to the gym after work, or go jogging – not quite as effective as expressing yourself at the time, but this will certainly go some way towards relieving the effects. They may play sport and perform other physical activities to dissipate the accumulated adrenalin and get the pressures out of their system. The autonomic accumulation can also be discharged through talking out the stresses, by crying, shouting or shaking. Or they might choose to deal with it in a therapeutic setting by hitting cushions – which is, of course, preferable to hitting wives, husbands or children, kicking the dog or the cat, or letting the accumulation of sympathetic stimulation build until you end up hitting out wildly in frustration over some minor irritation, getting into a fight, or exploding unreasonably over some minor incident, causing ever-increasing complications. Such reactions may dissipate the adrenalin in the moment, but invariably lead to further stresses, a continuing chain of conflicts and pressures, again perpetuating the cycle of sympathetic stimulation. The result of all this is disease.

Understanding

Persistent suppression of the sympathetic response leads to ill health. Inappropriate discharge of sympathetic response leads to conflict and ill health. So what is the solution?

As well as the appropriate discharge of autonomic stimulation and symptomatic relief, there is also a need for helping the patient towards a greater understanding – understanding of what is going on in their body and why.

Why is their body reacting the way it is with pain, strain, agitation, palpitations, ulcers, irritable bowel syndrome, headache, migraine, tinnitus, asthma, allergies, back pain, heart disease, digestive disturbance, menstrual disorders, sexual dysfunction, miscarriage, infertility, exhaustion, collapse, breakdown?

Why is their overall situation not improved, or at least only temporarily suppressed, by medication?

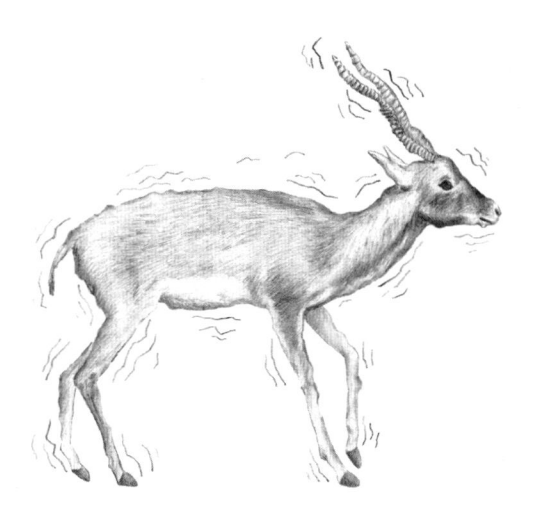

52.1 Autonomic discharge – even after the chase is over, an antelope may continue the process of autonomic discharge by shaking uncontrollably

The cranio-sacral therapist's role in dealing with these circumstances can be two-fold:

1. To *release the physical and physiological accumulations* of tension and disturbance in the body – but this in itself is clearly not enough if the patient is immediately returning to the same stressful conditions and habit patterns and a recurrence of those same tensions.

2. To *help the patient to understand the processes* involved, so that they can achieve lasting change, rather than mere relief of symptoms.

Once the patient understands the workings of the ANS, they can see where all these disturbances and dysfunctions are coming from, and through this understanding they can adapt to a life of health, fluency, ease and comfort. This doesn't mean a boring life of limitations and no fun. It means enjoying life all the more by being able to live it to the full through a more harmonious and integrated understanding of how the body-mind complex operates and through the ability to function optimally and feel healthy.

Clearly, it is not possible to eliminate pressures and stresses from life altogether – this is neither necessary nor desirable. Many people have highly active, busy, 'pressurised' lives and enjoy this enormously and thrive on it. With others, the slightest stress or pressure leads to physiological disturbance and physical dysfunctions.

So if different people are responding so differently to the same situations and stresses, what does this tell us about what is going on?

It is not the pressures themselves, but the *response* to the pressures which is most significant. So helping patients to find more effective ways of responding to pressure can be the most significant aspect of the therapeutic process.

How exactly you do that will vary from person to person; it is a very individual process, but it is all part of the process of effective cranio-sacral integration – seeing the cranio-sacal process in terms of treating, not merely a body with symptoms, but the whole person within the context of their life. A therapist with an appropriate understanding of the ANS will be better able to help a patient towards a clearer understanding of their health and the various factors affecting it and help them to discover what they want and how to get there.

Understanding the interaction between emotions and health is a key factor in maintaining health. The ANS gives us one of the most effective means of providing that understanding.

Physical causes of autonomic dysfunction

So far the emphasis has been primarily on stress and the psycho-emotional causes of autonomic disturbance. This is certainly a predominant factor. But as we have seen in previous chapters, the ANS can also be disturbed by factors that are more specifically physical (in so far as the two can be separated) – structural imbalances, vertebral restrictions, nerve impingement, neurological damage, physical injuries, visceral pathologies and infections.

Vertebral restrictions may impinge on the sympathetic nerves emanating from the spine, causing autonomic disturbance in the associated organ or area of the body, or agitation in the sympathetic plexi (with consequent emotional agitation) contributing to asthmatic conditions, menstrual disorders, agitation in the solar plexus, or persistent stimulation of the adrenal glands with consequent restlessness and hyperactivity – this could be the underlying factor in a hyperactive child, a delinquent teenager, a workaholic businessman, or an aggressive criminal.

Gastro-intestinal infections can be the source of persistent autonomic disturbance and could be the underlying explanation for inexplicable widespread symptoms – visceral, emotional and other – often dismissed as psychosomatic when no obvious explanation can be identified.

ANS dysfunction can very easily be attributed to psycho-emotional causes, sometimes inappropriately, so it is good to identify and eliminate any physical factors before attributing a patient's condition too readily to psycho-emotional factors. As always, physical and psycho-emotional cannot be separated – they invariably interact and one can't happen without the other – but an awareness of all the factors involved is helpful to the most effective therapeutic response.

Integration of ANS function

The vast majority of health issues involve autonomic disturbance. Addressing ANS dysfunction involves two main components:

- understanding the specific ANS associations involved in particular conditions
- recognising the fundamental need to bring the ANS as a whole into a more harmonious balanced state.

As always the first priority is overall integration – of the whole body, the body-mind, the whole person, the cranio-sacral system.

Whatever the condition, the first priority is integrated treatment:

- releasing the emotional centres of the heart centre and solar plexus with their important sympathetic plexi
- releasing the suboccipital area – so crucial to the superior cervical sympathetic ganglion, the sympathetic supply to the head and to the vagus nerve
- integrating the core
- bringing the whole system into balance and harmony.

Inevitably the overall effect of integration of the ANS and of the cranio-sacral system is in itself likely to bring profound effects of greater harmony and health to most patients – whatever their condition – from asthma to irritable bowel syndrome, palpitations to infertility.

Within the context of overall integration there are likely to be specific associations with specific areas and conditions, and an informed awareness of these relationships and associations will help to inform, guide and influence the therapeutic process, as shown in the following examples.

Autonomic associations

Cystitis

In many cases, cystitis is caused by an infectious organism. The infection is often recurrent but tests will sometimes reveal the absence of any infectious organism during these recurrent phases. The reasons for the recurrence and persistence of cystitis in the absence of any infectious organisms may lie in the setting up of a vicious cycle of activity within the autonomic nerve supply to the bladder and the other physical structures involved, such that, despite the lack of an infectious organism, the body continues to react as if there were a disturbance there.

Along with various other naturopathic means of treating the cystitis, and within the context of overall integrated treatment, it is helpful to maintain an awareness and understanding of how the autonomic nervous system may be contributing to and perpetuating the cycle of disturbance. This involves taking your attention to the following related structures, where you are likely to find evidence of disturbance – overstimulation, agitation, tension or restriction:

- *vertebral levels* T10 to L2 from where the sympathetic supply to the bladder emerges
- the pelvic *plexus* (inferior hypogastric plexus) where the sympathetic supply synapses
- *sacral* levels S2–4 from where the parasympathetic supply to the bladder emerges
- the penetration of these nerve pathways through the *dura*
- the *fascial* connections from the epineurium of the nerves to the surrounding fascia
- the *pathways* of the nerves
- the *organ* itself.

Ileo-caecal valve dysfunction

The ileo-caecal valve is the narrow junction between the ileum (the last section of the small intestine) and the caecum (the first portion of the large intestine) and is located in the lower abdomen on the right hand side. It is a common area of dysfunction, involving pain, tension, bloating and blockage of the digestive tract, potentially leading to appendicitis or other more serious conditions. Attempts to treat it are often merely local or through diet.

A common reason for these symptoms is excessive stimulation of the autonomic nervous system due to stress, and yet the autonomic involvement in the condition, even on a physiological level, is generally not taken into account and the psycho-emotional stresses and tensions are also not generally given attention. These emotional tensions are, of course, transmitted to the ileo-caecal valve through the autonomic nervous system.

As we have seen earlier, one of the functions of the sympathetic nervous system is to close down the digestive system ready for fight, flight or other action. One of the ways in which it does this is by contracting the sphincters. The ileo-caecal valve is one of these sphincters, so persistent stress leads to persistent contraction of the ileo-caecal valve with consequent dysfunction.

The sympathetic supply to the ileo-caecal valve arises from the spine at T10–12, synapsing in the solar plexus. The relevant connections to take into account are:

- the sympathetic supply, from vertebral levels around T10–12
- the solar plexus, involving the coeliac ganglia, the superior mesenteric plexus and the inferior mesenteric plexus through which the sympathetic nerves pass, and where the sympathetic neurons synapse on their pathway from the spinal column to the ileo-caecal valve
- the parasympathetic supply from the vagus nerve.

Emotional tensions are, of course, likely to affect the solar plexus and consequently create agitation of the sympathetic supply to the ileo-caecal valve. In any patient with an ileo-caecal disturbance, the solar plexus is likely to be a significant area to treat and any psycho-emotional factors contributing to that solar plexus stimulation will need to be identified and addressed in order to enhance the chances of a long-term resolution of the condition.

Irritable bowel syndrome

Irritable bowel syndrome (IBS), also known as spastic colon, has many similarities to ileo-caecal valve dysfunction and could be said to include ileo-caecal valve dysfunction. As its name suggests, the colon (or bowel) is in spasm or irritated due to excessive nerve stimulation. The nerve stimulation is autonomic nerve stimulation, and the reason for the excessive ANS stimulation may have physical causes but is most commonly due to stress.

Once again, although IBS is largely recognised as having a significant emotional component, the autonomic and emotional associations are rarely given sufficient attention; and once again, recognising and addressing the autonomic relations and associations can play a crucial part in resolving the situation.

One difference between ileo-caecal valve dysfunction and IBS is that ileo-caecal valve dysfunction is specifically on the right-hand side of the lower abdomen, whereas IBS may be in any part of the colon, and may often be found on the left-hand side of the lower abdomen. From the point of view of the sympathetic supply, this makes only a minor difference, extending the source of the nerve supply a little lower from T10–L2. However, from the point of view of parasympathetic supply, this makes a substantial difference, because the lower half of the colon on the left side of the abdomen receives its parasympathetic supply, not from the vagus, but from the sacrum. This distinction could be crucial, in that an ileo-caecal valve dysfunction might involve restriction to the vagus, particularly around the jugular foramen and suboccipital region (but would be unlikely to involve the sacrum), whereas the IBS on the left side might result from an injury to the sacrum – sitting down heavily, slipping on ice, horse-riding, or any other source of injury to the sacrum – presenting a very different picture and different requirements in terms of treatment. One might expect an experienced cranio-sacral therapist to identify the restriction wherever it might be – occiput or sacrum – but informed awareness is a powerful tool and enhances the therapist's effectiveness substantially.

Gastric and duodenal ulcers

The same principles can be applied to gastric and duodenal ulcers (notwithstanding the significance of helicobacter pylori and the very valuable benefits of appropriate treatment for any bacterial infection). The relevant autonomic associations here are:

- the sympathetic supply from vertebral levels T6 to T10
- the coeliac ganglia and solar plexus

- the parasympathetic supply from the vagus
- the likely involvement of psycho-emotional factors.

Similarly, the same principles can be applied to any condition, with an appropriate understanding of the autonomic relationships, thereby enhancing the therapeutic effectiveness through informed awareness and more comprehensive understanding.

Asthma

Asthma presents a prime example of a condition with a significant involvement of autonomic disturbance. Asthma may involve a combination of many different factors including allergies, immune system weakness, anxiety, lung dysfunctions and structural imbalances in the upper thoracic spine. The autonomic relationships are:

- the sympathetic supply to the lungs from vertebral levels T2 to T6
- the pulmonary plexus
- the parasympathetic supply from the vagus.

The emotional factors associated with asthma are often an important contributory factor to the autonomic disturbance, but are not generally given sufficient attention. Each case of asthma is individual, but certain typical features are often found:

- There may be an initial shock, perhaps in childhood, perhaps at birth, possibly involving difficulty breathing, such as falling into a pond, nearly drowning, loss of oxygen supply at birth, or prematurity. This might leave the body perpetually held in shock, with persistent consequences such as:
    - shallow breathing and holding of the breath
    - tension in the associated parts of the musculo-skeletal system around the upper thorax
    - tightness in the lungs.
- This may lead to:
    - a greater susceptibility and reactivity to allergens
    - a sensitised reactive facilitated emotional state, which is more readily aggravated and triggered by stress or anxiety
    - persistent anxiety – leading to holding the breath, holding the upper thorax in a constant state of contraction.

The solution in such cases is not to suppress the reaction with medication, but to release the underlying shock held in the system, thereby reducing the susceptibility and reactivity.

Patients with asthma almost invariably have a significant tightness and restriction in the upper thoracic spine around vertebral levels T2 to T6, reflecting the disturbance of autonomic nerve function.

Summary

In all these conditions, and all other such conditions, there is likely to be a complex interaction of many factors, involving:

- the viscera themselves
- the sensory nerve supply from the viscera
- the motor nerve supply to the viscera
- the associated vertebral levels and facilitated segments
- the nerve origins
- the dural associations
- the fascial connections
- the central nervous system connections
- psycho-emotional associations.

All of these can feed into each other creating cycles of physiological disturbance, and any combination of these can maintain or perpetuate the cycle.

All this information, whether regarding the ANS as a whole or regarding the specific conditions mentioned above, is not something to be used in isolation. It is all to be incorporated into the overall approach of cranio-sacral integration.

Within that context, specific awareness of ANS relationships will contribute to the understanding and effectiveness of the treatment – the very fact of your informed awareness will have an effect, by guiding your attention, consciously or unconsciously to relevant focal points; and the focus of your attention will influence the therapeutic process.

Unexpressed emotion

Emotion is clearly a major factor in creating disturbance in the ANS and consequent discomfort and disease in the body. This is not just a matter of pressure at work. Every emotion is affecting us – for better or for worse. Joy, love and happiness engender ease, fluency and harmony in the body and coherence in the cells and molecules and subatomic particles that make up our bodies. Emotional responses to work, play, relationships, life, current affairs, past events – recent or long gone, in adulthood or childhood, conscious or unconscious, are all affecting us all the time to a greater or lesser extent.

Everyone carries with them the emotional patterns and scars of the past – of childhood, of upbringing, of school, of relationships, of events and incidents throughout life. Much of this, particularly the unresolved difficult emotions, tends to be suppressed, forgotten (in so far as possible), hidden away under the surface where it may fester and lurk, creating underlying tensions and disruption. (It is of course the difficult emotions that tend to be suppressed; we don't generally feel any need to suppress happiness). Unexpressed emotion accumulating under the surface, whether it be bereavement or a broken relationship, anger, fear, sadness or any other emotional response, can play a significant part in causing autonomic dysfunction, including chemical changes, neurological changes, vascular changes and physical tensions – and therefore disease.

Human society does not on the whole cater adequately for the expression of these emotional responses. From an early age, habit patterns leading to autonomic disturbance can become deeply ingrained within the system – whether through emotional suppression, stressful lifestyle habits, work pressures or workaholism – leading to constant sympathetic stimulation, with the parasympathetic nervous system overworking in order to compensate for the excessive sympathetic stimulation, potentially leading to exhaustion of both divisions of the autonomic nervous system with all the consequent physical and physiological disturbances described previously and manifesting in a vast and varied array of different possible disturbances.

The results may be persistent ill-health, the gradual development of disease, or perhaps it may lead to the sudden breakdown of the system as a whole, with a wide variety of symptoms, as for instance in certain cases of ME (myalgic encephalomyelitis) or post-viral syndrome, and other such cases where the system under increasing pressure has eventually given way and broken down, perhaps in response to what seemed like a harmless viral infection.

Imagine a balloon, comfortably inflated to a standard sort of balloon pressure, contentedly living its life as a balloon. From time to time the pressure in the balloon might increase, and that's fine so long as the pressure is not excessive and the balloon is regularly deflated again back to its comfort zone. But if the pressure is increased excessively then the balloon will burst – and after that there is no going back. That balloon's ANS (if it had one) would have been excessively overstimulated.

Many people allow the pressure in their lives to accumulate excessively until eventually a point is reached when the system bursts or breaks down; and after that it is not easy to return to a balanced, manageable state. It needs time and careful reintegration.

Psychosomatics

The term psychosomatic sometimes seems to be used to mean:

- that the condition doesn't really exist
- that it's your fault, and you just need to pull yourself together
- that there's nothing to be done about it.

This is not generally helpful.

Medication may help to balance the chemical changes in the body, and in some cases may be helpful and very relevant, but on the whole it is not addressing the source of the problem.

Even when the psycho-emotional component is acknowledged and the patient is referred for psychotherapy, this may not be sufficient if it is only addressing the mind, not taking into account the ANS and the inextricable interaction between mind and body.

Through a more comprehensive understanding of the ANS, and of the inevitable interactions between body and mind, and through a comprehensive perspective on the cranio-sacral system – the whole person within the context of their environment – the cranio-sacral therapist can gain a clearer impression of the whole picture, so that they can not only relieve the physical and physiological patterns of discomfort and disturbance, but also help the patient towards a lasting resolution.

They can do this by:

- helping the patient towards a better understanding of their situation through which they can develop a more harmonious and coherent interaction with their environment
- integrating the whole system, the whole body-mind, the whole matrix, through cranio-sacral integration.

Part VIII
Further Contacts and Concepts

Chapter 53

The Throat

When would you treat the throat?

You might not treat the throat in every patient, but when it is relevant it can be crucial. It can be a site of severe trauma such as strangulation – whether accidental or deliberate – and the life-threatening sensations of strangulation can be deeply traumatising. Even without such specific severe trauma, it is a very common area for holding emotional tensions (it is another 'emotional centre') and both physical and emotional tensions in the throat can be very significant because of the many life-supporting structures passing through this area, enabling such essential functions as breathing, swallowing and blood supply to the brain, along with other significant structures such as the thyroid gland and the vagus nerve.

So you might treat the throat:

- for specific *local conditions* such as recurrent tonsillitis
- for *emotional tensions*
- for *systemic conditions* with a local focus such as a thyroid disorder
- for a specific life-affecting *trauma* to the throat
- because you are drawn there in the course of the cranio-sacral process
- because it is a significant factor in the overall integration of the person.

Local conditions

Local conditions involving the throat include loss of voice, difficulty swallowing, sore throat, tonsillitis, laryngitis, pharyngitis, ear infections (due to the drainage of the ear via the Eustachian tubes to the naso-pharynx), salivary gland disorders, lumps in the throat. Many of these may be transient, but if they persist or are recurrent, then further investigation and specific cranio-sacral treatment of the throat may be appropriate.

INFECTION

There may be an infectious organism involved and some patients, accustomed to the widespread prescription of antibiotics, might question how cranio-sacral therapy could counteract an infection. Along with this, one might also ask why some people are more susceptible to infection than others? Why do some people suffer from recurrent tonsillitis while others never get a sore throat?

INHERENT DEFENCES

The body has the inherent means to deal with infections; it has an immune system, mediated primarily through the vascular system and lymphatic system and through various communication systems such as the nervous system. If these are all functioning effectively, then the body should be able to deal with infectious organisms. When these systems are compromised, then the body may not be able to cope and infection can take hold and persist or recur. So the role of cranio-sacral integration in such situations is, as always, to enhance the body's natural resources by ensuring the free mobility and function of all these structures and the free flow of the vascular system and lymphatic systems.

DEPLETION

Why might the body's protective mechanisms not be working effectively? It could be because of physical blockages and restrictions to the blood supply, nerve supply and fluid pathways, perhaps arising from injuries to the neck and throat or postural tension, leading to contraction and compression of the area. It may also be due to emotional tensions held in the throat and neck, leading to muscular and soft tissue tensions causing tightness, blockage and congestion and consequent restriction to the flow of fluids and underlying vitality necessary to combat infection and maintain health. Whether the apparent cause is physical injury or emotional tension, appropriate cranio-sacral treatment to restore mobility and freely flowing function to the throat can help to resolve such conditions.

Angela came to me at the age of 25, having suffered recurrent tonsillitis since the age of nine, with several episodes each year since her early teens, developing into an almost continuous condition by this time. She was taking several courses of antibiotics each year, which brought temporary relief but each time the condition would recur within days. This continued year after year.

I treated her once, identifying a substantial degree of tension and restriction in her throat and neck. The antibiotics were clearly never going to address these restrictions – and yet these restrictions were the reason for her persistent susceptibility to recurrent infection and the essential factor that needed to be addressed. The tensions and restriction were cleared readily in that one treatment. Her tonsillitis disappeared immediately and she suffered no further episodes after that.

Emotional tensions

The throat is one of the principal areas through which we express ourselves – expressing our views, thoughts, beliefs and feelings in speech and sound – talking, shouting, screaming, shrieking, laughing, growling; words, feelings, noises, passion; fear, anger, frustration, joy, or love.

Suppression of expression – holding things in, holding yourself back when you want to say something or express your feelings – may therefore lead to constriction and restriction in the throat. And if this is a lifelong habit, then it may create a persistent pattern of tightness in the throat. Once again, this tightness can constrict the many vital structures passing through the throat – making it difficult to swallow or breathe – and restricting the vital resources necessary for the body's natural healthy function. Consequently, dysfunction and disease affecting the throat, transient or persistent, a minor illness or a severe pathology – whether it be recurrent tonsillitis, loss of voice, thyroid conditions, or tumours – may at least in part reflect suppressed expression or emotional tensions. Physical and emotional factors are inevitably inextricably intertwined, whether as cause or as reaction or both.

Systemic conditions with a local focus – the thyroid

Thyroid conditions are common, variable, potentially far-reaching and complex. A significant proportion of the population are under medication for thyroid conditions, often managing the condition very effectively with lifelong medication. But do they need to be on lifelong medication? The degree to which cranio-sacral treatment can affect thyroid conditions varies according to the underlying cause. There are those for whom the thyroid condition resolves completely and readily in response to cranio-sacral treatment; there are others for whom there is gradual and partial improvement; and there are those for whom medical treatment is the appropriate approach.

SHOCK

Many thyroid conditions arise following a significant shock (an accident or a bereavement) or a period of prolonged stress (final exams, break up of a relationship). In these circumstances the patient will generally respond very well to appropriate cranio-sacral treatment in which the shock effects are addressed, and the thyroid condition may resolve completely. If the start of a thyroid disturbance coincides with a significant physical or emotional event or period of stress, then it may be helpful to explore treatment through cranio-sacral integration rather than through immediate medication, allowing time for the disturbance to respond to the cranio-sacral process before becoming involved in the potentially disruptive vicious circle of medication.

As always, treatment involves addressing the whole person. Specific attention to the thyroid gland may not even be necessary – since the cause of the condition is in the shock, the matrix, the whole body-mind complex – but since the shock may at least partly be held in the throat, working on the throat may prove helpful to the release of any local effects of shock and tension, and to the enhanced flow of arterial, venous, lymphatic and neurological supply to the area; and specific attention to the thyroid gland along with its blood supply and nerve supply may be appropriate and beneficial.

There is an interesting question regarding thyroid conditions. They are common and are readily diagnosed through a blood test, yet a substantial number of thyroid conditions are misdiagnosed. Not only are many cases of thyroid disorder not recognised or identified, but also a surprising number of patients are diagnosed with thyroid conditions which they don't actually have.

Because thyroid dysfunction is so common, some further detail is included in Box 53.1 below.

Box 53.1 Thyroid dysfunction

Function
The principal function of the thyroid gland is the regulation of basal metabolic rate – maintaining our metabolism, keeping the body ticking over at the appropriate rate.

Action
The thyroid gland produces thyroxine (a hormone rich in iodine) also known as T4 (tetra iodo thyronine). T4 is de-iodised in the body's cells to form T3 (tri iodo thyronine), which produces the required physiological action.

Regulation
The thyroid gland is regulated by thyroid stimulating hormone (TSH) secreted by the anterior pituitary gland. (Any test for thyroid function therefore needs to include an assessment of TSH levels and the effective function of the pituitary gland.)

Dysfunctions
Dysfunctions of the thyroid gland can be broadly divided into two main categories:
- *hypothyroidism* – in which there is a deficiency of thyroid secretion
- *hyperthyroidism* – in which there is an excessive thyroid secretion.

HYPOTHYROIDISM
In hypothyroidism, the deficiency of thyroid secretion results in a decreased basal metabolic rate. This may or may not be accompanied by an enlargement of the thyroid gland (goitre).

Symptoms include increased weight, obesity, bowel changes (constipation or diarrhoea), dry coarse skin and hair (myxoedema), low blood pressure, a slow pulse, coldness, lethargy, decreased muscular activity and sluggishness of all functions. If the deficiency arises in childhood, it may lead to cretinism (failure to grow).

Medical treatment involves increasing iodine in the diet (if this is deficient), or replacement therapy with natural or synthetic thyroid hormone. With replacement therapy it is important to look out for signs of excessive thyroid activity (due to excessive dosage).

HYPERTHYROIDISM
In hyperthyroidism the excessive secretion of thyroid hormone leads to an increased basal metabolic rate.

The cause is unknown, but the condition is markedly more common in females than in males in a proportion of eight to one. There may be a constitutional predisposition and the condition is more prevalent in areas of low iodine. It can also be triggered or aggravated by shock, fear, fright, anxiety or stress and also by infectious diseases. It is more commonly, although not necessarily, associated with enlargement of the gland (goitre).

Symptoms include weight loss, altered bowel activity (vomiting and diarrhoea), nervousness, restlessness, irritability, a fine tremor, particularly in the fingers and hands, skin eruptions, heat, sweating, heat intolerance and an increased heart rate (tachycardia) with palpitation.

Hyperthyroidism may lead to an exophthalmic goitre (thyrotoxicosis, Graves disease).

Medical treatment involves anti-thyroid medication, or if this not sufficiently effective, surgery to remove up to seven-eighths of the gland.

GOITRE

Goitre is the term for any enlargement of the thyroid gland.

Causes include iodine deficiency, thyroiditis, inflammation due to infection, tumours, hyperthyroidism and hypothyroidism. (The thyroid gland is slightly larger in females than in males and may also enlarge slightly at the time of menstruation or during pregnancy.)

The goitre generally starts off as a soft enlargement, but may eventually develop cysts, nodules, deposits and hardness.

Simple goitre involves an enlargement of the gland with no disturbance of function (although gross enlargement may eventually lead to pressure on the trachea and may effect breathing and swallowing). Treatment involves increasing iodine intake.

Exophthalmic goitre involves an enlargement of the thyroid gland accompanied by disturbances of function as described under hyperthyroidism, with the development of bulging eyeballs, due to the deposit of fatty tissue behind the eyeball.

As mentioned above, thyroid dysfunctions are often initiated by shock or stressful events – and yet these are not generally given much consideration in conventional medical treatment. Addressing the shock or underlying stress can often eliminate the thyroid condition. This is something which is of course achieved, not simply through throat contacts, but through the total process of cranio-sacral integration.

Trauma to the throat

There are two particular forms of trauma to the throat which are both common and potentially severely life-disrupting.

Some people feel vulnerable, delicate or exceedingly sensitive around the throat, or apprehensive of any contact on the throat. Even the touch of a scarf can be too much for them, and they certainly don't want anyone touching their throat. This can be disruptive to intimate relationships and can be very disturbing, especially if no explanation can be identified. Sometimes it can be traced to a specific event, a known injury or incident. Sometimes it may be due to the chronic accumulation of suppressed expression.

UMBILICAL CORD

But often there is no obvious reason and in such cases the cause may lie in a rarely considered and generally neglected factor – the wrapping of the umbilical cord around the neck at birth, creating a deep-rooted but unconscious history of trauma and strangulation and consequent feelings of vulnerability in this area, as well as potential repercussions on the whole personality and nature of the patient.

When the umbilical cord is wound round the neck at birth, the cord will steadily tighten as the baby progresses down the birth canal, potentially strangling the baby. The baby's head needs to be delivered before the midwife can reach the cord in order to cut it, but for the baby's head to progress sufficiently far down the birth canal may involve excessive tightening of the cord around the neck. This requires prompt and exact timing on the part of the midwife to ensure that the cord is cut just at the right moment – gaining access to the cord as early as possible in order to allow the birth of the child without strangulation, while not cutting the cord so early that the baby is not yet able to breathe for itself. While this is quite a common situation, it is nevertheless delicate and potentially traumatic. The subconscious memory of this perhaps near-death experience at birth can be deeply embedded in the psyche, and retained, not only in the unconscious memory, but also in the tissues as tissue memory.

Trauma to the throat may arise from various other causes including wounds and accidental injuries, perhaps in childhood, perhaps in adulthood, perhaps in sport, perhaps during play, perhaps remembered, perhaps not remembered, which may lead to lifelong patterns of discomfort and reaction – difficult to cope with, but difficult to shake off. But there is one other type of trauma to the throat which requires particular attention and understanding.

STRANGULATION

Of particular significance is the severe trauma of strangulation, sometimes accidental, but most significantly in association with an attack or rape. This may lead to severe traumatic repercussions throughout the system, physically and emotionally. Working with severely traumatised patients, such as rape victims, is a profound, delicate, sensitive and complex process, requiring specific understanding for handling trauma. It is not something to be entered into lightly. We will look at this in more detail shortly, and in greater depth in a later volume.

In treating such situations, there is clearly much more to consider than just the throat, but for the moment let us consider the aspects which involve the throat. First, the patient may or may not tell you about the rape or the strangulation, so you may be picking up impressions from the cranio-sacral system without that verbalised information – impressions of shock, of trauma, and perhaps specific impressions around the throat. The patient may refuse to allow any contact on the throat, or even near the throat – which will of course always be respected, and which may also bring the story to light. Consequently, the whole approach to the throat and to the treatment as a whole will be determined by these circumstances, and will need to be approached with great care and sensitivity. Clearly the contacts for the throat described below would not simply be applied as a matter of course, just because there was a focus of trauma in the throat. The whole approach to the throat would be adapted accordingly, to take account of the severe repercussions of the trauma and the sensitivity of the patient's overall condition; and yet working with the throat, and the sensations and fears that they experience in association with their throat, exploring the reactions and repercussions and how to address them and resolve them – within a safe secure and supportive environment and at an appropriate point in the long term treatment process – may be a crucial and highly beneficial part of the therapeutic process of addressing the overall trauma for that patient.

The throat is clearly a very significant area, particularly for certain individuals. So we need to understand its structure, its associations, and how to treat it effectively.

Bone and cartilage

The throat contains three principal solid structures (see Figure 53.1):
- The *hyoid bone*.
- The *thyroid cartilage*.
- The *cricoid cartilage*.

The hyoid bone

The hyoid bone is a roughly horseshoe shaped bone, with its main body anteriorly, two greater cornua (large horns) projecting from the body posteriorly on each side of the throat (forming the horseshoe), and two lesser cornua (small horns) projecting superiorly from the junction between the body and the greater horns.

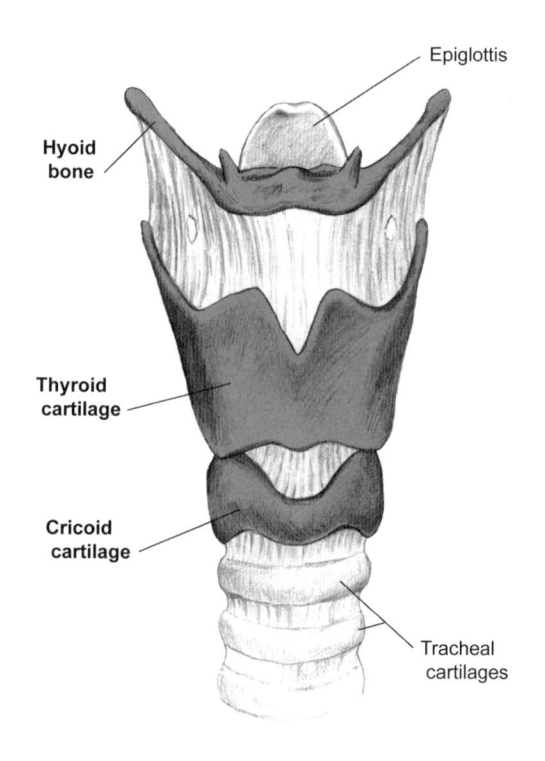

53.1 The throat contains three principal solid structures – the hyoid bone, the thyroid cartilage, the cricoid cartilage

It is unique in that it is the only bone that makes no direct articulations with any other bone in the body. It is tucked high up under the mandible, suspended by ligaments and between two groups of muscles – a suprahyoid group (above the hyoid) and an infrahyoid group (below the hyoid).

The two ends of the body of the hyoid bone can be palpated between finger and thumb, high in the upper throat. They can be distinguished from other lumps or protrusions in the throat by shifting the hyoid from side to side.

The thyroid cartilage

The thyroid cartilage, or laryngeal cartilage is the most prominent solid structure within the throat.

It is below the hyoid bone and is easily palpated, both anteriorly and laterally, but should be contacted gently and carefully to avoid discomfort and possible loss of voice, since it houses and protects the larynx or voice box.

It is also known as the Adam's apple and is significantly more prominent in men than in women.

The cricoid cartilage

The cricoid cartilage is situated below the thyroid cartilage and is the first and largest of the horseshoe-shaped cartilaginous rings which envelop the trachea, thereby maintaining an open airway. It can be palpated below the thyroid cartilage as a thin ridge of cartilage.

Below the cricoid cartilage are the remaining tracheal cartilages protecting the trachea, numbering twelve in total, of which the upper six are generally palpable above the manubrium.

Muscles

The *extrinsic muscles* of the throat can be divided into two main groups – supra-hyoid and infra-hyoid (see Figure 53.2):

- The *supra-hyoid muscles* attach from the hyoid bone up to the mandible and temporal bones.
- The *infra-hyoid muscles* attach from the hyoid bone down to the thyroid cartilage and the

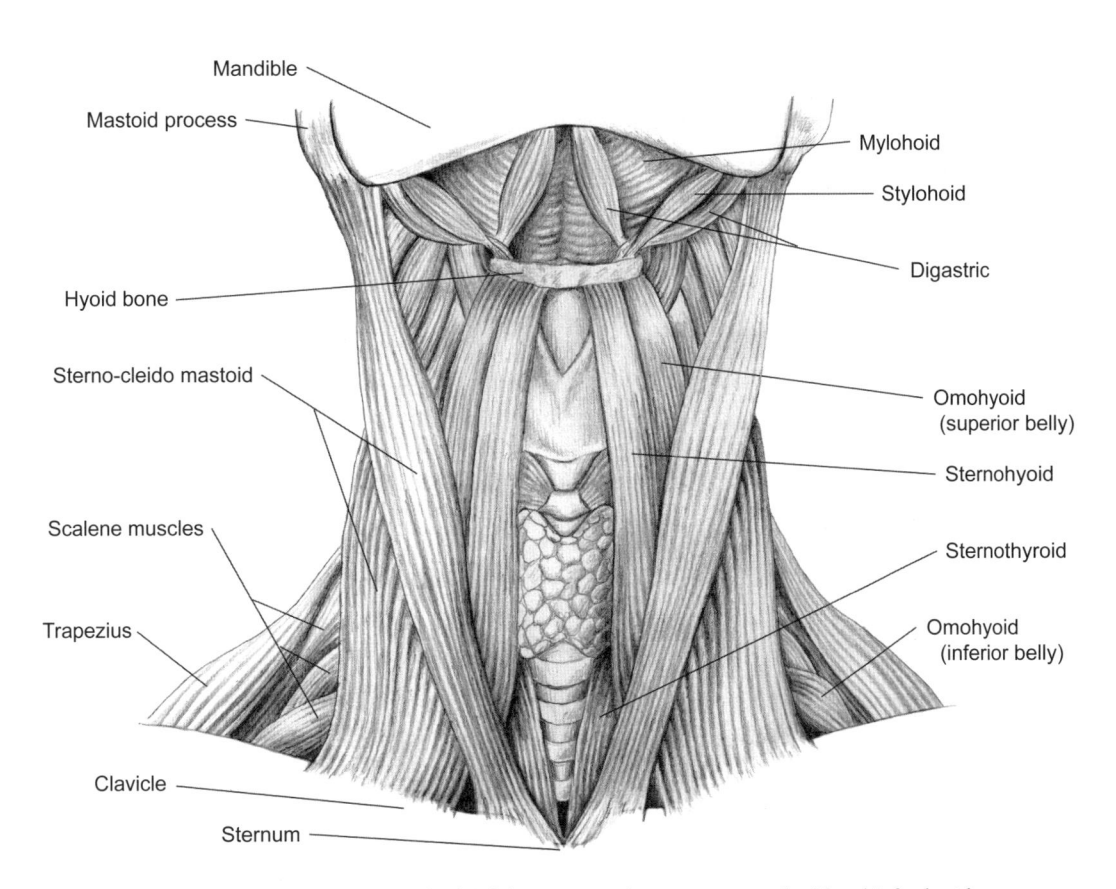

53.2 The extrinsic muscles of the throat can be divided into two main groups – supra-hyoid and infra-hyoid

sternum, with one curious diversion of the omohyoid muscle passing back to attach on to the superior border of the scapula – an interesting connection between throat and shoulder blade.

An association was drawn previously between the temporal bones and emotions, and it is relevant to note the association here between various structures, all particularly associated with emotions – the temporals, the throat, and the mandible (as often seen in jaw clenching and teeth grinding).

The *intrinsic muscles* consist of other, smaller muscles within the throat, which are involved in swallowing.

When working at the throat, certain *other prominent muscles* are likely to come to your attention, since they form a muscular frame around the throat area, and they may well be involved in conditions affecting the throat. These include:

- The *sterno-cleido-mastoid*, passing from the *sternum* and medial end of the *clavicle* to the *mastoid process of the temporal bone*.
- The *scalene muscles*, a group of three muscles (anterior, middle and posterior scalenes) on each side of the neck, passing from the lateral surface of the *cervical vertebrae* down to the *first rib*.

Nerve supply

Restrictions, tensions and dysfunctions of the throat may arise from impingement of the nerves supplying the various structures of the throat. Understanding the origins and pathways of these nerves may be significant in addressing these dysfunctions.

Supra-hyoid muscles	Cranial nerves V, VII and XII
Infra-hyoid muscles	Cervical plexus (C1–C4) and cranial nerve XII
Muscles of pharynx and larynx (swallowing)	Cranial nerves IX and X
Sterno-cleido-mastoid	Cranial nerve XI and C2
Scalene muscles	Cervical nerves C3–6
Thyroid gland	Sympathetic supply from T1–3, parasympathetic supply from laryngeal branches of vagus
Parotid glands	Cranial nerve IX – parasympathetic branch

Glands

Lymph glands

There is a substantial number of lymph glands in the throat and these may become enlarged and palpable as a result of infection in the area. Chronic infectious conditions such as glandular fever (mononucleosis) may result in permanently enlarged lymph glands.

Exocrine glands

The *parotid glands* (salivary glands) are large, soft glands located around the angle of the jaw and may be enlarged in cases of mumps. They receive nerve supply from the *parasympathetic branch* of cranial nerve IX.

The *submandibular glands* (salivary glands) are located under the inner surface of the mandible. They receive nerve supply from the *parasympathetic branch* of cranial nerve VII.

These glands are not generally palpable, due to their soft squashy nature. Dysfunctions of salivary gland secretion may benefit from cranio-sacral treatment to the gland itself (following appropriate investigations and taking into account any inflammatory condition), or to its nerve supply or blood supply, or to the surrounding area – always within the context of a broad understanding of the whole person.

Endocrine glands

The thyroid gland consists of two lobes, one on each side and slightly below the thyroid cartilage (roughly level with the cricoid cartilage) (see Figure 53.3), connected via an isthmus, running anteriorly below the level of the cricoid cartilage. The gland is generally soft and not palpable, except in thyroid disease, which may lead to a *goitre* (enlargement of the thyroid gland).

The parathyroid glands consist of four tiny glands located on the posterior surface of the thyroid lobes. They are not palpable.

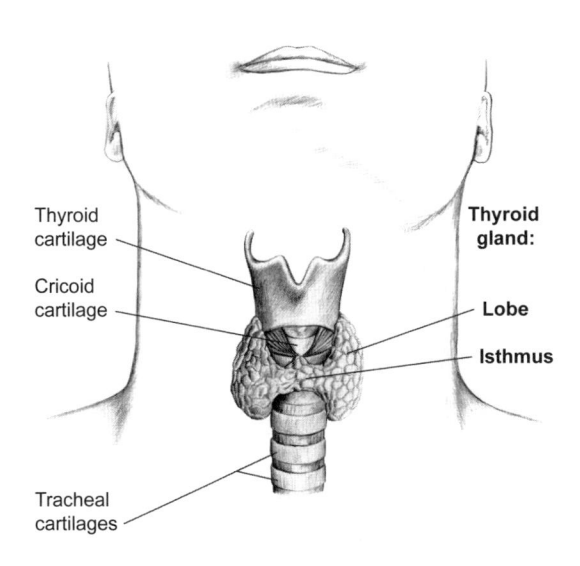

53.3 The thyroid gland consists of two lobes, one on each side, connected via an isthmus, approximately level with the cricoid cartilage

Lumps in the throat

Lumps in the throat of one kind or another are common. They are mostly harmless but they are a common cause of concern, raising the spectre of cancer of the throat – unidentified lumps always need to be investigated. It is helpful to be able to differentiate the various causes of such lumps in order to distinguish between those which are harmless and those which might require urgent attention. Some possible causes include:

- The two ends of the *hyoid bone* may protrude unevenly to one side more than the other, if the hyoid is unbalanced.
- *Lymph glands* may be transiently enlarged in an acute infection or in a transient allergic reaction (such as hay fever), or may be chronically enlarged from a past condition (such as glandular fever).

- A *bee sting* may lead to swelling of the throat, potentially leading to asphyxiation and death. As the throat swells over a period of several minutes, urgent medical attention should be sought if the bee sting is inside the throat.
- *Allergic reactions* of various kinds may lead to swelling in the throat and potential respiratory problems. Medical attention may be necessary if severe.
- *Goitre*, an enlargement of the thyroid gland.
- An *obstruction* in the throat, such as a fish bone, or a piece of nut shell, is perhaps more likely to be felt internally than palpated externally.
- *Tumours* can occur in various structures of the throat. Any concerns regarding an undiagnosed lump in the throat should be referred for medical investigation.
- *Globus hystericus* is one of the most common causes of an apparent lump in the throat in which, as the name suggests, the sensation of a lump is very real for the patient, but no lump is actually present. In any situation where a lump or apparent lump is perceived within the throat, medical investigation should be carried out – never be too ready to dismiss it as psychosomatic. However, if the sensation of a lump persists and medical investigations have been checked and double-checked without revealing any physical cause, then a psycho-emotional cause may be the likely diagnosis, and an appropriate whole person integrated cranio-sacral approach may be the most effective way to help the patient and address the condition. Some patients with *globus hystericus* will have been dismissed summararily by their doctors, and been told that there is nothing wrong with them. Some will have gone repeatedly for medical tests, plagued by persistent fears of cancer of the throat. An informed cranio-sacral therapist can be very effective in bringing both relief of the physical symptoms and release of the underlying emotional tension or trauma that may be at the root of the condition.

Practical approach to the throat
Integrated context
Any contact on the throat will, as always, be taken up within the context of an overall integrated treatment. A comprehensive understanding of the patient as a whole will have been reached, assessing the whole picture, settling, grounding and opening up the system, engaging with the core in whatever way is appropriate. Various areas specifically relevant to the throat may have been addressed as necessary – in particular perhaps the heart centre, the solar plexus, the neck, the suboccipital region and areas relevant to nerve supply and blood supply – in order to pave the way and prepare the ground for more effective work on the throat.

Apprehension
Since the throat is a sensitive and vulnerable area, an area around which many people may feel some concern about being touched, it is always best to talk about this with the patient before taking up contact, asking how they feel about having a contact on the throat. It is also helpful to remind them, and to keep reminding them, that they can always let you know if they feel any discomfort (physical or emotional) or if they would like you to remove your hand or lighten your touch.

Having said that, you don't want to create a climate of fear and apprehension. For most people the throat contact is perfectly comfortable. In fact many patients are pleasantly surprised at how much they enjoy throat work, finding it very comfortable and soothing – not only when a very light cranio-sacral contact is used, but perhaps even more so through gentle soft-tissue work and massage on the throat which can be very pleasant and very therapeutic, releasing superficial tensions and paving the way for a more profound response from the cranio-sacral work.

A gradual process
However, for any patient who has had severe trauma to the throat such as strangulation, or who for any reason feels apprehensive about a contact on the throat, a different preliminary approach is necessary – a gradual process of exploration and dialogue, exploring the patient's feelings, sensations and responses to a contact on the throat, or even the thought of a contact on the throat – all the time establishing and maintaining grounding. It will almost certainly be preferable to start with contacts away from the throat, gradually introducing contacts closer to the throat once the patient feels comfortable with that, all the time maintaining dialogue and communication, allowing the patient to express their feelings, responses and fears. In this way, it is possible gradually to address the throat, and their apprehension regarding their throat, and in due course – sometimes in a matter of minutes, sometimes over several sessions – move gently towards a subtle throat contact and eventually to the release of all fears and apprehension regarding the throat and the release of all trauma associated with the throat or with any traumatic incident that they may have experienced, often bringing a great sense of relief and freedom from long-standing suffering.

Having established whether it is appropriate to contact the throat, the following contacts can be used for addressing specific patterns within the throat.

Specific throat contacts
1. Throat contact – from the side
Sitting at the side of the throat and neck – level with the shoulder – place one hand (the hand nearest the patient's head) under the patient's neck, cradling the neck comfortably (see Figure 53.6).

Connect with and address patterns of restriction in the neck, cervical spine, musculature, and fascia, with an awareness of the nerve supply to the throat – the cervical plexus, the ansa cervicalis, and the relevant cranial nerves.

Allow your other hand to come in gently through the energy field to settle onto the front of the throat. The throat is a delicate and sensitive area; take care not to throttle your patient (!) nor to restrict, constrict or compress the throat; take care not to rest too heavily onto the front of the throat. In particular, take care not to rest on the thyroid cartilage at the front of the throat. However, a soft contact fully enveloping the throat can provide a very comforting and

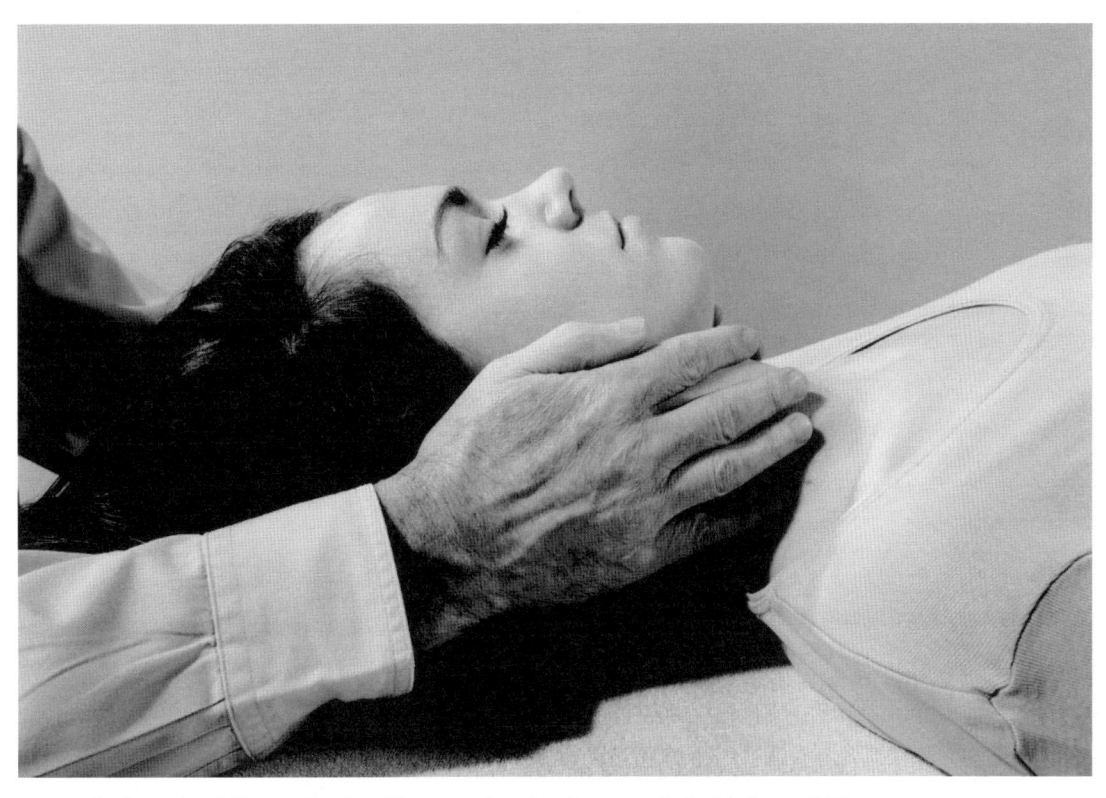

53.4 The throat is a delicate and vulnerable area and needs to be approached with due sensitivity

reassuring connection, even for patients who initially feel concerned about being contacted at the throat – whereas a tentative apprehensive contact, overconcerned about touching this delicate area can feel uncomfortable, uncertain, or ineffective.

LEVELS OF CONTACT

Be prepared to experiment with and to explore different degrees of comfort with various levels of contact; check with your patient which levels of contact feel most comfortable. Experience these contacts on yourself in order to identify and reassure yourself as to which contacts are most comfortable. A closer, firmer contact can be very effective in connecting with levels different from those involved in a light off-the-body contact and may be more effective in addressing various patterns of imbalance and restriction within the fascia, the musculature, and the throat structures as a whole, and in connecting with pulls throughout the body, above and below.

Keep checking that your patient is comfortable with the contact, particularly if you feel concerned that you may be imposing too much pressure on the throat, or if you notice any reaction in the patient. Check with them from time to time throughout the treatment.

It is of course possible to work off the body, with a very light, or off-the-body contact. This may be absolutely appropriate at times – if that is what the body demands. But if this is your only way of working with the throat, it may limit the range of levels on which you connect with the system. Be prepared to explore a more physical 'fascial unwinding' level of contact. The more physical levels of contact can be instrumental in helping the patient to connect with and release past trauma. You – and your patient – may also be surprised by how comfortable and comforting it can feel.

It is preferable to maintain a range of options at all times, in order to be able to respond appropriately to the body's needs with different levels of touch. It is not helpful to project any apprehension into the throat through an over-

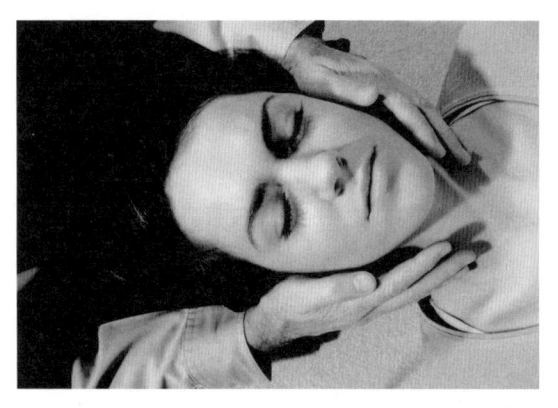

53.5 Take up contact with the pads of your index, middle and ring fingers resting lightly on the sides of the throat, close to but not touching the thyroid cartilage

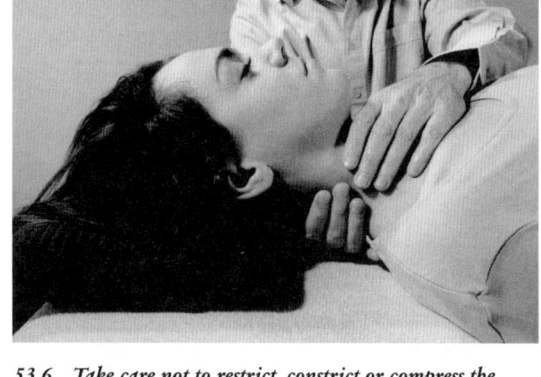

53.6 Take care not to restrict, constrict or compress the throat, or to rest too heavily onto the front of the throat

cautious contact. The appropriate level of contact needs to be established by the needs of the patient, rather than by the therapist's own apprehension about contacting the throat, or over-concern about being too firm, or by the therapist's limited range of contacts.

Having established an appropriate contact, it is helpful to start with some gentle soft tissue work, lightly but comprehensively massaging the whole throat area. You can then settle into stillness and allow the evolution of the inherent treatment process.

- Feel the increasing sense of engagement with the system – with both hands.
- Assess the quality, symmetry and motion in the throat and in the neck, front and back, left and right.
- Allow the system to express itself, leading to points of stillness and release.
- Maintain awareness, not only of the throat and neck, but also of patterns connecting to other parts of the body, and of the whole picture.
- Be aware, not only of physical pulls, but also of the significance, associations and interpretation of whatever you feel.
- Be open to adjusting your contact as necessary.
- Follow the process through to an increasing stillness and settledness, allowing the continuing subtle integration of the system.
- Take care to release your contact gently.

2. Throat contact – from the head

Sitting at the head, take up contact with the pads of your index, middle and ring fingers resting lightly on the sides of the throat, close to but not touching the thyroid cartilage (see Figures 54.3 and 54.5). The index fingers should be roughly level with the hyoid bone; the middle fingers roughly level with the thyroid cartilage; and the ring fingers roughly level with the cricoid cartilage.

Place your fingers far enough down to connect with the whole throat and place the pads of the fingers well round towards the front of the throat – but take care not to rest on the thyroid cartilage. Check with your patient that they are comfortable with this contact.

- Feel the increasing sense of engagement with the system.
- Allow the system to express itself and allow the evolution of the inherent treatment process.
- Allow your fingers and hands to float freely with the movements, following the fluidity of movement.

It may be appropriate simply to stay there with the system, allowing tensions and traumas to emerge, dissolve and release. Notice how the throat tissues may spontaneously lead you into patterns of side-shift, side-bending, rotation or complex combinations of all of these.

ENHANCING

If the throat is tightly held and unable to express itself freely, it might benefit from a gentle invitation or some encouragement, helping the system to uncover and initiate the release of hidden patterns (as with the spheno-basilar patterns). You could ask the throat if it would like to side-shift to the right or left, to rotate posteriorly to the right or left, side-bend inferiorly on the right or left – not imposing any physical force on the body, simply asking questions, offering options. If it takes up the option, let it lead you on a journey of exploration and discovery involving a complex mixture of twists turns and bends – from time to time reaching points of stillness, staying there for a while, eventually softening, releasing and returning to neutral. This may be unnecessary if the throat is already expressing itself freely.

As with the previous contact:

- Maintain awareness of the whole throat and of the whole body and of any associations, interpretations or emotional implications.
- Follow the process through to an increasing stillness and settledness, allowing the continuing subtle integration of the system.
- Take care to release your contact gently.

Following the completion of any treatment through the throat, carry on through the rest of your integrated treatment process as appropriate within the context of the whole person, integrating the rest of the system around any changes that have occurred in the throat, in order to bring the process to completion.

Addressing trauma

Addressing trauma is a huge subject and will be the subject of a whole volume later. It can't be addressed adequately within this context, but we can at least touch on the subject and establish a few basic guidelines. An appropriate approach to severe trauma is essential in any severely traumatised patient, whatever part of the body you may be working on, but it is particularly relevant to discuss the subject as we work with a sensitive area such as the throat – in order primarily to emphasise that it is not appropriate simply to proceed directly to treatment of the throat in such situations.

In patients who have experienced severe trauma associated with the throat, for example accidental strangulation, strangulation during rape, or similar experiences, the throat may remain a very sensitive and vulnerable area. Even if they have discomfort or other symptoms in the throat, it is clearly not generally a good idea to take up any direct contact on the throat. Probably, the last thing they want is anyone touching their throat. It may bring up vivid and traumatic memories of being attacked. In such circumstances, it is particularly vital to address the whole picture, the whole trauma – and addressing severe trauma is a process that requires specific awareness and understanding.

Brief guidelines for addressing trauma

- The first priority is for *the therapist to be suitably grounded*, centred, and balanced and to have the awareness, understanding and resources to respond appropriately to a severely traumatised patient.
- The next step is to establish *appropriate resources in the patient*:
  - resources of grounding and centering – creating an ability to respond positively and therapeutically to their situation and to the memories, sensations or emotions that may arise during the therapeutic process
  - resources of understanding the therapeutic process, and the nature of trauma release
  - resources of support that they may need in everyday life – friends, family, counsellors.
- Establish an appropriately *safe, secure and supportive environment* in which to address trauma.
- Establish the *understanding* that it is possible for them to move forward from their trauma and their traumatised state.
- Proceed *only at a pace for which the patient is ready*.
- The *initial stages* are likely to be concerned with coming to terms with the trauma, rather than addressing any specific areas (such as the throat).

- Maintain *constant communication* with your patient – open, clear, free and unrestricted – monitoring their response from moment to moment, maintaining their grounding and stability.
- Ensure *adequate grounding after each session*, in order to ensure that the patient is ready and able to go out into the world.
- Ensure *adequate support between sessions*, whether through your own availability at all times, or through other supportive contacts.

Retraumatisation

Some therapists are very concerned about 'retraumatisation', in which the emergence of suppressed trauma, instead of just arising, releasing and passing away, can result in further trauma and upset to the patient as they remember or re-experience previous trauma. Retraumatisation can be a possibility, but this possibility can be minimised by creating a safe, confident, reassuring environment in which the patient and the therapist are well-grounded, and in which the patient can feel secure and well-supported with a clear understanding of the nature of the therapeutic process.

Retraumatisation is more likely when the *therapist* is overly concerned and excessively anxious and puts too much emphasis on the risks of retraumatisation, thereby creating anxiety and fear in the patient. It is unlikely to arise when the therapist is well-grounded and has a good understanding of how to address trauma and is therefore able to provide an appropriate, reassuring environment for the patient.

Addressing throat trauma specifically

As has been made clear above, in a severely traumatised patient who has suffered strangulation or trauma to the throat, the emphasis of the treatment initially would be entirely on addressing the overall effects of shock in the system as a whole, and it would not be appropriate to take up specific contact on the throat. However, since this chapter is on the throat, let us jump ahead to the stage of treatment where the initial phases of coming to terms with and addressing the trauma have progressed well and the patient is ready to move forward further.

In order for them to release the effects of trauma from the throat and to relieve symptoms of discomfort, tightness, pain and restriction, along with their emotional associations, it may be very helpful to introduce specific contacts on the throat – but only when appropriate.

- This might start by *simply talking about the throat*, observing, exploring and addressing the sensations, feelings and reactions that arise in response to this.
- This could progress in due course to *talking about taking up contact on the throat*, observing, exploring and addressing the sensations, feelings and reactions that arise in response to this.
- This could eventually proceed to *taking up contacts somewhere near the throat*, observing, exploring and addressing the sensations, feelings and reactions that arise in response to this.
- This could eventually lead to *taking up actual contact on the throat*, observing, exploring and addressing the sensations, feelings and reactions that arise in response to this.

This process could proceed gradually, always ensuring appropriate grounding of the patient, allowing the patient to proceed step by step, addressing manageable portions of their traumatic response, until they have addressed and released all their traumatic response around the throat and are able to allow and even enjoy throat contact freely and uninhibitedly without any discomfort or disturbance.

This endpoint might seem completely unattainable to a severely traumatised patient, and even reading about the process might make the process sound unbearable, unthinkable and impossible, but with time and an appropriate therapeutic approach to trauma release, all this is possible.

Chapter 54

Energy Drive

The *energy drive* is a process for focusing and targeting cranio-sacral potency or energy, directing the body's inherent healing potential to wherever it may be needed.

While it can be used as a separate process in itself, the energy drive is more likely to be incorporated as an integral part of the treatment process, being introduced into the treatment from time to time as appropriate. Within the context of an overall treatment, it can be used for a wide variety of purposes: enhancing the release of resistant restrictions anywhere in the body – cranial sutures, vertebral articulations, peripheral joints; releasing tension in the soft tissues or in the solar plexus; dissolving blockages in the matrix; relieving congestion in the ears, liver, or elsewhere; enhancing the flow of energy or fluids; helping the body to address an infectious focus; assisting the healing of a fracture or wound. Its most frequent application is in assisting the release of particularly unresponsive resistances which may be encountered during treatment.

The energy drive is also known as *directing the tide, directing the fluid, direction of energy*, or *V-spread*. The term 'directing the fluid' reflects Sutherland's original concept that he was directing or channelling the cerebrospinal fluid (CSF) and the potency within the CSF. The concept of the V-spread reflects the fact that when Sutherland originally used this process he might often be applying it to a cranial suture and would form a V-shape with his index and middle fingers across the suture, directing the therapeutic process to the area within this V-shape. However, there are many applications of the energy drive which would not necessarily include this formation of the V-shape.

The process
The energy drive process consists of several stages, which can be summarised as follows:
1. Identifying the focus to be targeted.
2. Taking up contact at the *target point*.
3. Establishing the *drive point*.
4. Taking up contact at the drive point.
5. Initiating the energy drive.
6. Identifying and enhancing the pulsation.
7. Directing the energy drive towards the target.
8. Dissolving the resistances within the target area.
9. Allowing the process to come to a natural resolution.
10. Reassessing.

1. Identifying the focus
During a cranio-sacral treatment, there may be various times at which a particular point of resistance becomes apparent and the practitioner might decide to introduce an energy drive directed towards that focal point within the context of the integrated treatment. At other times, a particular injury or wound or other focal point might be selected as a target point, with the energy drive being carried out as a separate process. This target point could be anywhere in the body.

2. Taking up contact at the target point
The nature of the contact at the target point will vary according to the situation. If an energy drive is introduced as an integral part of the integrated treatment process, the hand contacts may remain where they are and the energy drive can simply be introduced within that contact. Alternatively, a specific contact may be taken up at the area to be targeted.

This contact is most commonly taken up at the target point either by forming a V-shape with the index and middle fingers across the target area where appropriate (as for instance in the case of a cranial suture) or by placing the palm of the hand under the target area in the case of a larger target area (as for instance the liver).

3. Establishing the drive point

The most appropriate point at which to establish the drive point is most commonly at the opposite pole of the cranium or the opposite aspect of the body. In order to harness as much potency as possible, it is helpful to be working through a substantial portion of the body and also to be including the cranium or the sacrum wherever appropriate.

While an energy drive can be carried out from any point, there will usually be specific points somewhere around the opposite pole which hold a particular resonance, as if there was already a natural line of energy flow from that point to the target area. With a contact already in place on the target point, these points of particular resonance can be identified by spreading a hand across the drive area and then initially thinking back from the *target area* towards the *drive area* (in the wrong direction, so to speak) feeling for the point of greatest resonance.

4. Taking up contact at the drive point

Having established your drive point, you can then take up contact at this drive point with bunched fingertips, the tip of a single finger, or the palm of your hand as appropriate. For a smaller, more specific area, a bunch of fingers or a single finger may be appropriate; for a wider area the palm of the hand is likely to be more appropriate.

5. Initiating the energy drive

Having taken up contact at the drive point you can then initiate the energy drive by visualising a stream of energy flowing from your drive point through the structures of the body to the target area. The exact nature of this stream of energy is not specific, but it may be helpful to visualise it as a stream of electrons, a stream of particles, a stream of photons, a beam of light, a laser beam, or a pulsating beam of radar. Attention always plays a significant part in determining subtle energy responses. The focus and direction of your attention are key factors in establishing and harnessing this flow of therapeutic energy.

6. Identifying and enhancing the pulsation

As you continue to visualise this beam of energy flowing towards the target area you may start to notice a subtle pulsation, as if your beam of energy were a pulsating radar beam. If it doesn't become apparent spontaneously, then allow your perception to open more widely, so that your attention can pick up any subtle impressions of pulsation more readily.

This pulsation is similar to an arterial pulse but you are likely to find that it fluctuates both in its intensity and in its speed, building up and fading away as resistances are encountered and dissolved. Having identified this pulsation, allow yourself to engage with the pulsation more fully, not doing anything, but becoming a part of it, becoming absorbed into it, as if the pulsation were passing through your hands as well. As you engage with it more fully, you may feel that the pulsation is enhanced, becoming clearer and stronger, pulsating more strongly towards the target area.

7. Directing the energy towards the target

As you proceed with the energy drive, you might visualise the beam passing though various body tissues on its way towards the target area, varying in intensity as it encounters different resistances.

As your attention reaches the target area, you can be aware of the energy reaching the surrounding structures and you can survey the various structures in the surrounding area (bones, sutures, muscles, fascia, membrane, ligament, fluid, nerve tissue etc.) to observe how they are affected. Your attention may be drawn to specific structures or specific areas of resistance. If not, you might again survey the surrounding structures to see if any of them draw your attention, or you might be aware of a specific structure towards which you wish to focus your attention.

8. Dissolving the resistances within the target area

The focus is likely to remain longer at areas of greater resistance, intensifying the power of the energy drive until the resistance dissolves and softens, while flowing more freely through areas of free mobility. As the energy drive intensifies in response to resistance, the pulsation is likely to increase, in both speed and strength; as the resistance gives way, the pulsation is likely to fade. As resistances and restrictions give way, you (and the patient) may feel an increasing warmth in the affected area and you may feel a sense of dissolving, melting and softening in the affected tissues. You may also feel an increase in fluid flow, increased energy flow and increased cranio-sacral motion in the area. In this way your attention may move from one resistance to another until the whole area has softened and dissolved. As the local area resolves, you may feel the repercussions throughout the body as the whole system adapts and reorganises around the local changes. Allowing your attention to expand out to be aware of the repercussions throughout the body will be helpful in enabling this to occur.

9. Allowing the process to come to a natural resolution

Once the resistance has given way and the area has softened, you are likely to feel the pulsation reducing in speed and in intensity and fading away. Once the softening is complete you can allow the process to come to natural resolution. Once it feels settled and resolved you can gently detach your consciousness from the area and then detach your contact.

10. Reassessing

You can then reassess the situation to see what changes have occurred and ensure that any changes have been fully integrated into the cranio-sacral system as a whole.

APPLICATIONS

The energy drive has a very wide range of applications and can be used in many different ways according to circumstances. It may be used very specifically in order to release a particular resistance. It may be incorporated into the treatment process in conjunction with other aspects of the cranio-sacral process, introducing an energy drive while holding at a point of stillness, or while projecting up the spine from the sacrum during a double contact, or while following into a spheno-basilar pattern, or while fascially unwinding a hip, or while working at the solar plexus. Some examples of situations which might benefit from an energy drive are:

- a restricted cranial suture
- a locked vertebral segment
- any joint restriction – from sacro-iliac to interphalangeal (finger joint)
- a focus of muscular tension
- strained or sprained ligaments (e.g. in the knee or the ankle)
- a focus of infection
- congestion within the ears
- a tight plexus (e.g. the solar plexus)
- any dysfunctioning organ (e.g. a spastic colon, congested liver, duodenal ulcer)
- the temporo-mandibular joint
- a restricted pterion or nasion
- the pituitary gland
- the orbit and the eye
- scar tissue
- fracture sites
- any area of inertia within the matrix.

Harnessing cranio-sacral potency

It is helpful to harness as much of the cranio-sacral potency as possible and it is therefore often helpful for the drive contact to be on the cranium or the sacrum.

The cranium is an appropriate contact point for cranial and intracranial restrictions, and also for carrying out an energy drive process through the vertebral column, in order to assist the release of restricted vertebral segments.

The sacrum is an appropriate contact point for carrying out energy drive processes throughout the pelvic area and the lower back, for scar tissue in the abdominal and pelvic areas, and particularly for projecting energy drives up through the spine, with or without a second hand at the target point. Energy drives can also be transmitted from the sacrum down through the lower limbs to the hips, the knees, the feet, or to fracture sites in the lower limbs.

You can also work straight through the thorax or abdomen, straight through a knee joint or an ankle as appropriate, either from front to back or from side to side.

Energy drives through the vertebral column are particularly valuable and effective and can be used to release vertebral restrictions and to ease facilitated segments. This process is described below.

In order to further clarify the energy drive process, here are two specific examples of energy drives described in greater detail, which can be used as practical exercises.

Energy drive to the occipito-mastoid suture

In the course of a treatment, you might encounter a cranium in which one of the occipito-mastoid sutures is particularly restricted – a common pattern often arising from birth and other injuries. If the resistance is not readily releasing in response to your other cranio-sacral work, you might choose to introduce an energy drive. You could then adjust your hand position as necessary (see Figure 54.1).

- Having identified the occipito-mastoid suture which needs attention, establish a V with index and middle fingers across the chosen occipito-mastoid suture, the index finger running along the mastoid process, the middle finger running along the occiput, the suture therefore located within the V.

- Establish the drive point at the opposite pole of the cranium, by placing the palm of the hand over the opposite pole and identifying the corresponding point of greatest resonance around the opposite pole.

- Take up contact on the drive point with the fingertips and thumb bunched together at the drive point.

- Initiate the energy drive process, visualising a beam of energy travelling from your fingers at the drive point towards the target area.

- Identify the pulsation, becoming absorbed into it and thereby enhancing the pulsation.

- Visualise your way through the various tissues of the cranium – bone, membrane, the nerve

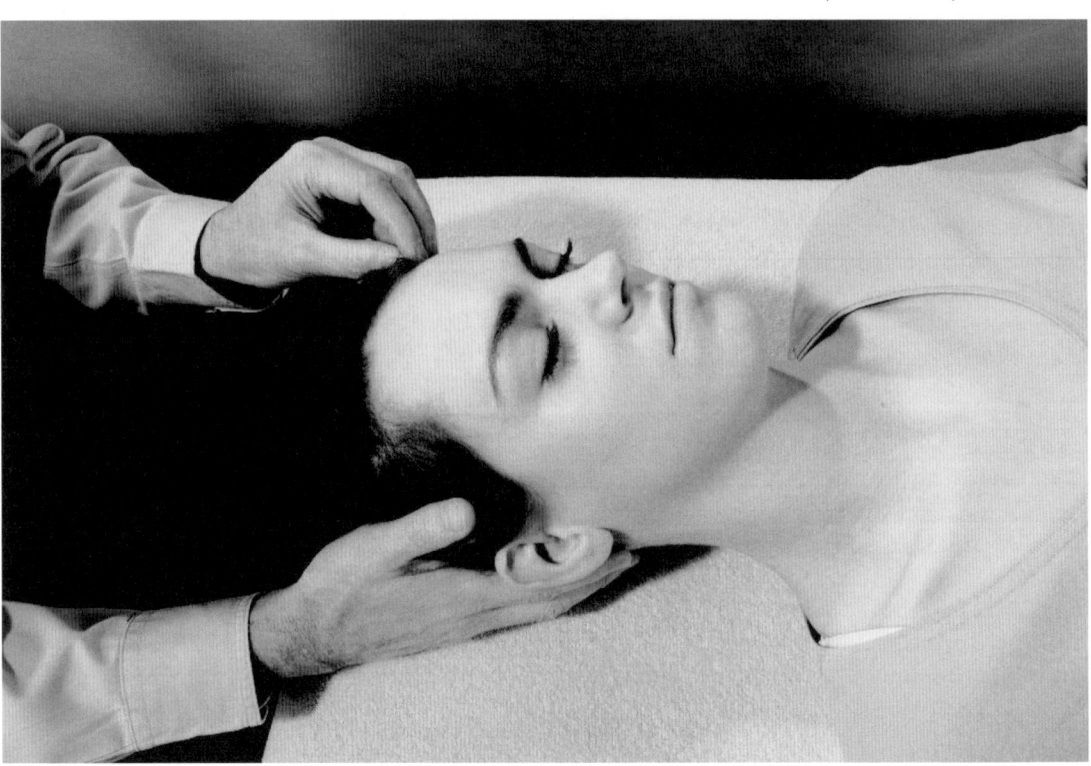

54.1 Contact for an energy drive to the occipito-mastoid suture on the right

tissue of the brain, across to the targeted occipito-mastoid suture.

- Allow your attention to be drawn to the specific areas of resistance.
- Survey the occipito-mastoid suture and the surrounding area including the jugular foramen, the surrounding bony structures, the membranes lining the cranium, the muscles surrounding the suture, the sterno-cleido-mastoid muscle attaching on each side of the suture and running diagonally down the side of the neck, the surrounding fascia.
- Identify focal points of resistance within all these tissues, allowing your attention to focus on particular areas of restriction as your attention passes from structure to structure.
- Follow the fluctuations in pulsation, with increasing intensity of speed and strength as the attention focuses on an area of resistance, and the pulsation generally fading away as resistance softens.
- Feel the resistances dissolving, softening and melting, often with an accompanying sense of warmth.
- Follow the process through until the resistances have dissolved and the pulsation has faded.
- Feel the repercussions of the release in the local area spreading throughout the rest of the system.
- Once the process has settled and resolved, gently release your attention from the area, then gently release your contact.
- Reassess the system, noting any changes which have occurred and ensuring that any local changes have been integrated into the cranio-sacral system as a whole and continuing with your overall integrated treatment process as appropriate.

Energy drive for the vertebral column

The spine, as we have seen, is a crucial area of the body. The spine is also a very common area of restriction – vertebral segments are often held into restricted mobility by the various components which contribute to a facilitated segment, as well as by postural strains, body mechanics, and emotional tensions.

Energy drives through the spine are often appropriate and beneficial. They are perhaps most commonly introduced within the context of working with double contacts from the sacrum, where the appropriate contacts at the target point and the drive point are already established. They can also be specifically introduced at any other time during a treatment, or carried out as a separate process.

During a treatment, with the patient lying supine and contacts already in place under the sacrum and a second contact somewhere up the spine, you might be aware of a particular resistance at this point of second contact. So you might choose to add an energy drive to whatever else might be happening at the time – thinking of your energy drive as a beam of energy from the drive point at the sacrum up through the spine towards the area of resistance at the second contact.

You might simultaneously be following the system to a point of stillness, release and reorganisation, or holding at a point of stillness waiting for release, or you might simply be projecting your attention up through the spine.

At whatever point you choose to introduce your energy drive, you can follow the same principles as described previously – initiating the energy drive up through the spine, visualising the beam of energy travelling up to the target area, feeling the pulsation, enhancing the pulsation, feeling the fluctuation in the pulsation as the energy drive encounters other points of resistance on its way, feeling the responses in the rest of the system – twists, turns, build-up of pressure, release – until your attention reaches the target area, drawn spontaneously to different structures within the target area – bone, muscles, membrane, nerves, surrounding muscles, fascia, or a more abstract sense of tightness or congestion – or surveying these structures more deliberately, feeling the build-up of intensity around a point of particular resistance, and the sense of softening and release, with an accompanying sense of warmth. Feel the repercussions through the system, the release of other resistances, the reflections through the body and the sense of the whole body settling into a balanced, settled symmetrical state. Allow the process to come to resolution, and continue with your integrated treatment process as appropriate.

The energy drive through the spine can also be carried out from the cranium. Possible contacts could include:

- sitting at the head, with one hand over the crown of the head and the other coming in under the back, between the scapulae down to T4 or T9 or wherever is appropriate
- sitting at the side with one hand over the crown and the other hand coming in from the side to whatever vertebral areas may be appropriate.

The energy drive though the spine can also be carried out as a separate process with the patient in a sitting position (see Figure 54.2).

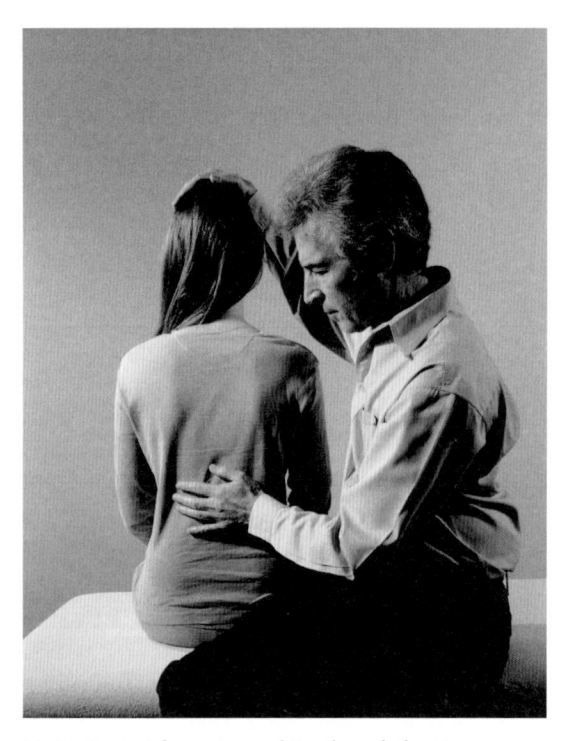

54.2 Contact for an energy drive through the spine

With your patient sitting, establish the vertebral level to be targeted. If this is not already apparent, then the spine can readily be assessed. This can be done on both an energetic and a structural level. First, run your hand down the spine, slightly *off the body* feeling for areas of warmth and coolness or for gaps in the aura or energy field (warmth perhaps indicating an area of more acute disturbance or inflammation, with increased energy, coolness perhaps indicating an area of chronic restriction, with depleted local energy). Next run your fingers down the vertebral column *on the body*, feeling for areas of tension, tightness and restriction. Both processes can help to identify the same area of greatest restriction within the vertebral column.

One hand can then be spread across the chosen vertebral segment, thereby gaining a sense of the whole local area – bony segment, surrounding muscles and fascia, etc.

- Bring your other hand gently to rest with the palm of the hand on the crown of the head ensuring that the very centre of the palm of your hand is resting on the very centre of the crown.
- From this drive point you can initiate the energy drive process from the palm of your hand through the crown, through the structures of the cranium – bony, membranous, neurological and fluid – down through the foramen magnum and visualising your way down through the vertebral column.
- As you work your way down the vertebral column, you can, as described previously, identify areas of resistance, feeling fluctuations in the pulsation. You may encounter a series of different resistances on the way down the vertebral column before you reach your chosen target area. You may feel the system expressing various subtle twists, turns, releases, intensifications and softenings.
- As you reach your target vertebral level, again follow the fluctuations in pulsation and the build-up of intensity as you focus your attention on this vertebral level, surveying the various structure– bony, muscular, ligamentous, capsular, membranous, fluid – allowing your attention to focus on the areas of resistance until they dissolve and soften.
- As the area softens, notice the pulsation fading away.
- Feel the repercussions of the release through the rest of the system.

- Once the process is complete, gently release any thought of transmitting an energy drive, release your consciousness from the area and release your contact.
- You can then reassess the area and check that any changes have been fully integrated into the cranio-sacral system as a whole.

The advantages of the sitting position are that various secondary resistances and restrictions are highlighted by the postural patterns brought into play by sitting; and as changes occur and restrictions release, a process of adaptation and integration on a postural level can take place. This transmits the therapeutic effect of the energy drive throughout the vertebral column and the rest of the body in a way that integrates the postural muscles and the whole body structure more effectively than is usually achieved in a lying position (where the postural muscles are not actively engaged). This can be particularly effective where the overall balance and integration of the back is weak, with postural misalignments and strains from various injuries and consequent back pain perhaps in various locations.

Chapter 55

The Emotional Body

How do we read the emotional state of the patient through the body?

The physical body and the psycho-emotional state are inextricably intertwined. Not only do they invariably affect each other; they are one – one body-mind complex, different manifestations of the same unified being, different aspects of the same matrix.

Everything that happens in the physical body is inevitably reflected in the psycho-emotional state on some level. Everything that happens on an emotional level is inevitably reflected in the physical body – and can be identified through the cranio-sacral system.

Emotions are held in the body in many ways, in various places, on different levels, some readily apparent, some deeply hidden, some obvious, some obscure, some clearly expressed, some deeply suppressed.

The degree to which you read the emotional state of your patients will depend on your perception. If you choose to explore emotion you will see it. If you don't, you won't, just as your breadth of perception will enable perception of anything else – rhythms and tides, subtle movement, tissues, fluids and energy fields.

If you visit a city, you will probably see the streets, buildings and other typical sights of the city, but you might not notice the wildlife. If however you take a particular interest in the wildlife and seek it out, you will almost certainly find a plentiful array – foxes, hedgehogs, birds and beasts of many kinds. They were always there, you just didn't notice them. In the same way with emotions, if you take an interest, you will find them and understand them.

When we are reading emotions in the body, we are not simply concerned with how the patient feels at that moment. We are engaging with the patterns of holding imposed by injuries, accidents, conflicts, pressures and stresses experienced throughout life:

- Deep patterns of emotional holding, perhaps imprinted from an early age by childhood, family life, upbringing, schooling, or from the various trials and tribulations of life.
- Deeply held unresolved grief, anger, resentment or hurt – from bereavement, broken relationships, attacks, perhaps long forgotten, but continuing to fester away inside, generating disease and dysfunction.
- Not just major incidents and events, but all the everyday aspects of life that affect everyone – the stresses and pressures of life which generate tension and disease, contributing to anything from tension headaches to cancer.
- The persistent influences in our lives which mould our nature and personality, and establish patterns of behaviour – reserved, contained, shy, withdrawn, depressed, assertive, irritable, angry, aggressive.

All of these factors affect the patient's health. They are probably the *most* significant factors affecting their health, yet they are largely disregarded. In order to understand a patient's state, we have to look at the whole person, to see every aspect of them, to understand how their emotional state is an intrinsic and fundamental aspect of their condition.

A happy relaxed person is more likely to be a healthy person. An unhappy, tense, stressed person is more likely to be unwell and develop disease – they are not just more likely to suffer from colds, digestive disturbances and back pain, but more likely to develop serious diseases like ulcers, arthritis, heart conditions and major pathologies.

READING EMOTIONS

There are various ways of reading emotions, including:

- *Observation.*
- *Symptoms.*
- *Case history.*
- *Palpation.*

Observation

We can observe the patient's demeanour, manner, posture, behaviour, breathing, facial expression, body language, mannerisms.

To some observers such 'body language' will be obvious, others find it very difficult to read. In some patients, their emotions are clearly evident, in others they can be hidden under layer upon layer of masking and armouring. And in everyone, both the expressive and the unexpressive, there are hidden depths.

Through attention and practice you can develop the skills to read the emotional state more and more accurately and perceptively. This can provide invaluable insight into your understanding of the person and their situation, enable you to recognise what part emotions play in their overall state and therefore enhance the effectiveness of your treatment.

Of course you need to take into account that what you are seeing is only the outer facade that the patient presents. Many patients will not be revealing their deepest emotions (or their emotions at all), particularly initially. What you are seeing on the surface may just be an outer mask – maintaining a front of some kind to cover insecurities, whether it be:

- a polite formal front to cover up feelings of anxiety and inadequacy
- a confident assertive front to cover up fear of failure
- a jokey front to cover up embarrassment or lack of confidence
- a person who is holding back the tears, putting on a brave face
- someone who has been putting on a brave face all their life
- a person who had a very traumatic childhood and has learnt to cope with life through various means, but still carries around the influence of that traumatic childhood in the behavioural patterns that they have developed in order to cope (e.g. polite smile, eagerness to please, resigned look, stoic indifference).

Symptoms

Every symptom and condition has psycho-emotional associations, as well as physical ones, even if it is just an emotional response to pain. If you hit yourself on the thumb while hammering a nail, the cause is ostensibly physical, but your emotional reaction to the pain as well as irritation with yourself could affect its recovery.

Even more so, if you are involved in a car accident, the injury might be seen as primarily physical, but the emotional components of shock and fear, anger towards the other driver, not to mention hopes of an insurance claim, may significantly influence the healing process.

Equally, many conditions generally thought of as primarily associated with emotional causes, or dismissed as psychosomatic, may have a primarily physical cause, as described in Chapter 49 on the autonomic nervous system.

Certain conditions and symptoms are commonly associated with emotional disturbance. These include asthma, irritable bowel syndrome, duodenal ulcers, globus hystericus, teeth grinding, many visceral disorders and the more obviously emotional symptoms such as palpitations and anxiety attacks.

Recognising this association may be helpful in tracing the cause, and above all in building the overall picture of the patient and therefore establishing the appropriate treatment approach.

If a child has asthma, you could just treat it as a physical condition and give them medication for the rest of their life. Or you could recognise that the symptoms of asthma suggest an underlying emotional factor, treat the patient accordingly, address the root cause, and the child could be free of asthma.

Cranio-sacral integration can be highly successful in treating childhood asthma – partly through recognising the emotional component and also through incorporating the various other aspects of cranio-sacral integration, such as an understanding of the autonomic nervous system. If a research project were set up to demonstrate the effectiveness of cranio-sacral integration, one of the conditions I would choose would be childhood asthma.

In order to enable more complete and comprehensive healing, it is necessary to acknowledge the emotional component as a matter of course, identifying in each patient the degree to which emotional factors need to be addressed (which does of course vary substantially from person to person), recognising the patients for whom the emotional element may be of particular significance, but always understanding every patient as a whole person in whom the physical and emotional are inextricably intertwined.

Case history

Taking a case history is an excellent opportunity to engage with your patient on many levels, not simply recording facts, but developing an interaction through which a comprehensive picture can emerge.

Patients may not necessarily mention or acknowledge emotional factors during a case history. They may not see them as relevant, may not recognise any connection between their emotions and their physical state. They may not be aware of them at all – because they have become accustomed to them, or because any emotionally significant event occurred so long ago, or because a particular trauma is so deeply buried under layers of protection, or perhaps because it occurred precognitively at birth.

Alternatively, they may not wish to mention such matters, at least initially. There are many different attitudes to emotions and many reasons why people may or may not want to talk about them – whether because they see them as private, or embarrassing, or as a sign of weakness, or something to be dismissed, or perhaps they just don't expect a doctor to take any interest in such things.

A detailed case history can reveal valuable insight into the emotional state and its relevance to the patient's condition, whether directly or indirectly, not just in what is said, but in the way it is said and the whole manner in which the patient presents their situation:

- in the way that they describe specific incidents – accidents, traumas, periods of stress
- whether or not they coincide with the onset of a condition
- in revealing background information which predisposes to stress or emotional disturbance (pressure at work, difficult personal relations, childhood trauma)
- simply in the manner in which the patient talks about (or doesn't talk about) various matters.

A case history, however, is only part of the story. It is not a reliable source. Patients seldom reveal the full story in a case history. What *is* reliable is cranio-sacral palpation.

Palpation

More than anything else, the key to recognising the relevance of psycho-emotional factors lies in the quality of the patient's cranio-sacral system. The cranio-sacral system never lies; it reveals everything; it carries the whole life story in every detail – the current emotional state, the deeper underlying personality, recent upsets, deeply embedded trauma – it is all there in the cranio-sacral system. These things can of course be hidden under layers of coping, pretence, therapy, and various other means, but not only will the underlying patterns of trauma be palpable, but also the various layers of masking or armouring will also be palpable and identifiable.

Specific indicators

Emotions are held everywhere in the body, but some areas are more significant indicators of emotion than others. In developing a greater awareness of emotions in the body, attention to these factors may be helpful:

General

- Quality – the overall quality of the system as a whole (e.g. tense, agitated, controlled, open, held in shock, frozen).
- Tissue tension.

- Fascia – the quality and response within the fascia.
- The sympathetic nervous system.
- Breathing – perhaps shallow, rapid, irregular.
- Responsiveness of the system.

Specific areas
- Sympathetic plexi (solar plexus; heart centre).
- The diaphragm.
- The suboccipital region.
- The shoulders.
- The neck.
- The jaw (clenching, teeth grinding).
- The throat.
- The viscera (digestive organs; heart and pericardium; lungs).

As always, it is primarily through the quality which you palpate within these structures that you can read and define the emotional component and state.

Emotion can also be held at a specific site of injury, for instance in the pelvic area as a result of rape or sexual abuse, in the throat following strangulation, or in the specific location of a blow, or the site of a fracture or sports injury. It can also be held in particular positions in which injury, abuse and trauma occurred, as we saw in the chapters on fascial unwinding.

Identifying the focal point of emotional tension within the body – whether it be a specific location or a quality held throughout the system – and working with that fulcrum can assist the release of deeply held trauma and tension and be crucial to the patient's progress.

Recognition, not just of the focal point, but also of the emotional component held there, is also crucial since, as always, informed awareness influences the response. Working with a particular fulcrum without recognising its emotional component might prove unproductive. As soon as you recognise the emotional component, this may enable release.

Visceral associations

Specific organs are often associated with specific emotions. This can provide a useful additional indicator of underlying emotional factors, but these associations are subtle impressions within an ocean of other relevant information and need to be viewed within the perspective of the overall picture, always seeking verification of impressions through other indications, and not jumping to immediate conclusions. Some of the main common associations are:

Liver	Anger
Gall bladder	Control
Kidneys	Fear
Heart	Grief
Lungs	Anxiety
Stomach	Insecurity

Bear in mind that it is suppressed emotions (rather than freely expressed emotions) which are likely to affect (or become embedded in) the associated organ. Someone who expresses their anger (appropriately) is less likely to hold it into their liver, whereas someone who suppresses their anger behind a polite exterior is perhaps more likely to accumulate the effects in their liver. Again it is the quality that informs you of the relevance and interpretation of your findings – for example, not only identifying a notable quality in the liver, but also distinguishing in a liver the difference between suppressed anger, hepatitis, or cirrhosis, although all of these may have become inextricably intertwined within the same liver.

Levels

A significant factor in reading the emotional state is recognising the many different levels on which it is being held. Initially, this can be one of the most deceptive and misleading factors in reading emotions – easily mistaking a settled outer state as indicating a lack of emotional disturbance.

An apparently calm, assured exterior may be masking an ocean of unprocessed trauma, or emotional turmoil deep inside.

A patient may appear to have everything under control, but be driven by emotional patterns of which they have no knowledge or understanding, and over which they have no control.

Some patients may have addressed their emotions at great length – through a multitude of therapies, personal development courses, trainings, and other activities – but still have deeper issues which they have not even recognised or touched upon, and which they are determinedly (though probably unconsciously) avoiding at all costs despite their incessant personal development work.

Patients may appear quite emotionally open and expressive on the surface, but may not be addressing deeper issues in their life, and may not be prepared to go anywhere near them.

Patients may appear to be emotionally volatile and in turmoil on the surface and in obvious need of emotional support, but because they are expressing their emotions, they may not be suppressing their emotions into their bodies, so their emotions may not be adversely affecting their physical health.

One of the great advantages of cranio-sacral integration is that it can read the body whatever the circumstances; it can penetrate through all the masking, armouring, hiding and pretence (assuming sufficient sensitivity and experience) and perceive everything that is happening on every level.

This is enabled by taking your perception to different levels of the patient's being, allowing your attention and your depth of contact to sink below the surface, connecting with ever deeper levels – whether in the physical tissues, in the various tidal levels – but above all identifying and defining the qualities that you encounter at different levels, and the differences in quality that reflect the deeper or more superficial patterns of emotion held at different levels.

You will still encounter (and potentially be deceived by) the calm, assured superficial layer (in the cranio-sacral system) masking the deeper layers of trauma and turmoil. But with insight, experience and understanding of the emotional body, you can penetrate beyond those superficial layers to identify and interpret the qualities at deeper levels.

A substantial portion, perhaps the vast majority, of physical disease and discomfort is caused or maintained by emotional factors. Identifying those emotional patterns and their repercussions held into the tissues of the body and enabling their release is a crucial part of the therapeutic process.

One of the major limitations of modern medicine is that it fails to acknowledge this as one of the most significant factors in maintaining pain and disease. And one of the major strengths of cranio-sacral integration is that it not only recognises the inextricable interaction between the physical and the emotional but also addresses them simultaneously as one unified process.

A great deal of disease and ill health – from back pain and peptic ulcers to heart disease and cancer – might be prevented through proper understanding of the whole person and the underlying emotional basis of disease, and through treating patients as whole people, taking into account their emotional state and needs.

Chapter 56

Personal Development

Coherence

The term coherence is used in biology to indicate the unified interaction of your cells, molecules, atoms, subatomic particles and waves, enabling the fluent flow of your own internal molecular web. Coherence means that everything is working in a cohesive integrated manner, essential for smooth function.

Cranio-sacral integration is an interaction. As has been emphasised throughout, the state of the practitioner is the most crucial element in the interaction of the cranio-sacral process, in other words: your calm, quiet presence; and your degree of coherence.

These elements are important for the practitioner to be able to engage effectively with the subtle forces and movements of the cranio-sacral process, so that what you bring to the therapeutic interaction is a positive, fluent, ordered, beneficial healing influence that can help to bring order and coherence to your patient's disordered system.

Genuine

Your presence needs to be genuine – not just a superficial impression of calmness, or a professional detachment, but genuine, profound connection with your own deeper nature, true integration of your own system, so that you can operate from the heart, from a well-grounded, centred state, from a position of true coherence.

In order to enable this, it is essential for the practitioner to work on their own development – constantly and continuously:

- in order to clear the clutter from their own system
- in order to address the effects of their own past traumas and tensions
- in order to clear out prejudices and preconceptions
- in order to develop the ability to maintain a constant state of grounding, centring, and balance.

A therapist is not aiming to be perfect, but is working constantly towards as high a level of clarity and balance as possible within the circumstances, in order to enhance their therapeutic interaction with others. Everyone will have their past traumas and tensions. The aim is to come to terms with your issues – genuinely, not just pushing them under the surface – so that they don't impinge on the therapeutic process, so that you can maintain an appropriate degree of clarity and grounding uncluttered by your own issues, a state of balance and integrity despite the traumas and tensions, so that you can operate from a position of ease and stability, rather than being driven by conscious or unconscious underlying patterns.

It is not enough simply to maintain a controlled professional manner. On the contrary, that is likely to create tension and conflict through the lack of awareness of your own issues and the probably unconscious struggle of suppressing unresolved inner conflict in order to maintain a superficial veneer of calmness – and this conflict and your own inner tensions will affect the therapeutic interaction. The cranio-sacral system is never fooled, so it is essential to be operating from a position of genuine clarity and coherence.

A personal journey

Personal development is an individual process. Each person has their own path to follow, their own journey to pursue, so we will not try to prescribe any particular approach, other than to say that common elements that cranio-sacral therapists may find useful include cranio-sacral treatment, other forms of therapy, counselling and psychotherapy, reflective practice, meditation, yoga, tai chi, alexander technique, and a wide range of continuing personal development groups and courses, with the aim of exploring one's own process of personal growth and development.

It also includes life experience – family, motherhood, fatherhood, relationships, community – all of which contribute to and play a part in personal development.

It also includes being happy, enjoying life, having fun, relaxing, allowing time for yourself, self-care, being at peace.

Challenging your comfort zone

It is not just a matter of remaining content on the surface, not just a superficially balanced life within your own comfort zone, not just being a 'good' person – charitable, well intentioned, caring – nor acting out of feelings of guilt, obligation or duty, but rather it is a matter of:

- clearing out past traumas and tension – truly, deeply, gladly
- coming to terms with your own deeper issues
- challenging your boundaries and preconceptions and comfort zone.

Bear in mind that the experiences that are most helpful to you may be the processes that are most challenging rather than the ones that you feel most comfortable with – so find a balance between comfort and challenge, and regard challenging situations as an opportunity to learn rather than as situations to avoid. It is often those who think that they don't need personal development who need it most. And of course it is not just a matter of more and more academic or technical learning (a common way of avoiding genuine personal development).

Balance of stability and exploration

There are many avenues to explore and much that can be learnt from many different sources. It can be helpful to explore as many different options as possible, to expand your horizons and gain a wider and deeper understanding of life and of yourself. It is also helpful to find a stable, consistent path to follow – without excessive attachment or dogma. Again there is a balance to be found between continuing exploration of new ideas for development and the stability of a stable consistent path.

For many people, practitioners and patients, it can be difficult to make changes, and many people will be reluctant to undergo any digging under the surface or inner exploration, leaving the underlying dissatisfactions to fester and grow, or not even acknowledging their existence – unless forced to by ill health or tragedy. Change can be challenging and frightening, especially inner change, and it often appears easier to stay with what's familiar – secure with the usual routine. But facing those fears and exploring new avenues can be transformative – not just for development as a cranio-sacral therapist but for every aspect of life. Such transformation can be an integral part of becoming an effective cranio-sacral therapist.

Summary

Personal development involves genuinely addressing your underlying personal processes so that you can operate from a position of true clarity, fluency and harmony, balance and integrity, coherence and fluency, in order to enable the most positive and beneficial therapeutic interaction with your patients.

Chapter 57

Further Contacts

There are many standard hand positions which are used fairly universally. There are good reasons for these hand positions, but we don't need to become too attached to specific hand contacts; they are only guidelines, or starting points. In the course of treatment, different situations will arise and you can take up contact anywhere, adapting hand positions as necessary.

If a contact under the sacrum doesn't feel quite right, then adjust it. If your contact under a particular vertebral level doesn't seem to be under the exact relevant spot for this patient then alter it. If you are engaging at the solar plexus centre and you feel drawn to the liver, you can move your front hand (or both hands) to the liver.

There are some contacts which do require more specific precision – the suboccipital release is a prime example – but for the most part there is infinite scope for adaptability. What matters is engagement, and you can adapt your hands in whatever way feels appropriate, improvising hand positions according to the needs of the moment.

Combined heart and solar plexus contact

In working with the emotional centres, we initially took up contact on the heart centre and the solar plexus centre separately. This is often relevant and useful and appropriate.

Another contact that can be very effective in engaging with these emotional centres is to combine these two contacts, with one hand under the back at the heart centre (as previously used for the heart centre) and the other hand over the solar plexus centre on the front of the body. This has the advantages firstly, of addressing both centres simultaneously, and secondly of feeling the interaction between them – the emotional responses in the heart centre and the control of the emotions from the solar plexus. There will often be a significant interaction.

This may become the contact of choice for engaging with these two centres. It can also be particularly appropriate when entering

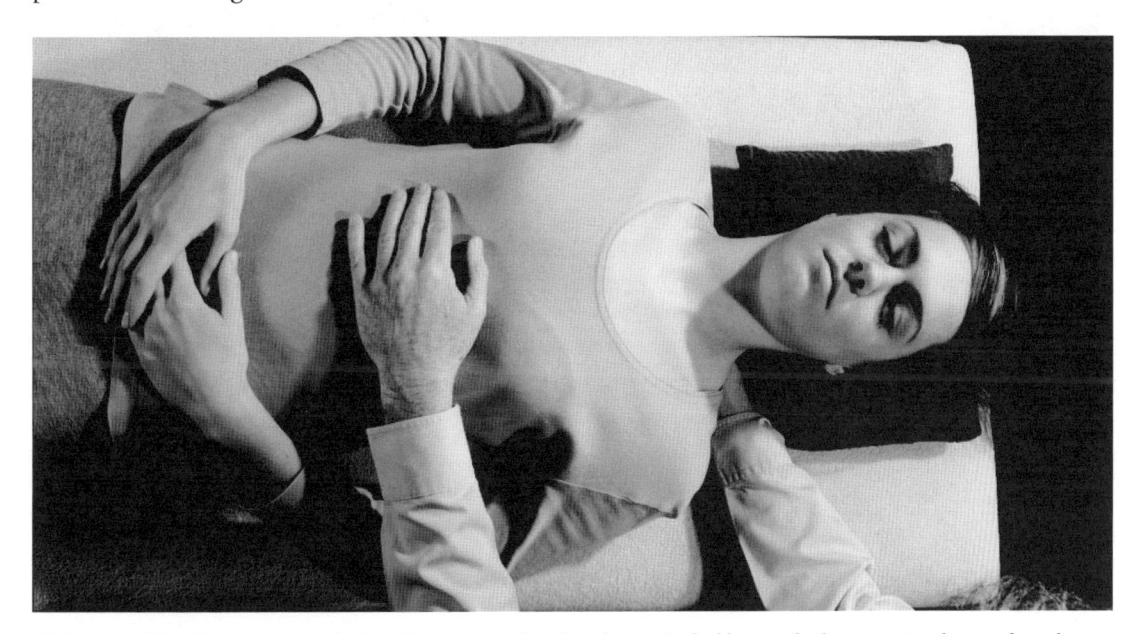

57.1   A combined heart centre and solar plexus contact has the advantage of addressing both centres simultaneously and feeling the interaction between them

into dialogue with the patient, as you can be positioned appropriately to engage with them face to face as you enter into conversation, while at the same time feeling what is happening in their heart and solar plexus.

From that position, you might also wish to respond to specific patterns within the body by introducing other variations, moving the solar plexus hand to the liver, the stomach or the gall bladder or wherever may be appropriate and monitoring the responses in the heart centre and upper thorax simultaneously.

You could also place both hands under the back, or both hands over the front of the body. The choice of position is primarily a matter of comfort and of what feels right, but there are also physiological reasons for this particular contact, since the sympathetic synapses for the cardiac plexus take place in the sympathetic chain at the back, whereas the sympathetic synapses for the solar plexus take place in the coeliac ganglia on the anterior surface of the aorta.

Rhomboid release

The name rhomboid release is a convenient title rather than an accurate description of this process. This contact is a variation which may often arise, or to which you may be drawn, as you work at the heart centre. With one hand under the back, at the upper thorax or heart centre, the other hand can come into contact on the shoulder. As with any contact, you can then engage with the system and follow the inherent treatment process, seeing how the system responds.

This contact has a variety of benefits, assisting the release of tension throughout the shoulder, shoulder girdle and upper thorax – with inevitable widespread repercussions throughout the body. It can engage more specifically with:

- the pericardium and heart
- the pleura and lungs
- the brachial plexus and arm

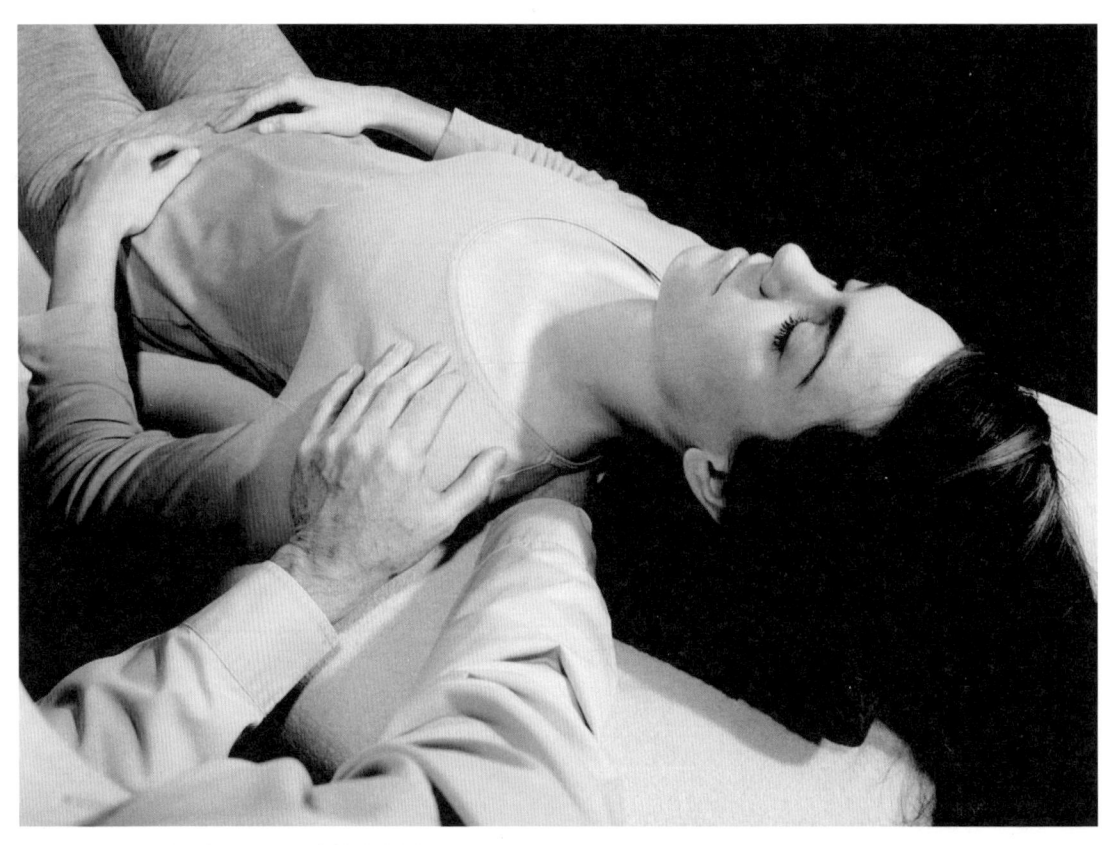

57.2 The 'rhomboid contact' can be helpful for engaging with the interaction of the many different factors which accumulate here – emotional holding, postural tensions, occupational tensions, physical injuries and the complex interaction of these various factors

- up through trapezius and levator scapulae into the head and neck
- through latissimus dorsi down to the pelvis
- through the rotator cuff muscles into the shoulder girdle
- through all the many other muscles and fascial sheaths in the area, addressing the specific tensions so commonly held in the neck and shoulders
- through all the individual patterns of tension and imbalance that are present in that individual patient, extending right through the body.

Physical and emotional interaction

It is a helpful contact for engaging with the interaction of the many different factors which accumulate here – emotional holding, postural tensions, occupational tensions, physical injuries and the complex interaction of these various factors – through its connection with, and informed awareness of, the soft tissues, fascia, muscles, neurological supply, vertebral segments, pericardium, viscera and the whole matrix, the accumulated interaction of which so often leads to intense contraction of the tissues in this area and a wide range of symptoms both local and distant. It can often enable very beneficial effects in the shoulder joint, in frozen shoulder, supraspinatus tendonitis, neck pain, upper back pain, brachial plexus disorders, or neurological disturbances in the arms, hands and fingers.

Through all of this it can enable release of a significant area of physical and emotional holding which can then enable profound release through the whole system.

Rhomboid contraction

Sometimes it may feel as if the practitioner's two hands are being drawn towards each other by contraction within the rhomboid muscles (a very common site of holding) and other tissues. Introducing containment by following into this pull can often enable the tissues, the fascia, the rhomboid muscles, the pericardium and the whole local matrix to build up in response to the containment to a point of contraction where they are able to unlatch, unhook, disentangle, thereby enabling them to slacken off into a relaxed released state, leading to reintegration, not only of the rhomboid muscles themselves, but also of the vertebral segments of the upper thoracic and cervico-thoracic spine, together with consequent repercussions through the whole area and throughout the whole body. This may sometimes be accompanied by a profound emotional release.

Exploring different levels of physical contact

This can be an interesting contact through which to explore the effects of different levels of physical contact – experimenting with simply being there with a very soft, light contact; and then very gradually introducing the possibility of slight compression – in response to contraction within the tissues – seeing how the system responds, then gradually increasing the level of contact very slowly, almost imperceptibly, monitoring the response in the tissues and in the matrix as you do so.

When practising with a practice partner, it can be interesting to discuss the responses at each moment, as felt by the 'patient' and by the therapist. It can also be interesting to treat the area very lightly on one occasion, and then treat the same area with a greater (although still very minor) physical input on another occasion on the same 'patient' and discuss the subsequent differences in response.

Using this contact on the *left side* has specific relationships to:

- the heart
- the pericardium
- left-sided patterns of tension and restriction through the arm shoulder, neck, back and down the left side of the body to the pelvis.

Using this contact on the *right-hand side* of the body has specific benefits for:

- the thymus chakra in the right upper thorax, affecting immune function
- the liver – with its pattern of referral up into the right shoulder
- all the corresponding structures throughout the right-hand side of the body.

This is a contact that can very readily be incorporated into an integrated treatment during the opening up process at the heart centre.

Cranial base and crown

A combined contact with one hand under the base of the cranium, supporting the occiput, subocciput and upper cervical area, and the other hand over the crown, is a valuable contact for addressing patterns throughout the cranium and particularly the very common area of complex restrictions around the occiput, occiput-atlas joint, subocciput, and upper cervical spine, as well as within the cranium around the falx cerebelli, the foramen magnum, the brainstem, the jugular foramina and many other structures. As always the inherent treatment process can be allowed to take its course, but again, containment can often be appropriate within this contact, particularly for responding to the strong contractions so often held in this area, both within the neck and within the membranes of the falx cerebri and falx cerebelli, and particularly for the compressive forces of birth. This contact is also useful following road traffic accidents and whiplash injuries in which the neck has been severely injured, and following many other head and neck injuries, and for a suboccipital area which is compressed or contracted and which is not responding readily to a standard subocciptal release.

Double contacts under the spine

As well as working with double contacts from the sacrum, it is often helpful to place both hands under the spine at different levels. These could be two areas of restriction, feeling the interaction between them. Or it could involve placing the hands on either side of a restricted area, sensing the flow of vitality between your hands and through the affected region, along with the various responses to your contact.

This contact enables a more specific focus on a particular area. It can of course be taken up anywhere along the spine, and usually involves sitting at the side of the patient, with both hands palm-upwards under the back.

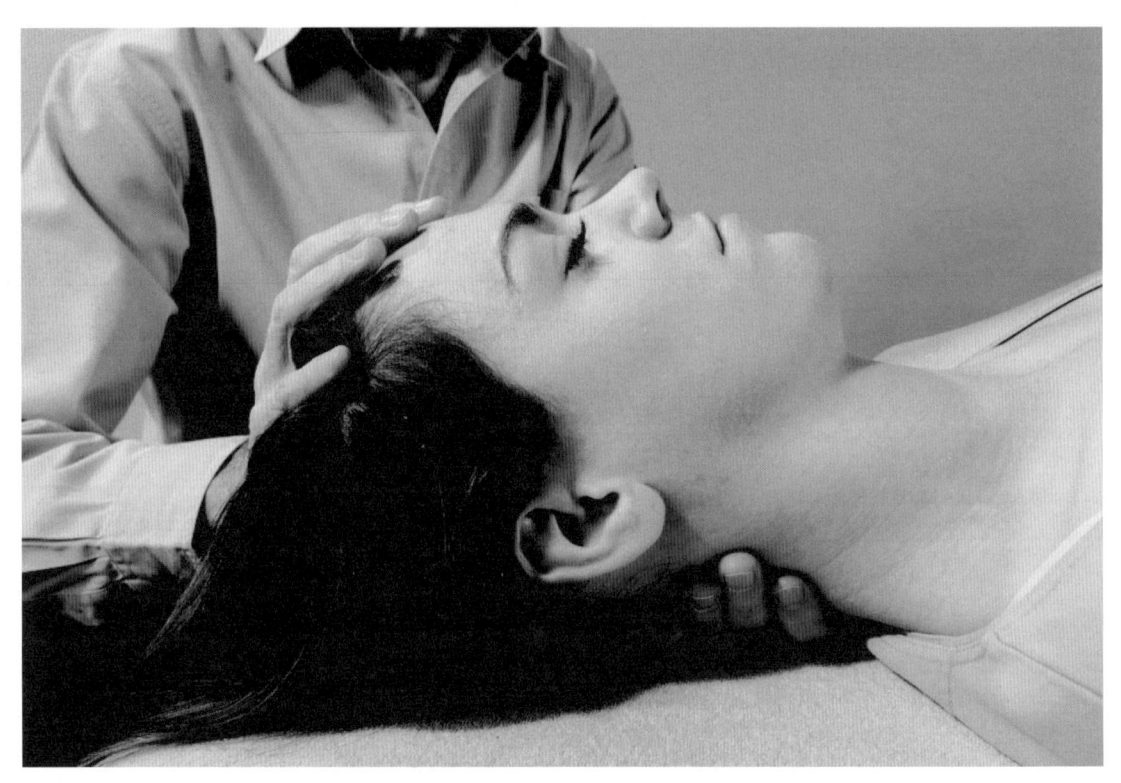

57.3 A combined contact for the cranial base and crown

Further Contacts / 425

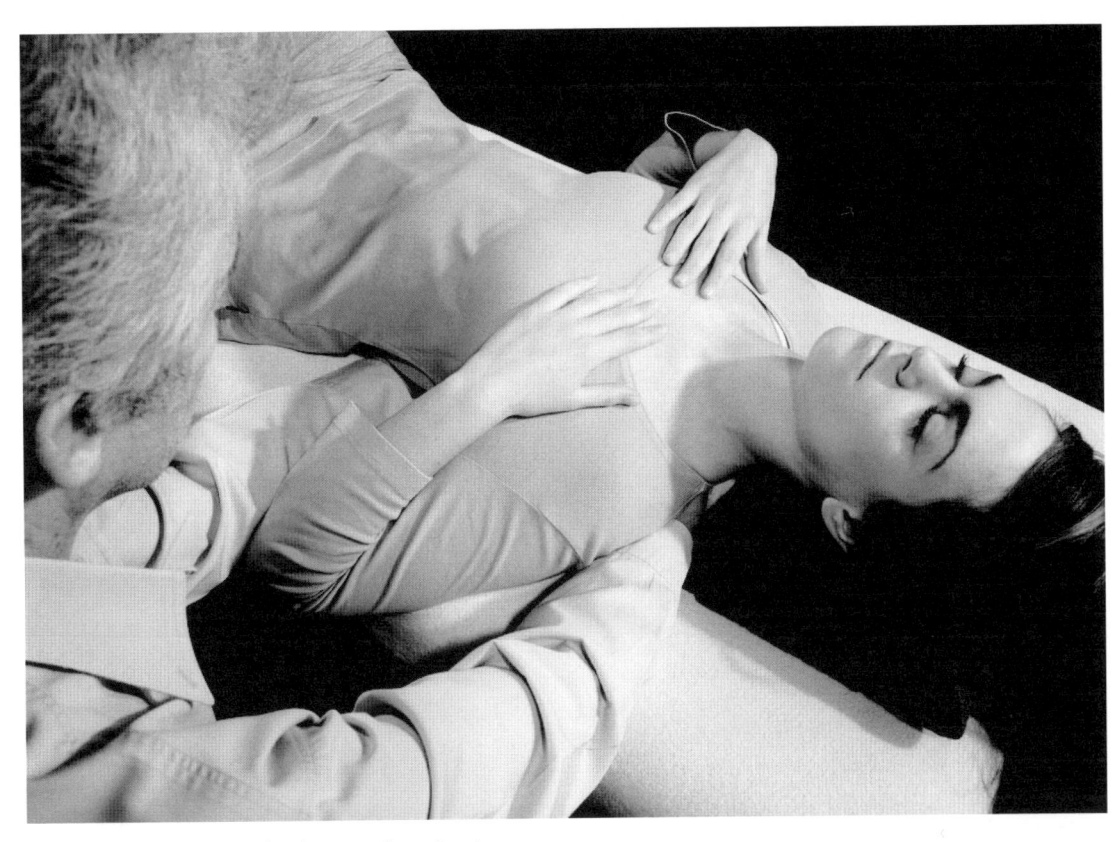

57.4   A double contact under the upper thoracic spine

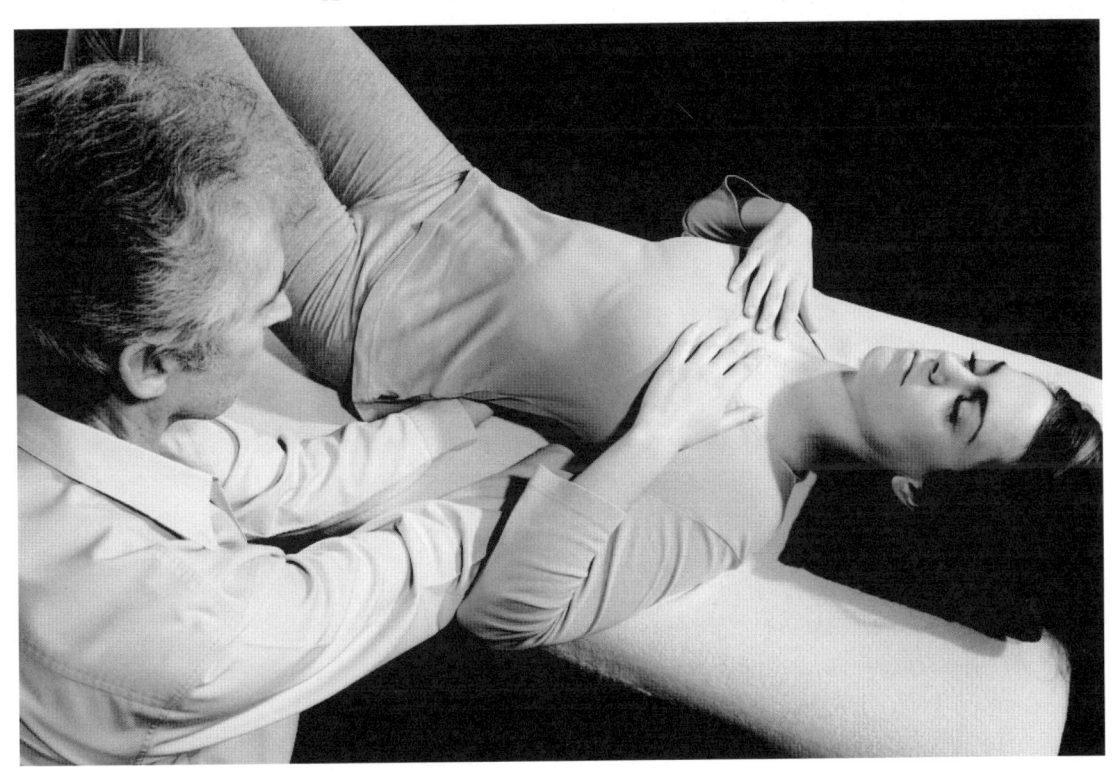

57.5   A double contact under the lower thoracic spine

Scapula contact

Once again the name is a convenient title rather than an accurate description. Sitting at the head, this contact involves asking the patient to arch their upper back and then sliding your hands under the back, palms facing upwards, coming to rest somewhere under the scapula area, and inviting your patient to rest back down again. From there you can as usual engage and allow the evolution of the inherent treatment process.

This is a beautifully symmetrical contact, in which the whole thorax, the whole trunk, the whole back, the spine, the shoulders and neck, the viscera, the heart, the lungs can all gently find their way into a more balanced integrated state around the fulcrum of your symmetrical bilateral contact.

You can remain there for prolonged periods, feeling the body gently reintegrating, your perception spreading through the whole person while at the same time observing the specific local responses from place to place, feeling the rhythmic motion (as the whole body externally rotates into expansion and internally rotates into contraction around the fulcrum of the spine); observing minor adjustments and releases occuring within the vertebral segments and surrounding spinal muscles; or feeling the whole body patterns drawing your attention and building to points of stillness and release, enabling the whole body to settle into a more balanced, integrated, neutral state.

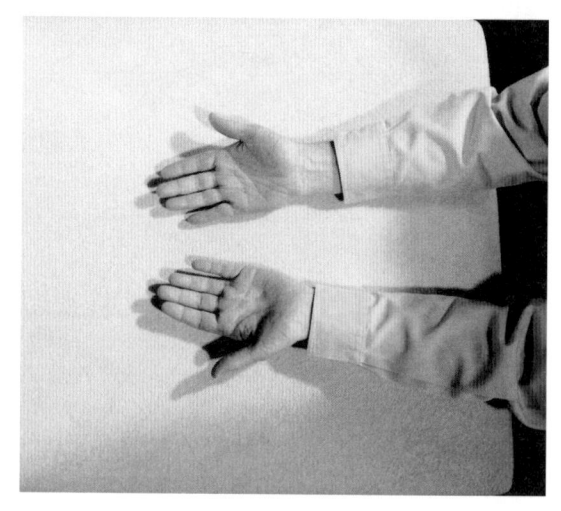

57.7 Hand position for a 'scapula contact'

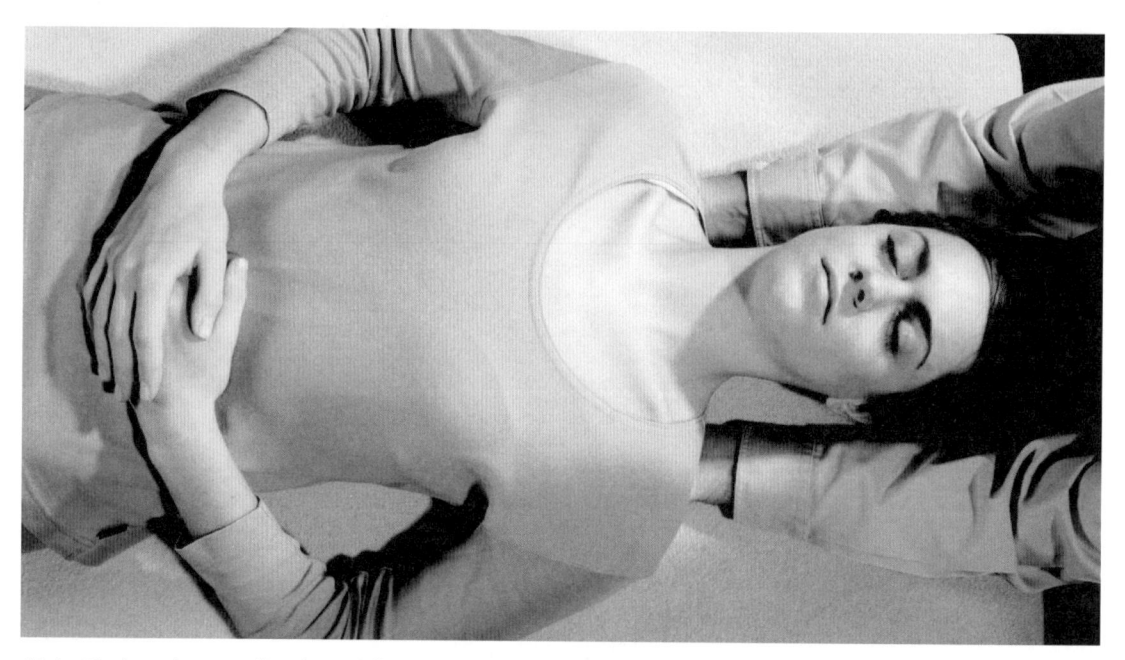

57.6 The 'scapula contact' is a beautifully symmetrical contact, in which the whole thorax and the whole matrix can gently find their way to a more balanced integrated state around the fulcrum of your symmetrical bilateral contact

The position of the hands under the back can, as always, be varied according to the needs of the patient. Most often a suitable location may be somewhere around the mid-thoracic level, under the scapulae, perhaps more medially under the rhomboids and close to the vertebral column – close to the spinal nerve outlets and the sympathetic chain and the main structures at the midline. Depending on the needs of the individual and the focal points of restriction, the hands may be placed further down the back, or further up towards the shoulders, or perhaps moving through a series of different contacts in different places. Particularly with babies and children it is easy to reach right down to the thoraco-lumbar region, the lumbar area, or even the pelvis. It can be a very comfortable and appropriate contact for babies and children.

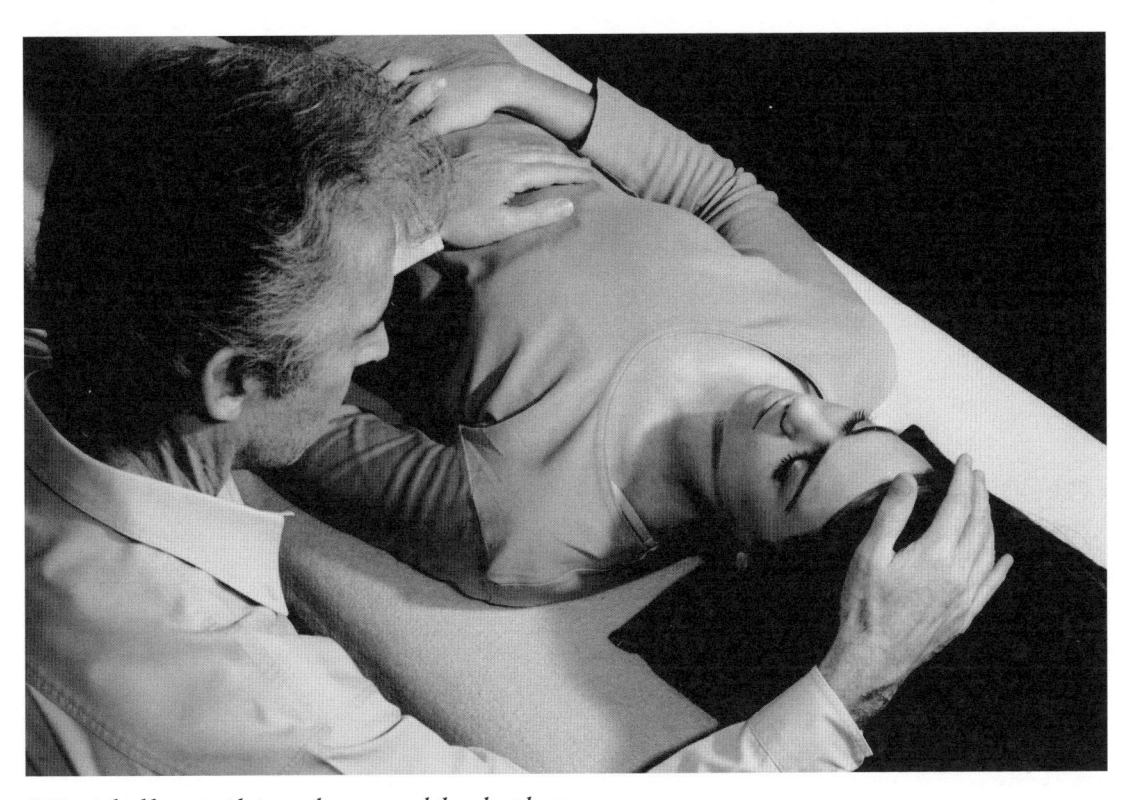

57.8 A double contact between the crown and the solar plexus

Further contacts for the sacrum

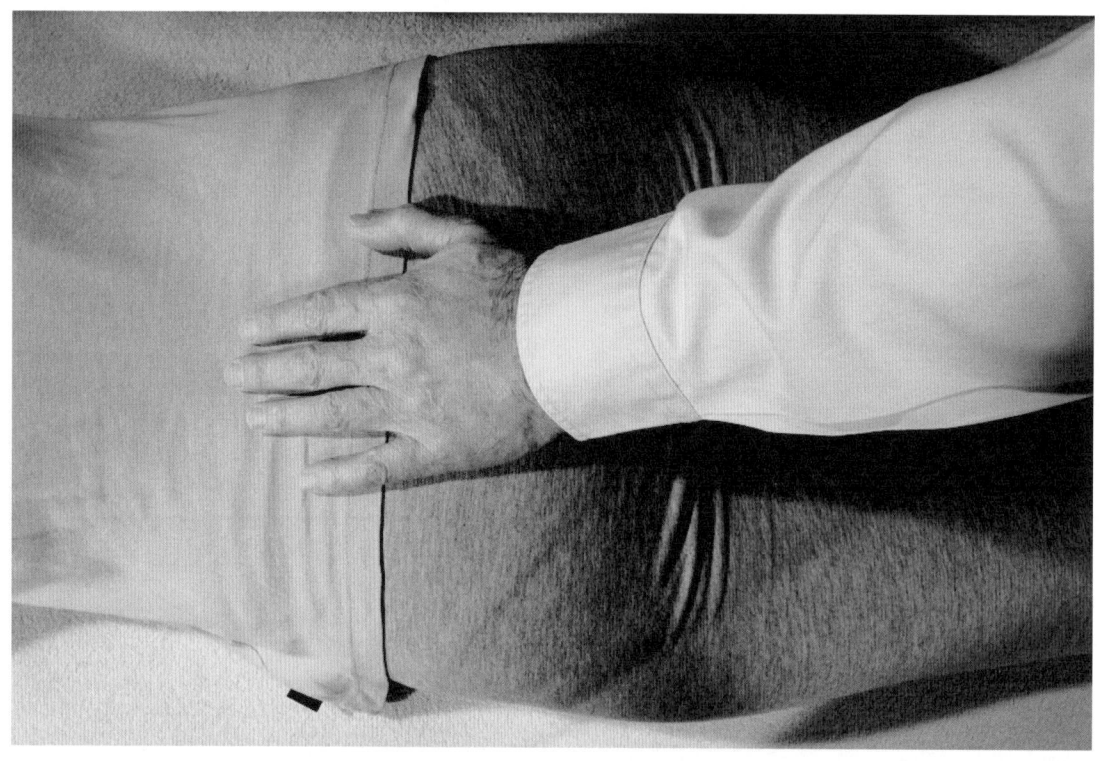

57.9 A contact on the sacrum in the prone position can gently allow the sacrum to release and bring the whole pelvis and spine (and consequently the whole system) into balance

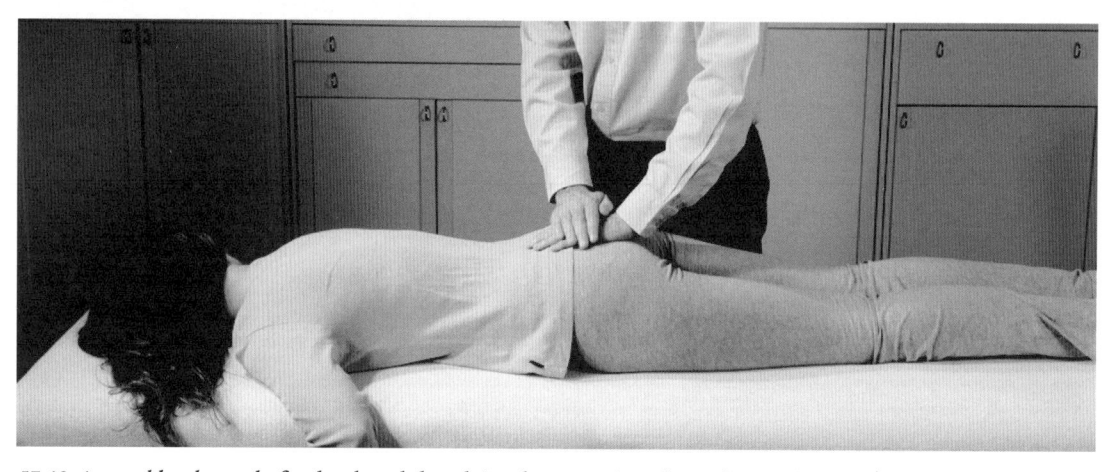

57.10 A second hand over the first hand can help to bring the sacrum into clearer focus and deeper release

Chapter 58

Diagnosis

Diagnosis has been an integral part of this book from the start, from the first mention of quality, through the identification of spheno-basilar patterns, to the piecing together of the whole picture. In Chapter 55 we touched on aspects of diagnosis including case history, symptom picture, observation, and palpation.

Diagnosis through palpation is an integral part of every moment of every cranio-sacral treatment, because everything that happens within the treatment process is a response to what you observe, a response to the conscious or unconscious diagnosis of the impressions under your hands.

Diagnosis includes identification of specific qualities, asymmetries and movements, assessment of the overall state, identification of specific fulcrums, and most of all diagnosis of the whole picture.

Levels of diagnosis

Diagnosis within the cranio-sacral process takes place on several different levels:

- Unconscious diagnosis of cranio-sacral patterns.
- Conscious diagnosis of cranio-sacral patterns.
- Specific diagnosis – interpreting cranio-sacral findings.
- Comprehensive diagnosis – describing the whole picture.

Unconscious diagnosis

In *unconscious diagnosis*, the hands are identifying and responding to patterns, enabling the whole cranio-sacral process to unfold, without necessarily ever being consciously identified or verbalised. This is a very substantial part of every moment of cranio-sacral treatment.

Conscious diagnosis

Conscious diagnosis of cranio-sacral patterns involves specific identification and description of the patterns emerging under the hands – qualities, asymmetries, focal points, levels of vitality, fluid drive, potency, whole body patterns, emotional states, specific membranous pulls, bony restrictions, facilitated segments, without necessarily relating them to specific causes or symptoms – just patterns within the cranio-sacral system. This specific identification influences the response and is therefore therapeutic in itself. It also provides a basis for more specific diagnosis.

Specific diagnosis

Specific diagnosis relates the patterns emerging within the cranio-sacral system to the symptoms, conditions, and history of the patient – identifying connections between areas of inertia and symptoms, between vertebral restrictions and visceral disturbances, between patterns of tension and accidents or injuries, between sites of emotional tension and the patient's experience, identifying chronicity, primary and secondary (or compensatory) patterns. It is based on interpretation of the cranio-sacral patterns.

Comprehensive diagnosis

Comprehensive diagnosis is an assessment of the overall picture of the patient, the total view of the whole person, physical, mental, emotional, spiritual, within the context of their life. It identifies the accumulation of everything that has happened to them throughout their life and is affecting them now and which has brought them to their present situation – as manifested through the cranio-sacral system. This picture can be formulated through piecing together the various aspects of the case history, observation, palpation and specific diagnosis.

Relevance of different levels of diagnosis

Significant therapeutic effect can be enabled simply through unconscious diagnosis – perhaps the most significant because this is allowing the inner wisdom of the body to determine the diagnosis and the treatment, which is the essence of cranio-sacral integration.

Other levels of diagnosis are, however, also useful:

- The conscious identification of cranio-sacral patterns enhances the therapeutic response through informed awareness.
- Specific diagnosis makes sense of the findings and provides an explanation for the patient, which in turn engenders confidence, which in turn contributes positively to the patient's response. It may also be significant in identifying pathologies which may need to be referred. It also helps to guide the overall treatment plan.
- Comprehensive diagnosis provides a clearer picture of the whole life situation, puts everything into perspective, and provides an understanding of timescales and prognosis, and plays a major part in establishing the overall treatment plan.

Informed awareness

As we have seen, when you diagnose a specific focal point of resistance, the fact of your attention being there alters the response. When you diagnose the specific tissues involved, it enhances the response. If you can diagnose the chronicity and the specific time fulcrum around which that restriction is revolving, that will further enhance the response. If you can gain a sense of the whole picture of the incident or circumstances that led to the patient's current situation, then the whole picture is more likely to change in response.

Variations in diagnosis

Diagnoses can vary substantially. They can be simple or complex. A diagnosis might identify one significant causative factor or may have a multitude of different components.

The diagnosis could be a specific physical injury. It could be a complex pattern of asymmetries and compensations throughout the body – perhaps revolving around one principal fulcrum.

It might involve the identification of an emotional basis underlying the patient's condition. It could be a reaction to a specific emotional event in the past – with multiple consequences. It could be a state of shock throughout the system.

It could be the identification of a severely traumatised system arising from a history of abuse as a child with all its ramifications on nature and personality and consequent physical and emotional tensions and symptoms and effects on social interactions and relationships.

It could be identifying the various physical and emotional reactions to a car accident – a restriction here, an imbalance there, a contraction there, shock throughout the system affecting responsiveness (maintaining the locked state and blocking healing) – all superimposed on previous patterns from earlier injuries and tensions.

It could be a birth pattern – both the physical forces and the shock element.

In most cases it will be the accumulation of factors throughout life leading to the present moment – the combination of birth, childhood, accidents, injuries, emotional tensions and traumas – all adding up to create the current situation with whatever symptoms or conditions may result.

In the final analysis, a comprehensive diagnosis within cranio-sacral integration is an assessment of the total picture of the whole person, the accumulation of everything that has happened to them throughout their life and which has brought them to their present situation – as manifested through the cranio-sacral system.

No point in treating

Understanding of the whole picture enables you to establish what level of treatment is appropriate. There is no point in treating a patient week after week on a physical level if the source of their discomfort is emotional and you are failing to identify and address that. Similarly, there is no point in treating a patient week after week if they are spending the rest of their week in a lifestyle that is destroying them – whether it be their work situation, their relationship, or their habit patterns. Cranio-sacral integration involves seeing the patient within the context of their life and helping them to understand and address their situation in so far as possible.

Differentiation

Patients may come to you with a variety of symptoms. It could be something as simple and common as a headache – but you need diagnosis to identify whether it is a life-threatening tumour of the brain (very rare), a transient tension in the neck (very common), or the result of being in a persistently stressful work situation which they resent – the treatment approach for each can be very different. It is not enough simply to engage with the cranio-sacral system.

A patient might arrive with multiple symptoms of palpitations, panic attacks, digestive disturbances, headaches – for which they have no explanation. They may have been given various medications for their assorted symptoms based on medical diagnosis, none of which are producing any lasting effect. A diagnosis of profound shock in their system (whether or not the original source of the shock is identified) and an appropriate cranio-sacral response to enable the release of that shock can be crucial to their recovery.

Diagnosis founded in knowledge of neurology can distinguish ulnar nerve symptoms from median nerve symptoms and potentially save a patient from an unnecessary operation for carpal tunnel syndrome (as described in Chapter 48).

Broad perspective

In cranio-sacral integration, we are looking at diagnosis from a broad perspective, including anything that might contribute to the picture. So cranio-sacral diagnosis can extend to factors beyond the immediate expressions of the cranio-sacral system:

Jim came to me with chronic pain in the right side of his neck and right shoulder. Looking at the whole picture, along with the case history and talking to him, my diagnosis was that he was spending most of his working day on the phone, with the phone tucked under his chin. I suggested that he buy a head set and his pain soon disappeared. To treat that patient week after week for chronic pain instead of diagnosing that simple factor would have been not only irrelevant and a waste of time and money for the patient, but also irresponsible.

Tanya had persistent pain in her left leg. Evaluating her situation I identified that she was sitting cross-legged in meditation every day with her left leg always folded inside the right leg. I suggested that she cross her legs the other way and her pain stopped.

I have mentioned previously (Chapter 12) the lady with the symptoms in her left arm arising from grief held in her heart. Diagnosis identified the fulcrum in her heart. Diagnosis identified the quality of grief held there. Diagnosis enabled engagement with that pattern and the consequent response.

You might identify a side-shifting pattern at the spheno-basilar synchondrosis. This is a diagnosis but what value does it have? If you merely see it in isolation, it is of little significance or value. You could use it to address that specific pattern at the SBS (in a biomechanical manner). You could also use that specific diagnosis to engage with the whole body pattern with its various fulcrums and primary source, as reflected through that particular window of the SBS, and this would enable a more comprehensive response. If you can diagnose the whole picture and the time fulcrum around which it revolves and the whole incident which led to it, the response will be most comprehensive. In this way diagnostic skills developed by exploration of SBS patterns are valuable.

You might find that the source of a patient's troubles is frustration with their life situation – their job, their marriage, their life.

I have seen many patients who wished to have a baby but were having difficulty conceiving. Most of them had had extensive (and often invasive) medical tests, usually culminating in various medical diagnoses such as blocked fallopian tubes or ovarian cysts. Cranio-sacral diagnosis was almost invariably different, and appropriate cranio-sacral treatment led to successful conception and birth. This is something we will explore further in a later volume.

An accurate diagnosis of birth trauma, identifying the typical signs and engaging with the appropriate time fulcrums again enables more effective transformation.

Fulcrums may also be located outside the body, in the external matrix, in the aura or beyond. This is not something unusual or esoteric. A car accident or a severe blow can create a fulcrum outside the body. If you are not aware of this possibility, you will probably fail to identify the fulcrum. Maintaining an awareness of this possibility enables accurate diagnosis of such fulcrums and consequent responses in the system.

For many patients, their physical symptoms might reflect autonomic nervous system (ANS) disturbance (one aspect of the diagnosis); this in turn might arise from stress (another aspect of diagnosis); this in turn might arise from their life situation (a further aspect of diagnosis). Effective cranio-sacral treatment can then be based on an understanding of the ANS, helping the patient to understand how stress leads to their symptoms through the ANS and how they can explore and alter their life circumstances to change their situation.

Most fundamentally, diagnosis includes an assessment of the underlying vitality and its potency. Inherent vitality lies at the source of all health, and identifying and addressing this fundamental factor is essential.

The whole picture

In cranio-sacral integration we are always looking to diagnose the whole person rather than any one specific cause. We may identify various specific factors that are relevant but these diagnoses are only made within the context of the whole. They are not made with a view to identifying a specific cause and fixing it, but rather towards integrating the whole person – because it is through integration that true health is obtained and maintained.

Diagnosis guides the treatment approach

Diagnosis guides us in how to approach treatment, identifying what stage of development the patient is at, what depth of treatment they are ready for. Depending on the diagnosis, different approaches might include:

- rapid resolution of a simple restriction and its associated symptoms
- addressing a transient superficial injury
- restoring balance following an accident
- releasing emotional holding
- referral elsewhere
- a need to talk
- settling and grounding
- physical body work
- working with breathing
- addressing profound trauma
- superficial settling
- general overall integration
- deeper engagement.

Dynamic diagnosis

Diagnosis also involves monitoring the response, the speed of response, and the reason for any lack of response or slow response. A cranio-sacral diagnosis is not absolute, it changes as the system progresses and reveals deeper layers, and cranio-sacral diagnosis is therefore all the more valid for being a dynamic diagnosis rather than a static fixed diagnosis.

Providing a diagnosis

With well-developed diagnostic skills, you could expect, by the end of the first session, to provide your patient with a diagnosis:

- what you have found, in terms of qualities, focal points, whole body patterns, chronicity of different fulcrums (not necessarily expressed in those terms) all adding up to provide a complete picture
- an explanation for their symptoms to which they can relate
- an explanation of how your findings relate to their history
- a treatment plan – including any other resources that might be helpful – together with a timescale
- a prognosis – together with a timescale.

Of course, not every detail will be clear and precise from the start. The diagnosis will evolve and progress over several sessions, as the system responds, changes and reveals deeper elements.

Diagnostic skills

Effective diagnosis and consequent effective responses from the cranio-sacral system arise from a secure foundation in diagnostic skills. These specific skills can only be developed through regular and consistent practice and application, until the process of diagnosis becomes second nature, intuitive and instinctive. Effective development of these skills requires not merely identification but also specific description, definition and refinement of definition, putting into words everything you identify. The process of putting it into words makes a substantial difference in identifying patterns more clearly and honing these diagnostic skills.

Engagement with inner wisdom through development of basic skills

In the final analysis, the most significant diagnosis is what the system in its wisdom identifies and reveals as the therapeutic process evolves – but your ability to engage with this inner wisdom is enabled through the consistent practice and development of comprehensive diagnostic skills.

As a means of practising and developing diagnostic skills, we will here present a practical exercise in diagnosis, while at the same time integrating intuitive and analytical levels of perception, energetic and tissue levels of the body, biodynamic and biomechanical levels of engagement.

A practical exercise in diagnosis – integrating intuitive and analytical levels of perception

In this practical we are seeking to further develop a balanced integration between engaging with the most subtle and profound levels of the whole matrix while at the same time understanding and assessing the detail within the anatomical structure – enhancing the underlying vitality of the system while at the same time identifying and addressing specific anatomical restrictions.

In this particular practical, we will work primarily through the sacrum, but the same principles could be applied to any contact. The intention is that each item should be specifically identified and defined, so that at the end of the session you can collate, write down and interpret your findings.

Take up contact at the *sacrum*, and establish engagement with the cranio-sacral system.

1. Initial impressions

a. Quality
- of the sacrum
- of the system as a whole

b. Mobility – free or restricted

c. Motion – expression of cranio-sacral motion – CSR, middle tide, long tide

d. Vitality – i.e. potency or fluid drive (e.g. powerful, feeble, strong, weak, fluent, contained, etc.).

Summarise your findings. Is the system, for example:

- strong on vitality, but tightly held, pent up, restricted
- soft, weak, feeble, lacking vitality
- full of vitality, but agitated, unsettled
- settled, with reasonable vitality, but asymmetrical?

2. Respond to individual circumstances

- If the system feels agitated, wait for calmness.
- If the system feels solid, wait for softening.
- If the system feels unbalanced, follow with your attention into any imbalances to points of stillness and release.

3. Symmetry of the sacrum

Maintaining engagement with the system and awareness of rhythmic motion:

- Define specifically any side-bending, rotation, or side-shift patterns in the sacrum (e.g. side-bent left or right, rotated left or right, side-shifted left or right).
- Define any preference or greater propensity towards flexion or extension of the sacrum or any combination of the above.

4. Identify the source of any restriction or imbalance

a. Is it:
- local (stuck, solid, immobile) – restricted locally
- remote (unbalanced but mobile and pliable) – pulled from elsewhere
- a combination of both?

b. Is it:
- a bony/joint restriction (hard, solid) – e.g. sacro-iliac restriction
- a soft tissue restriction (softer, more pliable) – e.g.
  - membranous pulls from the spinal dura
  - muscular pulls from the pelvic muscles
  - fascial pulls from elsewhere in the body?

c. Is it:
- chronic – resistant, unresponsive, solidified, deeply set
- acute – reactive, responsive, dynamic, active, agitated, vibrant?

(Notice that local, bony, and chronic can all feel more solid, whereas remote, soft tissue, and acute can all feel more soft and mobile – so you need to distinguish whether a sense of solidity is due to a local cause, a bony cause, a chronic cause, or a combination of all three. This is a skill which can develop steadily through practice and experience, and which is greatly helped by giving constant detailed attention to the essential concept of quality.)

d. Identify the specific location:
- follow with your attention into any pulls, twists or turns – to focal points
- project through the spine and through the body
  - to identify specific areas of restriction, solidity, intensity
  - to identify focal points

e. Evaluate any generalised causes of restriction:
- emotional holding – locally in the pelvic area or throughout the whole body
- systemic conditions (e.g. rheumatoid arthritis, multiple sclerosis).

Using the above observations, define the nature and location of the source or any imbalances, restrictions or focal points, as monitored from the sacrum.

5. Address the source

It is helpful to address local restrictions before addressing remote restrictions. So if you encounter any local restrictions at the sacrum, you could address them through sacro-iliac release and lumbo-sacral release.

With the sacrum free, you may find yourself spontaneously drawn to focal points elsewhere in the system, or you could project your attention to the source.

You might choose to introduce double contacts at any focal points that you encounter:
- feeling the response in each hand and between the two hands
- following the system to extremes of motion
- reaching points of stillness and release.

The exact way in which this occurs will vary according to the nature of the situation, but is essentially likely to involve engaging with the inherent treatment process.

If the system is not drawn spontaneously into points of stillness and release, or if you encounter particularly resistant restrictions, you might enhance its potential to do so by inviting the system to draw into the extreme of motion in the expansion phase (i.e. following the sacrum consistently into flexion).

The process could involve following through a series of focal points, settling through release and reorganisation into a neutral state between each stage.

6. Integrate the core of the system

Take up a *sacrum-crown* contact (one hand at the coccyx, the other hand over the frontal area):
- establishing a circuit of energy
- working with rhythmic waves of motion up and down the spine, following into extremes as appropriate

- surveying the spine from bottom to top and top to bottom, identifying any remaining focal points or pivots
- enhancing rhythmic motion.

7. Re-evaluate and enhance the fundamental vitality

The sense of vitality is likely to be revealed more clearly as restrictions are released and the system becomes more fluent.

The vitality can be enhanced by stimulating the motion:

- simply following the rhythmic motion with your attention
- rocking – enhancing the amplitude of rhythmic motion at each extreme
- following into the extremes of motion to points of stillness and release
- settling into long tide and dynamic stillness.

8. Completion

Following release and reorganisation, or a series of releases and reorganisations, as the system settles into a balanced neutral state:

- re-evaluate quality, symmetry, motion
- re-evaluate vitality
- stay with the system for a few cycles of easeful, settled, rhythmic motion, maintaining a centred balanced quality in yourself
- check that everything feels settled, balanced and complete.

Part IX
An Integrated Treatment Approach

Chapter 59

An Integrated Treatment Approach

Having established a fundamental understanding of the cranio-sacral process, developed some basic skills, outlined a framework for treatment, and added various other resources, we can now look at how all this fits together to form an integrated treatment approach.

The essential components of cranio-sacral integration are:
- Practitioner presence.
- Engagement.
- Patient grounding – settling superficial disturbances.
- Following the process through to deeper levels of engagement.
- Bringing the process to satisfactory completion.

Variations
A flexible framework
The broad four-stage treatment framework presented throughout this book:
- Tuning in (engagement)
- Opening up (settling and grounding)
- Core treatment
- Completion

provides a valuable context for all cranio-sacral treatment, but it is of course infinitely adaptable according to the individual needs of the patient. Patients arrive at different levels of development, and with different levels of previous cranio-sacral treatment. Some patients may need a whole session, or several sessions, of settling, grounding, opening up; they may need attention to their breathing; they may need to talk; others are already open to immediate access to deeper engagement with the core, so treatment sessions can take on very different forms accordingly.

Variations according to the patient's previous experience of cranio-sacral therapy
Patients who are unsettled or new to cranio-sacral integration are more likely to need superficial settling, involving the release and integration of multiple patterns throughout the whole system, rather than an immediate focus on one fulcrum or on deeper levels. This is likely to help them with settling and grounding and in feeling more comfortable. However, some patients coming for their first cranio-sacral treatment may be naturally settled and open, or may have received other forms of therapy, which may (or may not) have enabled a more settled state.

Patients who are settled, or who you have treated several times, or who have already received effective cranio-sacral integration, are likely to be able to move more readily into engagement with deeper patterns, moving through middle tide levels to long tide and dynamic stillness. It is worth bearing in mind, however, that patients may have received substantial previous cranio-sacral therapy – but only on certain levels. Significant aspects may have been neglected, so it is always necessary to make your own assessment. Commonly neglected areas (depending on the nature of any previous treatment) include: the emotional centres and the emotions; the suboccipital region; fascial unwinding; more profound engagement with deeper levels; breathing; grounding; talking; lifestyle.

Variation in time spent on each stage of a treatment
The amount of time spent on each stage of a treatment may vary substantially according to the state and needs of the patient:
- Engagement can happen instantly or take time.

- Settling and grounding may need a great deal of time in a patient who is unsettled, or it may be possible to progress immediately to engagement with deeper levels.
- Core treatment might generally be expected to be the most substantial part of the treatment, but if a patient is unsettled you might not even get to that stage at all.
- Completion can happen naturally, or may need time at the end of the session to ensure resolution.

Variation in time spent at each contact
The time spent at each contact is similarly infinitely adaptable. You may:
- use very few contacts, or several
- feel an immediate resolution and move on
- engage through a particular contact and feel that that area doesn't need attention at present
- remain engaged with a particular contact at great length, either because it is an area of chronic restriction that needs longer time to release, or because you have entered into deeper engagement.

However, it is always preferable to keep in mind the overall balance of the treatment session, rather than becoming too engrossed with one particular area, however significant, otherwise the treatment can be un-integrated and the patient can be left unbalanced and incomplete.

Variation in hand position
Within any contact, the hand position can be adapted to suit the needs of the moment:

As you contact the heart centre, you might be drawn to the heart, the pericardium, the lungs, the upper thoracic spine from which sympathetic nerve supply to these viscera emanates, or to an old fracture of the clavicle, or a chronic shoulder injury, or any other fulcrum of resistance – so you can adapt your hand position accordingly, moving your upper hand to the focal point of restriction, or moving your upper hand to a shoulder, as in the rhomboid contact.

Similarly at the solar plexus, you might be drawn to the liver on the right, the stomach on the left, an adrenal gland, a kidney, the diaphragm, the coeliac ganglia, or you might be drawn to a focal point or inertial fulcrum further up or down the body. So you can adapt your hand position accordingly – particularly your upper hand. The lower hand, because of its contact with the spine, plays an important anchoring role, in touch with the nerve centres and energy centres of the midline – but it may be appropriate to move the lower hand as well.

Similarly at the pelvis, you may be drawn to a sacro-iliac restriction, a lumbo-sacral restriction, a piriformis muscle contraction, the colon, the uterus, a focus of inertia around an ovary. So you can adapt accordingly, or you might introduce a double contact anywhere up the spine.

While engaging at the cranium, you can similarly adapt your hand positions according to the needs of the moment and the fulcrums that arise.

You don't necessarily need to move your hand to a focal point. In many cases, it may well be enough simply to let your focus of attention be drawn to the focal point of restriction – while still maintaining a broader perspective on the whole picture at all times.

With increasing experience and diagnostic skill, standard hand positions become less significant and you will let your hands be drawn to wherever is appropriate for the needs of the moment.

Overview
A well-integrated treatment will involve a fluent evolution – not four separate stages, but a continuous flow – with the various stages blending into each other – *tuning in*, flowing into *opening up*, deepening into *core treatment* and reaching its natural *completion*.

Develop and maintain an overall view of the whole person from the start. It is helpful to build a complete picture first, rather than jumping into the first significant fulcrum that draws your attention; and to ensure that the system is settled before progressing to deeper levels or specific focal points.

Tuning in

You can tune in anywhere. The feet provide a valuable perspective on the whole person and are also a non-invasive place to start. You can equally tune in elsewhere – heart, solar plexus, sacrum, shoulders, cranium – particularly with a patient whose system you already know, but it is generally preferable to establish connection through a less profound contact such as the shoulders or feet before entering into a deeper contact such as the sphenoid.

Opening up

Opening up is vital – it is very therapeutic in itself, it assists settling and grounding, it helps in gaining access to deeper levels, as already emphasised.

If the emotional centres are not addressed where necessary, they may block the progress of the treatment process, preventing access to deeper levels, or the emotions may erupt unpredictably.

Opening up also provides valuable insight into the overall picture – the emotional state, the tensions held in the heart, lungs, diaphragm, solar plexus, viscera, pelvic diaphragm, or pelvic organs, acknowledgement of the whole trunk area. It is not generally helpful to try to progress to core treatment and deeper engagement without addressing this level when it is needed. It is essential to devote appropriate time to this level as necessary. Also, take care not to be fooled by appearances with regard to settledness and groundedness. Be guided by what you feel within the system, rather than necessarily trusting what the patient presents outwardly.

Core contacts

Certain core contacts are generally experienced as being more significant than others.

Sacrum

- Its free mobility is fundamental to the free and potent expression of vitality through the whole system.
- It is a powerhouse of cranio-sacral potency.
- It is one of the principal avenues of access to the spine, the midline, and the deepest core of the system.
- It is often used in conjunction with various double contacts.

Subocciput

- Its free mobility is again essential to the free flow of vitality through the rest of the system.
- Failure to address a restricted subocciput can block progress on all other levels (particularly any other work on the cranium) and is a potential cause of uncomfortable side-effects in response to other contacts, which may be unable to resolve satisfactorily due to restriction at the subocciput.

Cranium

- Each therapist will develop their own preferred contacts, but certain contacts are commonly found to be most effective in engaging deeply with the core, notably:
  - Mastoid tip contact.
  - Falx contact.
  - Sphenoid (in particular).
  - Temporals.
- There is also a natural fluent progression from subocciput through mastoid tips through falx to sphenoid and temporals.

Core treatment might be expected to be the deepest part of the treatment and this may often be the case. However, it is preferable not to be too single-mindedly focused on deep treatment. Deepest isn't necessarily best.

Responding to the patient at the appropriate level for their particular needs at that moment is more relevant and significant. Also, extremely profound responses can arise from addressing other levels such as the emotional centres, opening up the system, or fascial unwinding.

Clinical choices

Within the context of this framework, there will inevitably be a variety of specific responses to individual circumstances. These could include being drawn to a different part of the body, adapting a hand position, working at the throat, introducing fascial unwinding as appropriate, introducing a further specific contact as appropriate, exploring the system through the spheno-basilar patterns, or any other variation.

If, as you work at the heart centre, you are drawn to an old shoulder injury, you might not only adapt your contact to address the shoulder as described above, but also decide that it would be helpful to introduce fascial unwinding of the shoulder and arm.

You have clinical choices to make here: Do you enter into that now or later? Do you have a sufficiently comprehensive view of the whole picture to make an informed decision? Does the system feel ready? Is the patient sufficiently settled, relaxed and open:

- to respond positively to fascial unwinding of the arm at this point
- to avoid stirring up treatment reactions.

Every patient will respond more profoundly to cranio-sacral treatment when they are relaxed and open.

For example, a patient might have a tight left arm and shoulder, which feel as if they could benefit from fascial unwinding. But that tightness might be related to grief following a bereavement. If you move into fascial unwinding too quickly or too soon, then either it may not be responsive, or that grief might erupt in a manner that could be alarming for the patient if they are not ready. If, on the other hand, you take the time to explore the whole picture, recognise the underlying emotion through the quality of the system, and take time to establish a firmer grounding – then the unwinding of the arm may help the patient greatly in enabling the release of grief and the physical tensions and symptoms associated with that grief – in a calm, quiet manageable manner – and the patient is likely to feel a great sense of relief and resolution, calmness and lightness, having shifted that burden of grief that was weighing heavily upon them.

So adapt accordingly, moving into an arm unwinding if the whole picture suggests that it is appropriate, or making a mental note to come back to it later in the treatment, once the system is more settled and open, or in a subsequent session.

Similarly, as you work at the pelvis, a similar scenario might develop. You might sense that a hip or knee injury or compressive injury up one leg is impinging into the pelvis and restricting mobility. Again, you make a clinical choice. If the hip or knee restriction is significantly affecting the pelvis and the ability of the system to respond, it may be appropriate to address that now, through fascial unwinding of the lower limb, in order to enable a greater degree of freedom and mobility in the pelvis and sacrum, and consequent deeper transition into core treatment. Alternatively, you might decide that a greater degree of overall balance of the pelvis and of the system as a whole needs to be established before the body can respond effectively to the leg unwinding.

Similarly at the subocciput, as you settle into a suboccipital release, you might feel that the neck wishes to move into a fascial unwinding process. This can arise spontaneously and may be very appropriate and you can allow the process to flow fluently from one to the other, from suboccipital release into fascial unwinding of the neck without interruption, maintaining contact with the subocciput even as you allow the unwinding, and then settling into the suboccipital release again once the unwinding has reached completion.

But again you need to make a clinical choice. Is this appropriate at this point in the treatment or would maintaining focus on the suboccipital release be more suitable? Both scenarios can be appropriate in the right circumstances. You need to evaluate from your understanding of the whole picture, which option is most appropriate for this patient at this moment within the context of the optimum progress of the treatment session.

In some cases, the unwinding process is the best option as it clears superficial tensions, releases patterns of trauma and holding in the muscles and fascia of the neck, and opens the way to a much deeper and more effective suboccipital release, with consequent deepening of the whole subsequent treatment. Unwinding of the neck can often bring about a deep sense of release, physically and emotionally, not only locally in the neck but throughout the whole system, so it may also help the patient to settle into a more comfortable and relaxed state, which can again deepen the whole subsequent treatment.

At other times, particularly if the system repeatedly enters into unwinding whenever you approach the suboccipital area, and where the neck has already been through unwinding previously or doesn't particularly need unwinding, then the unwinding can be an avoidance, a way of avoiding engaging with deeper elements of the therapeutic process, conscious or unconscious; and in such cases it may be more productive to discourage the unwinding and maintain focus on the suboccipital release and whatever arises from engaging more deeply with that crucial area.

Total integration

Within all of this, throughout every moment of each treatment, you can be maintaining your awareness of the whole picture and all the elements that contribute to that picture. This will involve incorporating into the picture your understanding of the nervous system, the autonomic nervous system, vertebral levels, visceral associations, spinal mechanics, emotional relations, time fulcrums, and many other resources – and seeing how they all fit together.

So as you treat each patient, you can maintain awareness of:

- the overall *quality* of the whole person, the local qualities in different areas, and what these tell you about the state of the patient
- the underlying level of *vitality*
- *sites* of injury, consequences of trauma
- *focal points* of resistance anywhere in the matrix
- the *emotional state* and emotional holding in particular areas
- the *overall balance* of the body – structurally, posturally, fascially, energetically
- *whole body patterns*
- focal points, fulcrums, the *neurological significance* of these, the visceral significance
- the *interactions* of viscera, vertebral levels, emotional factors, and facilitated segments.

You can gain an overall perspective, seeing how all this fits in with the patient's case history:

- injuries, illness, operations, car accidents, falls
- periods of stress, traumatic events, birth, childhood, giving birth
- the chronicity of different focal points, identified through the use of time fulcrums
- recognising primary and secondary fulcrums, adaptations and compensations

- identifying the root source, the underlying factors and the various interactions on every level
- making sense of all the different elements and interweaving strands
- putting the whole picture together.

This is not merely for intellectual diagnosis; its principal value is that through recognising the picture and focusing your informed awareness on the whole picture, you can enhance the therapeutic process. The cranio-sacral process is guided primarily by the inherent forces within the body under the influence of the subtle forces of nature around us, but your presence and your informed awareness play a significant role in enabling this process.

You can be aware of:

- bones, membranes, fluids, energy
- tissue levels, cellular levels, molecular levels, subatomic levels
- the whole person
- the whole energy field
- the whole energetic matrix – internal and external
- cranio-sacral rhythm, middle tide, long tide, dynamic stillness
- settling into deeper and deeper absorption.

It is impossible to describe a typical treatment, since there is no standard format, and each patient's needs are different, and so much will vary according to the patient's state and previous experience, but it may at least be helpful for beginners to set out an example of a possible initial treatment.

Sample initial treatment

Establish your own practitioner fulcrums. *Engage* wherever it feels comfortable to do so:

- The feet are a good place for initial engagement, but you can also engage elsewhere.
- Allow the process of engagement to develop in its own time, allowing whatever time it takes:

- which might be immediate, or might take several minutes, or longer
  - or might need some other resource or approach such as talking, or attention to breathing in order to facilitate engagement.
- Allow the superficial expressions of disturbance to resolve and settle into whatever level of engagement is appropriate for the patient at that moment.

Settle and ground the patient as necessary, depending on the patient's state. This will most probably involve working at the emotional centres, perhaps combined with attention to breathing:

- Take up contact at the emotional centres as appropriate:
  - whether at each individual centre
  - or perhaps using a combined heart and solar plexus contact.
- Adapt your hand positions as necessary, branching off to other fulcrums according to demands.
- Allow whatever time is necessary at each emotional centre and on the opening up process as a whole – which could be no time at all, or the whole session.
- At each contact, and as you progress through the different contacts, feel the system progressing to greater settledness and deeper engagement.

Core treatment

Once settled (this could be instantly, or the patient may need time):

- Allow the treatment process to evolve naturally:
  - through a smooth transition to deeper engagement with the core
  - moving fluently into contact with the sacrum.

SACRUM

Assess the state of this crucial area, enhancing release as necessary through various contacts – sacro-iliac, a single ilium, lumbo-sacral. As always, the sacrum may need attention, or may not. Once the sacrum is settled and freely mobile, move on to deeper engagement with the core – perhaps simply through your contact at the sacrum, or perhaps introducing double contacts as appropriate, adapting to the needs of the patient. Allow whatever time is necessary, perhaps staying at the sacrum for a long time, settling into greater depth, or perhaps incorporating a sacrum-cranium contact. This can be a particularly significant part of the treatment, remaining at the sacrum for a considerable time, settling into deep engagement with the long tide, subtle integration and dynamic stillness.

Whatever may be happening at the sacrum, it is generally a good idea within every treatment session to check and integrate the cranium as well, not getting so caught up in the response at the sacrum, or with some deeply ingrained pattern, that you lose sight of the overall integration of the patient and neglect the cranium, potentially leaving the system as a whole un-integrated, which can potentially leave the patient unsettled and with disturbance both in the head and elsewhere.

SUBOCCIPUT

Check this crucial area and address it as necessary – it may need attention, it may not (it usually does). Allow whatever time is necessary, which may be none at all. Treatment may involve releasing transient superficial tensions; addressing deeply ingrained patterns of trauma and restriction, allowing the system to branch off as necessary; and may develop into a neck unwinding, or adapting your contact according to demands.

CRANIUM

Continue to settle into deeper engagement. Continue to engage with the core through whatever cranial contacts may be appropriate for the individual needs of the patient, perhaps identifying one particularly relevant contact, or perhaps following the fluent natural evolution through the powerful contacts of the mastoid tip contact, the falx release, the sphenoid, the temporals. Allow time for deeper and deeper engagement – stay with each contact for long enough to settle into subtle integration, long tide, dynamic stillness. In an unsettled system which has not received much cranio-sacral treatment, it may be preferable to use several different contacts, in order to address the various different disturbances. In a more settled system which has received more previous treatments, it may be more productive to settle into one contact at great length, settling deeply into subtle integration and dynamic stillness.

Completion
Completion will usually occur naturally, but be sure to check for proper resolution, allowing adequate time for a suitably settled conclusion.

Subsequent treatments
As mentioned, there is no standard format, this is just an example.

We can appreciate the value of keeping in mind the four-stage treatment framework that we have established, acknowledging when specific aspects of the framework are necessary for particular individuals and when they may be redundant. Within that context, there is infinite scope for adapting the treatment to the circumstances.

With a new patient, it might be appropriate to check through the whole system more systematically, addressing a multitude of disturbances, spending more time resolving superficial disturbances and settling the patient.

With subsequent treatments, you might engage more readily with deeper levels – as the patient's system becomes more amenable, and as you get to know their system better.

Subsequent treatments might therefore be very different:

- A treatment session might consist entirely of one contact at the head.
- It might involve just two or three contacts.
- It might involve moving immediately to deeper engagement with the core.
- It might involve many different resources.

It can take any number of different forms depending on the state and circumstances of the patient. It is a matter of finding the appropriate level and means of engagement for each patient at that particular moment and following the process through to satisfactory integration and completion.

Summary
Cranio-sacral integration is a fluent, continuous evolution, from whatever starting point may be appropriate, helping the patient to settle into deeper engagement by whatever means are suitable, progressing steadily through to the deepest levels of engagement that are possible within the circumstances, to enable the most profound healing and integration.

Part X
Conclusion

Chapter 60

Cranio-Sacral Integration
A Summary

Foundation

This book is subtitled 'Foundation'. It provides a fundamental understanding and an overall treatment approach. It builds a firm grounding in basic skills and the informed awareness that they engender, from which we can move on to develop an increasingly fluent and spontaneous approach and consequent more subtle and profound engagement. It constitutes a small initial part of a complete training in cranio-sacral integration, from which we can then move forward to explore in many directions:

- deeper engagement and understanding
- deeper exploration of the underlying concepts
- specialised areas of treatment
- specific clinical application
- deeper emotional release
- more profound personal and spiritual development.

A basis for further exploration

Subsequent volumes will provide a basis for this exploration:

Volume 2, *Face to Face with the Face*, will explore the face – the ears, nose and throat, the jaw, dentistry and the many other fascinating facets of the face – together with the cranial nerves which supply those areas and which also supply and affect the whole person.

Volume 3, *Birth, Babies, Children, Mothers, Fathers*, will explore a comprehensive and practical approach to treating babies and children – a fascinating and rewarding area with far-reaching consequences for those individuals fortunate enough to receive cranio-sacral integration at an early age, along with the often neglected areas of looking after mothers before, during and after childbirth – and not forgetting fathers.

In this volume we will also explore the birth process in depth – a process which affects us all profoundly in one way or another, an understanding of which is vital to the understanding of every one of us, child or adult, determining the progression of our lives, with huge possibilities for transformation.

Volume 4, *The Psycho-Neuro-Immuno-Viscero-Endocrine System*, will explore the complex interactions of these various intertwining systems which epitomise the understanding of whole body integration.

Volume 5, *Trauma*, will explore the highly significant subject of trauma, which again affects every one of us, whether through birth trauma, the accumulation of minor traumas throughout life, or the more dramatic traumas suffered by so many people – from sexual abuse, childhood abuse, rape, car accidents, major injuries, war, post-traumatic stress disorder and so many other factors. We will discover how cranio-sacral integration, with its profound understanding of whole person dynamics and engagement with the deepest levels of being, can provide the conditions and resources to address such profoundly disturbing experiences and the lifelong patterns and habits which they often engender, enabling the restoration of a balanced and harmonious state.

Training

A training in cranio-sacral integration is not a matter of reading a book, nor a matter of technique or method. It is a profound process of personal transformation, involving substantial practical experience, extensive therapeutic interaction with other aspiring cranio-sacral therapists, the practical guidance and insight of experienced cranio-sacral therapists, clinical experience in the irreplaceable environment of a teaching clinic, and commitment to one's own continuing process of treatment and personal development, in order to develop an appropriate practitioner presence.

Professional practice

Working with cranio-sacral integration can be a beautiful journey – not only helping others to feel better and often transforming their lives, but also spending your own life in a state of peace and tranquillity, giving constant attention to your own state of ease, balance and comfort, in order to help others more effectively. It can be a peaceful and deeply satisfying way to live your life.

Practical applications of cranio-sacral integration

We defined the cranio-sacral system earlier in the book as 'the whole person within the context of their lives'. Cranio-sacral integration addresses not only the cranio-sacral patterns that arise within the body, but everything about the person. Cranio-sacral integration is a profound therapeutic process. It brings together the whole spectrum of cranio-sacral approaches in order to respond most appropriately to each patient's needs. It is effective in many different situations, from all the common aches, pains and conditions encountered in everyday clinical practice, through severe physical and emotional trauma, through to the deepest levels of personal and spiritual development.

Overview

Through this foundation, we hope that you have gained a glimpse of the potential, and as we come to the end of this volume, we will finish with a succinct summary of the key concepts underlying cranio-sacral integration:

- There is a universal matrix which unifies all matter.
- Our own personal individual matrix is a small part within that wider matrix.
- There are forces of nature flowing through the universal matrix which influence our personal individual matrix, determining the natural process of growth, development, health, healing, balance and integration.
- By engaging with these forces we can enhance their potency.
- In order to engage with these forces we need to establish our own calm, quiet presence, simply being there in stillness.
- In order to enable the patient's maximum responsiveness, we need to establish a settled, grounded and receptive state in the patient.
- Through establishing appropriate levels of contact, attention and tissue awareness, we can engage with the subtle quantum levels of being which constitute the matrix.
- These will manifest as quality, symmetry and motion.
- The therapeutic process will be guided by the inherent forces within the matrix.
- This process will be enhanced by the therapist's presence and informed awareness.
- By settling into profound stillness, we can connect with deeper levels of consciousness.
- Through this profound stillness we can engage with the most profound levels of being.
- This can lead us to the deepest levels of healing.

Glossary

Words in ***bold italics*** are terms which are not generally used in this book, but may be useful in understanding other texts, bearing in mind that these words may be used differently by different sources.

Acute

(a) A recent or currently active injury or condition.

(b) An angle of less than 90 degrees.

Anatomical position A position of reference, in which the patient is assumed to be standing upright with the palms of the hands facing forwards and the toes pointing forwards. Whatever position the patient may actually be in (lying, sitting, standing, etc.), all positional and directional terms refer to the patient as if he or she were in the anatomical position.

Anatomy The structure of the body.

ANS The autonomic nervous system.

Ansa cervicalis A nerve loop in the neck, giving off branches to the muscles of the throat.

Anterior In front of, forwards, at or towards the front of the body.

Arachnoid villi Protrusions of arachnoid membrane through the dura of the venous sinuses, through which cerebrospinal fluid can return to the venous blood.

Articulation

(a) The active mobilisation of joints and their associated tissues by a therapist.

b) A joint.

Asking the system

(a) Asking questions of the body to see what response arises.

(b) Asking questions of yourself to assess more precisely what you are feeling.

Asterion The meeting point of the squamosal, lamdoid and occipito-mastoid sutures, and the junction between the occipital, temporal and parietal bones. It is located behind the ear on each side of the cranium.

Augmentation Adding input to a process which is already happening.

Automatic shift A release arising from within the cranio-sacral system.

Autonomic nervous system The part of the nervous system which regulates involuntary functions such as digestion, heartbeat, pupil constriction and dilation.

Aura The energy field or force field that surrounds, envelops and includes the body. Its innermost layer is the etheric body.

Axon A nerve fibre.

Bilateral On both sides of the body.

Breath of Life The natural force which pervades all living things, generating vitality or aliveness. It is expressed in the body as rhythmic motion on various levels, and determines the orderly progression of life, growth, development, health and healing.

Bregma The meeting point between the sagittal and coronal sutures, located at the top of the head between the frontal and parietal bones. This is the site of the anterior fontanelle (soft spot) in a baby.

Caudad Towards the patient's tail.

Cephalad Towards the patient's head.

Cerebrospinal fluid The pure fluid which surrounds and bathes the central nervous system.

Chakras Energy centres located in certain midline areas of the body.

Choroid plexi The vascular structures in the ventricles of the brain, where cerebrospinal fluid is produced.

Chronic Long established (e.g. a long-established condition).

Chronicity The length of time that something has existed.

Circumduction A circular movement or articulation, particularly of an arm or leg or around a joint.

Cisterna A site of accumulation of cerebrospinal fluid within the subarachnoid space (e.g. cisterna magna, lumbar cistern).

Cisternae Plural of cisterna.

CNS The central nervous system.

Coherence Operating as a unified whole.

Compression Pushed together by external forces.

Contraction Drawn together by internal forces.

Coronal Passing across the body from one side to the other (e.g. the coronal suture).

Coronal section A view of the body as if sliced vertically through the body from one side to the other.

Cranium The bony skull.

Cranial base The base of the skull, formed primarily by the occiput and sphenoid.

Cranial vault The upper part of the cranium, in contrast to the cranial base.

Cranio-sacral motion The rhythmic movement of the cranio-sacral system at various different rates, including cranio-sacral rhythm, middle tide, long tide.

Cranial rhythmic impulse (CRI) The cranio-sacral rhythm – also used by some sources to indicate all levels of cranio-sacral motion.

Cranio-sacral system

(a) The whole person – mind, body and spirit – within the context of their life.

(b) The anatomical components (bones, membranes, fluids and fascia) which constitute the anatomical cranio-sacral system.

CSF Cerebrospinal fluid.

CV4 Compression of the fourth ventricle – a process for helping the system to reach a still point in the contraction phase.

Decompression Release from compression.

Directing the tide Energy drive.

Dorsal Posterior, at the back, on or towards the back of the body.

Dorsum (of the feet) The upper (superior) surface of the feet.

Dorsiflexion Upward movement of the front of the foot (toes towards the shin).

Dura The outer layer of the three membranes surrounding the brain and spinal cord. The dura itself comprises two layers:

- endosteal dura: the outer layer of dura lining the bones and enveloping the cranial bones
- meningeal dura: the inner lining of dura enveloping the brain and spinal cord.

Dynamic stillness

(a) A point of stillness preceding a release, within which subtle dynamic movements such as vibrations, wriggling, or pulsation may be felt.

(b) A profound level of therapeutic stillness where everything becomes still – the deepest phase of the therapeutic process.

Endosteum The outer layer of dura lining the bones of the cranium and vertebral column.

Energy drive A process for focusing the body's therapeutic forces at a particular fulcrum.

Entrainment The phenomenon by which separate elements come into unified operation when in close proximity, e.g. the pendulums of grandfather clocks, cardiac cells pulsating in unison, cicadas chirping together, cranio-sacral rhythms operating in harmony, energy fields intertwining and interacting.

Ependyma The thin pia-like membrane which lines the ventricles.

Equanimity A state of mental, emotional and spiritual balance.

Etheric body The innermost layer of the aura or energy field surrounding the body.

Exhalation The contraction phase of cranio-sacral motion.

Extension

(a) The movement of midline structures during the contraction phase of cranio-sacral motion.

(b) The movement of the whole system during the contraction phase of cranio-sacral motion.

(c) Opening an angle, e.g. extending (straightening) the elbow.

Extension phase The contraction phase of cranio-sacral motion.

External Rotation

(a) The movement of bilateral structures and the body as a whole during the expansion phase of cranio-sacral motion.

(b) In the feet – turning the front of the foot outwards.

Eversion In the feet – turning the sole of the foot outwards.

EV4 Expansion of the fourth ventricle.

A process for helping the system to reach a still point in the expansion phase.

Facial Relating to the face.

Fascia The thin interconnected connective tissue which envelops everything in the body – surrounding bones, muscles, nerves, blood vessels, organs.

Fascial Relating to the fascia.

Fibrosis The hardening and excessive formation of fibrous tissues.

Flexion

(a) The movement of midline structures during the expansion phase of cranio-sacral motion.

(b) The movement of the whole system during the expansion phase of cranio-sacral motion.

(c) Closing an angle, e.g. flexing (bending) the elbow.

Flexion phase The expansion phase of cranio-sacral motion.

Fluid body The individual matrix, comprising the physical body and its surrounding energy field.

Fluids The various fluids of the body – blood, lymph, CSF, extracellular fluid, etc.

Fluids A term used for vital energy.

Fluid within the fluid Vital energy within the system, potency, life force within the body.

Fluid drive The strength and power of the underlying vitality, potency, the strength of rhythmic motion.

Foramen A hole within a bone or between bones.

Foramen magnum The large hole at the base of the skull, through which the spinal cord passes up to meet the brainstem and brain.

Foramina Holes, plural of foramen.

Fossa A dip, or shallow indentation in a bone, of variable shapes and sizes. (Latin for 'ditch'.)

Fulcrum A pivotal point around which a system operates, including:

- mechanical fulcrums
- mental and emotional fulcrums
- focal points of resistance around which movement revolves
- practitioner fulcrums – the state of physical, mental and emotional balance from which a practitioner operates.

Fulcra Plural of fulcrum.

Fundamental principles The natural series of stages through which the therapeutic response evolves during the cranio-sacral process.

The orderly process through which the cranio-sacral system enables therapeutic response.

The components which comprise the inherent treatment process.

Ganglion
 (a) A site of nerve junctions, at which neurological messages are passed from one neuron to another.
 (b) A fluid-filled lump on a tendon, most commonly found in the hand or wrist.

Health, The The underlying vitality; the inherent potential for health; the way that the life force is expressed within the individual.

Homeostasis A state of dynamic balance, constantly adapting in response to the environment.

Inertia Lack of movement.

Inertial fulcrum A focal point of restriction where rhythmic motion is limited.

Inferior Below, downwards, towards the soles of the patient's feet.

Informed awareness Awareness of, and engagement with, patterns expressed by the body, combined with understanding based on background knowledge of anatomy, physiology, pathology, case history, the cranio-sacral process, clinical experience, life experience, personal development and wisdom.

Inhalation The expansion phase of cranio-sacral motion.

Inherent Naturally present within.

Inherent treatment plan
 (a) The cranio-sacral system's inherent ability to heal itself.
 (b) The therapeutic process which the body itself reveals and expresses.
 (c) The order of events which the body chooses within the cranio-sacral process.

Inherent treatment process The inherent therapeutic response of the cranio-sacral system. The natural tendency of the body to heal itself through the orderly expression of its fundamental principles of therapeutic release. The natural evolution of the therapeutic process.

Integrins Molecules located within the cell membrane and nuclear membrane, connecting extracellular and intracellular matrices, and enabling continuous interconnection and communication from the surface of the skin to the interior of every cell and nucleus in the body via the molecular web.

Interphalangeal joints The joints between the individual phalanges of the fingers and toes.

Internal rotation
 (a) The movement of bilateral structures and the body as a whole during the contraction phase of cranio-sacral motion.
 (b) In the feet – turning the front of the foot inwards.

Inversion In the feet – turning the sole of the foot inwards.

Jugular foramina Two foramina in the base of the skull, antero-lateral to the foramen magnum, one on each side; formed between the occiput and the temporal bones; through which pass the internal jugular vein and cranial nerves IX, X and XI.

Kyphosis A forward bending curve of the spine; the natural curve of the spine in the thoracic spine and the sacrum.

Lamda The meeting point between the sagittal and lamdoid sutures; located at the top of the head between the occiput and parietal bones; often identifiable through a small indentation.

Lamina Terminalis The anterior wall of the third ventricle; the fulcrum around which the central nervous system moves in cranio-sacral motion.

Lateral At or towards or closer to the sides of the body, or outwards from the midline.

Lateral fluctuation
 (a) Any movements within the cranio-sacral process other than longitudinal fluctuation. Rocking, shaking, pulsating, vibrating, twisting, pulling. The multiplicity of movements expressed throughout the system, usually most evident during the early stages of a treatment. They are not necessarily lateral or fluctuating.

(b) Specific alternating lateral movement, such as rocking from side to side, or figure of eight pattern.

(c) A specific technique described by Sutherland involving inducing alternating movement of the temporal bones, with the intention of fluctuating the fluid from one side to the other.

(d) The same technique applied anywhere in the body or in the matrix.

Lesion Any disturbance to function, whether due to injury, disease, imbalance or any other cause.

Longitudinal fluctuation The expression of rhythmic motion throughout the system. It includes the longitudinal flow of vitality up and down the spine, but also includes the expansion/contraction movement throughout the body and in every cell of the body – so it is not necessarily longitudinal.

Lordosis A backward bending curve of the spine; The natural curve of the spine in the cervical and lumbar regions.

Matrices Plural of matrix.

Matrix A flexible environment within which something can grow, develop or exist; a coherent force field, including:

- The embryonic matrix – the force field within which the embyro develops.
- The individual matrix – the force field comprising the body and its surrounding aura, consisting of: internal matrix, the matrix within the body; external matrix, the field around the body.
- The universal matrix – the coherent field of forces within which the whole natural world operates as a unified cohesive system, and within which we all exist.

ME Myalgic encephalomyelitis – a persistent and debilitating post viral condition.

Medial At or towards or closer to the midline of the body.

Membrane system The membranes – dura, arachnoid and pia – which enclose the brain and spinal cord, and include the intracranial infoldings.

Meningeal dura The inner layer of dura mater.

Meninges The triple layered membranes – dura, arachnoid and pia – which surround the brain and spinal cord, and include the intracranial infoldings.

Meningism A milder, often unrecognised, form of meningitis.

Meningitis Inflammation of the meninges, usually as a result of bacterial or viral infection.

- Bacterial meningitis, due to bacterial infection, can be rapidly fatal unless treated with antibiotics.
- Viral meningitis, due to viral infection, is usually milder, sometimes persistent, and is not affected by antibiotics.
- The chronic, persistent long-term after-effects of meningitis or meningism are often very debilitating, involving severe headache, neck pain, pain behind the eyes, poor memory, poor concentration and extreme tiredness; and are usually very responsive to cranio-sacral integration.

Molecular web The interconnected network through which every molecule in the body is in continuous communication with every other molecule, enabling coordinated interaction and response, including healing responses, throughout the body.

Nasion The junction between the nasal bones and the frontal bone, at the top of the nose.

Neutral A balanced settled state in which the cranio-sacral system is resting comfortably.

- Open and receptive, with rhythmic motion being expressed freely and evenly.
- A state which indicates and enables engagement or deeper engagement.
- A state to which the cranio-sacral system generally returns following a release.

Neutral, The A point of balanced tension or stillness preceding a release.
- *Patient Neutral* – a state of settledness within the patient, enabling engagement.
- *Practitioner Neutral* – a state of settledness within the practitioner; calm, quiet presence.

Perineural system A communication system reaching to all parts of the body, in close anatomical relation to the nervous system, but functioning as a separate system; its communications are more generalised and widespread than the nervous system, and it plays a significant part in injury repair and restoration of health.

Periosteum The membrane (dura) which covers the external surface of bones. In the cranium, the perisoteum (on the outer surface) is continuous with the endosteum (on the inner surface) of the bones.

Physiology The function of the body.

Plantar Referring to the sole of the foot.

Plantarflexion Movement of the front of the foot downward (inferiorly), pointing the toes.

PNS The peripheral nervous system.

Posterior Behind, backwards, at or towards the back of the body.

Potency The power or strength of the vitality.

Potency
(a) The power within the system, the organising force, the fluid within the fluid the potential for therapeutic release.
(b) An alternative word for energy, particularly for those who don't like to use the term energy.

Practitioner fulcrums The state of physical, mental and emotional balance from which a practitioner operates.

Pressurestat Model John Upledger's concept of the cranio-sacral system as a semi-closed hydraulic system within which cranio-sacral motion is influenced by the pressure of cerebrospinal fluid contained within the membrane system.

Primary respiration The expression of the Breath of Life as rhythmic motion.

Primary respiratory system The cranio-sacral system.

Process
(a) A bony protrusion (e.g. the mastoid process).
(b) An interaction with the cranio-sacral system through a specific contact (as distinguished from the mere application of a technique).
(c) The whole therapeutic process that the patient is going through.
(d) Process work, working with a patient's whole life process – mental, emotional, spiritual, as well as physical.

Prone Lying on the front, face down.

Pterion The junction at which the frontal, parietal, temporal and sphenoid bones come together; located at the temple, behind the lateral corner of the eye on each side.

Quanta Plural of quantum.

Quantum The smallest unit of anything, such as photons of light.

Quantum science The basis of modern scientific thinking, initially conceived in the 1920s by Werner Heisenberg, Erwin Schrödinge and Paul Durak, recognising that everything in the universe (galaxies, planets, mountains, rocks, plants, animals, humans, oceans, fluids, air, heat, light, thought) is composed of quanta – elementary particles, waves and forces – in a state of constant interaction, through which everything influences everything else, including the observer and the observed.

Reflex arc A rapid response system which enables reflex reactions through connections between sensory and motor neurons at a local spinal cord level, as for instance when you touch something hot.

Reciprocal tension membrane system The system of continuously interconnected membranes (dura, arachnoid, pia) which surround the central nervous system and form the intracranial infoldings of the falx cerebri, falx cerebelli and tentorium cerebelli, and which attach to the bones of the cranium and to the sacrum. Tensions anywhere in the membrane system are transmitted reciprocally throughout the rest of the membrane system.

Rhythmic motion Cranio-sacral motion, including cranio-sacral rhythm, middle tide and long tide.

Sacrum The tail bone.

Sagittal Passing between front and back of the body (e.g. the sagittal suture).

Sagittal section A view of the body as if sliced vertically through the body from front to back.

SBJ Spheno-basilar joint (same as spheno-basilar synchondrosis).

SBS Spheno-basilar synchondrosis.

Scoliosis An abnormal lateral curvature of the spine – present in many people to some degree.
- Idiopathic scoliosis – a condition in which a severe and persistent scoliosis of the spine develops spontaneously, commonly starting in teenage and pre-teen years, particularly in girls.

Sclerosis Hardening.

Sinus A space.
- Air sinuses – air-filled spaces within the cranium, prone to infection leading to sinusitis.
- Venous sinuses – spaces within the dural membrane inside the cranium for the collection and drainage of venous blood.

Solar plexus The coeliac ganglia and associated neurological structures of the sympathetic nervous system.

An energy centre in the central upper abdomen

An area where emotion, stress and sympathetic stimulation are often felt.

Spheno-basilar synchondrosis The primary cartilaginous joint between the body of the sphenoid and the basilar portion of the occiput.

Sphincter A valve-like structure which closes through constriction in order to regulate the passage of food, etc. (e.g. pyloric sphincter, ilio-caecal valve).

Squamous Flat (e.g. the squamous portion of the temporal bone).

Superior Above, upwards, towards the top of the patient's head.

Supine Lying on the back, face up.

Sutherland's fulcrum A shifting fulcrum located within the straight sinus, at the junction of the falx cerebri, falx cerebelli and tentorium cerebelli, around which the rhythmic motion of the membrane system operates.

Suture A fibrous joint between bones of the cranium; the majority of joints between cranial bones are sutures.

Synchondrosis A primary cartilaginous joint, which ossifies gradually over several years (e.g. the spheno-basilar synchondrosis).

Synchronisation Engagement with the cranio-sacral process.

System, The The cranio-sacral system.

Therapeutic pulse A pulsation very similar to the arterial pulse, except that it is transient and varies both in intensity and in rate, and generally arises in relation to therapeutic releases.

TMJ Temporo-mandibular joint, the joint through which the lower jaw attaches to the cranium.

Tissue memory

(a) Patterns of injury or tension held in the tissues.

(b) Memories of past events arising in conjunction with releases in the tissues.

Torticollis A twist of the neck, also known as wry neck.
- Infant torticollis – occurs in babies, often associated with the birth process, and often responds well to the cranio-sacral process.
- Acute torticollis – an acute spasm in the neck at any age, frequently associated with sleeping awkwardly and often very responsive to cranio-sacral treatment.

Traction Stretching.

Transmutation

(a) A change of state (e.g. from solidity to fluidity, from hard to soft, tight to loose, from resistance to free mobility).

(b) A change in quality (e.g. softening or dissolving of a restriction).

(c) A release within the cranio-sacral process.

(d) A release of restrictions within the matrix.

Transverse Passing horizontally across the body (e.g. the transverse sinuses).

Transverse section A view of the body as if sliced horizontally through the body.

Vault hold Any contact on the cranium which embraces or contains the cranial vault (e.g. falx contact, temporal contact, sphenoid contact).

Vector A line of force passing through or within the body.

Venous Relating to veins and venous (de-oxygenated) blood.

Venous sinuses The system of sinuses (spaces) within the cranium through which venous blood collects in order to return to the heart for re-oxygenation.

Ventouse A vacuum machine for assisting the delivery of a baby.

Ventral Anterior – at the front, on or towards the front of the body.

Ventricles Cavities deep within the brain and spinal cord, filled with cerebrospinal fluid.

Ventricular system The system of cavities and canals, deep within the brain and spinal cord, where cerebrospinal fluid is formed and is contained.

Viscera The organs of the body (e.g. heart, lungs, digestive organs).

Viscus Singular of viscera.

References

Blechschmidt, E. and Gasser, R. (1978) *Biokinetics and Biodynamcis of Human Differentiation.* Springfield, IL: Charles C. Thomas.

Chaitow, L. (2005) *Cranial Manipulation – Theory and Practice, 2nd Edition.* London: Elsevier Churchill Livingstone.

Oschman, J.L. (2000) *Energy Medicine: The Scientific Basis.* London: Churchill Livingstone.

Seifriz, W. (1954) *Seifriz on Protoplasm* (film).

Still, A.T. (1977) *Philosophy of Osteopathy.* Indianapolis, IN: American Academy of Osteopathy. (Original work 1899.)

Sutherland, W.G. (1967) *Contributions of thought.* Fort Worth, TX: Sutherland Cranial Teaching Foundation.

Upledger, J. (1990) *Somato Emotional Release and Beyond.* Palm Beach, CA: UI Publishing.

Wernham, S.G.J. (1956) *Mechanics of the Spine.* Maidstone: Osteopathic Institute of Applied Technique.

Index

Note: page references to illustrations are given in *italics*; page references in **bold** refer to terms included in the glossary

accessibility of impressions 98
accessory nerves 137
accidents 138, 262, 263
accumulation of imbalances 53
adults, relevance of treatment 16
aggression 139
alertness 73
allergic reactions 401
Amy's case 10, 12
anatomical cranio-sacral system 25
  bones 34–9
  cerebrospinal fluid 39–46
  fascia 46–7
  membrane system 26–33
anger 79, 417
ankle
  articulation 292, *293*
  contact 292, *293*
  following process 292–3
  practitioner fulcrums 292
  projection through body 293–4
ansa cervicalis 402, **448**
anterior rami 352
application of therapy 13
apprehension 402
Aqueduct of Sylvius *see* cerebral aqueduct
arachnoid mater 26, *32*, 164, 346
arachnoid villi 42, *43*, **448**
arms 279–80
  active process 280–2
  aiding finishing 288
  completion 287
  concluding 286–7
  contact 284
  distinction between articulation and unwinding 283–4
  encouraging process start 287
  establishing practitioner fulcrums 284
  holding at balanced tension point 286
  identifying focal points 285
  maintaining focus 286
  moving body fluently 285
  pain 288–9
  preparatory articulation 282–3
  principles of fascial unwinding 280
  stillness 284, 285–6
  unwinding process *283*, 284–5
  using traction 287–8
  whole person assessment 280
arterial blood 39
articulation (mobilisation of joints) 309, **448**
  ankle 292, *293*
  arms 282–4
  fascial unwinding 310
  hips 299
  knee 294
  neck 304–5
articulations (joints) **448**
  frontal bone 202
  occipital bone (occiput) 155–6
  parietal area 211
  sacrum 162, *163*, 164
  sphenoid bone 177
  temporal bones 190–1
asking the system 184, 192, 198, 208, 320, 335, **448**
asterion 215, **448**
asthma 139, 389
atlas vertebra 136, 137, 143, 154
attention
  divided 103
  to energy drive 408–9, 411
  establishing levels of 56–7, 83
  exploring levels of 120–1, 123–4
  focusing 82
  to frontal area 209
  to leg 293–4, 296
  to parietal area 215
  practising 233–4
  to practitioner fulcrums 96
  projecting 103–5, *117*, 234, 268–9
  to self-awareness 310
  spaciousness of 58
  to sphenoid 182–3, 187
  to spine 159–60, 172–3
  still points 226–7
  to suboccipital region 141–2
  to temporal area 199
  use in treating knee 296
  to whole person 336
aura 22, 23, 412, 431, **448**
autonomic discharge 385
autonomic nervous system (ANS) 343, 359, *360*, **448**
  associations 387–90
  causes of disturbance 366–7
  causes of dysfunction 386
  dynamic balance 366, 384–5
  dysfunctional imbalance 366
  ganglia 362
  general anatomy 361
  integration of function 387
  nerve root origins 369
  parasympathetic function 365–6
  psychosomatics 390–1
  relationships with vertebral levels 367
  summary of 368, *369*
  sympathetic function 366
  two neuron pathway 361
  understanding 385–6
  unexpressed emotion 390
axon 341, 363, **448**

babies
  consequences of restriction 138
  relevance of treatment 14–15
balanced tension point 286
basilar portion 155, 156, 159, 316
bee sting 401
bike accidents 262

biodynamic approach 244–8
biodynamic model 17, 244–6, 247
biomagnetic fields 24, 99, *100*, 101
biomechanical approach 244–8
birth trauma 10, 12, 14, 138
Blechschmidt, E. 244
blood supply to cranium 33
body as integrated unit 148
bones of cranial-sacral system 34, *34–8*
  disturbances to 38
  movement of 20, 39
bony attachments 30–1
bony ridges 31
brachial plexus 352, *353*, 354–7
brain 348–50, *349*
  development in babies 138
brainstem 349
Breath of Life 19, 22, 52, 244, 246, **448**
breathing 69, 105, 115
  assisting release 250–1
  depth of relaxation 250
  diagnosis 249
  and habit patterns 251–2
  letting go 250
  pain in treatment session 252
  responding to sensations 251
  response to trauma 249
  for therapist 252–3
bregma 219, **448**

calm, quiet presence 55, 67, *68*, 76, 99–106
car accidents 262, 303
carotid arteries 136
carotid nerves 137
cartilaginous joint 177, 316, 454
cavernous sinus *44*, 45–6
central canal 39, 42, 152
central nervous system (CNS) 342, 346–8, **449**
  associations 348–50
  cerebral aqueduct *40–1*, 42

cerebrospinal fluid (CSF) 20, 39, **448**
   distribution through ventricular system 39–42
   emergence from ventricular system 43
   formation from arterial blood 39
   reabsorption into venous blood 43–6
   seeping through brain 46
   volume 46
cervical nerves 352, *353*
cervical plexus 352, *353*, 354
Chaitow, L. 39
chakras 127, **448**
children, relevance of treatment 15
choroid plexi 39, 42, 46, **448**
chronicity 82, **449**
circular sinus *44*, 45
circumduction 282, 292, *293*, 299, **449**
cisternae 43, 347, **449**
clinical choices 440–2
coccygeal nerve *347*, 348, 352, *353*
coccyx 29, *30*, 31, 38, 145, *163*, 164, 347–8
coherence 419, **449**
cold sensation 69–70
colic 138
collateral ganglia 362, 365
comfort zone 420
completion 61, 113, 186, 223–4
   in diagnosis 435
   fascial unwinding 311
   integrated treatment 439, 444
   practising 233, 234
   sphenoid 119
   still points 230
   treatment of arms 287
   treatment of hips 301–2
   treatment of legs 294
   treatment of neck 307–8
   treatment of throat 405
compression **449**
   frontal area 206, 208, *209*
   lumbo-sacral 171–2
   spheno-basilar 184–6, *185*, 327–8
concluding treatment 223
   arms 286–7, 288
   fascial unwinding 311
   legs 297, 299

see also completion
conclusions, jumping to 84–5
condylar portions 155
confluence of sinuses 30, *44*, *46*, 156–7, 217
conscious recall 97
contact
   ear hold 196–200, *197*
   exploring levels of 120, 122–3, 423–4
   hand 318–319
   time spent on 439
contact, taking up 55–7, 76
   ankle 292, *293*
   arms 284
   combined cranial base and crown 424
   combined heart & solar plexus centres 421–2
   cranium 117–18, 124, 376–7, 440, 443–4
   double 370–8, 424, *425*, *427*
   drive point 408
   emotional centres *129*, *132*, 133–4
   falx 218–20, *219*
   feet 265–7
   frontal area 205–8, *207*
   hips *299*, 300–1
   knee 294–6, *295*, *298*
   legs 291–2
   listening posts 270–5
   lumbo-sacral *169*–70
   mastoid tip 192, 194–5
   neck 305
   occipital 157, *158*
   parietal area 212–14, *213*
   pelvic centre *133*–4
   sacro-iliac joints 168, *169*–70
   sacrum *134*, 164–5, *169*–70, 370–8, *428*, 440
   scapula 426, *427*
   shoulder 115–16
   sphenoid 179–80, *180*–*1*
   still points 228
   suboccipital 140–1, 440
   target point 407–8
   temporal area 192–200
   throat 398, 402–5, *403*–*4*, 406
   trunk region 276, *277*
   vertebral column 411–12
containment 67
continuation 61, 186
continuous unified sheath 26–7

contra-indications
   for beginners 74–5
   for experienced therapists 74
contraction of rhomboid 423
contraction phase (of motion) 11, 49–51, 166, 191–2, 205, 228–9, **450**
core contacts 440
core treatment 113, 145–6
   individual processes 148–9
   integrated treatment 439, 443
coronal section *27*, **449**
coronal suture 202, 209, 211–13, 215, **449**
cranial base 36–7, *176*, *190*, *203*, 424, **449**
cranial dura 26–7, *30*
cranial nerves 350–1, 363, 365
cranial osteopathy 17, 247
cranial rhythmic impulse (CRI) 48, 52, **449**
cranial vault **449**
cranio-sacral fulcrums 91
cranio-sacral integration 17–18, 76
   basis of 65
   benefits of 14–16
   essence of 53–4
   fundamental principles 57–62
   interactive process 99
   practising 232–4
   process of 54–5
   summary 444, 446–7
cranio-sacral motion 48–9, **449**
   expression of rhythmic motion 50–1
   falx *221*
   feet/legs 268
   frontal area 204–5
   interaction of rhythms 51–2
   layers of rhythmic motion 48
   occipital region 159
   parietal area 212
   rhythmic terminology 52
   sacrum 166
   slime mould 52
   sphenoid 179
   stability of rhythm 51
   a state of being 49
   temporal bones *191*

two phases of motion 49–50
see also motion; rhythmic motion
cranio-sacral rhythm 48–9, 51, 52, 87, 119, 238–43, 246
cranio-sacral system **449**
   anatomy of 25–47
   blockages 139
   constituents 20–4
   expression of 58–9
   following 59, 62
   opening up 113, 126–35, 440
   relations with nervous system 346–58
cranio-sacral therapy
   approaches to 17–18
   basics 13–14
   as biodynamic 245
   broad spectrum of care 18
   and cranial osteopathy 247
   development of skills 103–5
   evolution 18
   monitoring through quality 82
   origins 17, 20
   patient's previous experience of 438
   responses to 69–73, 251
cranium 20, *34*–*5*, *38*, 375–6, **449**
   bones of *34*–*5*, *38*, 191–2
   contact on 117–18, 124, 376–8, 440, 443–4
   membranous contraction within 33
   movement of bones 39
   sample initial treatment 443–4
cricoid cartilage *398*, 399
crown 424
crying 70–1
currents 59, 87, 89
CV4 (compression of fourth ventricle) 228–9, *230*, **449**
cystitis 374, 387

dandelion analogy 259–60
decompression **449**
   following compression 328
   lumbo-sacral 172
   spheno-basilar 186–8, *187*, 329
depression 139

depth, patient, levels of 83
diagnosis
    diagnostic skills 433
    dynamic 432
    guiding treatment
        approach 432
    integrating perception
        levels 433–5
    levels of 429–30
    observation of breathing
        249
    providing 432
    and rhythmic motion 241
    through SBS 336–8
    variations in 430–2
diaphragma sellae 28, 29, 30,
    178–9
directing the tide 407, **449**
dorsiflexion 292, 293, **449**
dorsum 104, 265, 267, 270,
    292, 294, 407
double contacts 370–8, 424,
    425, 427
drive points 408
drugs
    medicinal 80
    recreational 81
duodenal ulcers 388–9
dura **449**
    contact with bones 31
    subdivisions of 26–7
dura mater 26, *32*, 164, 346
Durak, P. 23, **453**
dural membrane 30, 346
dynamic balance 366, 384–5
dynamic diagnosis 432
dynamic stillness 63, 108,
    109, 188, **449**
dysfunctional imbalance 366

ear hold contact 196–200,
    197
earhole 190
elderly people, relevance of
    treatment 16
embryonic matrix 22, 452
emotional balance 95
emotional body
    determining emotional
        states 414
    emotional levels 417–18
    observation 415
    palpation 416
    specific indicators 416–18
    symptoms 415–16
    taking case history 416
emotional centres 126–7,
    128–35, 382, 421–2,
    443

emotional effects
    on matrix 22–3
    on throat 394–5
emotional factors 333–4
emotional fulcrums 92
emotional links to fascia
    262–3
emotional patterns, chronic
    263–4
emotional responses 63,
    70–1, 79, 206
emotional tension 138, 144,
    388, 395
emotions
    in fascial unwinding 312
    opening up 440
    and physical interaction
        423
    temporal area 200–1
    unexpressed 390
endocrine glands 127,
    400–1
endosteal layer 27, 152
energy 25
    centres *see* chakras
    fields 101, 182
    matrix 20, 22
energy drive 62, **449**
    applications 409
    harnessing cranio-sacral
        potency 409–10
    to occipito-mastoid suture
        410–11
    process 407–9
    for vertical column
        411–13
energy fields 101, 182
engagement 11, 76, 114
    with cranial-sacral system
        57–8, 112
    deepening 63, 120–5
    with deeper tides 241–3
    with fascia 264
    with inner wisdom 433
    integrated treatment
        439–40
    levels of 62, 238–9, 240
    with matrix 20
    practical process of
        114–19
    practising 232–3
    with rhythmic motion
        224, 239–41
    sample initial treatment
        442–3
    through the sacrum
        164–72
    through the sphenoid
        179–83

trunk region 278
    of whole system 149
enhancement 65–6
entrainment 51–2, 99–100,
    238, **449**
entunement 99
environmental awareness 107
ependyma 42, **449**
epilepsy 14–15, 350
epineurium 32, 46, *47*, 257,
    367
equanimity 55, 95, 102,
    105, **449**
etheric body 22, 23, **450**
ethmoid bone *34–5, 37*, 177
EV4 (expansion of fourth
    ventricle) 228–9, **450**
eversion (of feet) *293*, **450**
exhalation 51, **450**
exocrine glands 359, 400
exophthalmic goitre 396,
    397
expansion phase (of motion)
    11, 49–51, 159,
    191–2, 205, 221,
    228–9, **450**
exploration 420
expression
    of rhythmic motion 50–1
    of system 58–9
extension 50, 166, 177–8,
    318, 319–20, **450**
extension phase *see*
    contraction phase (of
    motion)
external auditory meatus *see*
    earhole
external face 83–4
external matrix 11, 20, *21*
external occipital
    protuberance 156
external rotation 50, *268,
    293*, **450**
extraneous movements 66–7,
    243

facilitated segments 379–83
falx cerebelli *27*, 29, 30,
    152, *212*, 217–18
falx cerebri *27, 28*, 29, 30,
    157, 204, *212*, 217
falx cerebri and falx release
    216–17, 234
    connections through
        reciprocal tension
        membrane system
        218
    contact 218–20, *219*
    falx cerebelli 217–18

falx cerebri 217
    rhythmic motion 221
    subtle integration 222
    taking up the slack
        218–19
fascia 46–7, 127–8, 256,
    450
    causes of fascial restriction
        46–7, 260–4
    engagement with 264
    fascial unwinding
        258–60, 310–13
    functions 258
    penetration 257–8
    whole body
        interconnection
        256–7
fascial evaluation
    building picture of whole
        person 273–5
    contact at feet 265–7
    cranio-sacral motion 268
    hands floating freely 268
    identifying focal points
        269
    interpreting impressions
        269
    listening posts 270–3
    maintaining self-awareness
        269
    projection 268–9
    quality, symmetry and
        motion 267
fascial nerve sheath *see*
    epineurium
fascial restrictions 46–7,
    256, 260–1
    car and bike accidents 262
    chronic emotional patterns
        263–4
    long-lying symptoms 263
    lumbo-sacral plexus
        357–8
    operation scars 261
    physical and emotional
        links 262–3
    RSI, writer's and
        musician's cramp
        261–2
    severe trauma 262
    sprains and strains 261
fascial unwinding
    of the arm 279–89
    articulation 310
    attention to self-awareness
        310
    benefits of 256
    distinction with
        articulation 283–4

fascial unwinding *cont.*
  emotions 312
  ending 311
  integrating 312–13
  of the leg 290–302
  main factors of 313
  maintaining focus 311
  maintaining overview 311
  memories 311–12
  of the neck 303–9
  principles 258–60, 310
  starting 310–11
  stillness 311
  within the trunk region 276–8
fear 79, 333, 402
feet
  contact 265–7
  cranial-sacral motion 268
  hands floating freely 268
  projecting up through body 268–9
  quality, symmetry and motion 267
fibrosis 261, **450**
fight/flight response 384–5
filum terminale *30*, 31, 152, 164
finger curling 141–2, 196
flexion 50, 166, 177–8, 318, 319–20, **450**
  of hip 300
flexion phase *see* expansion phase (of motion)
floating freely 187, 209–10, 268, 329
fluency 285, 319, **450**
fluent fluidic flow 378
fluid analogies
  beyond fluids 88
  fluidic progression of treatment 87
  forces and fields 89
  treatment 88–9
  value of 87–8
fluid drive 153, 241, 433, **450**
fluidic matrix *117*
fluidity 118, 242
foramen magnum *27*, 30–1, 217–18, **450**
foramen of Magendie *40–1*, 42, 43
foramina 42, **450**
foramina of Luschka *40*, 42, 43
fossa 176, 190, 350, **450**
frontal area
  articulations 202

compression and lift 206, 208–9
contact 205–8, *207*
cranio-sacral motion 204–5
effects of injury 205–6
floating freely 209–10
informed awareness 209
location 202
membranous relations 204
stimuli 206
subtle integration 210
frontal bone *34–5, 37–8*, 177, *202–3*, 204
fulcrums *90*, **450**
  cranio-sacral 91
  emotional 92
  establishing appropriate 95–6
  as main focal points 93–4
  mechanical pivots 90
  mental 91–2, 94–5
  natural and unnatural 93
  practitioner 94–6, 292, 296, 305–6
  Sutherland's 91, 93, 94
  time 92–3, 96–8
fundamental principles **450**
  of cranio-sacral integration 57–62

ganglia 362, 364–5, 368, **450–1**
Gasser, R. 244
gastric ulcers 388–9
gentleness of therapy 12, 14, 16, 56
glial cells (neuroglia) 340, 341–2
globus hystericus 401
glossopharyngeal nerves 137
goitre 396, 397, 401
grey matter 342
grounding 96, 113, 126–35, 443

habit patterns 251–2, 390
hands
  contact 318–19
  floating freely 268
  softness of 120, 142
  variation in position 439
happiness 79
head and neck injuries 138, 303
headaches 139, 308
health
  depleted 53
  true 13
  underlying 16, 241

heart centre 126, 127, 128–31, 421–2
heart conditions 139
Heisenberg, W. 23, 453
hips
  articulation 299
  contact *299*, 300–1
  establishing focus 299–300
  integration and completion 301–2
holistic therapy 12, 79–80, 337
homeostasis 54, 225, 366, **451**
hot sensation 69–70
hyoid bone 398–9, 401
hyperthyroidism 396
hypothyroidism 396

ileo-caecal valve dysfunction 387–8
ilia, release of sacrum between 168
iliac crests 270, 271, *272*, 273
imbalances
  accumulation of 53
  dysfunctional 366
  imperfect 319
  spontaneous 159
  structural & postural 138
incompleteness 224
individual matrix *21*, 22, 23, 248, 447, 452
individual processes 148–9, 233
inertia 85, 94, 320, 334, **451**
inertial fulcrum 94, 96–8, 258, 439, **451**
infection
  lingering effects 15
  throat 394
inferior petrosal sinus *44*, 46
inferior sagittal sinus *44*, 45, *46*
informed awareness 98, 199, 209, 332, 430, **451**
infra-hyoid muscles 399–400
inhalation 51, **451**
inherent treatment plan **451**
inherent treatment process 11–12, 76, **451**
  fundamental principles 57–62
  variations in 62–4
inion 156
inner stillness 107

innervation, rich 258
integrated treatment 112–13
  autonomic nervous system (ANS) 384–91
  clinical choices 440–2
  fascial unwinding 312–13
  framework for 234–5
  hips 301–2
  neck 307–8
  overview 439–40
  practising 232–4
  sample initial treatment 442–4
  spheno-basilar 331–8
  throat 402
  total integration 442
  variations in practice 438–9
integrins 340, **451**
internal jugular veins 45–6, 136
internal matrix 11, *21*, 22
internal occipital protuberance 156
internal rotation 50, *268*, *293*, **451**
interphalangeal joints 141, **451**
interventricular foramen *40–1*, 42
intracranial membranes *27*, *28*
inversion (of feet) *293*, **451**
irritability 139
irritable bowel syndrome 388

Jealous, J. 17, 244
jugular foramina 45, 137, 199, **451**

knee
  articulation 294
  concluding 297–9
  contact 294–6, *295*, *298*
  holding into resistances 297
  maintaining practitioner fulcrums 296
  moving body fluently 296–7
  process 296
  use of attention 296
kyphosis 373, **451**

L3 (third lumbar vertebra) 373
L5 (fifth lumbar vertebra)
  mechanical associations 372

Index

neurological associations 372–3
lamina terminalis 91, 93, 94, **451**
lateral fluctuation 66, **451–2**
lateral motion 159, 205
lateral pterygoid plate 176
lateral shift *166*, 324–5, 335
lateral ventricles *40–1*, 42
laughter 70–1
legs 290–1
   completion 294
   contact 291–2
   principles of fascial unwinding 291–2
   projection 293–4
   reassessment 294
   resistances 294
   weight of 291
letting go 71, 250
lift
   frontal area 206, 208–9
   parietal area 214–15
light-headedness 72, 224
lightness of touch 58, 120
listening posts 270–5
Littlejohn's triangles *373*, 375
living matrix 24, 101
long tide 48, 49, 52, 83, 87, 119, 242–3, 246, 259
longitudinal fluctuation 153, **452**
longitudinal motion 159, 205
lordosis 373, **452**
lumbar nerves *353*
lumbar plexus 352, *353*
lumbar vertebrae 372–4
lumbo-sacral compression 171–2
lumbo-sacral contact *169–70*
lumbo-sacral decompression 172
lumbo-sacral joint 164
lumbo-sacral plexus 357–8
lumbo-sacral release 171
lymph glands 400, 401

mandibular fossa 190
mastoid portion 189, 191–2
mastoid tip contact 192, 194–5
matrix 11, 20–2, *21*, 76, **452**
   effect of emotions 22–3
   in science 24
ME (myalgic encephalomyelitis) 13, 98, 229, 390, **452**

medial **452**
medial epicondyle 355, 357
medial pterygoid plate 176
median nerve *356*
membrane system **452**
   arachnoid mater 26
   bony attachments to 30–1
   disturbances to 32–3
   dura mater 26–7
   membranous infoldings 29
   pia mater 26
   spinal membranes 31–2
   triple layered *26*
membranous attachments
   frontal area 204
   occipital bone (occiput) 157
   parietal area 212
   sacrum 164
   sphenoid 178–9
   temporal area 191
membranous infoldings 27, 29, 157
memories 71, 311–12
meningeal dura 152–3, 449, **452**
meningeal layer 27, 31, 152
meninges 26, 31, **452**
meningism 81, **452**
meningitis 33, 81, 217, **452**
mental fulcrums 91–2, 94–5
middle tide 48, 49, 52, 83, 87, 119, 167, 238–9, 243, 246, 259
migraine 139
molecular web 148, 340, 419, **452**
motion 19, 116–17, 130–1, 221–2, 267
   and fascial unwinding 260
   repetitive patterns of 306–7
   see also cranio-sacral motion; rhythmic motion
motor neurons 343–4
muscles
   suboccipital 137–8
   throat 399–400
musician's cramp 261–2

nasion 202, 409, **452**
natural fulcrums 93
neck
   articulation 304–5
   common trauma site 304
   contact 305
   extension down to T4 304
   extreme positions 306

holding into deeper patterns 307
integration and completion 307–8
placement of head 308
practitioner fulcrums 305–6
principles of fascial unwinding 304, 306
repetitive patterns of motion 306–7
significance of treating 303–4
specific applications 303
standing or sitting 308–9
stillness 307
unwinding process 305
nerve supply to throat 400
nerve tissue 340
nervous system
   anatomy of 342–3
   glial cells (neuroglia) 341–2
   nerve tissue 340
   neurons (nerve cells) 340–1
   perineural system 345
   physiology of 343
   sensory and motor neurons 343–5
   synapse 341
   white and grey matter 342
neurological irritation 153
neurons (nerve cells) 340–1
neutral state 11, 60–1, 186, 187–8, 318, **452**
nothingness, feelings of 85
nuclei of the vagus 137

occipital bone (occiput) 30, *34*, *36*, *38*, 191, 234
   articulations 155–6
   cranial-sacral motion 159
   features 156–7
   integration of spine 159
   location 155
   membranous attachments 157
   occipital contact 157, *158*
   preparatory suboccipital release 157
   spontaneous imbalances 159
   still point induction at 230–1, 234
occipital sinus *44*, 45, *46*, 217
occipito-mastoid suture, energy drive to 410–11
oceanic waves 87

opening up 113, 126–35, 440
operation scars 261
Oschman, J.L. 24, 57, 101, 345
overview, maintaining 311

pain 70, 252, 288–9
palpation 416
parasympathetic distribution 368
parasympathetic division 343, 359, *360*, 363, 368
parasympathetic function 365–6
parathyroid glands 401
paravertebral ganglia 362, *363*, 364
parietal area
   articulations 211
   contact 212–14, *213*
   cranio-sacral motion 212
   lift 214–15
   location 211
   membranous relations 212
parietal bone *34–8*, 211
parotid glands 400
pathologies, identifying 80
patient preparation 114
patient stillness 107–8
pelvic centre 127, 133–5
pelvic diaphragm *see* pelvic centre
penetration of therapy 12
perceptions
   defining and refining 85
   false 84–5
   of quality 85–6
perfect body 19
perfection 102
perineural system 345, **452**
periosteum 27, 257, **453**
peripheral nervous system (PNS) 342–3, 348
   associations 350–4
personal development
   balance of stability and exploration 420
   challenging comfort zone 420
   coherence 419
   genuine presence 419
   personal journey 419–20
personal matrix *see individual matrix*
petrous portion 190
physical and emotional interaction 423
physical awareness 94

physical contact
  establishing levels of 56
  exploring different levels 120, 122–3, 423–4
physical links to fascia 262–3
physiological processes, influencing 54–5
pia mater 26, *32*, 164
pivots, mechanical 90
plantarflexion 267, 292, *293*, **453**
pleasantness 73
plexi
  somatic 354–8
  sympathetic 127, 352, 362, 365, 368
posterior rami 352
postural imbalances 138
postural shift 72
potency 88, 153, **453**
  harnessing 11, 371, 409–10
practice, daily 105
practising treatment 232–5
practitioner fulcrums 94–8, 292, 296, 305–6, **453**
practitioner quality 84
practitioner, state of 99–106
pregnant women, relevance of treatment 15–16
preparatory release
  sacrum 370–1
  suboccipital 157
presence
  benefits of 102–3
  calm, quiet 55, 67, *68*
  development of skills 103–5
  establishing 105
  genuine 419
  quality of 99
pressurestat conceptual model 17, **453**
primary respiration 17, 19, 52, 244, 246, **453**
professional approach 102–3
professional practice 447
profundity of therapy 12
projection
  as inherent part of process 103
  practical exercise in 104–5
  through legs 293–4
  through SBS 336
protective defensive mechanisms 54
psychosomatics 390–1

pterions (temples) 175, *177*, 202, 209, **453**
pudendal plexus 352, *353*, *358*
pulsation 61–2, 408–9

quality 19, 116–17, 130–1
  concept of 78–86
  as emotion indicator 416–17
  evaluation 267
  of presence 99
  of stillness 108–9, 227
quantum model 248
quantum science 23, **453**

radiation, extremely low frequency (ELF) 99, *100*
reciprocal tension membrane system *29*, 33, 218, **453**
reflective practice 105
reflex arc 344–5, **453**
relaxation 69, 72, 73, 250
release 11–12, 60
  breathing 250–1
  importance of 139
  reluctance to 144
  rhomboid 422–4
  sacral 168, 171, 370–1
  sphenoid 183–8
  suboccipital 140–4, 157
  trunk region 278
reorganisation 60, 186
resistance 11
  dissolving 408–9
  holding into 297
  identifying points of 285
  persistent 370
  stubborn 294
responses to treatment 69–73, 251
restriction
  consequences of 138–9
  fascial 256, 260–4
  and fulcrums 93–4
  identifying source of 434
  membranous 33, 217
  release from 11–12
  sacrum 164, 167–8
  tissue 82, 96
retraumatisation 406
rhomboid contraction 423
rhomboid release 422–4
rhythmic motion 11, 19, **453**
  deeper tides 241–3
  in diagnosis 241
  engaging with 224

falx cerebri and falx release 221
  identifying remaining 226
  layers of *48*
  as part of engagement 118–19
  in temporal area 191–2
  value of engagement with 239–41
  working with different rhythms 243
  see also cranio-sacral motion; motion
ripples 87
RSI (repetitive strain injury) 261–2
rumbling 69

sacral nerves *353*, 363, 365
sacral plexus 352, *353*
sacro-iliac joints 164, 167–8, *169–70*
sacrum 162, *163*, **453**
  articulations 162, 164
  asymmetries of *166*
  compression 171–2
  contact *134*, 164–5, *169–70*, 370–8, *428*, 440
  cranio-sacral motion 166
  decompression 172
  initial impressions 165
  injury to 38
  integration of spine through 172–4
  membranous attachments 164
  release 168, 171, 370–1
  response to impressions 167
  restriction 164, 167–8
  sample initial treatment 443
  shifting to deeper levels 167
  subtle integration 174
  symmetry of 433
sagittal **453**
sagittal section 29, 41, 212, **454**
sagittal suture 30, 211, *212*, 217
scalene muscles 400
scapula contact 426, *427*
scars 261
Schrödinge, E. 23, **453**
sciatic nerve 348, *358*, 372–3
sclerosis 32, 81, 261, 263, **454**

scoliosis 322, 339, **454**
segments *see* facilitated segments
Seifriz, W. 52
self-awareness 95, 114, 116, 310
self-preparation 114–15
sella turcica 29, 176, 178
sensations, response to 251
sensitivity 74
sensory neurons 343–4
settling 113, 126–35, 443
shock, effect on throat 395–6
shoulder contact 115–16, 288
side-bending *166*, 322–4
side-shift *see* lateral shift
sigmoid sinus 44, 45, *46*
simple goitre 397
sleep 69
  waking from deep 72
slime mould 52
softness of hands 120, 142
solar plexus centre 127, 131–3, 421–2, **454**
somatic nervous system 343, 344
somatic plexi 354–8
spacious perception 336–7
spaciousness
  of attention 58, 123–4
  balance with grounding 96
spheno-basilar compression 184–6
spheno-basilar decompression 186–8, *187*, 329
spheno-basilar integration 331–2
  diagnosis and treatment of whole person 336–8
  emotional factors 333–4
  informed awareness 332
  intertwinement 333
  jammed up system 334
  opposing forces 335
  into overall treatment session 335–6
  patterns 332–3
  stacking 333
spheno-basilar release 184
spheno-basilar synchondrosis (SBS) 177–8, **454**
  basic building blocks 318
  compression 327–9
  decompression 329
  flexion/extension 319–20

hand contact 318–19
importance of 316–17
lateral shift 324–5
patterns 317–18, 319–30, *330*
practical application 318
reflecting whole system 318
side-bending 322–4
torsion 321–2
vertical shift 325–7
sphenoid bone 30–1, *34–7*, 175–6
   allowing expression 182
   articulations 177
   awareness of whole person 182–3
   contact 179–80, *180–1*
   cranio-sacral motion 179
   dynamic stillness 188
   engagement 180, 182
   importance of 316
   impressions 180, 182
   location 176
   membranous attachments 178–9
   release of 183–8
   responding to energy field changes 182
   shifting to deeper levels 183
   spheno-basilar synchondrosis 177–8
   subtle integration 183
sphincters 388, **454**
spinal cord 31, *32*, 39, 42, 152–3, 342–8
spinal dura 26–7, *30*, 31, 32
spinal membranes 31–2, 152–3, 164
spinal nerves *32*, 347, 351–4, *353*
spine *150–1*, 152, 371
   accessing 153–4
   double contacts 424, *425*
   flow of vitality 153
   importance of 371
   integration through occiput 159
   integration through sacrum 172–4
   segments 160
   spinal membranes 152–3
   surveying 159–60
   viscera and periphery 160–1
   see also vertebral column
spontaneous imbalances 159
spontaneous still points 225

spontaneous time fulcrums 96
sprains and strains 261
squamous portion 155, 189, **454**
stability
   balance with exploration 420
   of rhythm 51
stacking 333, 334
steadying influence 102
Steiner, R. 244
sterno-cleido-mastoid muscle 400
Still, A.T. 256
still points 11, 108, 311
   completing treatment process 230
   contact points 228
   CV4 and EV4 228–9, *230*
   duration 227–8
   expansion and contraction 228
   induction 66, 225–6, 227, 229, 230–1
   spontaneous 225
   variations and observations 226–7
stillness 59–60, 87
   dynamic 63, 108, 109, 188, **449**
   and engagement 114, 182
   environmental awareness 107
   inner 107
   motion and movement 107–8
   patient 107
   qualities of 108–9
   staying with 311
   still points 108
   in treatment of arms 284, 285–6
   in treatment of neck 307
stimulus 65–8, 183–4
stormy seas 88
straight sinus 29, *44*, 45, *46*, 199
strangulation 397–8
strength, underlying 13
structural imbalances 138
styloid process 190
subarachnoid space 26, 39, *41*, 42, 43
submandibular glands 400
suboccipital muscles 137–8
suboccipital region 127
   consequences of restriction 138–9

contact 140–1, 440
   reluctance to release 144
   sample initial treatment 443
   significance of 136
   structures in 136–8
   suboccipital release 140–4, 157
subsequent treatments 444
subtle integration 61
   falx cerebri and falx release 222
   frontal area 210
   sacrum and spine region 174
   sphenoid 183
   suboccipital region 143–4
   temporal area 201
Superconducting Quantum Interference Device (SQUID) 24, 101
superior cervical sympathetic ganglia 137, 368
superior petrosal sinus *44*, 45
superior sagittal sinus 43, *44*, 45, *46*, 212, 217
suppression 95
supra-hyoid muscles 399, 400
Sutherland, W.G. 17, 18, 19, 20, 49, 50, 51, 52, 88, 91, 177, 228, 229, 244, 317, 318, 319, 323, 407, **451**
Sutherland's fulcrum 91, 93, 94, **454**
sutures **454**
symmetry 19, 116–17, 130–1
   evaluation of 267
   of sacrum 433
sympathetic distribution 368
sympathetic division 343, 359, *360*, 368
   anatomy of 363–5
   sympathetic chain *363*, *364*
sympathetic function 366
sympathetic ganglia 137, 368
sympathetic nerve pathways *361*
sympathetic plexi 127, 352, 362, 365, 368
synapse 341, 365
synchondrosis **454**
   see also spheno-basilar synchondrosis (SBS)

T4 (fourth thoracic vertebra) 304, 378
   contact 377
   mechanical associations 375
   neurological associations 375–6
   syndrome 382–3
   tension at 337–8
T9 (ninth thoracic vertebra)
   mechanical associations 374
   neurological associations 374–5
T12/L1 (thoraco-lumbar junction)
   mechanical associations 373–4
   neurological associations 374
tailbone *see* sacrum
target point 407–8
temporal area
   articulations 190–1
   contacts 192–200
   emotions 200–1
   location 189–90
   membranous attachments 191
   rhythmic motion 191–2
   subtle integration 201
   temporal bone *34–7*, *189–90*
temporo-mandibular joint (TMJ) *189*, 191, **454**
tentorium cerebelli *27–8*, 29–31, *30*, 157, 178, *191*, 200, 249
terminal ganglia 362
thenar eminences 231
therapeutic energy fields 101
therapeutic intention 57
therapeutic pain 70
therapeutic pulse 61–2, **454**
therapeutic response 72, 98
therapists
   breathing for 252–3
   fulcrums 94–8
   professionalism 102–3
thoracic diaphragm *see* solar plexus centre
thoracic inlet *see* heart centre
thoracic nerves *353*
thoracic vertebrae 374–6
throat
   bone and cartilage 398–9
   contacts 398, 402–5, *403–4*, 406
   emotional tension 395

throat *cont.*
　glands 400–1
　infection 394
　lumps within 401
　muscles 399–400
　nerve supply 400
　practical approach to 402
　reasons for treating 394–5
　thyroid conditions 395–7
　trauma to 397–8, 405–6
thumbs 184–5, 231
thyroid cartilage 399
thyroid conditions 395–7
thyroid gland 396–7, 400, *401*
tides 87, 241–3, 407
time
　quality of 81–2
　spent at each contact 439
　spent on treatment 438–9
　tracing back through 97–8
time fulcrums 92–3, 96–8
tissue health 81
tissue levels 121, 124–5
tissue memory 71, 96, **454**

torsion *166*, 321–2
torticollis 137, 195, 256, 303, **454**
traction 66, 287–8, **454**
training 446–7
transverse diaphragms *see* fascia
transverse sinuses *44*, 45, *46*, 199
transverse structures 200, 249, **455**
trauma
　handling 71–2
　neck, common site of 304
　retraumatisation 406
　severe 262
　to throat 397–8, 405–6
trunk region
　contact 276, *277*
　engagement 278
　identifying focal point 276
　release 278
tumour, throat 401
tuning in *see* engagement

Turkish saddle *see* sella turcica
two neuron pathway 361

ulnar nerve 348, 355, *356*
umbilical cord 397
universal matrix *21*, 22, 447, 452
unlatching 62
unnatural fulcrums 93
Upledger, J. 17, 312
urination 70

vagus nerves 136–7
vectors 38, 281, **455**
venous drainage 27, 29
venous sinuses 27, 29, 43, *44*, 45–6, 454, **455**
ventouse 16, **455**
ventricles 39, *40–1*, 42, **455**
ventricular system 39, *40–1*, 42–3, **455**
vertebral arteries 136
vertebral canal 31, *32*, 152–3, 164
vertebral column *150–1*
　energy drive for 411–13

see also spine
vertebral levels 367, *369*
vertebro-basilar insufficiency 138–9
vertical shift 325–7
viscera 160–1, 260–1, 263, 361, 369, **455**
visceral associations 417
visceral efferent neurons 344
vitality 11, 19, 76
　enhancing 240, 435
　evaluation of 83, 116, 433
　flow of 153

waves and wavelets 87, 248
white matter 342
whole person 12
　assessment 280
　awareness of 182–3
　building picture of 273–5
　reintegration of 53
　treatment through SBS 336–8
writer's cramp 261–2

zygomatic process 190, 202